Introduction to
Chinese Materia Medica

World Century Compendium to TCM

World Century Compendium to TCM – Vol. 3

Introduction to
Chinese
Materia Medica

Jin Yang
Huang Huang
Li-jiang Zhu

Nanjing University of Chinese Medicine, China

translated by

Yun-hui Chen

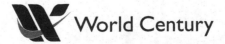
World Century

Published by

World Century Publishing Corporation
27 Warren Street
Suite 401-402
Hackensack, NJ 07601

Distributed by

World Scientific Publishing Co. Pte. Ltd.
5 Toh Tuck Link, Singapore 596224
USA office: 27 Warren Street, Suite 401-402, Hackensack, NJ 07601
UK office: 57 Shelton Street, Covent Garden, London WC2H 9HE

Library of Congress Control Number: 2013930712

British Library Cataloguing-in-Publication Data
A catalogue record for this book is available from the British Library.

World Century Compendium to TCM
A 7-Volume Set

INTRODUCTION TO CHINESE MATERIA MEDICA
Volume 3

Copyright © 2013 by World Century Publishing Corporation

Published by arrangement with Shanghai Century Publishing Co. Ltd.

ISBN 978-1-938134-34-0 (Set)
ISBN 978-1-938134-16-6 (pbk)

Typeset by Stallion Press
Email: enquiries@stallionpress.com

Printed in Singapore

Contents

Preface

AUTHOR'S REMARKS

In order to make the majority of readers understand the theory of traditional Chinese medicine and its methods of diagnosing and treating diseases in a relatively short period of time, in 1991, *Learn to Prescribe Chinese Medical Formulas in 100 days* was compiled and published by Shanghai Scientific & Technical Publisher and The Commercial Press (Hong Kong) Limited. It provided a brief introduction to the basic characteristics and theory of traditional Chinese medicine, and a detailed schedule of learning a commonly-seen diseases and patterns and their corresponding around 60 prescriptions. This is a great attempt to let more people initially know how to use the theory of traditional Chinese medicine to diagnose and treat common diseases and provide corresponding formulas.

Twenty-one years after its publication, the book remains immensely popular and has been widely regarded as the easy-to-use guide for the beginners. However, to study traditional Chinese medicine in depth, grasp its essence, and apply its theories for both prevention and treatment of disorders, the readers need to learn more than just the basics and should first have a deep understanding of Chinese materia medica, the powerful weapon in the treatment of disorders. Hereby, we compile this book as a supplementary to *Learn to Prescribe Chinese Medical Formulas in 100 days* and give a reference to the readers who are strongly interested in traditional Chinese medicine. Readers will be exposed to the theories of Chinese materia medica, detailed information on more than 200 kinds of herbs, and further interpretation of *Learn to Prescribe Chinese Medical Formulas in 100 days*.

This book aims at facilitating readers with the clinical application and is in line with the principle of "correspondence of Chinese medicinals and patterns". It contains a brief introduction to relative theories, divides these medicinals by actions into exterior-releasing, heat-clearing, purgative, dampness-dispelling, fluid retention-disinhibiting, interior-warming, qi-regulating, blood-invigorating, blood-stanching, food accumulation-relieving, phlegm, cough and wheezing-arresting, mind-tranquilizing, liver-calming, orifices-opening, tonifying, astringing, and worm-dispelling categorizes, and elaborate each herb in terms of actions, quality, indications, usage, and dosage. Furthermore, mnemonics and simple and effective formulas are provided to help readers know more practical applications, and precautions and daily practices are specifically designed to help readers to digest the content easier.

It continues to build the contents page on the chosen styles of *Learn to Prescribe Chinese Medical Formulas in 100 days*, one section one day, six days a week, fourteen weeks one hundred days.

Same as *Learn to Prescribe Chinese Medical Formulas in 100 days,* readers are expected to carry out day-to-day and week-to-week tasks following the order of the medicinal listed in this book. Progresses can really be accomplished with one hour a day and few more minutes to recite Mnemonics, patience and perseverance are two essential qualities for success.

Statement of revised edition of *Learn Chinese Materia Medica in 100 Days*

It has been 9 years since the first *Collection of Mastering Traditional Chinese Medicine in 100 days* came out in 1996. This series is popular among readers because of its distinctive compile style, profound contents written in simple and easy-to-master approaches, and pragmatic explanation conducive to clinical application. Eleven different kinds of books are available at the market and have been reprinted again and again, among which the best seller has been reprinted up to 100,000 copies.

Between the end of 20th century and the beginning of 21st century, disease spectrum has witnessed tremendous changes; correspondingly, clinical application of traditional Chinese medicine has also been changed in terms of indications and methods. In a bid to provide latest information and techniques concerned, meticulous revisions are made by experts, original style and format are kept, techniques and contents that are outdated and no longer frequently-used are deleted, and new disease species and therapeutic methods are supplemented. We sincerely hope this re-edited series will make due contributions to the promotion of Chinese culture, further publicity of traditional Chinese medicine, and popularization of medical knowledge.

Shanghai Scientific & Technical Publisher
May 2005

First Week

1

I. General Information

Chinese materia medica and its science

Chinese materia medica refers to the botanical, mineral, and zoological substances applied by traditional Chinese medicine as a primary weapon for preventing and treating diseases.

Some people are of the wrong impression that Chinese materia medica are all produced in China. However, some medical substances, known as imported goods *"Bó Lái Pǐn"* in ancient time, are either from other parts of the world such as *Shā Rén* (Fructus Amomi, villous amomum fruit), *Xuè Jié* (Sanguis Draconis, dragon's blood), and *Pàng Dà Hǎi* (Semen Sterculiae Lychnophorae, sterculia seed), or have been introduced and planted in China, such as *Shā Rén* (Fructus Amomi, villous amomum fruit). The antibiotics and biological products that made in China are called western medicine instead of Chinese materia medica.

Back in early history when people relied on collecting plants and hunting animals as their main source of food, they gradually recognized the beneficial or harmful effects of those plants or animals on human body. This is the original knowledge of Chinese materia medica. With a time-honored history of civilization tracing back to 6000 years ago, China has a large population, vast territory, and abundant resources, and Chinese people have accumulated rich medical experiences in fighting for survival and disease prevention and treatment, and gradually built up the theoretical knowledge of Chinese materia medica. About 2000 years ago when *The Yellow Emperor's Inner Classic* (黄帝内经, *Huáng Dì Nèi Jīng*) (including *Basic Questions* and *the Spiritual Pivot*) and *Shen Nong's Classic of the Materia Medica* (神农本草经, *Shén Nóng Běn Cǎo Jīng*) have been compiled, a comprehensive theoretical system of Chinese materia medica has formed. The former is a systematical expression of the correlative theories of Chinese materia medica and principles of their application, such as four natures, five flavors, relations between the five-*zang* organs and medical natures and flavors, and medicinal selection for five-*zang* organs' diseases, while the latter focuses on the detailed description of 365 herbs in terms of natures, flavors, actions, and indications.

Science of Chinese Materia Medica, as one of the primary disciplines of traditional Chinese medicine, mainly expounds the basic knowledge of Chinese medicine in terms of source, nature, processing, actions, indications, as well as its basic theories and administration.

In ancient China, Science of Chinese Materia Medica and correlative works were called "materia medica" (Běn Cǎo, 本草) because herbal medicine is a major component. There are abundant books on materia medica in history with a continuous accretion of new herbs together with a revaluation and addition of new uses. For instance, *Shen Nong's Classic of the Materia Medica* (神农本草经, *Shén Nóng Běn Cǎo Jīng*) is the source and archetype of Chinese material medica, from this beginning, the literatures developed in terms of theories of traditional Chinese medicine and addition of new herbs. For instances, *Newly Revised Materia Medica* (新修本草, *Xīn Xīu Běn Cǎo*) in Tang dynasty records 844 entries, *Materia Medica Arranged According to Pattern* (证类本草, *Zhèng Lèi Běn Cǎo*) in Song dynasty embraces 1558 items, *The Grand Compendium of Materia Medica* (本草纲目, *Běn Cǎo Gāng Mù*) in Ming dynasty contains 1892 species, and contemporary *Encyclopedia of Materia Medica* (中药大辞典, *Zhōng Yào Dà Cí Diǎn*) and *Chinese Materia Medica* (*Zhōng Huá Běn Cǎo*) list 5767 and 8980 entries, respectively. On the one hand, it is a reflection of China's wealth of China is rich in Chinese medicinals resources, and on the other hand, Science of Chinese Materia Medica is rich in content with great numbers of Chinese medicinals. The learner should also remember that Chinese materia medica is not easy to learn.

With great achievements, Science of Chinese Materia Medica not only plays an essential role in the historical development of traditional Chinese medicine in China and medicine in neighboring countries, but also has exerted important influences on the development of medicine across the world. Studies on Chinese materia medica, especially crude medicinals, become one of the hotspots in the international medical fields and new products are extracted from Chinese medicinals every year. For instance, medicines prepared from active ingredients extracted from Yín Xìng Yè (Folium Ginkgo, ginkgo leaf), which is known for its excellent actions of preventing and treating cardiovascular diseases, bring great profits to European pharmaceutical companies.

How to learn science of Chinese materia medica

Science of Chinese Materia Medica is the compulsory professional course, students need to have a solid grasp of basic knowledge of Chinese medicinals before they continue with further studies in formulas, internal and external medicines, gynecology, and pediatrics of traditional Chinese medicine. Chinese materia medica is the major tool in preventing and treating disorders and a practitioner of Traditional Chinese medicine must have profound knowledge on its theories and medicinals, just like someone cannot be a soldier if he does not know how to use weapons. However, so many books about Chinese materia medica covering extremely enormous contents are available now, how should we study it?

The first step is to understand the basic theories of traditional Chinese medicine, such as visceral manifestation, etiology, pathogenesis, principles of pattern differentiation, and treatment principles and methods, as Chinese materia medica theory is an important component of traditional Chinese medicine theories, and theories, methods, formulas and medicinals are inseparable. Without knowing the basic theories of traditional Chinese medicine, students cannot understand actions and indications of Chinese medicinals with a failure to apply. From this perspective, Western medicine and traditional Chinese medicine are greatly different from each other. If a clear diagnosis is made, the former is used directly to treat the disease in most cases, which is relatively easy to understand and master. While the latter aims at treatment based on a pattern, which must be identified by differentiating the nature of disease, yin or yang, exterior or interior, cold or heat, and deficiency or excess. There are also a few formulas that contain only one medicinal. The absence of the basic theories of traditional Chinese medicine will make it impossible to study Science of Chinese Materia Medica, let alone applying it in prevention and treatment of diseases. Hereby, Shanghai Scientific and Technical Publisher and The Commercial Press (Hong Kong) Limited compiled and published *Learn to Prescribe Chinese Medical Formulas in 100 days* that covers the basic theories of traditional Chinese medicine. Reading it or other theoretic books of traditional Chinese medicine first will facilitate your understanding of this book; mastery of traditional Chinese medicine theories will make it easier to understand theories of Science of Chinese Materia Medica.

When studying Chinese materia medica, one needs to focus on correlative basic theories, and the properties, actions and indications of commonly used medicinals. This book aims to help learners to master the properties, actions and indications of around 200 commonly-used Chinese medicinals in just 100 days. The learners are required to create summaries and make comparisons among medicinals with similar actions to identify their similarity and differences, which will make it easier to memorize, and also lays a foundation for clinical application. The column of Mnemonicsis is designed to assist the learners to remember the properties, actions and indications of medicinals, the column of Simple and Effective Formulas aims to provide references for the reader to understand the actions and indications of medicinals, and the column of Daily Practices at the end of each section covers questions that are worth thinking over and beneficial for good comprehension.

Undoubtedly, students are supposed to develop their skills of Chinese medicinal both theoretically and practically in treatment of various diseases, and they will be really impressed with the actions and indications of medicinal when certain disorders are cured by applying those medicinal plants.

Classification of Chinese medicinals

There are several different methods to classify traditional Chinese medicinals. In ancient materia medica works, they are classified by:

1. The properties and actions of medicinals.
   For instance, *Shen Nong's Classic of the Materia Medica* (神农本草经, *Shén Nóng Běn Cǎo Jīng*) listed medicinals with mild nature and

boosting effect as the upper grade, those with drastic nature and purgative effect as the lower grade, and others are the middle grade.

2. Sources of medicinals.

For instance, *The Grand Compendium of Materia Medica* (本草纲目, *Běn Cǎo Gāng Mù*) recorded the type of water, fire, earth, golden stone, grass, grain, vegetable, fruit, wood, tool, insect, scale, shell, bird, beast, and human being.

3. Medicinal parts.

For instance, *The Quality and Rational Application of Chinese Materia Medica* (中药的质量及其合理应用, *Zhōng Yào De Zhì Liàng Jí Qí Hé Lǐ Yìng Yòng*) has divided Chinese medicinals into root and rhizome, stem, peel, leaf, whole plant, flower, fruit and seed, animal, and mineral categorizes.

4. Actions of medicinals.

In modern and contemporary Chinese medicine works, medicinals are classified by actions into exterior-releasing, heat-clearing, purgation, wind-dispelling and dampness-eliminating, dampness-eliminating, qi-rectifying, digestion-promoting, worm-expelling, blood-regulating, phlegm, cough and panting-relieving, mind-calming, liver-calming and wind-distinguishing, orifices-opening, tonic, astringent, emetic, and external-application types. Each method has its advantages and disadvantages; classification based on source of medicinal cannot reflect its actions, whereas classification method employing certain predominant action cannot objectively reflect its overall actions, although it is helpful for memorizing and comparison. For instance, Má Huáng (Herba Ephedrae, ephedra herb) is capable of both releasing the exterior and arresting panting but is categorized into the medicinal that release the exterior. In this book, medicinals are classified by actions and learners are expected to pay more attention to make comparison between medicinals that have similar actions.

Daily practice

1. What is Chinese materia medica? What are the main contents of Science of Chinese Materia Medica?
2. What are the good ways to study Chinese materia medica?
3. How is Chinese materia medica classified?

2

II. Property Theory of Chinese Materia Medica

The "Property theory" section in this book includes information about three aspects of Chinese medicinals that explained and interpreted with unique theories of traditional Chinese medicine. One is the four qi and five flavors (四气五味, Sì Qì Wǔ Wèi), one is the ascending, descending, floating, and sinking, the other is channel entry. Property theory of Chinese materia medica and other basic theories of traditional Chinese medicine are closely related and constitute theoretical system of traditional Chinese medicine.

The four Qi and five flavors (四气五味, Sì Qì Wǔ Wèi)

Also known as Qì Wèi 气味 or Xìng Wèi 性味, it is a basic theory used to illustrate the actions of medicinals and also the core of property theory. From the perspective of Traditional Chinese medicine, medicinals have different natures and flavors that determine their therapeutic effects, and therefore they can rectify and treat various pathogenic visceral changes either functionally or organically. That is to say, learners should know the natures and flavors of medicinals before learning their actions. This theory includes two aspects, one is the four qi and the other is the five flavors.

[Four Qi] Four qi is also called "四性 Sì Xìng", cold, hot, warm, and cool are the four natures of Chinese medicinal. It is one of the characteristics of traditional Chinese medicine in understanding medicinal properties. The cold, hot, warm, or cool nature does not refer to the temperature of medicinal, but a designation based on a patient's reaction to the medical substances. For instance, medicinals that generate hot sensation and relieve cold symptoms such as abdominal pain relieved by warmth, watery diarrhea or diarrhea with undigested food, absence of thirst, ice-cold hands and feet, white moist tongue coating, pale tongue, and deep thin pulse are warm or hot in nature. These medicinals include Fù Zǐ (Radix Aconiti Lateralis Praeparata, Monkshood), Ròu Guì (Cortex Cinnamomi, Cassia Bark), Gān Jiāng (Rhizoma Zingiberis, Dried Ginger Rhizome), Jú Pí (Pericarpium Citri Reticulatae, Tangerine Pericarp), and Shēng Jiāng (Rhizoma Zingiberis Recens, Fresh Ginger). Whereas, medicinals that eliminate heat symptoms such as high fever, thirsty with a desire for cold drink, restlessness, yellow and dry tongue coating, red tongue, and slippery rapid pulse are cold or cool in nature. These medicinals include Huáng Lián (Rhizoma Coptidis, golden thread), Dà Huáng (Radix et Rhizoma Rhei, rhubarb root and rhizome), Shí Gāo (Gypsum Fibrosum, gypsum), Jú Huā (Flos Chrysanthemi, chrysanthemun flower), and Sāng Yè (Folium Mori, mulberry leaf).

That is to say, these four qi are summaries based on patient's reactions to the medicinal substances. *Shen Nong's Classic of the Materia Medica* (神农本草经, *Shén Nóng Běn Cǎo Jīng*) noted that "cold diseases must be treated with hot medicinals, and hot diseases must be treated with cold medicinals", indicating the basic principle of traditional Chinese medicine treatment is to correct imbalance of yin and yang as well as of qi and blood with properties of different medicinals. Meanwhile, medicinal properties are credited by long-term observation of its therapeutic effects on imbalance of yin and yang as well as qi and blood. Medicinals effective for cold pattern are considered hot in nature, and medicinals effective for heat pattern are cold natured. Property theory is closely associated with etiology, pathogenesis and treatment based on pattern differentiation.

[Five Flavors] Five flavors refer to the degree to which a medicinal has a taste, namely acrid, sweet, sour, bitter, and salty. In traditional Chinese medicine, the taste of foods or medicinals has specific effects on the body. *Basic Questions* (素问, *Sù Wèn*) stated the basic summary of "acrid substances scatter, sour substances astringe, sweet substances moderate, bitter substances drain, and salty substances soften". Together, five flavors and four qi constitute the unique theoretical pharmacology system of Science of Chinese Materia Medica.

Acrid substances move and disperse. Dispersing means to scatter and dissipate the exterior pathogens, while moving refers to remove qi stagnation, and unblock the obstructed channels, collaterals, and orifices. Therefore, medicinals that used to relieve the exterior such as Má Huáng (Herba Ephedrae, Ephedra Herb), Guì Zhī (Ramulus Cinnamomi, Cassia Twig), Zǐ Sū Yè (Folium Perillae, Perilla Leaf), and Bò He (Herba Menthae, Field Mint) are acrid, while medicinals that regulate qi such as Jú Pí (Pericarpium Citri Reticulatae, Tangerine Pericarp), Mù Xiāng (Radix Aucklandiae, Common Aucklandia Root), Shā Rén (Fructus

Amomi, Villous Amomum Fruit), and Xiāng Fù (Rhizoma Cyperi, Nutgrass Galingale Rhizome) are also acrid.

Bitter substances dry and drain. Drying means to eliminate dampness, and draining refers to dispel pathogenic heat outward and drain pathogenic toxins downward. For this reason, medicinals that used for relieve dampness such as Hòu Pò (Cortex Magnoliae Officinalis, Magnolia Bark) and Dú Huó (Radix Angelicae Pubescentis, Double Teeth Pubescent Angelica Root) are bitter; and medicinals that clear heat and resolve toxins or subdue fire, such as Huáng Lián (Rhizoma Coptidis, Coptis Rhizome), Lóng Dǎn Cǎo (Radix et Rhizoma Gentianae, Chinese Gentian), Zhī Zǐ (Fructus Gardeniae, Cape Jasmine Fruit), and Huáng Bǎi (Cortex Phellodendri Chinensis, Amur Cork-tree Bark) are also bitter.

Sweet substances tonify qi, blood, yin, and yang, harmonize and relax tension, and moderate the effects of other medicinals. That is why most tonics are sweet, such as *Gān Cǎo* (Radix et Rhizoma Glycyrrhizae, Liquorice Root), *Fēng Mì* (Mel, Honey), and *Dà Zǎo* (Fructus Jujubae, Chinese Date), they can also be used in relax tension. Besides, medicinals that nourish, moisten the intestines to promote defecation, and moisten the lung to dissolve phlegm are also sweet.

Sour substances astringe fluid and qi and prevent or reverse the abnormal leakage, such as cough, sweating, seminal emission, enuresis, and diarrhea. Medicinals with sour taste include Wǔ Wèi Zǐ (Fructus Schisandrae Chinensis, Chinese Magnolivine Fruit), Wū Méi (Fructus Mume, Smoked Plum), and Shí Liú Pí (Pericarpium Granati, Pomegranate Husk).

Salty substances soften hard masses, fixed abdominal masses of definite shape, or movable abdominal masses of indefinite shape, such as lumps (benign or malignant tumor), scrofula (tuberculosis of lymph nodes), and Yīng Líu (goiter). These salty medicinals include Mǔ Lì (Concha Ostreae, Oyster Shell), Kūn Bù (Thallus Laminariae, Kelp), and Hǎi Zǎo (Sargassum, Seaweed). Besides, owning to their effects on softening hard masses, they are also commonly used for constipation with dry stools in the intestines, and sores and masses of external diseases.

Astringent taste and sour taste have similar actions of astringing and are usually part of the same medicinal. Such medicinals include Jīn Yīng Zǐ (Fructus Rosae Laevigatae, Cherokee Rose Fruit) and Shí Liú Pí

(Pericarpium Granati, Pomegranate Husk). However, some medicinals are astringent but not sour, such as Lóng Gǔ (Os Draconis, Dragon Bones), Qiàn Shí (Semen Euryales, Euryale Seed), and Lián Zǐ (Semen Nelumbinis, Lotus Seed). Substances that have none of these tastes are said to be bland, "bland taste affiliated to sweet taste" mainly acts to promote urination and percolate dampness, and medicinals that disinhibit water retention such as Fú Líng (Poria, Indian Bread) and Zhū Líng (Polyporus, Polyporus) are bland-tasted.

The concept of flavor is complicated, as different medicinals have different tastes or distinctive taste even though with similar actions, some medicinals may taste the same but be variously thick or thin; and some have multiple flavors, such as sour sweet, pungent bitter, and pungent sweet. Medicinals with multiple tastes also have multiple actions, for instance, sour and sweet substances such as Shān Zhū Yú (Fructus Corni, cornus) can tonify and astringe.

In theories of Science of Chinese Materia Medica, the flavor of a medicinal partly determines its therapeutic effects. They are precious inheritance from our ancestors, and most of them are practical. However, it has certain one-sided limits due to historical conditions, and modern researches reveal that Chinese medicinals contain multiple active ingredients, which have shown different pharmacological effects, the flavor of its effective component contributes partially to its actions. For instance, tonics contain saccharides that taste sweet, exterior-releasing and qi-rectifying medicinals contain volatile oil that taste acrid, heat-clearing and toxin-relieving medicinals contain alkaloid that taste bitter, and astringents contain organic acid that taste sour. However, for some active ingredients, flavors are not inevitably connected to actions. Therefore, in Science of Chinese Materia Medica, the flavor of medicinal refers to its original taste and also the taste that deductively grouped taking into account its actions. Bái Sháo (Radix Paeoniae Alba, White Peony Root), for instance, does not taste sour but is grouped into medicinal with sour flavor based on its actions of astringing yin and softening the liver. In this way, the flavor of medicinal and its actions are most closely related to each other, that is to say, knowing the flavor provides a preliminary clue regarding its actions; however, on the other hand, the original taste of few medicinals is different from that recorded in *Science of Chinese Materia Medica*.

[Relationship between four qi and five flavors] Each medicinal has four qi (cold, hot, warm, and cool) and five flavors (acrid, sweet, sour, bitter, and salty). Understanding the properties of medicinals should take both qi and flavors into account. This book elaborates upon the qi and flavor of every medicinal, which are regarded as necessary foundations for further analysis of their actions. For instance, Huáng Lián (Rhizoma Coptidis, Coptis Rhizome) is cold in qi and bitter in flavor and therefore capable of clearing heat, drying dampness, and draining downward; Hòu Pò (Cortex Magnoliae Officinalis, Magnolia Bark) is warm in qi and pungent-bitter in flavor and therefore effective in warming the middle *jiao* and moving qi to dry dampness.

In *Science of Chinese Materia Medica*, the action of medicinal can be distinguished by certain qi and flavors. Medicinals with the same flavor (acrid, sweet, sour, bitter, or salty) can present with different qi (cold, hot, warm, or cool); and vise versa. For this reason, different medicinals may act differently. Má Huáng (Herba Ephedrae, Eph Edra) and Bò He (Herba Menthae, Field Mint), for instance, are both acrid in flavor and can release the exterior and induce sweating, but the former is warm in nature and therefore suitable for wind-cold exterior pattern, and the latter is cool in nature and therefore appropriate for wind-heat exterior pattern; Huáng Lián (Rhizoma Coptidis, Coptis Rhizome) and Shēng Dì (Radix Rehmanniae, rehmannia root) both are cold in nature and can clear heat, but the former is bitter in flavor and therefore capable of clearing heat and drying dampness and suitable for damp-heat disorders, while the latter is sweet in flavor and hereby effective in nourishing yin, engendering fluid, and cooling blood and appropriate for yin fluids deficiency, yin deficiency resulting in vigorous fire, and blood heat. The actions of every medicinal are predominated by either four qi or five flavors, which are heavily dependent on the specific situation.

Daily practices

1. What is the theory of medicinal property of Chinese materia medica? What are the best ways to master them comprehensively?
2. What is the concept of four qi and five flavors? What are their actions?
3. What are the relationships between four qi and five flavors?

3

Ascending and descending, floating and sinking

the theory of ascending, descending, floating and sinking refers to four directions or trends of medicinal actions. Complementary to four qi and five flavors theories, it plays an essential role in comprehensively understanding properties of Chinese medicinal and in guiding its clinical applications.

[Definition of ascending and descending, floating and sinking]
Ascending and floating refer to the upward and outward movement of medicinal action, while descending and sinking mean the downward and inward flow of medicinal action. Pathologically, the disease may lodge in the superior, inferior, exterior, or interior part of the body; and may develop inward or outward. Therefore, medicinals that tend to ascend, descend, float, or sink should be prescribed in line with affected area and pathogenesis, as echoed by "treat adverse rising by inhibition, treat fallen by raising" in *The Yellow Emperor's Inner Classic* (黄帝内经, *Huáng Dì Nèi Jīng*).

Ascending medicinals, capable of raising and lifting, are mainly used for sinking patterns. Huáng Qí (Radix Astragali, Astragalus Root), and Shēng Má (Rhizoma Cimicifugae, Black Cohosh Rhizome), for instance, both can raise qi in the middle *jiao* and are therefore applicable for gastroptosis, hysteroptosis, and proctoptosis due to enduring diarrhea.

Descending medicinals, capable of downbearing and suppressing, are mainly used for disorders due to ascending counterflow of qi, and pathogenic fire flaming upward. For instance, Dài Zhě Shí (Hematitum, Hematite) is effective in descending adverse flow of stomach qi and lung qi and therefore considered suitable for vomiting and panting, and Lóng Dǎn Cǎo (Radix et Rhizoma Gentianae, Chinese Gentian) is potent in subduing liver fire and hereby appropriate for diseases caused by fire-heat of the liver and gallbladder flaming upward.

Floating medicinals, capable of ascending upward and dispersing, are mainly used for diseases located exteriorly and superiorly in the body. For instance, Bò He (Herba Menthae, Field Mint) and Chán Tuì (Periostracum

Cicadae, Cicada Moulting) both are floating and dispersing in nature and thus applicable for cases of exterior pattern and pathogenic changes in the head or face.

Sinking medicinals, capable of downbearing and promoting defecation and urination, are mainly used for diseases affected the interior or lower part of the body. For instance, Dà Huáng (Radix et Rhizoma Rhei, Rhubarb Root and Rhizome) that promotes defecation and Mù Tōng (Caulis Akebiae, Akebia Stem) that disinhibits urination are both sinking in nature.

All in all, each medicinal has a functional tendency to either rise, fall, float, or sink, which is also indicative of the clinical situation in which it can be effectively used. These trends of medicinal actions and their clinical applications are complementary and supplementary to each other. It is worth to note that a few medicinal substances have shown a tendency to both float and rise, or both sink and descend. Jú Huā (Flos Chrysanthemi, Chrysanthemum Flower), for instance, scatters and dissipates wind-heat exteriorly, and also clears and subdues liver fire interiorly; and Fú Píng (Herba Spirodelae, Duckweed) induces sweating to release the exterior pathogen and meanwhile disinhibits internal water retention to relieve edema.

[Influential factors on ascending, descending, floating, and sinking]
Many factors influence the ascending, descending, floating, and sinking of medicinals. The primary cause is medicinal property such as qi, flavor, and texture. Generally, medicinals that are pungent and sweet in flavor and warm and heat in nature tend to ascend and float; while those that are bitter, sour, and salty in flavor and cold and cool in nature are prone to descend and sink. Medicinals originating from flowers, leaves or lightweight substances are primarily ascending and floating; the ones from seed and heavyweight substances like mineral and shell are mostly descending and sinking. However, there are some exceptions, for instance, Xuán Fù Huā (Flos Inulae, Inula Flower) and Yuán Huā (Flos Genkwa, Lilac Daphne Flower Bud) both are from flowers, but the former descends and sinks, and the latter drains downward; Niú Bàng Zǐ (Fructus Arctii, great burdock achene), originated from seed, acts to scatter and dissipate by ascending and floating.

Additionally, the functional tendency of medicinal is found associated with its processing and combination. For instance, medicinals treated with ginger, vinegar, and wine have shown dispersing, astringing, and ascending-floating property, respectively. Suppression occurs when a medicinal that tends to float and rise is combined with a group of sinking and descending substances, and vise versa.

Channel tropism

Another branch of medicinal property theory is channel tropism. Based on *zang-fu* theory and channel and collateral doctrine, it is an attempt to sum up the actions of medicinals and describe the selective therapeutic effects of a medicinal on a certain part of the body. In *Science of Chinese Materia Medica*, an herb is said to have specific actions because of the *zang-fu* organ and channel it enters. For instance, medicinals that clear heat can be subdivided by targeted organs into stomach-heat clearing, gallbladder-heat draining, lung-heat relieving, and large intestines-heat removing category; and among the tonics, some strengthen the lung, some reinforce the spleen, while others may supplement the liver or kidney. To understand this theory comprehensively, learners should know *zang-fu* theory and channel and collateral theory, especially the running routes of channels and collaterals. For instance, some medicinals that relieve chest and rib-side pain are inferred with liver and gallbladder channel tropism because these two channels run through the above-mentioned areas. The theory of channel tropism is summed up through clinical outcomes. Therefore, only when attention is paid to the different aspects of medicinals such as actions and indications, can its channel tropism be comprehended.

Each of the above discussed theories tries to explain the properties and actions of medicinals from different aspects. Among them, the theory of four qi and five flavors is the core and also the key concepts for students. The theories of the four qi and five flavors, and actions of lifting, lowering, floating and sinking of herbs, and channel tropism, should be associated with each other to be comprehensively analyzed and thoroughly understood.

Daily practice

1. What is the meaning of ascending, descending, floating and sinking? What are their influencial factors?
2. What are the relationships between four qi and five flavors and actions of ascending, descending, floating, and sinking?
3. What is the essence of channel tropism of a medicinal?

4

III. Influencing Factors of Chinese Medicinal Therapeutic Effects

Chinese medicinals have been used as major tools in traditional Chinese medicine to treat disorders, and doctors and patients and their family members share a common concern about therapeutic effects. Clinically, formulas and medicinals that are appropriately prescribed can sometimes fail to produce optimal outcomes, or medicinals provided by different pharmacies may have different therapeutic effects. Therefore, it is necessary to know the factors that influence the therapeutic effects of Chinese medicinal.

Quality of Chinese medicinal

Doctors and patients are both greatly concerned about the quality of Chinese medicinal, and it will be helpful if they know how to identify. Quality is undoubtedly the primary factor affecting therapeutic effects, the scales and grades that identified and licensed by Department of Commerce is considered the major standard for quality evaluation.

[Specification of Chinese Materia Medical] The specifications of medicines are categorized in the following ways:

1. Clarity and methods of processing
   Take Shān Yào (Rhizoma Dioscoreae, Common Yam Rhizome) as an example, those with skin are known as 毛山药, Máo Shān Yào, whereas those without peel and prepared into round shapes are known

as 光山药 Guāng Shān Yào. Other examples include Máo Xiāng Fù (Nutgrass Galingale Rhizome with root hair) and Guāng Xiāng Fù (Nutgrass Galingale Rhizome without root hair), Yuǎn Zhì Tǒng (Thin-leaf Milkwort Root without core) and Yuǎn Zhì Ròu (fleshy Thin-leaf Milkwort Root), and Shēng Shài Shēn (Radix et Rhizoma Ginseng Cruda, Sun-dried Ginseng) and Hóng Shēn (Radix et Rhizoma Ginseng Rubra, Red Ginseng).

2. Harvest time

Take Sān Qī (Radix et Rhizoma Notoginseng, Pseudoginseng Root) as an example; 春七 Chūn Qī that harvested before blooming in spring are full-grown and with better quality, while 冬七 Dōng Qí that collected after seed setting in autumn and winter are of loose texture and poor quality. Another example is Tiān Má (Rhizoma Gastrodiae, Tall Gastrodis Tuber), 春麻 Chūn Má that harvested upon sprouting in summer are lightweight with a hollow-centered cross section and poor quality, while 冬麻 Dōng Má that harvested in autumn are solid and heavyweight with better quality.

3. Growth period

Lián Qiào (Fructus Forsythiae, Weeping Forsythia Capsule) is categorized by the maturity of the fruit into 黄连翘 Huáng (yellow) Lián Qiào and 青连翘 Qīng (green) Lián Qiào. Another example is Bò He (Herba Menthae, Field Mint), the first harvested is known as 头刀薄荷 Tóu Dāo Bò He, and the second is 二刀薄荷 Èr Dāo Bò He, has the content of peppermint essential oil is most plentiful in pre-bud period, and the greatest percentage of menthol crystal is yielded in full flowering stage.

4. Production area

Bái Sháo (Radix Paeoniae Alba, White Peony Root) produced in Zhejiang, Anhui, and Sichuan is known as 杭白芍 Háng Bái Sháo, 亳白芍 Bó Bái Sháo, and 川白芍 Chuān Bái Sháo, respectively. Hòu Pò (Cortex Magnoliae Officinalis, Magnolia Bark) from Sichuan and Wenzhou of Zhejiang are named as 川朴 Chuān Pò and 温朴 Wēn Pò, respectively.

5. Medicinal parts and morphology

Different parts from the same Chinese materia medica can be used as medicinal; however, their actions are different or even opposite. Take Má Huáng (Herba Ephedrae, Eph Edra) as an example, its stem and leaf induce sweating, whereas its root arrests sweating. For Dāng Guī (Radix Angelicae Sinensis, Chinese Angelica), different functions are ascribed to 归头 Guī Tóu (the head-uppermost part), Guī Wěi (the tail part deepest in the soil), 归身 Guī Shēn (the body part in-between), and Quán Dāng Guī 全当归 (the whole medical plant). The head is considered most potent in invigorating blood and the body is for harmonizing blood.

[Grading of Chinese materia medica] Medicinals with the same specification or name are divided by quality into grade A, B, C, D, and so forth, where grade A is for the best. All of the rankings undergo specific ranking criteria, take Sān Qī (Radix et Rhizoma Notoginseng, Pseudoginseng Root) as an example; grade A refers to less than 20 pieces with an aggregate weight of 500 g, and grade B refers to less than 30 pieces with an aggregate weight of 500 g.

Gradeless goods (统货, Tǒng Huò) refers to the Chinese medicinals that have no specifications and grades, as there is no big difference in their quality. These medicinals include Yì Mǔ Cǎo (Herba Leonuri, Motherwort Herb), Pí Pá Yè (Folium Eriobotryae, Loquat Leaf), and Bǎi Zǐ Rén (Semen Platycladi, Oriental Arborvitael).

Specifications and grades can to some extent reflect the quality and appearance of medicinal, but the appearance quality is not always in line with the inner quality. For instance, the primary criterion for selecting Rén Shēn (Radix et Rhizoma Ginseng, Ginseng) is the thick root in terms of appearance quality, however, the clinical efficacy of the thinner root is as good as that of the thicker.

Production area and harvesting of Chinese materia medica

Dated back to ancient China, people already realized that medicinals produced in different areas have different quality. Each medicinal needs a certain amount of sunlight, proper climate, and moisture optimal soil conditions, the highest quality herbs with best therapeutic effects come from the most suitable areas and are known as genuine regional medicinals (地道药材, Dì Dào Yào Cái). This has been proven by both clinical practice and modern experiments. Owing to differences in climate, soils, and water quality in production areas, there are certain differences in the content of active ingredients and ratio of the components.

[Production area and genuine regional medicinals] The well-known genuine regional medicinals include Huáng Lián (Rhizoma Coptidis, Coptis Rhizome), Fù Zǐ (Radix Aconiti Lateralis Praeparata, Monkshood), Bèi Mǔ *(Bulbus Fritillaria, Fritillary Bulb)*, and Chuān Xiōng (Rhizoma Chuanxiong, Sichuan Lovage Root) from Sichuan; Sān Qī (Radix et Rhizoma Notoginseng, Pseudoginseng Root) from Yunnan; Dāng Guī (Radix Angelicae Sinensis, Chinese Angelica) and Gǒu Qǐ Zǐ (Fructus Lycii, Chinese Wolfberry Fruit) from Gansu; Gān Cǎo (Radix et Rhizoma Glycyrrhizae, Licorice Root) from Inner Mongolia; Rén Shēn (Radix et Rhizoma Ginseng, Ginseng) from Jilin; Huáng Qí (Radix Astragali, Astragalus Root) and Dǎng Shēn (Radix Codonopsis, Codonopsis Root) from Shanxi; Dì Huáng (Radix Rehmanniae, Rehmannia), Shān Yào (Rhizoma Dioscoreae, Common Yam Rhizome), and Niú Xī (Radix Achyranthis Bidentatae, Two-toothed Achyranthes Root) from Henan; Mǔ Dān Pí (Cortex Moutan, Tree Peony Bark) and Mù Guā (Fructus Chaenomelis, Chinese Quince Fruit) from Anhui; Zhè Bèi Mǔ (Bulbus Fritillariae Thunbergii, Thunberg Fritillary Bulb), Xuán Shēn (Radix Scrophulariae, Figwort Root), and Yán Hú Suǒ (Rhizoma Corydalis, Corydalis Rhizome) from Zhejiang; Zé Xiè (Rhizoma Alismatis, Water Plantain Rhizome) from Fujian; Huò Xiāng (Herba Agastachis, Agastache), Chén Pí (Pericarpium Citri Reticulatae, Aged Tangerine Peel) from Guangdong; Gé Jiè (Gecko, Gecko) and Ròu Guì (Cortex Cinnamomi, Cinnamon Bark) from Guangxi; Zhǐ Shí (Fructus Aurantii Immaturus, Immature Bitter Orange) from Jiangxi; and Bò He (Herba Menthae, Field Mint), Xià Kū Cǎo (Spica Prunellae, Common Self-heal Fruit-spike), Tài Zǐ Shēn (Radix Pseudostellariae, Heterophylly False Satarwort Root), and Cāng Zhú (Rhizoma Atractylodis, Atractylodes Rhizome) from Jiangsu. Genuine regional medicinals are preferable in the clinic and the source of the herb is often incorporated into its name, such as Guǎng Mù Xiāng (Radix Aucklandiae, Saussurae Root), Chuān Bèi Mǔ (Bulbus Fritillariae Cirrhosae, Sichuan fritillaria bulb), and Lù Dǎng Shēn (Radix Codonopsis from Lu'an, Lu'an Codonopsis). Demand for Chinese medicinals has increased both domestically and abroad, therefore more efforts should be paid to develop genuine regional medicinals, and on the other hand the introduction and domestication should be carried out. Some introduced species have been cultivated successfully in China, and their quality are as good as genuine regional ones, such as Mù Xiāng (Radix Aucklandiae, Common Aucklandia Root), Ròu Dòu Kòu (Semen Myristicae, Nutmeg), Mǎ Qián Zǐ (Semen Strychni, Nux Vomica Seed), Dīng Xiāng (Flos Caryophylli, Clove Flower), Ròu Guì (Cortex Cinnamomi Cinnamon Bark), and Xī Yáng Shēn (Radix Panacis Quinquefolii, American ginseng).

[Harvesting of Chinese materia medica] The quality of medicinal is closely related to the season, time, and method of collection. Take harvest season for an example, the content of alkaloid in Cǎo Má Huáng (Herba Ephedrae, Ephedra) is extremely low in spring, increases dramatically in summer, reaches its peak in August and September, and then decreases significantly; active ingredients of Fān Xiè Yè (Folium Sennae, Senna Leaf) are most plentiful on 90th day; and Yáng Jīn Huā (Flos Daturae, Datura Flower) should be harvested from 10 a.m. to 2 p.m. as its total alkaloid content is richest when blossoms are falling. Herbs should be collected at the time when their active ingredients are most plentiful, specifically, the entire plant, stems, branches, and leaves usually in the period when stems and leaves are blooming or blossoming, except for some leaves that are harvested in autumn (such as Sāng Yè (Folium Mori, Mulberry Leaf) and Pí Pá Yè (Folium Eriobotryae, Loquat Leaf)); root or rhizome just before sprouting in early spring or in late fall when aerial part is withered, except for some roots that are harvested in summer when their stems and leaves wither (such as Tài Zǐ Shēn (Radix Pseudostellariae, Heterophylly False Satarwort Root), Yán Hú Suǒ (Rhizoma Corydalis, Corydalis Rhizome), and Bàn Xià (Rhizoma Pinelliae, Pinellia Rhizome); the bark in late summer or early autumn when sap is most plentiful and it is most peelable; flowers before opening or just opening when the petals are intact and fragrance is easy to preserve; and fruits and seeds upon ripening, except for some that are harvested when immature (such as Wū Méi (Fructus Mume, Smoked Plum), Qīng Pí (Pericarpium Citri Reticulatae Viride, Green Tangerine Peel), and Zhǐ Shí (Fructus Aurantii Immaturus, Immature Bitter Orange)). When insect species are used for medicinal purposes, the physician should know their hatching, growth, and development season: the whole body usually in the most active period; flying insects in early morning (before the dew dries out); and ootheca before hatching (steaming the ova until dead).

Processing of Chinese materia medica

Processing of Chinese materia medica is to adapt it to the needs of a particular medical care, prescription, preparation, and storage under the guidance of theories of traditional Chinese medicine. It is also known as an important characteristic of Chinese materia medica, can directly influence the therapeutic effects and therefore is helpful to know some general knowledge.

[Purpose of processing] The medicinal is processed for the following purposes:

1. To reduce or eliminate side-effects.
   Some medicinals have toxicity or cause side-effects. For example, ingesting untreated Rǔ Xiāng (Olibanum, Frankincense) and Mò Yào (Myrrha, Myrrh) may easily cause nausea and vomiting, but stir-frying eliminates their tendency.
2. To alter a medicinal properties for a particular clinical condition.
   For instance, Shēng Dì Huáng (Radix Rehmanniae, Rehmannia) is cool in nature and used for clearing blood, after processing it becomes Shú Dì Huáng (Radix Rehmanniae Praeparata, Prepared Rehmannia Root), which is warming in nature and used as a tonic. Another example is Shēng Hé Shǒu Wū (Radix Polygoni Multiflori, Fleece Flower Root), which is used for moistening the intestines to promote defecation, after processing it becomes Zhì Hé Shǒu Wū (Radix Polygoni Multiflori Praeparata cum Succo Glycines Sotae, Prepared Fleeceflower Root) that is usually used to nourish the liver and kidney.
3. To improve therapeutic effects: For example, using vinegar to process Yán Hú Suǒ (Rhizoma Corydalis, Corydalis Rhizome) can increase its potency of relieving pain, and charred Dì Yú (Radix Sanguisorbae, Garden Burnet Root) is considered more effective in stopping bleeding.

Additionally, processing can make medicinals clean and render them more suitable for preparation and storage.

[Methods of Processing] Many processing methods and general knowledge are available in our sources.

Generally, processing methods of Chinese medicinals are categorized into 修治 Xiū Zhì and 炮炙 Páo Zhì. The former refers to removing ashes, soils, impurities, and non-medicinal portions of a substance, soaking and rinsing in water, cutting into segments, slices, and slivers, or grinding into powder; while the latter refers to stir-frying, frying with liquid, quick-frying, calcining, roasting in ashes, steaming, boiling, frosting (removing seed-oil by pressing and making the residue into frostlike powder), fermenting, and sprouting.

Clinically, the processing of medicinal is conducted to the needs of treatment, and the method adopted is often included into its name. For instance, 姜半夏 Jiāng Bàn Xià refers to the Bàn Xià (Rhizoma Pinelliae Praeparatum, Pinellia Rhizome) processed with ginger juice (姜, Jiāng), 胆南星 Dǎn Nán Xīng (Arisaema cum Bile, Bile Arisaema) indicates the substance been treated with bile of pig or cow (胆, Dǎn), and Cù Chái Hú (vinegar-fried thotowax root) refers to the Chái Hú (Radix Bupleuri, Bupleurum) prepared by vinegar (醋, Cù). Processing is a special technique that has many operational methods and been expounded by monographs. This book provides you with the preliminary knowledge.

Daily practice

1. How to identify the quality of Chinese materia medica?
2. What is the genuine regional medicinal? Could you please explain the relationship between harvesting and quality with examples of medicinals?
3. What are the purposes and major methods of processing?

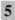

5

Usage of Chinese materia medica

Appropriate usage is another important factor that influences the therapeutic response. Generally, it includes oral administration (usually prepared into decoction, pill, powder, decocted extract, and medicinal wine) and external application (including moxa-compression, medicinal bath, laryngeal insufflation, eye dropping, warm medicated compression, and suppository). Proper usage is determined based on a particular clinical condition and the need of treatment. However, some medicinals should not be used in decoction, such as Gān Suì (Radix Kansui, gansui root) containing water-insoluble active ingredients and Shè Xiāng (Moschus, Musk) and Bīng Piàn (Borneolum Syntheticum, Borneol) containing aromatic compounds that are easily volatilized after being heated.

Generally, decoction is considered most appropriate for acute disorders, and pills and powders are used primarily for chronic diseases. Therefore, there is a saying in traditional Chinese medicine that "decoction takes effect quickly and drastically, while pills slowly and moderately". There are a few details that should be noted when taking medicinals.

[Decocting methods] Decoction (Tāng) is by far the most common way by which Chinese medicinal is taken. Correct method of decocting can improve therapeutic effects.

Earthenware pots are preferred, and porcelain utensil is acceptable when the former is not available, but the cooking utensil made of aluminium and iron should not be used as the interaction between these metals and medicinals may influence the therapeutic effects.

Medicinals should be soaked in cold water for 30 minutes before decocting, the liquid should at most cover the herbs in the cooking utensil. Usually, one dose should be decocted for two times, three times if it is a tonic, 250–300 ml medicinal juice each time.

Flame in cooking medicinals may either be strong fire (武火, Màn Huǒ) or slow fire (文火, Wén Huǒ), the former is fierce with high heat, while the latter is gentle with low heat. Usually when there are exterior-releasing or aromatic medicinals in the decoction, it is first brought to a boil using strong fire and then cooked over slow fire for several minutes to avoid the loss of volatile active ingredients. Tonics are cooked over slow fire for long periods to get the full effect of active ingredients.

Hard minerals and shells demand prolonged cooking to facilitate active ingredient extraction, such as Shí Gāo (Gypsum Fibrosum, Gypsum), Cí Shí (Magnetitum, Magnetite), Mǔ Lì (Concha Ostreae, Oyster Shell), and Lóng Gǔ (Fossilia Ossis Mastodi, dragon bones). They are boiled first for over 10 minutes before other medicinals are added to the decoction. This method, known as decocting first "先煎, Xiān Jiān", is also applied in cooking certain toxic herbs to reduce its toxicity.

It is easy for medicinals such as Bò He (Herba Menthae, Field Mint), Shā Rén (Fructus Amomi, Villous Amomum Fruit), and Bái Dòu Kòu (Fructus Amomi Kravanh, Round Cardamon) to lose their active ingredients during the course of prolonged decocting. They should be added to a decoction only a few minutes before the cooking is finished; this method is known as add near end "后下, Hòu Xià".

Tiny, powdery, and hairy medicinals are usually decocted in gauze as they float on the surface of decoction or make the the liquid sticky or irritate the throat. This method is noted as decocted in gauze "包煎, Bāo Jiān" in doctor's prescription.

Extremely expensive medicinals such as Rén Shēn (Radix et Rhizoma Ginseng, Ginseng) and Lù Róng (Cornu Cervi Pantotrichum, Deer Velvet) are often simmered separately in a double boiler (known as 另炖, Lìng Dùn) or cooked individually (known as 另煎, Lìng Jiān) for a long period of time to get the full effect of active ingredients and avoid loss of efficacy caused by decocting together with other medicinals. Some gelatine substances such as Ē Jiāo (Colla Corii Asini, Donkey-hide Gelatin) should be separately steamed in a small bowl until melted and the resulting solution added to the strained decoction of other ingredients before ingestion, or directly added into the strained decoction of other ingredients and melted by stirring. This method, known as melting (烊化, Yáng Huà), prevents such medicinals from sticking to the pot or other medicinals.

[Methods of taking medicine] Appropriate precautions should be taken for oral administration of Chinese medicinals in different forms. For instance, a decoction should be taken as one dose and twice a day; two doses and once every 4–6 hours in emergent and severe cases. Tonics should be taken before meals; irritants to the stomach should be taken after meals; mind-calming medicinals should be taken before sleep; worm-expelling substances should be taken on an empty stomach; malaria-relieving herbs should be taken two hours before the onset. Ignorance of the above-mentioned precautions may cause decreased clinical outcomes.

Storage of Chinese materia medica

Chinese materia medica is featured by extensive sources, various species, large amount, complicated properties and actions, and differences in active constituent. During the storage, various external factors may impact the quality of medicinals and eventually affect their therapeutic effects. Some general guidelines of the storage are necessary for practitioners to identify the quality of Chinese materia medica.

[Deterioration of Chinese materia medica] The common deterioration phenomena of Chinese materia medica during storage are as follows:

1. Damage caused by worms: worms can settle in the medicinal, resulting in deterioration phenomena such as fleck, holes or even powdery texture. It will reduce the medicinal value to different degrees, and neutralize the effect or generate toxicity in severe cases.
2. Mildew damage: mildew will grow on or inside any medicinal surface, as long as it has moisture. It will cause decomposition and deterioration of the medicinals, reducing or depriving their positive effects, even generating toxins and being a health hazard. A common example is the toxin generated by aspergillus flavus.
3. Color change: it is related with damage caused by worms, mildew damage, solarization, and long-term storage of the medicinal. It will result in deterioration and invalidity.
4. Oil leakage: it, also known as extensive diffusion of oil, is a deterioration phenomenon that caused by the spilling over of oil ingredients of oily medicinals, or leakage of oil-like substances from sugar or mucilage-containing medicinals.

Other types of deterioration include volatilization and vapidity of the aromatic medicinal, fusion, efflorescence, deliquescence, and decomposition.

[Method of Storing Chinese materia medica] The storage of Chinese medicinal is a complex subject that depends on many factors, professional knowledge, specific techniques, and methods. Still, doctors or patients should know the general storing methods of Chinese medicinals. For medicinals that easily to be damaged by worms, they should be dried by solarization or baking before storage; or method of killing insects by low temperature and isolation. In addition, medicinals with special components or fragrance have been traditionally used to kill or expel worms and prevent other medicinals from damage caused by worms. Two examples are storing Huā Jiāo (Pericarpium Zanthoxyli, Pricklyash Peel), Xì Xīn (Radix et Rhizoma Asari, Manchurian Wild Ginger), and Zhāng Nǎo (Camphora, Camphor) with animal species used for medicinal purpose or medicinals most likely to be damaged by worms; or putting 70% ethanol at the bottom of the container, and tightly covering it to protect against worms and inhibit bacteria. Another preferred worm-resisting approach is to keep certain medicianls together, a common example is storing Mǔ Dān Pí (Cortex Moutan, Tree Peony Bark) with Zé Xiè (Rhizoma Alismatis, Water Plantain Rhizome), and Chén Pí (Pericarpium Citri Reticulatae, Tangerine Pericarp) with Gāo Liáng Jiāng (Rhizoma Alpiniae Officinarum, Galangal) to improve their resistance to worms and maintain their original color, luster, and aroma. Medicinals susceptible to mildew need sun exposure in a timely manner, temperature regulation, and good ventilation.

Medicinals prone to color change and smell and taste loss should be stored away from high temperatures but in a less-ventilated area. Medicinals susceptible to discoloration upon sun exposure should be stored away from direct sunlight. Easily deliquescent and efflorescent medicinals need to be kept in a sealed container. Small amounts of medicinal stored at home should be kept in a cool and shady place for no more than six month. Precious and expensive medicinals, such as Rén Shēn (Radix et Rhizoma Ginseng, Ginseng) and Lù Róng (Cornu Cervi Pantotrichum, Deer Velvet), should be completely dried and then kept well sealed; or stored with scorched fried rice in a sealed container; and Shè Xiāng (Moschus, Musk) and Niú Huáng (Calculus Bovis, Cow Bezoar) should be wrapped in oiled paper, stored in sealed containers, and then kept away from light and high temperatures. Chinese patent medicine should be stored beyond the expiration date on the package.

IV. Combination and its Contraindication of Chinese Materia Medica

When applying Chinese materia medica, practitioners are supposed to know the natures, flavors, actions, indications, contraindications of every medicinal and precautions of certain toxic medicinals. When organizing a prescription, the principle of combining medicinal substances should be followed. These aspects are closely related with the therapeutic effects.

Combination of Chinese materia medica

Combination is an art that uses two or more medicinals together for clinical purpose and is based on the action of the ingredients employed. It is one of the essential characteristics of traditional Chinese medication, the primary form of clinical medication, and also the basis of the organization of prescription. Combination of medicinals reflects the experience accumulated by numerous practitioners over the ages, and the concrete treatment method based upon the theories of traditional Chinese medicine. Only when the principles of combining medicinals became familiar to the practitioners can they become proficiently in treating various diseases with Chinese materia medica.

[Effects of combination of medicinals] Medicinals have been combined to

1. Accommodate complicated clinical conditions
   In the clinic, simple case can be cured with a single medicinal, however there are many complex cases that need to be treated with the combination of medicinals, such as diseases involving both the exterior and interior, diseases involving several *zang* organs, disorders affecting both the upper and lower part of the body, deficiency-excess complex, or cold-heat complex.
2. Increase therapeutic effectiveness
   Combination of several medicinals with similar actions can accentuate their therapeutic functions. Sometimes, for a certain disease or pattern, combination of two or more medicinals with different actions can improve their clinical outcomes as the ingredients employed act on different aspects.
3. Reduce the toxicity and side effects
   Some medicinals generate toxic and side effects while treating disease. If that is the case, it is necessary to combine some medicinals that counteract these undesirable effects.

[Categories of combination of medicinals] Traditionally the seven relations of medicinal compatibility (七情, Qī Qíng) were first mentioned in *Shen Nong's Classic of the Materia Medica* (神农本草经, Shén Nóng Běn Cǎo Jīng), namely use of a single medicinal (单行, Dān Xíng), mutual reinforcement (相须, Xiāng Xū), mutual assistance (相使, Xiāng Shǐ), mutual restraint (相畏, Xiāng Wèi), mutual inhibition (相杀, Xiāng Shā), mutual antagonism (相恶, Xiāng Wù), and mutual incompatibility (相反, Xiāng Fǎn). Mutual reinforcement (相须, Xiāng Xū) refers to the combination of medicinals with similar actions to generate synergistic effect and improve therapeutic effectiveness. Two examples are combining Huáng Lián (Rhizoma Coptidis, Coptis Rhizome), Huáng Qín (Radix Astragali, Milk-vetch Root), and Huáng Bǎi (Cortex Phellodendri Chinensis, Amur Cork-tree Bark) to improve their potency of clearing heat and relieving toxin; and combining Jīng Jiè (Herba Schizonepetae, Schizonepeta) and Fáng Fēng (Radix Saposhnikoviae, Ledebouriella Root) to highlight their actions of dispelling exterior cold pathogen; mutual assistance (相使, Xiāng Shǐ) means the combination of medicinals with different actions in which one substance enhances the effect of the principal ingredients to enhance therapeutic effectiveness. Examples are combining qi-tonifying Huáng Qí (Radix Astragali, Astragalus Root) and exterior-dispersing Fáng Fēng (Radix Saposhnikoviae, Siler) to improve the former's ability of consolidating the exterior; or heat-clearing Shí Gāo (Gypsum Fibrosum, Gypsum) and downward-running Niú Xī (Radix Achyranthis Bidentatae, Two-toothed Achyranthes Root) to direct stomach-fire downward; mutual restraint (相畏, Xiāng Wèi) refers to a combination in which the toxicity or side effects of one medicinal are reduced or eliminated by another medicinal. Traditional examples are that the toxicity of Dīng Xiāng (Flos Caryophylli, Clove Flower) is reduced by Yù Jīn (Radix Curcumae, Turmeric Root Tuber); and the toxicity of Bàn Xià (Rhizoma Pinelliae, Pinellia Rhizome) and Dǎn Nán Xīng (Arisaema cum Bile, Bile Arisaema) are alleviated by Shēng Jiāng (Rhizoma Zingiberis Recens, Fresh Ginger); mutual inhibition (相杀, Xiāng Shā) is the converse of mutual restraint in that here one medicinal also reduces or eliminates the toxicity or side effects of another; mutual antagonism (相恶, Xiāng Wù) means the ability of two medicinals to minimize or neutralize each other's original effects. A common example is that Lái Fú Zǐ (Semen Raphani, Radish Seed) antagonizes Rén Shēn (Radix et Rhizoma Ginseng, Ginseng) and weakens the latter's effect; and mutual incompatibility (相反, Xiāng Fǎn) occurs when the combination of two medicinals gives rise to toxicity or side effects. Traditional example is that Gān Cǎo (Radix et Rhizoma Glycyrrhizae, Licorice Root) is incompatible with Gān Suì (Radix Kansui, Gansui Root).

[Prohibited combination] In ancient Chinese materia medica works, there are many records about prohibited combination like mutual antagonism (相恶, Xiāng Wù) and mutual incompatibility (相反, Xiāng Fǎn) mentioned above. Meanwhile, two sets of prohibited combinations known as nineteen antagonisms (十九畏, Shí Jiǔ Wèi) and eighteen incompatibilities (十八反, Shí Bā Fǎn) gained the widest recognition. Nineteen antagonisms (十九畏, Shí Jiǔ Wèi) means a combination in which one medicinal minimize the positive effect of another, such as Liú Huáng (Sulphur, Sulphur) antagonizes Pò Xiāo (Mirabilitum, Mirabilite), Shuǐ Yín (Hydrargyrum, Mercury) antagonizes Pī Shuāng (Arsenic Trioxide), Láng Dú (Radix Euphorbiae Fischerianae, Wolf's Bane) antagonizes Mì Tuó Sēng (Lithargyrum, Galena), Bā Dòu (Fructus Crotonis, Croton Seed) antagonizes Qiān Niú Zǐ (Semen Pharbitidis, pharbitidis seed), Dīng Xiāng (Flos Caryophylli, Clove Flower) antagonizes Yù Jīn (Radix Curcumae, Turmeric Root Tuber), Yá Xiāo (Crystalline Sodium Sulfate) antagonizes Sān Léng (Rhizoma Sparganii, Common Burr Reed Tuber), Chuān Wū (Radix Aconiti, Common Monkshood Mother Root) and Cǎo Wū (Radix Aconiti Kusnezoffii, Kusnezoff Monkshood Root) antagonizes Xī Jiǎo (Cornu Rhinocerotis, Rhinoceros Horn), Rén Shēn (Radix et Rhizoma Ginseng, Ginseng) antagonizes Wǔ Líng Zhī (Feces Trogopterori, Flying Squirrel Feces), and Guān Guì (Cortex Cinnamomi, Cinnamon Bark) antagonizes Chì Shí Zhī (Halloysitum Rubrum, Halloysite). Eighteen incompatibilities (十八反, Shí Bā Fǎn) occurs when the combination of two medicinals generate toxicity or side effects, such as Wū Tóu (Radix Aconiti) is incompatible with Bàn Xià (Rhizoma Pinelliae, Pinellia

Rhizome), Guā Lóu (Fructus Trichosanthis, Snakegourd Fruit), Bèi Mǔ (Bulbus Fritillaria, Fritillary Bulb), Bái Liǎn (Radix Ampelopsis, Ampelopsis), and Bái Jí (Rhizoma Bletillae, Bletilla Rhizome); Gān Cǎo (Radix et Rhizoma Glycyrrhizae, Licorice Root) is incompatible with Hǎi Zǎo (Sargassum, Seaweed), Dà Jǐ (Radix Euphorbiae Pekinensis, Euphorbia Root), Gān Suì (Radix Kansui, Gansui Root), and Yuán Huā (Flos Genkwa, Lilac Daphne Flower Bud); Lí Lú (Radix et Rhizoma Veratri Nigri, Veratrum Root and Rhizome) is incompatible with Rén Shēn (Radix et Rhizoma Ginseng, Ginseng), Shā Shēn (Radix Adenophorae seu Glehniae), Dān Shēn (Radix et Rhizoma Salviae Miltiorrhizae, Danshen Root), Xuán Shēn (Radix Scrophulariae, Figwort root), Kǔ Shēn (Radix Sophorae Flavescentis, Light Yellow Sophora Root), Xì Xīn (Radix et Rhizoma Asari, Manchurian Wild Ginger), and Sháo Yào (Radix Paeoniae, peony root). The understanding of above-mentioned "antagonisms" and "incompatibilities" has been under dispute over the ages, and there are many ancient formulas that those incompatible or antagonistic medicinals are prescribed together. Modern researches have no exact conclusions yet, however, they should be used with more cautions.

[Addendum] Eighteen incompatibilities (十八反, Shí Bā Fǎn), so called because they are composed of three set with a total of eighteen incompatible substances:

Wū Tóu (Radix Aconiti) is incompatible with:
  Bàn Xià (Rhizoma Pinelliae, Pinellia Rhizome)
  Guā Lóu (Fructus Trichosanthis, Snakegourd Fruit)
  Bèi Mǔ (Bulbus Fritillaria, Fritillary Bulb)
  Bái Liǎn (Radix Ampelopsis, Ampelopsis)
  Bái Jí (Rhizoma Bletillae, Bletilla Rhizome);

Gān Cǎo (Radix et Rhizoma Glycyrrhizae, Licorice Root) is incompatible with:
  Hǎi Zǎo (Sargassum, Seaweed)
  Dà Jǐ (Radix Euphorbiae Pekinensis, Euphorbia Root)
  Gān Suì (Radix Kansui, Gansui Root)
  Yuán Huā (Flos Genkwa, Lilac Daphne Flower Bud);

Lí Lú (Radix et Rhizoma Veratri Nigri, Veratrum Root and Rhizome) is incompatible with:

Rén Shēn (Radix et Rhizoma Ginseng, Ginseng)

Shā Shēn (Radix Adenophorae seu Glehniae)

Dān Shēn (Radix et Rhizoma Salviae Miltiorrhizae, Danshen Root)

Xuán Shēn (Radix Scrophulariae, Figwort root)

Kǔ Shēn (Radix Sophorae Flavescentis, Light Yellow Sophora Root)

Xì Xīn (Radix et Rhizoma Asari, Manchurian Wild Ginger)

Sháo Yào (Radix Paeoniae, peony root).

Nineteen antagonisms (十九畏, Shí Jiǔ Wèi)

Liú Huáng (Sulphur, Sulphur) antagonizes Pò Xiāo (Mirabilitum, Mirabilite)

Shuǐ Yín (Hydrargyrum, Mercury) antagonizes Pī Shuāng (Arsenic Trioxide)

Láng Dú (Radix Euphorbiae Fischerianae, Wolf's Bane) antagonizes Mì Tuó Sēng (Lithargyrum, Galena)

Bā Dòu (Fructus Crotonis, Croton Seed) antagonizes Qiān Niú Zǐ (Semen Pharbitidis, pharbitidis seed)

Dīng Xiāng (Flos Caryophylli, Clove Flower) antagonizes Yù Jīn (Radix Curcumae, Turmeric Root Tuber)

Yá Xiāo (Crystalline Sodium Sulfate) antagonizes Sān Léng (Rhizoma Sparganii, Common Burr Reed Tuber)

Chuān Wū (Radix Aconiti, Common Monkshood Mother Root) and Cǎo Wū (Radix Aconiti Kusnezoffii, Kusnezoff Monkshood Root) antagonizes Xī Jiǎo (Cornu Rhinocerotis, Rhinoceros Horn)

Rén Shēn (Radix et Rhizoma Ginseng, Ginseng) antagonizes Wǔ Líng Zhī (Feces Trogopterori, Flying Squirrel Feces)

Guān Guì (Cortex Cinnamomi, Cinnamon Bark) antagonizes Chì Shí Zhī (Halloysitum Rubrum, Halloysite)

Daily practice

1. What precautions should be taken when decocting Chinese materia medica?

2. What are the main deterioration phenomena of Chiense materia medica, what precautions should be taken for storage?

3. What are the actions and categories of Chinese materia medica combination?

6

Prevention of adverse reactions of Chinese materia medica

Chinese medicinals are in general safe to use with few side effects, however, they may cause negative results if applied inappropriately. Therefore, comprehensive understanding of their contraindications is necessary to prevent those adverse reactions.

[Knowing the properties of Chinese materia medica] Chinese materia medica can treat diseases but also create undesirable effects. Cold or cool agents, for instance, can clear heat but also injure yang qi; hot or warm ingredients can dispel cold but also exhaust yin fluids; tonics can assist healthy qi but also retain pathogens or hinder digestion if applied inappropriately; and pathogen-dispersing medicinals are necessary approaches for treatment but prone to damage healthy qi. In addition, wrong patterns of differentiation can lead to improper administration of medication with negative therapeutic effectiveness. Huáng Lián (Rhizoma Coptidis, Coptis Rhizome), for instance, owning to its bitter flavor and cold nature, is considered suitable for damp-heat dysentery, and may injure spleen qi and exacerbate the disorder when misused for diarrhea due to spleen deficiency. These known adverse reactions are avoidable only when physicians know the properties including both advantages and disadvantages of Chinese medicinal well.

[Using toxic Chinese materia medica with cautions] Some Chinese materia medica have different levels of toxicity, namely Dà Dú (大毒, strong toxicity) and Xiǎo Dú (小毒, mild toxicity). Improper, high doses, or long term use of these poisonous compounds are harmful to the human body. The following precautions for administration are advised

1. Dosage: the dosage of toxic medicinals, especially strong toxics, must be strictly controlled. Commonly used dosage of these poisonous

ingredients has been elaborated in Chinese materia medica works. They should be started from small dose, and gradually increased until optimum efficacy is achieved. Larger dosage should be based on a particular clinical condition. Precautions should be taken to prevent poisoning due to accumulation of toxicity, even for patients who use small amount for a long period of time. External application of toxic medicinals should be localized (limited to one part of the body) for a short period of time to avoid poisoning due to over-absorption.

2. Strict processing: toxic medicinals should be processed under the strict requirements to eliminate their toxicities. For instance, deep-frying can reduce the toxicity of Mǎ Qián Zǐ (Semen Strychni, Nux Vomica Seed), partially destroying its primary toxic ingredient brucine; preparing Bā Dòu (Fructus Crotonis, Croton Seed) into Bā Dòu Shuāng (Semen Crotonis Pulveratum, Defatted Croton Seed Powder) or Bā Dòu Tàn (Semen Crotonis Carbonisatum, Carbonized Croton Seed) to reduce its toxicity due to drastic purgative.

   Usage: different toxic medicinals have different methods of administration, and therefore should be used with more cautions. Some should only be used externally, such as Shēng Yào (Hydrargyrum Oxydatum Crudum, Mercuric Oxide) and Máo Liáng (Ranunculus japonicus Thunb, Buttercup); some should only be used in the form of pill or powder, such as Niú Huáng (Calculus Bovis, Cow Bezoar), Chán Sū (Venenum Bufonis, Toad Venom), and Bān Máo (Mylabris, Cantharide); and others can be used in decoction but should not be prepared into medicated wine, such as Wū Tóu (Radix Aconiti, Common Monkshood Mother Root). Combination of medicinals, as an important approach to prevent or reduce toxic reaction, can help attenuate the toxicity of certain poisonous ingredients, such as combining Fù Zǐ (Radix Aconiti Lateralis Praeparata, Monkshood) with Gān Jiāng (Rhizoma Zingiberis, Dried Ginger Rhizome) and Gān Cǎo (Radix et Rhizoma Glycyrrhizae, Licorice Root), and combining Wū Tóu (Aconite Main Tuber) with Fēng Mì (Mel, Honey).

3. Species: the species of Chinese materia medica are complex and diversified. The medicinals with the same name may come from a variety of species, in which some are toxic, some are non-toxic, some are with strong toxicity, and others are of mild toxicity. It is therefore helpful to

know elementary knowledge of medicinal species and make species identification when using these medicinals. Wǔ Jiā Pí (Cortex Acanthopanacis, Eleutherococcus Root Bark) that dispel wind-damp, for instance, has two species, namely 南五加 Nán Wǔ Jiā, toxic, is root and bark of Eleutherococcus nodiflorus and 北五加 Wǔ Jiā Beǐ, non-toxic, is root and bark of Periploca sepium Bunge, family Asclepiadaceae. Another example is that urination-promoting and strangury-relieving Mù Tōng (Caulis Akebiae, Akebia Stem) has three species, namely Bái Mù Tōng (Akebia Trifoliata Varaustralis), Chuān Mù Tōng (Caulis Clematidis Armandii, Clematidis Caulis), and toxic Guān Mù Tōng (Caulis Aristolochiae Manshuriensis, Manchurian Dutchmans Pipe Stem) that now forbidden to be used for medicinal purposes.

[Contraindications during pregnancy] Medicinals should be used with more cautions during pregnancy, as modern research indicate that improper medication may cause fetal deformity or even miscarriage. Generally, Chinese mediicnals are safe to the fetus, but some may generate side effects or lead to problems for the fetus, even causing miscarriage. Our ancestors have accumulated abundant experiences on contraindications during pregnancy, which are categorized into the following aspects:

1. Drastic toxicants such as Bān Máo (Mylabris, Cantharide) cantharide, Yuán Qīng (Lytta Caraganae), Wū Tóu (Aconite Main Tuber), Mǎ Qián Zǐ (Semen Strychni, Nux Vomica Seed), and Chán Sū (Venenum Bufonis, Toad Venom) are harmful to the fetus and may cause miscarriage.
2. Drastic purgatives such as Bā Dòu (Fructus Crotonis, croton seed), Dà Huáng (Radix et Rhizoma Rhei, Rhubarb Root and Rhizome), Gān Suì (Radix Kansui, Gansui Root), Dà Jǐ (Radix Euphorbiae Pekinensis, Peking Euphorbia Root), Yuán Huā (Flos Genkwa, Lilac Daphne Flower Bud), and Qiān Niú Zǐ (Semen Pharbitidis, Pharbitidis Seed) may result in miscarriage.
3. Blood-activating and blood stasis-relieving medicinals such as Niú Xī (Radix Achyranthis Bidentatae, Two-toothed Achyranthes Root), Shuǐ Zhì (Hirudo, leech), Méng Chóng (Tabanus, gradfly), Sān Léng (Rhizoma Sparganii, Common Burr Reed Tuber), É Zhú (Rhizoma

Curcumae, Curcumae Rhizome), and Táo Rén (Semen Persicae, Peach Seed) can promote blood circulation, strengthen uterine contraction, and eventually cause miscarriage.

4. Acrid, aromatic, and scattering medicines such as Shè Xiāng (Moschus, Cow Bezoar) may excite uterus and lead to miscarriage.
5. Acrid-hot medicinals such as Fù Zǐ (Radix Aconiti Lateralis Praeparata, Monkshood), Ròu Guì (Cortex Cinnamomi Cinnamon Bark), and Gān Jiāng (Rhizoma Zingiberis, Dried Ginger Rhizome) are harsh substances and easy to influence the fetus, or even cause miscarriage.

In the opinion of the ancients, medicinals such as Bàn Xià (Rhizoma Pinelliae, Pinellia Rhizome), Chán Tuì (Periostracum Cicadae, Cicada Moulting), Yì Yǐ Rén (Semen Coicis, Coix Seed), Dài Zhě Shí (Haematitum, Hematite), Zào Jiǎo (Fructus Gleditsiae, Chinese Honeylocust), Tōng Cǎo (Medulla Tetrapanacis, Rice Paper Plant Pith), Qú Mài (Herba Dianthi, Lilac Pink Herb), and Bái Máo Gēn (Rhizoma Imperatae, Woolly Grass) are generally contraindicated during pregnancy. However, they can be prescribed with the utmost caution and only for carefully selected patients, as *The Yellow Emperor's Inner Classic* (黄帝内经, *Huáng Dì Nèi Jīng*) stated "toxicants are applicable only when they are used carefully and for the right pathogenic changes". Some of the above mentioned medicinals may not be harmful to the fetus and still need further research.

Dosage of Chinese materia medica

[Dosage of Chinese materia medica] Dosage is of great importance for the treatment of disease, especially when composing a right prescription. Traditionally it was a secret reserved for doctors and was not discussed publicly, which also indicates its importance for improving therapeutic effect and reducing side effects.

Compared with chemicals, dosage of Chinese materia medica is featured by (1) mild nature. These moderate medicinals are used in the maximum safe dose or even higher when necessary; and (2) flexibility of use especially for decoction. Under the guidance of theories of traditional Chinese medicine, the variables governing dosage include the state of illness, patient's constitution, and different usage.

Now, metric measurements are used for the dosage, gram for weight, and milliliter for volume. To convert back to the traditional measurement, one Liǎng is equal to 30 g, and one Qián is equal to 3 g.

Dosage of Chinese materia medica is determined by medicinal properties and combination, usage, state of illness, and patient's constitution and age. For instance, moderate medicinals are used in high doses with a large dosage range; heavy and fresh substances are usually prescribed in larger doses; toxic and violent medicinals are used with cautions as the old saying goes "Má Huáng (Herba Ephedrae, Ephedra) should be less than 9 g, and Xì Xīn (Radix et Rhizoma Asari, Manchurian Wild Ginger) less than 3 g". If a medicinal is prescribed by itself or with just a few other medicinals, a larger dose is preferred. For instance, Mǎ Chǐ Xiàn (Herba Portulacae, Purslane Herb) is prescribed alone over 150 g for treating dysentery. If a substance is used as a principal substance in formula, a larger dose is prescribed. For instance, Yì Mǔ Cǎo (Herba Leonuri, Motherwort) is used as a chief medicinal over 60 g in the treatment of nephritis edema, and its dose is decreased to 10–15 g in other formulas. Other important factors are the kind of preparation used, severity of disorder, patient's constitution, and age. The dosage is usually less for pills and powders than for decoction; severe and emergent problems usually require a larger dose, Rén Shēn (Radix et Rhizoma Ginseng, Ginseng), for instance, is used up to over 20 g for rescuing collapse, and reduced to 5 g as a general tonic; strong patients need a larger dosage; and the young cannot tolerate too large a dose (e.g., 1/4 of adult dosage for patient less than one year old, 1/3 for 1–3 years old, 1/2 for 4–6 years old, 3/4 for 7–10 years old, and adult dosage for above 10 years old). Dosage also depends on climate and region.

To sum up, dosage prescription is with flexibility, practitioners are expected to integrate traditional Chinese medicine literatures with their own clinical experiences in an effort of improving therapeutic effect and reducing side effects.

Daily practice

1. How to prevent the adverse reactions of Chinese materia medica?
2. What are the factors influencing the dose of Chinese materia medica?

Second Week

1

MEDICINALS THAT RELEASE THE EXTERIOR

Exterior pattern refers to a disorder that caused by an invasion of the body's exterior by exogenous pathogens. It is common in early stage of externally-contracted disorder and characterized by fever, chills, headache, body ache, white thin tongue coating, and floating pulse. From the perspective of traditional Chinese medicine, *Exterior* (表, Biaǒ) refers to a disease manifesting in the superficial layers of the body-skin, hair, flesh, and meridians. Exterior-releasing herbs are those that dissipate external pathogen and release exterior pattern. They have some common features, namely pungent in flavor, light-weight in texture, and ascending and dispersing in nature, most of these herbs are diaphoretics, i.e., they release or expel the external pathogenic influence through sweating. Some of the herbs that release the exterior have additional functions resulting from their dispersing effect: diffusing the lung to stop cough and wheezing, venting and promoting eruption of measles, promoting urination to reduce swelling, dispersing wind to arrest pain, and dissipating carbuncles and swellings. Exterior-releasing medicinals are therefore not only applicable for exterior pattern, but also cough and wheezing, measles, edema, muscle and joint pain, and carbuncles and swelling in early stage.

In the clinic, medicinals that release the exterior should be selected according to the nature of exogenous pathogen. The warm and acrid herbs that release the exterior (known as release the exterior with acrid-warm medicinals) are used for exterior disorders caused by wind-cold and wind-damp pathogen. Cool and acrid substances that release the exterior (known as release the exterior with acrid-cool medicinals) are used in treatment of wind-heat patterns. Clinically, the herbs are often combined in prescriptions with other herbs in accordance with patient's condition. For instance, these substances are combined with medicinals that clear heat and resolve toxins for intense wind-heat exterior pattern; with dampness-dispelling medicinals for wind pathogen binding with dampness; with phlegm-dissolving herbs for cough and wheezing with profuse sputum; with herbs that move qi and harmonize the stomach when accompanied with chest oppression and vomiting; with yin-nourishing medicinals for constitutionally yin deficiency with exterior pattern; with yang-warming herbs for constitutionally yang qi deficiency with exterior pattern; and with qi-boosting medicinals for constitutionally qi deficiency with exterior pattern.

Generally, exterior-releasing medicinals are neutral in moderate and applicable for mild cases, but may cause adverse reactions when applied inappropriately. Selection of warm or cool herbs for clinical use is based on the nature of disorder, namely heat or cold; medicinals with strong diaphoretic effect should not be overused, especially for patient with sweating; and high doses are not recommended. Slight sweating is expected after using diaphoretics, if there is lack of sweating, patients can take warm water or congee, or increase sweating with aid of more coats and quilts, but profuse sweating is discouraged as it can consume yin fluid and healthy qi. These medicinals should be used with caution for constitutionally weak patient, people who always have a higher tendency towards sweating, or in cases of profuse bleeding.

Most of these herbs are aromatic and rich in volatile components and must not be overcooked when used in decoction to prevent loss of active ingredients.

I. Acrid-Warm Medicinals that Release the Exterior

麻黄 Má Huáng *herba ephedrae ephedra*

The source is from the stem of herbaceous perennial *Ephedra sinica* stapf, *E. equisetina* Bunge, or *E. intermedia* schrenk et Mey. family Ephedraceae. Acrid and slightly bitter in flavor and warm in nature.

[Actions] Promote sweating to disperse cold, diffuse the lung to relieve wheezing, and promote urination to reduce swelling. It is applicable to common cold of wind-cold pattern, chest oppression, cough, wheezing, and wind edema. Modern pharmacological researches reveals that ephedra contains a variety of ephedrine and volatile oil with multiple effects of inducing sweating, relaxing bronchial smooth muscle, vasoconstriction, stimulating the central nervous system, raising blood pressure, diuretic, anti-inflammation, fighting against allergy, and resisting influenza virus.

[Quality] Ephedra is native to northern China. The herb grown in Shanxi, Gansu, Shaanxi, and Qinghai provinces is of the high quality and called 西麻黄 Xī Má Huáng. Good quality is dry, light green, and bitter and acrid, and has a thick stem and solid center.

[Indications] It is a typical herb for wind-cold common cold and wind-cold-damp obstructing the fleshy exterior with absence of sweating, fever with aversion to cold, edema, and wheezing. Absence of sweating indicates the dry skin and difficulty sweating, patients may also present with aversion to cold, joint pain, and different levels of edema (swelling all over the body in some cases, superficial swelling with a heavy body in some cases, and swelling in a combination with yellow darkish complexion and floating loose muscle in other cases). Má Huáng (Herba Ephedrae) is one of the principal herbs used to treat different kinds of wheezing due to excess pattern, sometimes accompanied with aversion to cold, absence of sweating, edema, nasal congestion, or clear nasal discharge. Its indications are as follows:

1. Wind-cold exterior excess pattern: this pattern is caused by the invasion of wind-cold pathogen, manifested as aversion to cold, absence of sweating, and muscle and joint pain. People's fleshy exterior will be invaded by the wind, cold and damp pathogen when they are attacked by wind-cold, having excessive wading, drinking cold too much, and living or working long-term in the gloomy, cold and moist environment. Clinical manifestations include absence of sweating, aversion to cold, joint pain, muscle aching pain, heavy sensation all over the body, lassitude, and fatigue. In most cases, the tongue is white moist and the pulse is moderate and powerful. Those symptoms can be slightly alleviated when patients move to a warmer place, have a heating bath, or get sweating upon exercises. Herein, Má Huáng (Herba Ephedrae) is not only applicable to common cold and influenza in a combination with

such herbs as Guì Zhī (Ramulus Cinnamomi), Gān Jiāng (Rhizoma Zingiberis), and Fù Zǐ (Radix Aconiti Lateralis Praeparata), but also diseases like arthritis, muscle pain, sciatica due to its effect of dissipating cold and relieving pain.

2. Cough and wheezing: manifestations include cough and wheezing with thin and clear sputum and puffing and blowing sound in the throat with accompanying chest oppression, nasal congestion, absence of sweating or slight sweating caused by cough and wheezing, aversion to cold, and listlessness. Auscultation revealed wheezing rales over both lung fields. Má Huáng (Herba Ephedrae) is not suitable when patient present persistent wheezing, profuse sweating, and fast but feeble pulse. It is usually combined with Xìng Rén (Semen Armeniacae Amarum) and Gān Cǎo (Radix et Rhizoma Glycyrrhizae) for cough and wheezing in such diseases as bronchitis, asthma, pneumonia, and pollinosis; and Xìng Rén (Semen Armeniacae Amarum), Pí Pá Yè (Folium Eriobotryae), and Jié Gěng (Radix Platycodonis) to disperse wind-cold and diffuse lung qi with a purpose of arresting cough with itching throat and scanty sputum when the invasion of exogenous wind-cold pathogen make lung fail to diffuse and govern descent.

3. Edema: it is featured by sudden onset of swelling all over the body and combined with heavy feeling in the body and scanty urine. It is most likely to be found in the cases of acute and chronic nephritis, angioneurotic edema. Má Huáng (Herba Ephedrae) is often combined with Shí Gāo (Gypsum Fibrosum), Lián Qiào (Fructus Forsythiae), and Jīn Yín Huā (Flos Lonicerae Japonicae) for throat pain and skin infection via clearing heat and resolving toxins; with Shí Gāo (Gypsum Fibrosum), Xìng Rén (Semen Armeniacae Amarum), and Gān Cǎo (Radix et Rhizoma Glycyrrhizae) for restlessness, thirst, and slight sweating; and with Fù Zǐ (Radix Aconiti Lateralis Praeparata), Bái Zhú (Rhizoma Atractylodis Macrocephalae), and Fú Líng (Poria) to warm yang and promote urination for yang-deficiency cold pattern manifested as chronic edema, poker face, heavy sensation all over the body, absence of sweating, aversion to cold, thirst, and deep pulse.

[Usage and Dosage] The raw herb is an effective diaphoretic used for exterior excess patterns with the manifestations of wind-cold fettering the exterior, absence of sweating, and aversion to cold; while the honey-fried herb is better at relieving wheezing and cough, mild in promoting sweating, and more preferred for the elderly, weak, and young. Use 3–10 g in decoction, and decrease the dosage as in powder.

[Mnemonics] Má Huáng (Herba Ephedrae, Eph edra): pungent and warm; induce sweating to release the exterior, promote urination to relieve edema, and diffuse the lung to reduce wheezing.

[Simple and Effective Formulas]

1. 麻黄汤 Má Huáng Tāng — Ephedra Decoction from the *Treatise on Cold Damage* (伤寒论 Shāng Hán Lùn): Má Huáng (Herba Ephedrae) 6g, Guì Zhī (Ramulus Cinnamomi) 6g, Xìng Rén (Semen Armeniacae Amarum) 10g, and Gān Cǎo (Radix et Rhizoma Glycyrrhizae) 3g; decoct in water for oral administration to treat patients suffering from wheezing without sweating, body pain without sweating, and floating powerful pulse. Also applicable for wind-cold exterior-excess pattern in diseases such as influenza, arthritis, and bronchial asthma.
2. 三拗汤 Sān Ào Tāng — Rough and Ready Three Decoction from the *Formulas from the Imperial Pharmacy* (和剂局方, Hé Jì Jú Fāng): Má Huáng (Herba Ephedrae) 6g, Xìng Rén (Semen Armeniacae Amarum)10g, and Gān Cǎo (Radix et Rhizoma Glycyrrhizae) 3g for patient with stuffy nose, aversion to cold, headache, and wheezing without sweating. Also applicable for asthma due to wind-cold invading the lung.
3. 麻杏石甘汤 Má Xìng Shí Gān Tāng — Ephedra, Apricot Kernel, Gypsum and Licorice Decoction from the *Treatise on Cold Damage* (伤寒论, Shāng Hán Lùn): Má Huáng (Herba Ephedrae) 6g, Xìng Rén (Semen Armeniacae Amarum) 10g, Shí Gāo (Gypsum Fibrosum) 15g, and Gān Cǎo (Radix et Rhizoma Glycyrrhizae) 3g; decoct in water for oral administration to relieve asthma with slight sweating and floating fast pulse. Also applicable for different types of bronchial pneumonia.
4. 小青龙汤 Xiǎo Qīng Lóng Tāng — Minor Green Dragon Decoction from the *Treatise on Cold Damage* (伤寒论, Shāng Hán Lùn): Má Huáng (Herba Ephedrae) 5g, Gān Cǎo (Radix et Rhizoma Glycyrrhizae) 3g, Gān Jiāng (Rhizoma Zingiberis) 10g, Xì Xīn (Radix et Rhizoma

Asari) 6g, Wŭ Wèi Zǐ (Fructus Schisandrae Chinensis) 10g, Guì Zhī (Ramulus Cinnamomi) 10g, Bàn Xià (Rhizoma Pinelliae) 10g, and Sháo Yào (Radix Paeoniae) 10g; decoct in water for oral administration to treat patient with cough, wheezing, and vomiting clear phlegm-drool due to cold-rheum retention. Also applicable for chronic bronchitis due to retention of cold fluid in the lung.

[Precautions] Má Huáng (Herba Ephedrae) is a strong diaphoretic, do not overdose. Avoid prescribing it to patients who have weak constitution, sweat easily, or suffer from deficiency-type asthma. It is also a powerful blood pressure and cardiac stimulant and must be used with caution by people with hypertension and heart disorders especially tachycardia. Clinical application requires a careful identification of the constitution of patients. It is generally usable for patients who have yellow darkish complexion, dry and rough skin, floating loose muscle, more likelihood to get edema; aversion to cold with preference for heat, susceptibility to the common cold, muscle aches from the common cold, and fever without sweating; stuffy nose and asthma; susceptibility to edema with scanty urine, thirst with little water intake; heavy sensation in the body with slow response; enlarged tongue body with white moist coating, and floating powerful pulse. It should be used with caution by people with white complexion, emaciation, sweating easily, and tachycardia.

Daily practices

1. What are the different types of exterior pattern and how to select the corresponding exterior-releasing medicinals?
2. What are the actions and indications of exterior-releasing medicinals?
3. What are the actions and indications of Má Huáng (Herba Ephedrae)?

2

桂枝 Guì Zhī *ramulus cinnamomi cinnamon twig*

[Addendum] 肉桂 Ròu Guì Cortex Cinnamomi Cinnamon Bark
   The source is from the tender branch of *Cinnamomum cassia* Presel, family Lauraceae. Pungent and sweet in taste and warm in nature.

[Actions] Dredge the exterior and release the flesh, warm and open the channels and collaterals, unblock yang and transfer qi, and calm surging and direct counterflow downward. It is applicable to wind-cold type of common cold, cold obstruction in the channels and collaterals, unsmooth movement of yang qi, and ascending counterflow of qi. From the perspective of modern pharmacological research, the major constituent of this herb is the volatile oil that contains ingredients such as cinnamaldehyde and cinnamic acid. Cassia oil is an effective substance to dilate central and peripheral blood vessels and promote blood circulation, which can direct enhanced blood flow to the skin and is conducive to the diaphoresis and fever-relief. Cinnamaldehyde has shown mild analgesic and sedative effects. Guì Zhī (Ramulus Cinnamomi) also can control convulsion, relieve allergy, and improve stomach function.

[Quality] Soaked in water until softened and moistened, cut into segments or slices, and dried in the air. Good quality is tender, thin, even in size, and intensely fragrant and has a brownish red color. Also known as 桂枝尖 Guì Zhī Jiān.

[Indications] Guì Zhī (Ramulus Cinnamomi) is important to relieve the exterior, warm yang, and dissipate cold. In addition to treat wind-cold exterior pattern, it is used widely for the diseases and patterns of yang deficiency with excessive cold. The yang deficiency mainly involves exterior-yang and heart-yang with such major symptoms as spontaneous sweating, aversion to wind, joint pain, palpitation, and qi rushing up.

1. Wind-cold exterior pattern: Guì Zhī (Ramulus Cinnamomi), pungent and dissipating, is capable of dispersing exterior cold to treat different types of wind-cold exterior pattern. It is often prescribed together with Bái Sháo (Radix Paeoniae Alba), Shēng Jiāng (Rhizoma Zingiberis Recens), and Dà Zǎo (Fructus Jujubae) for wind-cold exterior-deficiency pattern manifested by spontaneous sweating, aversion to wind, and floating slow pulse; and with Má Huáng (Herba Ephedrae) for wind-cold exterior-excess pattern featured by aversion to cold, absence of sweating, and floating tight pulse.

2. Qi counterflow pattern: *Treatise on Cold Damage* (伤寒论, Shāng Hán Lùn) called it qi rushing up to the chest, which is a subjective feeling

of the patient. Patients may feel the sense of rushing up, that is to say, qi rushing up from the lower abdomen to the chest causes a sensation of suffocation and distending pain in the throat, chest and abdomen, or sometimes even leads to wheezing; on the other hand, patients may have a throbbing sensation, palpitation ameliorated upon pressing, throbbing sensation all over the body, or obvious throbbing sensation in the umbilical region, usually combined with spontaneous sweating, aversion to wind, and floating, moderate, deficient, and relatively-enlarged pulse. Other chief complaints may not include the rushing-up sensation of qi but spontaneous sweating, aversion to wind, frequent sweating even not in a hot weather or taking any diaphoretic. This pattern is commonly found in cardiovascular and neurotic diseases. Guì Zhī (Ramulus Cinnamomi) is often combined with Gān Cǎo (Radix et Rhizoma Glycyrrhizae), Dà Zǎo (Fructus Jujubae), Bái Sháo (Radix Paeoniae Alba), Lóng Gǔ (Os Draconis), and Mǔ Lì (Concha Ostreae).

3. Spontaneous sweating: it refers to sweating not due to hot weather, excessive physical exertion, or administration of diaphoretic medicinals. Spontaneous sweating is very often combined with aversion to wind, fear of cold, joint pain, and sensation of throbbing and palpitation. Patients prefer to wear thick clothing and quilt when sweating, but have a feeling of vexing heat after. It is most likely to be found in vegetative nerve functional disturbances, cardiovascular diseases, common cold, arthritis, allergic diseases, and postpartum. In this case, Guì Zhī (Ramulus Cinnamomi) is often combined with Huáng Qí (Radix Astragali), Duàn Mǔ Lì (calcined Concha Ostreae), and Bái Sháo (Radix Paeoniae Alba).

4. Pain: it refers to paroxysmal abdominal pain combined with qi rushing-up and throbbing; pain in the joint, waist and lower extremities with accompanying aversion to cold, spontaneous sweating, and cold sensation aggravated by exposure to wind; and dysmenorrhea complicated with dark menorrhea, joint pain or cold sensation in the lower abdomen.

[Usage and Dosage] Use 5–12g, decoct in water for oral administration.

[Mnemonics] Guì Zhī (Ramulus Cinnamomi, Cinnamon Twig): pungent and sweet; relieve the exterior and dissipate cold, calm surging and direct counterflow downward, and eliminate spontaneous sweating.

[Simple and Effective Formulas]

1. 桂枝甘草汤 — Guì Zhī Gān Cǎo Tāng — Cinnamon Twig and Licorice Decoction from the *Treatise on Cold Damage* (伤寒论, Shāng Hán Lùn): Guì Zhī (Ramulus Cinnamomi) 10g and Gān Cǎo (Radix et Rhizoma Glycyrrhizae) 5g; mainly for patients with throbbing in the epigastrium with a preference for pressing and rushing-up qi movement. Also applicable to hypertension, heart diseases, and neurasthenia with the above-mentioned symptoms.

2. 桂枝汤 — Guì Zhī Tāng — Cinnamon Twig Decoction from the *Treatise on Cold Damage* (伤寒论, Shāng Hán Lùn): Guì Zhī (Ramulus Cinnamomi) 10g, Sháo Yào (Radix Paeoniae) 10g, Gān Cǎo (Radix et Rhizoma Glycyrrhizae) 5g, Shēng Jiāng (Rhizoma Zingiberis Recens) three pieces, and ten Dà Zǎo (Fructus Jujubae); mainly for fever, headache, spontaneous sweating, aversion to wind, nasal sound, body pain, and moderate floating pulse, or with accompanying abdominal pain and qi rushing-up pattern in some cases. Also applicable to abnormal sweating, deficiency common cold, cardiovascular diseases, skin problems, nerve system diseases, orthopedic disorders, and allergic ailments.

3. 桂枝加附子汤 — Guì Zhī Jiā Fù Zǐ Tāng — Cinnamon Twig Decoction plus Aconite from the *Treatise on Cold Damage* (伤寒论, Shāng Hán Lùn): Guì Zhī (Ramulus Cinnamomi) 10g, Sháo Yào (Radix Paeoniae) 12g, Gān Cǎo (Radix et Rhizoma Glycyrrhizae) 5g, Shēng Jiāng (Rhizoma Zingiberis Recens) three pieces, twelve Dà Zǎo (Fructus Jujubae), and Fù Zǐ (Radix Aconiti Lateralis Praeparata) 10g, mainly for patients with sweating, aversion to cold and joint pain. Also applicable for common cold, allergic rhinitis, neuralgia, and arthritis.

4. 桂枝加龙骨牡蛎汤 — Guì Zhī Jiā Lóng Gǔ Mǔ Lì Tāng — Cinnamon Twig Decoction plus Dragon Bones and Oyster Shell from the *Essentials from the Golden Cabinet* (金匮要略, Jīn Guì Yào Lüè): Guì Zhī (Ramulus Cinnamomi) 10g, Sháo Yào (Radix Paeoniae) 12g, Gān Cǎo (Radix et Rhizoma Glycyrrhizae) 5g, Shēng Jiāng (Rhizoma Zingiberis Recens) three pieces, twelve Dà Zǎo (Fructus Jujubae), Lóng Gǔ (Os Draconis) 15g, and Mǔ Lì (Concha Ostreae) 20g; mainly for qi rushing-up pattern marked by loss of essence, spontaneous

sweating, night sweating, deficiency asthma, and hollow throbbing pulse. Also applicable for diseases like neurasthenia and rickets.

5. 桂苓五味甘草汤 Guì Líng Wǔ Wèi Gān Cǎo Tāng — Cinnamon, Poria, Schisandra, and Licorice Decoction from the *Essentials from the Golden Cabinet* (金匮要略, Jīn Guì Yào Lüè): Guì Zhī (Ramulus Cinnamomi) 10g, Fú Líng (Poria) 15g, Wǔ Wèi Zǐ (Fructus Schisandrae Chinensis) 10g, and Gān Cǎo (Radix et Rhizoma Glycyrrhizae) 5g; mainly for qi rushing-up pattern indicated by cough, wheezing, dizziness, and spontaneous sweating. Also applicable for such disorders as bronchial asthma, emphysema, and neurasthenia.

[Precautions] Guì Zhī (Ramulus Cinnamomi) has been widely used to treat various disorders, but its clinical application requires a close identification of a particular patient's constitution. The most important indicators are white moist thin skin, emaciated body, floating and relatively enlarged pulse with moderate or slow rate, reddish or darkish soft and flexible tongue body, and thin white and moist tongue coating. Its contraindications include red tough tongue with greasy and thick coating. Owning to its acrid and warm properties, it may easily damage yin and cause bleeding and must be used with cautions by people with internal heat depleting yin or bleeding due to blood-heat.

[Addendum] 肉桂 Ròu Guì Cortex Cinnamomi Cinnamon Bark

The source is from the stem and branch bark of *Cinnamomum cassia* Presel, family Lauraceae. It has almost the same indications as Guì Zhī (Ramulus Cinnamomi), but is more effective in warming up the interior. It, known as one of the important interior-warming medicinals, is frequently used for cold pain in umbilical region. Good quality is oily, fragrant, thick, sweet, and slightly-pungent, and has a fine skin, amaranth section, and no chewing residue. Use 5g in decoction and decrease the dosage as in powder.

紫苏叶 Zǐ Sū Yè *folium perillae perilla leaf*

[Addendum] 苏梗 Zǐ Sū Gěng Caulis Perillae Perilla Stem

The source is from the dried tender branch and leaf of annual herbaceous *Perilla frutescens* (L.) Britt. Var. *acuta* (Thunb.) Kudo., family Labiatae. Pungent in flavor and warm in nature.

[Actions] Relieve the exterior to dissipate cold, rectify qi and harmonize the stomach, and remove fish and crab poisoning. It is applicable to either wind-cold common cold manifested as fever and aversion to cold with accompanying chest oppression, or the spleen and stomach qi stagnation manifested as vomiting and diarrhea. Its volatile oil contains perillalde-hyde and l-Limonene as the major components. Oral administration of its decoction and infusion has a slight antipyretic effect on rabbit and can promote the secretion of digestive fluid and gastrointestinal motility.

[Quality] Collected in summer, chopped, and sun-dried. Good quality is large, purple, tender, and fragrant, especially the one collected on sunny days, easy to be dried with intense fragrance and best quality.

[Indications] Zǐ Sū Yè (Folium Perillae), capable of not only relieving the exterior to dissipate cold but also rectifying qi and harmonizing the stomach, is most appropriate for exterior wind-cold pattern accompanied with interior qi stagnation.

1. Wind-cold exterior pattern: Zǐ Sū Yè (Folium Perillae) is especially suitable for patients who first have improper diet or emotional problem and then suffer from wind-cold invasion with the manifestation of aversion to cold, absence of sweating, headache, fever, nausea, vomiting, abdominal distention, loose stool, cough with sputum, and white greasy tongue coating. It is often used together with Xìng Rén (Semen Armeniacae Amarum), Fáng Fēng (Radix Saposhnikoviae), Hòu Pò (Cortex Magnoliae Officinalis), Bàn Xià (Rhizoma Pinelliae), and Shēng Jiāng (Rhizoma Zingiberis Recens) to induce slight sweating to improve the general condition. Wind-cold exterior pattern is most likely to be found in common cold, tracheitis, and gastroenteritis.
2. Vomiting due to qi counterflow: Zǐ Sū Yè (Folium Perillae) is combined with Bàn Xià (Rhizoma Pinelliae), Hòu Pò (Cortex Magnoliae Officinalis), and Shēng Jiāng (Rhizoma Zingiberis Recens) for either morning sickness and vomiting during pregnancy or vomiting due to qi stagnation with accompanying chest oppression, abdominal distention, poor appetite, and greasy tongue coating. It is often used together with Huáng Lián (Rhizoma Coptidis) when patients suffer from frequent vomiting, vexation, bitter taste in the mouth, and yellow greasy tongue coating, and the decoction should be taken in small portions at frequent intervals.

It can also relieve fish and crab poisoning, and oral administration of its decoction is effective for such poisoning symptoms as vomiting, diarrhea, and abdominal pain. Applying its decoction for external wash can treat scrotum eczema. Rubbing a wart with the fresh herb to rub the wart can relieve verruca vulgaris.

[Usage and Dosage] Use raw, 6–12g in decoction.

[Mnemonics] Zǐ Sū Yè (Folium Perillae, Perilla Leaf): pungent and warm; relieve the exterior to dissipate cold, and harmonize the stomach to eliminate vomiting and diarrhea.

[Simple and Effective Formulas]

1. 半夏厚朴汤 — Bàn Xià Hòu Pò Tāng — Pinellia and Officinal Magnolia Bark Decoction from *Essentials from the Golden Cabinet* (金匮要略, Jīn Guì Yào Lüè): Zǐ Sū Gěng (Caulis Perillae) 10g, Bàn Xià (Rhizoma Pinelliae) 10g, Hòu Pò (Cortex Magnoliae Officinalis) 6g, Fú Líng (Poria) 10g, and Shēng Jiāng (Rhizoma Zingiberis Recens) 10g; mainly for foreign body sensation in the throat, chest oppression, abdominal distention, and cough. Also applicable for digestive system diseases, neurosis, and tracheitis with the above mentioned symptoms.
2. 连苏饮 Lián Sū Yǐn — Coptis and Perilla Leaf Decoction from *Treatise on Damp-heat Induced Diseases* (湿热病篇, Shī Rè Bìng Piān): Zǐ Sū Yè (Folium Perillae) 6g and Huáng Lián (Rhizoma Coptidis) 5g; decoct in water for oral administration and take in frequent intervals to treat patients with unremitting vomiting, restlessness, and epigastric *pǐ*. Also applicable for morning sickness during pregnancy and digestive system diseases.

[Precautions] It is appropriate to use Zǐ Sū (Folium Perillae) when the tongue coating is white thin or greasy, whereas it must be used with caution by people suffering from vomiting and abdominal distention but presenting red tongue without coating.

[Addendum] 苏梗 Sū Gěng Caulis Perillae Perilla Stem
Sū Gěng (Caulis Perillae), the old stem of Folium Perillae, is acrid and warm, can move qi and harmonize the center, and mainly functions to treat qi stagnation in the spleen and stomach, liver constraint, and fetal irritability. It should be combined with Hòu Pò (Cortex Magnoliae

Officinalis), Bàn Xià (Rhizoma Pinelliae), Fú Líng (Poria), Zhǐ Qiào (Fructus Aurantii), and Jú Pí (Pericarpium Citri Reticulatae) for foreign body sensation in the throat, belching, constipation, cough, wheezing, chest pain, anxiety, insomnia, palpitations, restlessness, menstrual irregularities, and distending pain in the lower abdomen.

Daily practices

1. What are the actions and indications of Guì Zhī (Ramulus Cinnamomi)?
2. What are the other actions of Zǐ Sū Yè (Folium Perillae) apart from relieving the exterior and what are the similarity and difference between Zǐ Sū Yè (Folium Perillae) and Guì Zhī (Ramulus Cinnamomi) in terms of actions and indications?

生姜 **Shēng Jiāng** *rhizoma zingiberis recens fresh ginger*

The source is from the fresh rhizome of perennial herbaceous *Zingiber officinale* Rosc., family Zingiberaceae. Pungent in flavor and warm in nature.

[Actions] Disperse the exterior, dissipate cold, warm the center, arrest vomiting, dissolve phlegm, and resolve toxins. It is applicable to relieve wind-cold type of common cold, eliminate abdominal pain and vomit induced by interior-cold, and remove fish and crab toxin. Its volatile oil and gingerol can invigorate blood circulation, stimulate gastric secretion and gastrointestinal tract, and promote digestion.

[Quality] Collected in summer, washed and dirt removed, and cut into slices before use. Good quality is large, full-grown, and tender.

[Indications]

1. Wind-cold exterior pattern: manifestations include aversion to cold, absence of sweating, abdominal distention, vomiting, clear saliva, clear and profuse urine, and white thick tongue coating. In this case, patient may take warm decoction of Shēng Jiāng (Rhizoma Zingiberis Recens)

or with brown sugar, then lie in bed quietly with quilt, get mild hot sensation over the body, and eventually induce sweating with relief of wind-cold. Shēng Jiāng (Rhizoma Zingiberis Recens) can be used either alone or together with acrid and warm medicinals such as Má Huáng (Herba Ephedrae), Guì Zhī (Ramulus Cinnamomi), and Fù Zǐ (Radix Aconiti Lateralis Praeparata).

2. Vomiting: Shēng Jiāng (Rhizoma Zingiberis Recens) is mainly used to treat nausea, vomiting, increased salivation, lack of thirst, and white greasy or white glossy tongue coating (which is the point of identification), or thirst with little water intake and non-red tongue with greasy coating. For people suffering from severe vomiting or who feel nausea upon the smell of herbs and have difficulty in swallowing herbal decoction, a recommended approach is to drip Shēng Jiāng (Rhizoma Zingiberis Recens) juice on the tongue or rub the tongue surface with ginger slices, and then take the decoction slowly so as to prevent subsequent episodes of vomiting.

The decoction or juice of Shēng Jiāng (Rhizoma Zingiberis Recens) can help remove toxicity of fish, crab, Bàn Xià (Rhizoma Pinelliae), Tiān Nán Xīng (Rhizoma Arisaematis) and a variety of mushrooms.

[Usage and Dosage] Wēi Jiāng (Rhizoma Zingiberis Rosc., Roasted Ginger, 煨姜), made by roasting the ginger until it is cooked, is moderate in pungent flavor and less effective in dissipating, but more potent for warming the center and arresting vomiting, and mainly functions to treat vomiting and abdominal pain. Pounding fresh ginger into juice is more convenient for urgent need, oral administration, and nasal feeding. Fresh ginger skin is most likely to be used for relieving edema, distention and fullness. Use raw in general, 3–12g in decoction, and 3–10 drops/time in juice.

[Mnemonics] Shēng Jiāng (Rhizoma Zingiberis Recens, Fresh Ginger): stop vomiting and dissipate wind-cold; the key point of identification is the white glossy tongue coating.

[Simple and Effective Formulas]

1. 小半夏汤 — Xiǎo Bàn Xià Tāng — Minor Pinellia Decoction from *Essentials from the Golden Cabinet* (金匮要略, Jīn Guì Yào Lüè):

Shēng Jiāng (Rhizoma Zingiberis Recens) three pieces and Bàn Xià (Rhizoma Pinelliae) 12g for patients with nausea, vomiting, and vomiting drool without thirst. Also applicable for vomiting during pregnancy, neurotic vomiting, and aural vertigo.

2. 橘皮汤 — Jú Pí Tāng — Tangerine Peel Decoction from *Essentials from the Golden Cabinet* (金匮要略, Jīn Guì Yào Lüè): Shēng Jiāng (Rhizoma Zingiberis Recens) three pieces and Jú Pí (Pericarpium Citri Reticulatae) 10g; decoct in water for oral administration to treat patients with hiccup, belching, and nausea. Also applicable for vomiting and hiccup during pregnancy.

3. 姜枣汤 — Jiāng Zǎo Tāng — Ginger and Jujube Decoction from *Empirical Formulas* (经验方, Jīng Yàn Fāng): decoct Shēng Jiāng (Rhizoma Zingiberis Recens) five pieces and ten Dà Zǎo (Fructus Jujubae); decoct in water and take hot for oral administration to treat wind-cold pattern manifested as aversion to cold, absence of sweating, nausea, poor appetite, and absence of thirst. Also applicable for common cold and digestive system diseases with above-mentioned symptoms.

[Precautions] Shēng Jiāng (Rhizoma Zingiberis Recens), pungent in flavor and warm in nature, is suitable for cold pattern manifested as profuse clear drool in the mouth without thirst, but inappropriate for patients with dry red tongue and thirst with desire for cold drink.

荆芥 Jīng Jiè *herba schizonepetae schizonepeta*

The source is from the aerial part with inflorescence of the annual herbaceous *Schizonepeta tenuifolia* Briq., family Labiatae. Pungent in flavor and warm in nature.

[Actions] Expel wind and relieve the exterior, promote eruption of papules, relieve itching, and stanch bleeding. It is applicable for externally-contracted wind-cold, rubella with itching, inhibited eruption of measles, and ulcers and sores in the early stage with exterior pattern. This substance contains volatile oil, and oral administration of its decoction has shown diaphoretic, skin blood circulation-reinforcer, mild antipyretic, antiallergic, and spasmolytic effect. Jīng Jiè Tàn (Herba Schizonepetae Carbonisatum) can shorten bleeding time and clotting time.

[Quality] Impurity removed, soaked in water for a while, cut into segments, and sun-dried. Good quality is fragrant, dry, and green with a thin stem and dense spikes.

[Indications]

1. Exterior pattern: Jīng Jiè (Herba Schizonepetae), neutral in nature with an action of dissipating wind, can be used to treat either wind-cold or wind-heat exterior pattern, especially for the exterior pattern with blur-minded vertigo and forehead and bi-temple headache. Usually, patients will present with other symptoms such as aversion to wind, fever, itching and red eyes, stuffy nose, sneezing, itching and painful throat, and thin white tongue coating in most cases. This pattern is most likely to be found in patients with common cold, rhinitis, infection of the upper respiratory tract, and angioneurotic headache. This medicinal is usually combined with Jīn Yín Huā (Flos Lonicerae Japonicae) and Lián Qiào (Fructus Forsythiae) for wind-heat, and Fáng Fēng (Radix Saposhnikoviae), Qiāng Huó (Rhizoma et Radix Notopterygii) and Zǐ Sū Yè (Folium Perillae) for wind-cold exterior pattern.

2. Itching skin: Jīng Jiè (Herba Schizonepetae) is particularly suitable in cases of red papule with itching. According to a report, Jīng Jiè (Herba Schizonepetae) powder has been applied externally for acute and chronic urticaria and different types of skin itching. It is spread equably over the affected area and then rubbed with palm back and forth until the skin get off heat, one or two times in mild case, and two to four times in severe cases. It is often prescribed together with Chán Tuì (Periostracum Cicadae), Bò He (Herba Menthae) and Dì Fū Zǐ (Fructus Kochiae) when used in decoction for oral administration. It can also be combined with Fáng Fēng (Radix Saposhnikoviae) and Bái Zhǐ (Radix Angelicae Dahuricae) to treat early stage sores or dysentery with exterior symptoms such as aversion to cold with fever.

[Usage and Dosage] Use raw in general, the herb is stir-fried to charred-black ash and is called Jīng Jiè Tàn (Herba Schizonepetae Carbonisatum, Charred Schizonepeta) when used for such hemorrhagic disorders as epistaxis, stool with blood, profuse uterine bleeding, and prolonged scanty uterine bleeding of variable intervals. Use 10–15g in decoction.

[Mnemonics] Jīng Jiè (Herba Schizonepetae, Schizonepeta): pungent; clear the head and eyes, dispel wind to stop itching, and arrest bleeding when charred.

[Simple and Effective Formulas]

1. 荆防汤 — Jīng Fáng Tāng — Schizonepeta and Saposhnikovia Decoction from *Empirical Formulas* (经验方, Jīng Yàn Fāng): Jīng Jiè (Herba Schizonepetae) 10g and Fáng Fēng (Radix Saposhnikoviae) 10g; decoct in water for oral administration to treat wind exterior pattern with vertigo, headache, skin itching, body spasms, and muscle soreness and pain. Also applicable for such diseases as urticaria, pruritus, common cold, and neuralgia.
2. 荆薄汤 — Jīng Bò Tāng — Schizonepeta and Mint Decoction from *Empirical Formulas* (经验方, Jīng Yàn Fāng): Jīng Jiè (Herba Schizonepetae) 10g and Bò He (Herba Menthae) 5g; decoct in water for oral administration to treat wind-heat exterior pattern manifested as fever, vertigo, headache, itchy and red eyes, fever, and sweating without improvement of the condition. Also applicable for such diseases as common cold and infection of the upper respiratory tract.
3. 荆槐散 — Jīng Huái Sǎn — Schizonepeta and Pagoda Tree Flower Powder from *Ren-zhai's Direct Guidance on Formulas* (仁斋直指, Rén Zhāi Zhí Zhǐ Fāng): Jīng Jiè (Herba Schizonepetae) 10g and Huái Huā (Flos Sophorae) 10g; decoct in water for oral administration to treat bleeding gums and nosebleed. Also applicable for periodontitis, epistaxis, and other hemorrhagic disorders.

[Precautions] As a diaphoretic, Jīng Jiè (Herba Schizonepetae) requires that the patients has a relatively good constitution with strong and tight muscle and red tongue, and therefore its prescription should be avoided for patient with spontaneous sweating, aversion to wind or cold, and light tongue. Owning to its acrid and dissipating properties, it is hereby contraindicated for spontaneous sweating due to exterior deficiency or headache caused by yin-deficiency heat.

防风 **Fáng Fēng** *radix saposhnikoviae siler*

The source is from the root of perennial herbaceous *Saposhnikoviae divaricata* (Turcz.) Schischk, family Umbelliferae. It is named after its function of fighting against exogenous pathogenic wind. Pungent and sweet in flavor and warm in nature.

[Actions] Dispel wind and dampness, release the exterior, and stanch spasm and arrest pain. It is applicable for headache due to common cold, wind-damp *bì* pain, rubella, itching, and tetanus. This substance contains volatile oil, mannitol, phenolic compounds, polysaccharide and organic acid. Pharmacological experiments show that its decoction and infusion have an antipyretic effect on artificially-induced fever of rabbits, its ethanol infusion has antalgic and anti-inflammatory effects. Frequent gavage of high dose has shown inhibitory effects on electric shock in mice, indicating Fáng Fēng (Radix Saposhnikoviae) has certain antiepileptic effect.

[Quality] Soaked in water, moistened thoroughly, sliced, and dried under sunshine. Good quality is thick, strong, and aromatic with a light brown cortex and light yellow rings on cross section. 关防风 Guān Fáng Fēng native in northeast China is the best, it is thick, glutinous, soft, light-weight, fleshy, and moist and therefore also known as 软防风 Ruǎn Fáng Fēng. 西防风 Xi Fáng Fēng produced in Hebei and Shanxi and 青防风 Qīng Fáng Fēng produced in Shandong are of ordinary quality. 川防风 Chuān Fáng Fēng from Sichuan and 云防风 Yún Fáng Fēng from Yunnan are poor in quality.

[Indications]

1. Wind-cold exterior pattern: Fáng Fēng (Radix Saposhnikoviae), warm in nature and good at dispelling wind pathogen, is suitable for wind-cold exterior pattern in a combination with Jīng Jiè (Herba Schizonepetae) and Qiāng Huó (Rhizoma et Radix Notopterygii).
2. Wind-damp painful *bì*: manifestations include soreness and pain of the muscle all over the body and spasms of the joints with accompanying aversion to cold and spontaneous sweating. Fáng Fēng (Radix Saposhnikoviae) is often combined with Gé Gēn (Radix Puerariae Lobatae) and Chuān Xiōng (Rhizoma Chuanxiong) for problems of the upper extremities

weakness failing to stretch and stiffness of the shoulder and back, and with Dú Huó (Radix Angelicae Pubescentis), Dāng Guī (Radix Angelicae Sinensis), and Chì Sháo (Radix Paeoniae Rubra) for lower extremities disorders of difficulty walking.

3. Spontaneous sweating: Fáng Fēng (Radix Saposhnikoviae) is used together with Huáng Qí (Radix Astragali) and Bái Zhú (Rhizoma Atractylodis Macrocephalae) to form Jade Wind-Barrier Powder (玉屏风散, Yù Píng Fēng Sǎn) to treat the accompanying symptoms of spontaneous sweating, vertigo, nasal congestion, heaviness of the body, limited range of motion, or even muscle soreness and pain.

4. Headache: Fáng Fēng (Radix Saposhnikoviae) is usually combined with Gé Gēn (Radix Puerariae Lobatae), Chuān Xiōng (Rhizoma Chuanxiong), Huáng Qí (Radix Astragali), Bái Sháo (Radix Paeoniae Alba), and Bái Zhǐ (Radix Angelicae Dahuricae) to relieve pressing or tightening headache with vertigo and stiffness of the nape and back, which are commonly occurred in neurogenic headache, hypertension, and cervical osteoarthritis.

[Usage and Dosage] Use raw in general, when used for patients with weak constitution and chronic diseases, this herb is stir-fried to reduce its dry nature and moderate its effect. Use 6–12g in decoction.

[Mnemonics] Fáng Fēng (Radix Saposhnikoviae, Siler): pungent and warm; good at dispelling wind-cold; and capable of treating headache and arresting sweating.

[Simple and Effective Formulas]

1. 防芷汤 — Fáng Zhǐ Tāng — Ledebouriella and Angelica Root Decoction from *Formulas for Universal Relief* (普济方, Pǔ Jì Fāng): Fáng Fēng (Radix Saposhnikoviae) 10g and Bái Zhǐ (Radix Angelicae Dahuricae) 10g for unbearable headache.

2. 玉屏风散 — Yù Píng Fēng Sǎn — Jade Wind-Barrier Powder from *Teachings of Dan-xi* (丹溪心法, Dān Xī Xīn Fǎ): Fáng Fēng (Radix Saposhnikoviae) 10g, Bái Zhú (Rhizoma Atractylodis Macrocephalae) 10g, and Huáng Qí (Radix Astragali) 15g to treat patients with spontaneous sweating, a higher risk of catching common cold and nasal congestion. Also applicable for chronic rhinitis and allergic rhinitis.

3. 二防汤 — Èr Fáng Tāng — Ledebouriella and Stephania Root Decoction from *Empirical Formulas* (经验方, Jīng Yàn Fāng): Fáng Fēng (Radix Saposhnikoviae) 10g and Fáng Jǐ (Radix Stephaniae Tetrandrae) 12g for joint pain and edema. Also applicable for deformative arthritis and rheumatic diseases.

[Precautions] Fáng Fēng (Radix Saposhnikoviae), known as the medicinal for dispersing wind but with moisturizing effect, is still pungent in flavor and warm in nature. It is suitable for patients bigger in body size with darkish complexion and contraindicated to joint pain patients presenting emaciation and red tongue without coating due to yin and blood deficiency. It is also not advised in cases of headache resulting from yin deficiency and liver wind and night sweating caused by internal heat.

Daily practices

1. What are the similarities and differences among Shēng Jiāng (Rhizoma Zingiberis Recens), Jīng Jiè (Herba Schizonepetae) and Fáng Fēng (Radix Saposhnikoviae) in terms of actions and indications?
2. What are the similarities among Jīng Jiè (Herba Schizonepetae), Fáng Fēng (Radix Saposhnikoviae), Má Huáng (Herba Ephedrae), Guì Zhī (Ramulus Cinnamomi), and Zǐ Sū Yè (Folium Perillae) in terms of relieving the exterior pathogen? What are their differences in terms of other actions and indications?

羌活 Qiāng Huó *rhizoma et radix notopterygii notoptetygium root*

The source is from the dried rhizome and root of the perennial herbaceous *Notopterygium incisum* Ting ex H.T. Chang or N. *forbesii* Boiss., family Umbelliferae. Pungent and bitter in flavor and warm in nature.

[Actions] Release the exterior and dissipate cold, and eliminate dampness and arrest pain. It is applicable to wind-cold type of common cold, headache, body pain, wind-damp *bì* pain, and soreness and pain in the shoulder and back. This substance contains volatile oil, alkaloid, and organic acid and has shown antipyretic, antalgic, and diaphoretic effects.

[Quality] Impurities removed, washed clean, moistened thoroughly, cut into slices, and dried in the air. It includes many varieties, good quality is thick, coarse, and aromatic, and has a dense cross section with many red spots.

[Indications]

1. Externally-contracted wind-cold-dampness: Qiāng Huó (Rhizoma et Radix Notopterygii) is commonly used together with Fáng Fēng (Radix Saposhnikoviae), Dú Huó (Radix Angelicae Pubescentis), and Cāng Zhú (Rhizoma Atractylodis) for exterior wind-cold-dampness pattern with such symptoms as aversion to cold, absence of sweating, stiffness and pain in the head and neck, joint pain and soreness, and white greasy tongue coating.
2. Muscle and joint pain: Qiāng Huó (Rhizoma et Radix Notopterygii) is suitable for eliminating headache affecting the nape and back or pain in the upper extremities due to invasion of exogenous pathogenic factors. It is combined with Fù Zǐ (Radix Aconiti Lateralis Praeparata), Bái Zhú (Rhizoma Atractylodis Macrocephalae), Cāng Zhú (Rhizoma Atractylodis), and Gān Jiāng (Rhizoma Zingiberis) for the accompanying symptoms of aversion to cold, absence of sweating, and white greasy tongue coating.

[Usage and Dosage] Use raw in general, 3–10g in decoction.

[Mnemonics] Qiāng Huó (Rhizoma et Radix Notopterygii, Notoptetygium Root): pungent and warm; relieve the exterior, induce sweating, arrest body pain, and dissipate cold-damp.

[Simple and Effective Formulas]

1. 九味羌活汤 — Jiǔ Wèi Qiāng Huó Tāng — Nine Ingredients Notopterygium Decoction from *Medical Works* (此事难知, Cǐ Shì Nán Zhī): Qiāng Huó (Rhizoma et Radix Notopterygii) 10g, Fáng Fēng (Radix Saposhnikoviae) 10g, Cāng Zhú (Rhizoma Atractylodis) 8g, Xì Xīn (Radix et Rhizoma Asari) 3g, Chuān Xiōng (Rhizoma Chuanxiong) 8g, Bái Zhǐ (Radix Angelicae Dahuricae) 8g, Shēng Dì (Radix Rehmanniae) 10g, Huáng Qín (Radix Scutellariae) 10g, and Gān Cǎo (Radix et

Rhizoma Glycyrrhizae) 3g; decoct in water for oral administration to treat exterior pattern of wind-cold-dampness with the manifestation of aversion to cold, fever, absence of sweating, headache, soreness and pain of the extremities, bitter taste in the mouth with slightly thirst, white tongue coating, and floating pulse.

2. 羌黄汤 — Qiāng Huáng Tāng — Notopterygium and Turmeric Root Tuber Decoction from *Empirical Formulas* (经验方, Jīng Yàn Fāng): Qiāng Huó (Rhizoma et Radix Notopterygii) 10g and Jiāng Huáng (Rhizoma Curcumae Longae, Turmeric Root Tuber) 10g; decoct in water for oral administration to treat pain in the shoulder, back, and joints of upper extremities and reduced mobility of the joints. Also applicable for periarthritis of shoulder, cervical osteoarthritis, and stiff neck.

3. 感冒退热方 — Gǎn Mào Tuì Rè Fāng — Curing Common cold and Relieving Fever from *Empirical Formulas from Longhua Hospital of Shanghai TCM Hospital* (上海中医院龙华医院验方, Shànghǎi Zhōng Yī Yuàn Lóng Huá Yī Yuàn Yàn Fāng): Qiāng Huó (Rhizoma et Radix Notopterygii) 12g, Bǎn Lán Gēn (Radix Isatidis) 30g, and Pú Gōng Yīng (Herba Taraxaci) 30g; decoct in water for oral administration to treat common cold with fever and tonsillitis.

4. 羌附汤 — Qiāng Fù Tāng — Notopterygium and Aconite Decoction from *Formulas to Aid the Living* (济生方, Jì Shēng Fāng): Qiāng Huó (Rhizoma et Radix Notopterygii) 10g, Fù Zǐ (Radix Aconiti Lateralis Praeparata) 10g, Bái Zhú (Rhizoma Atractylodis Macrocephalae) 10g, and Gān Cǎo (Radix et Rhizoma Glycyrrhizae) 6g; decoct in water for oral administration to treat contention between wind and dampness manifested as body vexing pain, pulling pain with failure to bend and stretch, and mild body swelling with numbness. Also applicable for arthritis and sciatica.

[Precautions] Qiāng Huó (Rhizoma et Radix Notopterygii), pungent in flavor and warm in nature, is suitable for cold-damp pattern manifested as aversion to cold, absence of sweating, pale tongue with white greasy coating, and floating, tight and moderate pulse and patients who have strong muscle and darkish complexion. It, however, should be used with caution for patients with fever, vexation and agitation, sweating, yellow urine or blood deficiency. The herb is not recommended in cases of exterior heat pattern because it is potent in releasing the exterior, but drying in nature and prone to assist heat damaging yin further.

白芷 **Bái Zhǐ** *radix angelicae dahuricae angelica root*

The source is from the root of herbaceous perennial *Angelica dahurica* (fisth. Ex Hoffm.) Benth. Et Hook. F. or *A. dahurica* (fish, ex Hoffm) Benth. Et Hook. *f. var. formosana* (Boiss.) Shan et Yuan, family Umbelliferae. Pungent in flavor and warm in nature.

[Actions] Disperse wind and eliminate dampness, open the orifices and arrest pain, and reduce swelling and expel pus. It is applicable to headache in common cold, orbital pain, nasal congestion, sinusitis, toothache, leukorrhagia, sores, ulcers, swellings, and pain. This herb contains volatile oil and coumarin compounds and has shown an antalgic effect. Pharmacological researches reveal small-dose angelicotoxin has an excitatory effect on respiratory center, vasomotor center, and vagus, and can reinforce respiration, raise blood pressure, and slow down pulse rate. Injection of angelicin has shown sedative and antipyretic effects on mice. This Chinese medicinal has shown an inhibitory effect against such organisms as shigella dysenteriae, typhoid bacillus, and human type tubercle bacillus.

[Quality] Impurity removed, washed clean, soaked and moistened thoroughly, cut into slices, and dried in the air. It includes many varieties; good quality is long, thin-skinned, heavy, powdery, and aromatic. 库页白 芷 Kù Yè Bái Zhǐ, produced in northeastern China, and Inner Mongolia is toxic and should not be used.

[Indications]

1. Wind-cold or wind-damp exterior pattern: Warm-natured Bái Zhǐ (Radix Angelicae Dahuricae) is capable of dispelling wind to arrest pain and therefore effective in relieving headache, especially for the forehead and orbital headache. It is often in a combination with Qiāng Huó (Rhizoma et Radix Notopterygii) and Fáng Fēng (Radix Saposhnikoviae).

2. Deep-source nasal congestion: it is a disorder marked by repeatedly occurrence of nasal congestion, nasal itching with sneezing, runny nose, and headache involving the forehead, orbit and maxilla. This is most likely to be found in acute and chronic rhinitis and paranasal sinusitis. Bái Zhǐ (Radix Angelicae Dahuricae), capable of improving the nasal air passage and arresting pain, is usually prescribed together with Cāng Ěr Zǐ (Fructus Xanthii), Xīn Yí (Flos Magnoliae), and Xì Xīn (Radix et Rhizoma Asari).

3. Carbuncles in the early stage: during this stage, carbuncles appear to be red, swollen and painful with a hot sensation, Bái Zhǐ (Radix Angelicae Dahuricae) is used together with Dà Huáng (Radix et Rhizoma Rhei), Lián Qiào (Fructus Forsythiae), and Jīn Yín Huā (Flos Lonicerae Japonicae) for either oral administration or external application when ground into powder and mixed with vinegar.

4. Abnormal vaginal discharge: owning to its drying nature and ability of dispersing dampness, Bái Zhǐ (Radix Angelicae Dahuricae) can be used to relieve abnormal vaginal discharge. It should be combined with Bái Zhú (Rhizoma Atractylodis Macrocephalae) and Hǎi Piāo Xiāo (Endoconcha Sepiae) for the problem caused by damp-cold in the lower *jiao*, and with Huáng Bǎi (Cortex Phellodendri Chinensis), Chūn Gēn pí (Cortex Ailanthi), and Chūn Bái Pí (Cortex Toonae Sinensis Radicis) for the damp-heat.

[Usage and Dosage] Use raw in general, 3–6g in decoction, also be used as pill and powder.

[Mnemonics] Bái Zhǐ (Radix Angelicae Dahuricae, Angelica Root): pungent and dissipating; good at curing sinusitis; capable of unblocking the orifices, removing pain, relieving abscesses, and arresting abnormal vaginal discharge.

[Simple and Effective Formulas]

1. 白芷细辛吹鼻散 — Bái Zhǐ Xì Xīn Chuī Bí Sǎn — Angelica Root and Asarum Nose Blowing Powder from *Fine Formulas of Zhong Fu Tang Gong* (种福堂公选良方, Zhǒng Fú Táng Gōng Xuǎn Liáng Fāng): Bái Zhǐ (Radix Angelicae Dahuricae), Xì Xīn (Radix et Rhizoma Asari),

Shí Gāo (Gypsum Fibrosum), Rǔ Xiāng (Olibanum), and Mò Yào (Myrrha) (oil deprived) in equal dosage; prepare into fine powder to treat migraine, brew the powder into the left nasal cavity for the migraine on the right side, and right cavity for the left.

2. 鼻渊方 — Bí Yuān Fāng — Sinusitis Formula from *The Complete Compendium of Sores* (疡医大全, Yáng Yī Dà Quán): Xīn Yí (Flos Magnoliae) 2.4g, Bái Zhǐ (Radix Angelicae Dahuricae) 2.4g, Fáng Fēng (Radix Saposhnikoviae) 2.4g, Cāng Ěr Zǐ (Fructus Xanthii) 3.6g, Chuān Xiōng (Rhizoma Chuanxiong) 1.5g, Xì Xīn (Radix et Rhizoma Asari) 2.1g, and Gān Cǎo (Radix et Rhizoma Glycyrrhizae) 0.9g; decoct in water for oral administration to treat acute or chronic sinusitis and rhinitis.

3. 芷黄饮 — Zhǐ Huáng Yǐn — Angelica Root and Rhubarb Beverage from *Empirical Formula* (经验方, Jīng Yàn Fāng): Bái Zhǐ (Radix Angelicae Dahuricae) and Dà Huáng (Radix et Rhizoma Rhei) in equal dosage; grind into powder and take 6g/time with rice soup to treat red swollen sores and carbuncles.

[Precautions] Bái Zhǐ (Radix Angelicae Dahuricae), pungent and warm, shares similar contraindications with Qiāng Huó (Rhizoma et Radix Notopterygii) and Fáng Fēng (Radix Saposhnikoviae).

苍耳子 **Cāng Ěr Zǐ** *fructus xanthii cockleburr fruit*

The source is from the fruit with involucre of *Xanthium sibiricum* Patr., family Compositae. Pungent and bitter in flavor and warm in nature with mild toxicity.

[Actions] Dispel wind-damp, open the nasal passage, and arrest pain. It is applicable to sinusitis with headache, loss of smell, and turbid nasal discharge, wind-damp *bì* pain and contracture in the muscle and extremities.

[Quality] Impurities removed, stir-fried until thorn is brown and fruit is deep-yellow, thorn removed, and sifted. Good quality is dry, large, full-grown, and yellow-green without impurities.

[Indications]

1. Nasal congestion and runny nose: Cāng Ěr Zǐ (Fructus Xanthii) is often combined with Xīn Yí (Flos Magnoliae), Bái Zhǐ (Radix Angelicae Dahuricae), and Bò He (Herba Menthae) for nasal congestion and runny nose with accompanying loss of smelling and headache due to wind-pathogen attacking the upper part of the body.
2. Skin itching: Cāng Ěr Zǐ (Fructus Xanthii) is usually used together with Dì Fū Zǐ (Fructus Kochiae), Bái Xiān Pí (Cortex Dictamni), Fáng Fēng (Radix Saposhnikoviae), and Jīng Jiè (Herba Schizonepetae) for stubborn dermatitis or tinea manifested as itching, coarse and thickened skin.

[Usage and Dosage] Use raw in most cases, or use stir-fried after its thorns have been removed. Use 3–10g in decoction, and proper dosage for external application.

[Mnemonics] Cāng Ěr Zǐ (Fructus Xanthii, Cockleburr Fruit): acrid and bitter; best for wind dissipation; capable of resolving skin itching and unblocking nasal congestion.

[Simple and Effective Formulas]

苍耳散 — Cāng Ěr Sǎn — Cockleburr Fruit Powder from *Formulas to Aid the Living* (济生方, Jì Shēng Fāng): Cāng Ěr Zǐ (Fructus Xanthii) 10g, Xīn Yí (Flos Magnoliae) 10g, Bái Zhǐ (Radix Angelicae Dahuricae) 6g, and Bò He (Herba Menthae) 5g; decoct in water for oral administration to treat nasal congestion, constant runny nose, headache, acute and chronic rhinitis, and allergic rhinitis.

[Precautions] Cāng Ěr Zǐ (Fructus Xanthii) is toxic and should not be used overdose. It should be prescribed cautiously for people with yin and blood deficiency manifested as emaciation, white complexion, fever, sweating easily, and nasal congestion.

辛夷 Xīn Yí *flos magnoliae blond magnolia flower*

The source is from the flower bud of *Magnolia biondii* Pamp, *M. denudate* Desr.,or *M.sprengeri* Pamp., family Magoliaceae. Pungent in flavor and warm in nature.

[Actions] Disperse wind-cold and unblock the nasal orifices. It is applicable to wind-cold type of common cold, headache, nasal congestion, and sinusitis-induced headache. Its volatile oil can contract nasal mucosa and vessel, and has an anti-histaminic effect.

[Quality] Impurities, branches, and stems removed, and pounded into pieces. Good quality is acrid, cool, slight bitter, aromatic, and hairy; has large, dry and green buds that have not opened; and with tight inner valves and without stems or branches. The dried flower bud of *Magnolia grandiflora* Linn., family Magoliaceae is also available at the market, but bigger in size, more attention should be paid to identify.

[Indications] Xīn Yí (Flos Magnoliae) is primarily used to treat various nasal problems depending on the other herbs in prescription. Specifically, it is combined with Bái Zhǐ (Radix Angelicae Dahuricae), Fáng Fēng (Radix Saposhnikoviae), Cāng ěr Zǐ (Fructus Xanthii), Chuān Xiōng (Rhizoma Chuanxiong), and Xì Xīn (Radix et Rhizoma Asari) for nasal congestion, clear nasal discharge, and loss of smell due to wind-cold invasion; while with Cāng Ěr Zǐ (Fructus Xanthii), Huáng Qín (Radix Scutellariae), and Shí Gāo (Gypsum Fibrosum) for sinusitis with yellow, smelly, and thick nasal discharge caused by wind-heat attacking.

Dripping its preparation of oiling agent and emulsion into the nasal cavity or brewing its powder into the nasal cavity, or applying its ointment externally is also helpful for the treatment of the above diseases.

[Usage and Dosage] Use raw in general, 3–10g in decoction, and proper amount for external application.

[Mnemonics] Xīn Yí (Flos Magnoliae, Blond Magnolia Flower): unblock the nasal passage, important for any nasal problems, and essential for stuffy and running nose.

[Simple and Effective Formulas]

芎䓖散 Xiōng Qióng Sǎn — Chuanxiong Powder from *Standards for Diagnosis and Treatment* (证治准绳, Zhèng Zhì Zhǔn Shéng): Xīn Yí (Flos Magnoliae) 10g, Chuān Xiōng (Rhizoma Chuanxiong) 6g, and Xì Xīn (Radix et Rhizoma Asari) 5g; decoct in water for oral administration to treat nasal congestion. Also applicable for acute and chronic rhinitis, allergic rhinitis, and pollinosis.

[Precautions] The hairy texture of Xīn Yí (Flos Magnoliae) may cause irritation of the throat and should therefore be placed in a cheesecloth bag before decocting.

Daily practices

1. Qiāng Huó (Rhizoma et Radix Notopterygii), Bái Zhǐ (Radix Angelicae Dahuricae), Cāng ěr Zǐ (Fructus Xanthii), and Xīn Yí (Flos Magnoliae) are all medicinals that release exterior with acrid-warm properties. What are the similarity and differences among them in terms of actions and indications?
2. Some exterior-relieving medicinals can also arrest headache. What are the differences among those herbs in terms of action and indications?

香薷 **Xiāng Rú** *herba moslae aromatic madder*

The source is from the herb with flower of herbaceous perennial *Elsholtzia splendens* Nakai ex F. Maekawa, family Labiatae. Pungent in flavor and slightly warm in nature.

[Actions] Induce sweating to release the exterior, dispel summerheat and remove dampness, and promote urination to reduce swelling. It is applicable for the externally-contracted cold with accompanying summerheat-damp in summer manifested as fever, aversion to cold, headache, absence of sweating, abdominal pain, vomiting and diarrhea, edema, and inhibited urination. This herb contains volatile oil and has diaphoretic and antipyretic effects. It can also stimulate secretion of digestive glands and gastro-intestinal motility, and has diuretic effect as it stimulates renal blood vessel to make glomerulus congested and increase filtration pressure when it is excreted by the kidney.

[Quality] Impurity removed, softened by spraying water, residue root removed, cut into segments, and sun-dried. Good quality is tender and dry with light purple stems, green leaves, intense fragrance, and lots of flower spikes.

[Indications]

1. Cold invasion in summer: Xiāng Rú (Herba Moslae) is commonly combined with Hòu Pò (Cortex Magnoliae Officinalis), Jīn Yín Huā (Flos Lonicerae Japonicae), and Biǎn Dòu Huā (Flos Lablab Album) for aversion to cold with fever, headache, absence of sweating, abdominal pain, and vomiting with diarrhea resulted from externally-contracted summerheat-dampness binding with turbid dampness in the interior due to drinking too much cold beverage.

2. Edema: Xiāng Rú (Herba Moslae) is used together with Bái Zhú (Rhizoma Atractylodis Macrocephalae) for the sudden onset of edema especially on the head, scanty urine, and scanty or absence of sweating.

Rinsing the mouth with Xiāng Rú (Herba Moslae) decoction is helpful for removing bad breath.

[Usage and Dosage] Use raw in general, 3–10g in decoction.

[Mnemonics] Xiāng Rú (Herba Moslae, Aromatic Madder): together with Hòu Pò (Cortex Magnoliae Officinalis) to resolve summerheat; with Bái Zhú (Rhizoma Atractylodis Macrocephalae) to remove edema.

[Simple and Effective Formulas]

1. 新加香薷散 — Xīn Jiā Xiāng Rú Sǎn — Newly-Supplemented Mosla Powder from *Systematic Differentiation of Warm Diseases* (温病条辨, Wēn Bìng Tiáo Biàn): Xiāng Rú (Herba Moslae) 10g, Jīn Yín Huā (Flos Lonicerae Japonicae) 12g, Lián Qiào (Fructus Forsythiae) 12g, Hòu Pò (Cortex Magnoliae Officinalis) 6g, and Biǎn Dòu Huā (Flos Lablab Album) 12g; decoct in water for oral administration to treat patients suffering from fever in the summer with slight aversion to cold, absence of sweating, headache, vexation, red complexion, abdominal distention, vomiting, diarrhea, and red tongue with white coating. Also applicable for common cold, sunstroke, and gastroenteritis.

2. 香薷术丸 — Xiāng Rú Zhú Wán — Mosla and Atractylodes Macrocephala from *Seng Shen's Formula Collection* (僧深集方, Sēng Shēn Jí Fāng): Xiāng Rú (Herba Moslae) 10g and Bái Zhú (Rhizoma Atractylodis Macrocephalae) 12g; decoct in water for oral administration to treat

swelling throughout the body. Also applicable for acute nephritis and idiopathic edema.

[Precautions] Xiāng Rú (Herba Moslae), pungent, warm, and diaphoretic, is effective in treating externally-contracted cold pattern in summer, whereas inappropriate in cases of high fever, vexation and agitation, thirst, and profuse sweating due to working under high temperature environment. Xiāng Rú (Herba Moslae) has an effect of relieving summerheat, but still not a panacea for all the disorders occurred in summer.

ACRID-COOL

Medicinals that Release the Exterior

薄荷 **Bò He** *herba menthae field mint*

The source is from the dried branch and leaf of *Mentha haplocalyx* Briqi, family Labiata. Pungent in flavor and cool in nature.

[Actions] Disperse wind-heat, clear the head and eyes, and benefit the throat. It is applicable to wind-heat type of common cold and wind-warmth in the early stage with symptoms and sighs of headache, red eyes, throat pain, aphtha, urticaria, measles, and distention and fullness sensation in the chest and rib-side. Its volatile oil contains such major ingredients as menthol and menthone and can cause irritation of the skin. This substance has anti-inflammatory and antalgic effect through touching nerve ending receptor in the skin, first generating cold sensation and slight stabbing and burning sensation, then slowly penetrating into the skin, and eventually increasing topical blood flow. Menthone can also promote respiratory tract mucous secretion and relieve topical inflammatory response.

[Quality] Impurity and residue root removed, leaves shaked off, stem moistened thoroughly by spraying water, cut into segments, dried under sunshine, and mixed with leaves. Good quality has many leaves with intense fragrance, the herb produced in Jiangsu is the best.

[Indications]

1. Wind-heat exterior pattern: Bò He (Herba Menthae) is frequently used together with Jīng Jiè (Herba Schizonepetae), Jié Gěng (Radix

Platycodonis), Lián Qiào (Fructus Forsythiae), Jīn Yín Huā (Flos Lonicerae Japonicae), and Gān Cǎo (Radix et Rhizoma Glycyrrhizae) for externally-contract wind-heat pattern with symptoms of fever, slight aversion to wind-cold, headache, itchy and red eyes, red throat, nasal congestion, runny nose, red margins and tip of the tongue with white thin coating, rapid pulse, or itchy skin in some cases.

2. Headache and sore throat: Bò He (Herba Menthae) is often combined with Jié Gěng (Radix Platycodonis), Niú Bàng Zǐ (Fructus Arctii), Bái Jiāng Cán (Bombyx Batryticatus), and Gān Cǎo (Radix et Rhizoma Glycyrrhizae) to relieve externally-contracted wind-heat pattern with headache and dry, red and sore throat.

3. Pruritus: Bò He (Herba Menthae) is prescribed together with Chán Tuì (Periostracum Cicadae) and Jīng Jiè (Herba Schizonepetae) to relieve red rashes or wheal all over the body with accompanying aversion to wind, sweating but without any improvement in the condition, and dizziness.

[Usage and Dosage] Use raw, 3–6g in decoction, add at the end of decoction, and do not overcook.

[Mnemonics] Bò He (Herba Menthae, Field Mint): pungent and cool; best at promoting eruption of papules; and capable of dispelling wind-heat and clearing the head and eyes.

[Simple and Effective Formulas]

1. 鸡苏散 Jī Sū Sǎn — Ji Su Powder from *Direct Investigation of Cold Damage* (伤寒直格, Shāng Hán Zhí Gé): Bò He (Herba Menthae) 5g, Huá Shí (Talcum) 12g, and Gān Cǎo (Radix et Rhizoma Glycyrrhizae) 2g; decoct in water for oral administration to disperse wind and relieve summerheat for summerheat-damp pattern with manifestations of slight aversion to wind-cold, headache, feeling of fullness in the head, and cough. Also applicable for common cold, gastroenteritis, and urinary tract infection in the summer caused by the invasion of external summerheat-damp pathogen and with manifestations of fever, sweating without improvement of the condition, and inhibited and yellow urination.

2. 薄蝉煎 Bò Chán Jiān — Mint and Cicada Moulting Decoction from *Empirical Formulas* (经验方, Jīng Yàn Fāng): Bò He (Herba Menthae) 6g and Chán Tuì (Periostracum Cicadae) 6g; decoct in water for oral administration to treat skin itching of summer dermatitis and urticaria.

[Precautions] Bò He (Herba Menthae) has a diaphoretic effect and is contraindicated in cases of spontaneous sweating due to yang deficiency.

蝉蜕 Chán Tuì *periostracum cicadae cicada moulting*

The source is from the slough shed by the cicada, *Cryptotympana pustulata* Fabricius or *C. atrata* Fabr., family Cicadidae. Alternate names include 蝉衣 Chán Yī and 蝉退 Chán Tuì. Sweet and salty in flavor and cool in nature.

[Actions] Disperse wind-heat, vent rashes, extinguish wind and calm spasm, and remove nebula to improve vision. It is applicable to either externally-contracted wind-heat pattern with accompanying fever, headache, and early stage of measles with an incomplete expression of the rash, or wind-heat in the liver channel manifested as red eyes, nebula, profuse tears, child night terrors, convulsions, and spasms. Experiments reveal this substance can prolong the life of tetanus experiment rabbits and reduce the convulsions and deaths of mice induced by strychnine. It has shown central nervous system-sedative and antipyretic effects.

[Quality] Washed clean and sun-dried. Good quality is yellow, lightweight, and complete without soils, sands, and impurities.

[Indications]

1. Wind-heat exterior pattern: Chán Tuì (Periostracum Cicadae), cool and lightweight, can clear heat and disperse wind. This substance is frequently combined with Bò He (Herba Menthae), Niú Bàng Zǐ (Fructus Arctii), and Jú Huā (Flos Chrysanthemi) for wind-heat invading the exterior pattern.
2. Loss of voice: Chán Tuì (Periostracum Cicadae) can be used together with Bò He (Herba Menthae), Jié Gěng (Radix Platycodonis), and Gān Cǎo (Radix et Rhizoma Glycyrrhizae) to relieve sudden hoarseness of

voice with accompanying sore throat, cough, and headache due to externally-contracted wind-heat.

3. Red eyes with nebula: Chán Tuì (Periostracum Cicadae) is combined with Jú Huā (Flos Chrysanthemi) and Mù Zéi Cǎo (Herba Equiseti Hiemalis) for wind-heat induced eyes problems such as blurred vision, red and itchy eyes, and nebula.

4. Pediatric convulsions: Chán Tuì (Periostracum Cicadae) is often pre-scribed with Gōu Téng (Ramulus Uncariae Cum Uncis), Wú Gōng (Scolopendra), and Quán Xiē (Scorpio) to control convulsions. This medicinal is also used as an auxiliary substance in treating childhood night terrors and tetanus via arresting convulsion. It can be ground into fine powder and applied topically to the afflicted area of tetanus.

5. Skin itching: Chán Tuì (Periostracum Cicadae) is combined with Bò He (Herba Menthae), Bái Jí Lí (Fructus Tribuli), Fáng Fēng (Radix Saposhnikoviae), and Jīng Jiè (Herba Schizonepetae) for itchy skin.

6. Unsmooth eruption of measles and rubella: Chán Tuì (Periostracum Cicadae) is conducive to vent rashes and therefore used together with Gé Gēn (Radix Puerariae Lobatae) and Niú Bàng Zǐ (Fructus Arctii) for inhibited eruption in the early stage of measles.

[Usage and Dosage] Use raw in general, 3–10g in decoction; if used for tetanus, grind 15–30g into powder for oral administration, twice a day; traditional usage requires the removal of its head and feet, however recent researches reveal that the body is more effective in relieving convulsion and syncope, and the head and feet is a powerful antipyretic. Thereby, the head and feet should also be used.

[Mnemonics] Chán Tuì (Periostracum Cicadae, Cicada Moulting): cool; clear wind-heat, relieve dry eyes and skin itching, improve night crying, and cure loss of voice.

[Simple and Effective Formulas]

1. 辛凉解表法 Xīn Liáng Jiě Biǎo — Release the Exterior with Acrid Cool Method from *Treatise on Seasonal Diseases* (时病论, Shí Bìng Lùn): Chán Tuì (Periostracum Cicadae) 3g, Bò He (Herba Menthae) 4.5g, Qián Hú (Radix Peucedani) 4.5g, Niú Bàng Zǐ (Fructus Arctii)

4.5g, Dàn Dòu Chǐ (Semen Sojae Praeparatum) 12g, and Guā Lóu Pí (Pericarpium Trichosanthis) 6g; decoct in water for oral administration to treat wind-warmth in the early stage, initial state of wind-heat invasion, winter-warmth invading the lung, and cough.

2. 止啼煎 Zhǐ Tí Jiān — Arresting Crying Decoction from *Empirical Formulas* (经验方, Jīng Yàn Fāng): Chán Tuì (Periostracum Cicadae) 5g, Bò He (Herba Menthae) 5g, and Gōu Téng (Ramulus Uncariae Cum Uncis) 10g; decoct in water for oral administration to treat pediatric night-crying.

[Precautions] Use with caution during pregnancy, and contraindicated in cases of inhibited eruption of measles due to deficiency.

Daily practices

1. Compared with the exterior-relieving madicinals that we learn before, what are the differences between Bò He (Herba Menthae) and Chán Tuì (Periostracum Cicadae) and those in terms of the nature and indications of medicinals?
2. What are the differences between Xiāng Rú (Herba Moslae) and general medicinals that release the exterior with acrid and warm property in terms of actions and indications?
3. What are the similarities and differences between Bò He (Herba Menthae) and Chán Tuì (Periostracum Cicadae) in terms of actions and indications?

牛蒡子 Niú Bàng zǐ *fructus arctii great burdock achene*

The source is from the fruit of herbaceous biennial *Arctum lappa* L., family Compositae. Pungent and bitter in flavor and cold in nature. Alternate names include Niú Zǐ 牛子, Shǔ Zhān Zǐ 鼠粘子, and Dà Lì Zǐ 大力子.

[Actions] Scatter and dissipate wind-heat, resolve toxins and vent measles, and benefit the throat and relieve swelling. It is applicable for externally-contracted wind-heat, cough with sputum difficult to expectorate, swollen and painful throat, inhibited eruption of measles in the initial stage, wind-heat rashes, and heat-toxin sores. This substance contains arctiin, its decoction has shown an *in vitro* inhibitory effect against staphylococcus aureus, and its infusion has shown an inhibitory effect against a variety of pathogenic fungus. Its extractives have shown a significant and prolonged hypoglycemic effect on rats.

[Quality] Good quality is even fruit, full-grown, and rich in oiliness without impurities. The herb produced in Tongxiang village in Zhejiang province is the best and called 杜大力子 Dù Dà Lì Zhǐ.

[Indications]

1. Wind-heat exterior pattern: Niú Bàng Zǐ (Fructus Arctii) can treat externally-contracted wind-heat patterns manifested as fever, cough, and throat pain, and is especially suitable for patients with accompanying constipation due to its effect of moistening the intestine to promote defecation. It is commonly combined with Bò He (Herba Menthae), Jīn Yín Huā (Flos Lonicerae Japonicae), Lián Qiào (Fructus Forsythiae), and Jié Gěng (Radix Platycodonis).
2. Measles and rubella: Niú Bàng Zǐ (Fructus Arctii), capable of dispersing wind and relieving toxins, is usually used together with Bò He (Herba Menthae) and Yán Suī (Chinese Parsley) for eruptive disorders when there is a inhibited expression of the rashes or itching skin.
3. Heat-toxin patterns: owning to its ability of dissipating heat-masses and reducing swelling, Niú Bàng Zǐ (Fructus Arctii) is often combined with Dà Qīng Yè (Folium Isatidis), Lián Qiào (Fructus Forsythiae), Yě Jú Huā (Flos Chrysanthemi Indici), and Bái Jiāng Cán (Bombyx Batryticatus) for carbuncle, swelling, and mumps caused by heat-toxin.

[Usage and Dosage] Raw herb is potent in dispersing with its pungent flavor; stir-frying to reduce its cold and slippery nature to prevent diarrhea; and preparing with wine to treat facial and eye swelling and pain. Use 6–15g in decoction, crush into pieces before decocting.

[Mnemonics] Niú Bàng Zǐ (Fructus Arctii, Great Burdock Achene): cold; disperse wind-heat, clear the throat, and dissipate swellings and toxins.

[Simple and Effective Formulas]

1. 启关散 Qǐ Guān Sàn — Opening Gate Powder from *Formulas for Universal Relief* (普济方, Pǔ Jì Fāng): Niú Bàng Zǐ (Fructus Arctii) (stir-fried) 30g and raw Gān Cǎo (Radix et Rhizoma Glycyrrhizae) 30g; grind into powder and decoct 5g/time in water for oral administration to treat swollen and painful tonsil and throat due to wind-heat invasion.

2. 透疹散 — Tòu Zhěn Sàn — Promoting Eruption of Papules Powder from *Essential Formulas of Health Cultivation* (养生必用方, Yǎng Shēng Bì Yòng Fāng): Niú Bàng Zǐ (Fructus Arctii) and Fú Píng (Herba Spirodelae, Duckweed) in equal dosage; take 6g/time with Bò He (Herba Menthae) decoction for oral administration, twice a day to treat urticaria all over the body caused by wind-heat invasion.

[Precautions] Niú Bàng Zǐ (Fructus Arctii) is contraindicated in cases of spleen deficiency with loose stools, as it is cold in nature and capable of moistening the large intestine.

菊花 Jú Huā *flos chrysanthemi chrysanthemum flower*

The source is from the capitulum of herbaceous perennial *Chrysanthemum morifolium* Ramat, family Compositae. Sweet and slightly bitter in flavor and cool in nature.

[Actions] Disperse wind and clear heat, and calm the liver and improve vision. It is used in the treatment of wind-heat type of common cold, headache, vertigo, dizziness, red, swollen and painful eyes, and blurred vision. This substance contains a variety of volatile oil and such major ingredients as chrysanthemum glycosides, cosmosiin, luteolin-7-gluco-side, robinin, choline, and stachydrine. Its decoction and ethanol precipi-tation have shown an *in vitro* dilatory effect on coronary artery of animal to reinforce myocardial contraction. It has shown an *in vitro* inhibitory effect against a variety of pathogenic bacteria.

[Quality] They are many varieties, such as 白菊花 Bái Jú Huā, 滁菊花 Chú Jú Huā, 贡菊花 Gòng Jú Huā, 杭菊花 Háng Jú Huā, 怀菊花 Huái Jú Huā, 川菊花 Chuān Jú Huā, and 野菊花 Yě Jú Huā. Good quality is dry, soft, fragrant, and bright in color, has a good shape and white-like or yellow ligulate flower with less stems and leaves.

[Indications]

1. Wind-heat exterior pattern: Jú Huā (Flos Chrysanthemi), lightweight in texture and potent in clearing wind-heat pathogen, is commonly used in the treatment of for wind-heat type of common cold in early stage with such symptoms as fever, aversion to cold, throat pain, and cough. It is frequently in a combination with Sāng Yè (Folium Mori), Bò He (Herba Menthae), and Jīn Yín Huā (Flos Lonicerae Japonicae).

2. Eye problems and vertigo: owning to its actions of clearing wind-heat in the liver channel and calming liver yang, Jú Huā (Flos Chrysanthemi) is applicable for red, swollen, and painful eyes or vertigo caused by either exterior wind-heat pattern or liver-heat pattern. It is often combined with Sāng Yè (Folium Mori) and Bái Jí Lí (Fructus Tribuli) for the problems caused by exterior wind-heat; with Jué Míng Zǐ (Semen Cassiae) and Xià Kū Cǎo (Spica Prunellae) for heat in the liver channel; and with Gōu Téng (Ramulus Uncariae Cum Uncis), Shí Jué Míng (Concha Haliotidis), Shú Dì Huáng (Radix Rehmanniae Praeparata), and Gǒu Qǐ Zǐ (Fructus Lycii) for dry eyes and dizzy vision due to liver-kidney yin deficiency.

This herb has recently been used to treat hypertension and coronary heart diseases.

[Usage and Dosage] Use raw in general. The ability of 白菊花 Bái Jú Huā (moderate in nature) to nourish the liver and improve vision is superior to the other varieties; 黄菊花 Huáng Jú Huā (extremely bitter) has a greater wind-heat dispersing capacity, and 野菊花 Yě Jú Huā (bitter and cold) is more effective in clearing heat and relieving toxin and most often used in treating sores, ulcers, swelling, and pain. Use 5–9g in decoction

[Mnemonics] Jú Huā (Flos Chrysanthemi, Chrysanthemum Flower): sweet and cool; strong at calming the liver, good at dispersing wind, and capable of relieving red eyes and headache.

[Simple and Effective Formulas]

1. 菊花散 Jú Huā Sǎn — Chrysanthemum Powder from *Comprehensive Recording of Divine Assistance* (圣济总录, Shèng Jì Zǒng Lù): Jú Huā (Flos Chrysanthemi) (baked) 30g, Pái Fēng Zǐ (Ailanthus vilmoriniana Dode) (also known as Guǐ Mù and capable of clearing heat and improvingvision) (baked) 30g, and Gān Cǎo (Radix et Rhizoma Glycyrrhizae) (blast-fried) 30g; grind into fine powder and take 5g/time with warm water at bedtime to treat red eyes, dizziness, blurred vision, and swollen face due to heat-toxin attacking the head and face.

2. 桑菊饮 Sāng Jú Yǐn — Mulberry Leaf and Chrysanthemum Beverage from *Systematic Differentiation of Warm Diseases* (温病条辨, Wēn Bìng Tiáo Biàn): Sāng Yè (Folium Mori) 7.5g, Jú Huā (Flos Chrysanthemi) 3g, Xìng Rén (Semen Armeniacae Amarum) 6g, Lián Qiào (Fructus Forsythiae) 4.5g, Bò He (Herba Menthae) 2.4g, Jié Gěng (Radix Platycodonis) 6g, Gān Cǎo (Radix et Rhizoma Glycyrrhizae) 2.4g, and Lú Gēn (Rhizoma Phragmitis) 6g; decoct in water for oral administration, three times a day to treat patients with cough, mild fever, and slight thirst due to wind-heat attacking the lung-*wei*.

3. 菊睛丸, Jú Jing Wán — Chrysanthemum for Eye Pill from *Formulas from the Imperial Pharmacy* (局方, Jú Fāng): Gān Jú Huā (Flos Chrysanthemi Indici) 120g, Bā Jǐ Tiān (Radix Morindae Officinalis) (plumule removed) 30g, Ròu Cōng Róng (Herba Cistanches) (soaked in wine, peel removed, stir-fried, cut, baked) 60g, and Gǒu Qǐ Zǐ (Fructus Lycii) 90g; grind into fine powder, make into phoenix tree seed-sized pill with honey, and take 30–50 pills/time with warm wine or salt solution before meal to treat blurry and dim vision due to liver and kidney insufficiency.

[Precautions] Although primarily used for exterior wind-heat pattern, Jú Huā (Flos Chrysanthemi) is less potent in dissipating and often combined in prescriptions with herbs that dissipate wind-heat and those that clear heat and resolve toxicity. Few patients will present with abdominal pain or diarrhea after taking extract tablet, long-term high dose use is not recommended to protect gastrointestinal functions.

葛根 Gé Gēn *radix puerariae lobatae kudzuvine root*

The source is the root of sprawling herbaceous perennial *Pueraria lobata* (Willd.) ohwi, family Leguminosae. Alternate names include 粉葛根 Fěn Gé Gēn. Sweet and pungent in flavor and neutral in nature.

[Actions] Release the muscle and relieve fever, uplift yang to eliminate diarrhea, engender fluid to alleviate thirst, and hasten recovery from measles with incomplete expression of the rash. It is applicable for exteriorly-contracted headache, stiffness of the neck, thirst, wasting-thirst, incomplete expression of measles, dysentery, diarrhea, hypertension, and cervical osteoarthritis. It contains flavonoid glycoside and puerarin, and has cardiac and cerebral vasodilator, hypoglycemic, and potent antipyretic effects.

[Quality] Impurity removed, washed clean, soaked in water and moistened thoroughly, cut into slices, and sun-dried. Good quality is big, heavy, solid, white, and powdery with a coarse section. It should not be very fibrous.

[Indications]

1. Painful and stiff nape and back: it is defined by contracture, stiffness and pain in the muscle from the occiput to the back, involving the waist in some cases and accompanied with headache and vertigo in most cases. Patients' chief complaints cover stiffness and pain of the head and nape, soreness and pain in the waist and back, or dizziness and headache. Doctors feel the muscle is coagulated and contracted when they press fingers on the paravertebral musculature region from the Fēng Chí (GB 20) down, meanwhile patients feel pain. This occurs most often in patients with hypertension, cervical osteoarthritis, cerebral artery blood supply insufficiency, diabetes, cardiovascular diseases, and chronic digestive system diseases. Gé Gēn (Radix Puerariae Lobatae), effective in promoting fluid production and releasing the flesh, can relieve or eliminate pain and stiffness in the nape and back that attribute to sinking clear yang failing to distribute body fluid to the sinews. It is combined with Huáng Qí (Radix Astragali), Bái Zhú (Rhizoma Atractylodis Macrocephalae), Chuān Xiōng (Rhizoma

Chuanxiong), Sháo Yào (Radix Paeoniae), Huáng Lián (Rhizoma Coptidis), and Huáng Qín (Radix Scutellariae) according to different concurrent patterns.

2. Fever due to exogenous pathogenic factors: Gé Gēn (Radix Puerariae Lobatae), lightweight and ascending in nature with the action of relieving fever, can treat exterior pattern manifested as fever, aversion to cold, headache, sore limbs, thirst, and dry nose, especially for the headache in the back of the head. It is commonly combined with Chái Hú (Radix Bupleuri) and Zǐ Sū Yè (Folium Perillae).

3. Wasting-thirst: it is a disorder featured by excessive thirst that cannot be relieved even after intensive drinking of water. The thirst relieved by Gé Gēn (Radix Puerariae Lobatae) is accompanied with stiffness and pain in the nape and back, diarrhea, and dysentery. And it is not caused by insufficiency of body fluid but failure of yang qi to ascend. Gé Gēn (Radix Puerariae Lobatae) can relieve the thirst via uplifting yang qi to prompt body fluid upward and is frequently combined with Huáng Qí (Radix Astragali), Bái Zhú (Rhizoma Atractylodis Macrocephalae), Mài Dōng (Radix Ophiopogonis), Tiān Huā Fěn (Radix Trichosanthis), Dì Huáng (Radix Rehmanniae), Cāng Zhú (Rhizoma Atractylodis), and Shān Yào (Rhizoma Dioscoreae).

4. Diarrhea and dysentery: Gé Gēn (Radix Puerariae Lobatae) is often used together with Huáng Qín (Radix Scutellariae), Huáng Lián (Rhizoma Coptidis), and raw Gān Cǎo (Radix et Rhizoma Glycyrrhizae) for damp-heat diarrhea and dysentery with accompanying abdominal pain, yellow watery stool, and burning sensation in the anus; and with Rén Shēn (Radix et Rhizoma Ginseng), Bái Zhú (Rhizoma Atractylodis Macrocephalae), Fú Líng (Poria), and Shān Yào (Rhizoma Dioscoreae) for chronic diarrhea of spleen deficiency with loose stool, or stinky smell in few cases, and obscure abdominal distention and pain.

[Usage and Dosage] Raw substance is more effective to uplift yang, generate fluid, and release the flesh; roast the herb until it turns into yellow to invigorate stomach qi and treat diarrhea due to spleen-stomach weakness. Use 10–15g in decoction, up to 30–60g for curing prolapsed organs.

[Mnemonics] Gé Gēn (Radix Pucrariae Lobatae, Kudzuvine Root): sweet and neutral; best at releasing the flesh; capable of arresting fever, promoting fluid production to quench thirst, and relieving neck rigidity.

[Simple and Effective Formulas]

1. 葛根汤 Gé Gēn Tāng — Pueraria Decoction from *Treatise on Cold Damage* (伤寒论, Shāng Hán Lùn): Gé Gēn (Radix Puerariae Lobatae) 12g, Má Huáng (Herba Ephedrae) 6g, Guì Zhī (Ramulus Cinnamomi) 6g, Shēng Jiāng (Rhizoma Zingiberis Recens) 6g, Gān Cǎo (Radix et Rhizoma Glycyrrhizae) 4g, Sháo Yào (Radix Paeoniae) 6g, and Dà Zǎo (Fructus Jujubae) six pieces; decoct in water for oral administration to treat wind-cold invading the exterior pattern with manifestations of fever, aversion to wind, absence of sweating, and stiffness and spasm of the nape and back.
2. 葛根黄芩黄连汤 Gé Gēn Huáng Qín Huáng Lián Tāng Pueraria, Scutellaria, and Coptis Decoction from *Treatise on Cold Damage* (伤寒论, Shāng Hán Lùn): Gé Gēn (Radix Puerariae Lobatae) 20g, Gān Cǎo (Radix et Rhizoma Glycyrrhizae) 5g, Huáng Qín (Radix Scutellariae) 10g, and Huáng Lián (Rhizoma Coptidis) 6g; decoct in water for oral administration to treat intestinal heat-induced dysentery or diarrhea with yellow watery stool and burning sensation in the anus.

[Precautions] Gé Gēn (Radix Puerariae Lobatae), sweet and neutral, is still relatively cool in nature with a function of uplifting and therefore should be used with caution for patients with the spleen and stomach deficiency-cold or more likelihood of getting vomiting. It is contraindicated in cases of macules and papules entering *ying*-blood.

柴胡 Chái Hú *radix bupleuri bupleurum*

The source is from the rhizome or herb of herbaceous perennial *Bulpleurum chinense* Dc. or *B. scorzonerifolium* Willd., family Umbelliferae. Alternate names include 茈胡 Zǐ Hú. Bitter in flavor and cool in nature.

[Actions] Resolve lesser yang disorders to reduce fever, spread liver qi to relieve stagnation, and raise center qi. It is applicable for common cold, alternating chills and fever, malaria, chest and rib-side distending pain, menstrual irregularities, prolapse of uterine, and prolapse of anusains volatile oil, sterol, and saponin. Pharmaceutical research reports state it has antipyretic, sedative, antalgic, anticonvulsive, antibechic, choleretic, liver-protective, biliary tract sphincter-relaxative, gastric secretion-inhibitory, and antiallergic effects. It can also increase gastric-pH value and improve humoral and cellular immunity.

[Quality] It includes many varieties and now the most commonly-used are 北柴胡 Běi Chái Hú, 南柴胡 Nán Chái Hú and 竹叶柴胡 Zhú Yè Chái Hú. The first two are from the root, and the last is from the whole plant. 北柴胡 Běi Chái Hú is light brown to rustic brown outside, solid, pliable, slightly aromatic, and bland tasted, and has a cylinder-shaped or conical root; 南柴胡 *Nán Chái Hú* has a dried, thin, cylinder-shaped or conical root with few branches, and is curving, yellow brown or rustic brown outside, lightweight, brittle easy to be broken off, slightly aromatic, bland tasted, and certain oily; and 竹叶柴胡 Zhú Yè Chái Hú is the whole plant with root and has dried, thin, cylinder-shaped or conical root, grayish green to light green stem leaves, brittle stem easy to be broken off, and soft leaves. Among these herbs, 北柴胡 Běi Chái Hú is the best.

[Indications]

1. Chest and rib-side fullness and discomfort: from the perspective of traditional Chinese medicine, it refers not only to the fullness, oppression, distending pain, and stuffiness in the chest and rib-side, but also the distending pain and masses of the breasts in women, gall bladder pain, and intercostal neuralgia. Fullness and discomfort in the chest and rib-side are subjective symptom in most cases; the doctor, however, sometimes can notice the sensations of resistance when press their fingers inward along ach of the ribs, meanwhile patients can feel pronounced heavy pressure and pressing pain. This has been defined as a symptom complex as it is often in a companion with alternating chills and fever, poor appetite, nausea, vomiting, abdominal pain, insomnia, headache, and menstrual irregularities. It is most likely to be found in biliary tract disease, gastrointestinal disease, neuropsychiatric disorders and urogenital system diseases. Most of these cases are caused by constrained

liver qi and stagnated qi movement. Chái Hú (Radix Bupleuri), owning to its effect of soothing the liver and relieving stagnation, is capable of moderating chest and rib-side fullness and discomfort and frequently combined with Sháo Yào (Radix Paeoniae), Zhǐ Shí (Fructus Aurantii Immaturus), Gān Cǎo (Radix et Rhizoma Glycyrrhizae), Chuān Xiōng (Rhizoma Chuanxiong), Qīng Pí (Pericarpium Citri Reticulatae Viride), and Jú Pí (Pericarpium Citri Reticulatae).

2. Fever due to exogenous pathogenic factors and alternating chills and fever: Chái Hú (Radix Bupleuri), ascending and dispersing in nature, is applicable for either wind-cold or wind-heat exterior pattern. It is combined with Qiāng Huó (Rhizoma et Radix Notopterygii), Dú Huó (Radix Angelicae Pubescentis), Chuān Xiōng (Rhizoma Chuanxiong), and Zǐ Sū Yè (Folium Perillae) for the wind-cold; and with Gé Gēn (Radix Puerariae Lobatae), Jīn Yín Huā (Flos Lonicerae Japonicae), and Lián Qiào (Fructus Forsythiae) for the wind-heat. Alternating chills and fever, most likely to be found in acute infectious diseases, is a subjective symptom of patient that caused by remittent change of temperature and usually accompanied with bitter taste in the mouth and discomfort in the chest and rib-side.

3. Sinking of clear qi: it refers to lassitude, lack of strength, chronic diarrhea, or even prolapse of anus, uterine, or other organs resulting from severe deficiency of center qi. Chái Hú (Radix Bupleuri) is often prescribed together with Shēng Má (Rhizoma Cimicifugae) and Huáng Qí (Radix Astragali).

[Usage and Dosage] Use raw medicinal to dispel half-exterior half-interior pathogens, relieve heat, and sooth the liver and resolve constraint; stir-frying with vinegar to increase its ability of soothing the liver and resolving constraint as sour enters the liver; when used for qi stagnation and blood stasis and menstrual irregularities due to constrained liver qi, stir-frying with turtle blood to strengthen its capacity of clearing the liver, relieving heat, nourishing the blood, and removing blood stasis. Use 5–10g in decoction, small-dosage to soothe the liver and resolve constraint, and 2–3g to uplift yang; increase dosage to relieve fever. It has been recently prepared into injection to treat fever, cough, and headache caused by many different conditions.

[Mnemonics] Chái Hú (Radix Bupleuri, Bupleurum): bitter and cool; good at relieving fever, and capable of soothing the liver to resolve constraint, and raising and lifting clear yang.

[Simple and Effective Formulas]

1. 小柴胡汤 — Xiǎo Chái Hú Yǐn — Minor Bupleurum Decoction from *Treatise on Cold Damage* (伤寒论, Shāng Hán Lùn): Chái Hú (Radix Bupleuri) 10g, Huáng Qín (Radix Scutellariae) 10g, Rén Shēn (Radix et Rhizoma Ginseng) 10g, Bàn Xià (Rhizoma Pinelliae) 9g, Zhì Gān Cǎo (Radix et Rhizoma Glycyrrhizae Praeparata cum Melle) 6g, Shēng Jiāng (Rhizoma Zingiberis Recens) 6g, and Dà Zǎo (Fructus Jujubae) five pieces; decoct in water for oral administration to treat patients with alternating chills and fever, chest and rib-side fullness and discomfort, vexation, and vomiting.

2. 正柴胡饮 — Zhèng Chái Hú Yǐn — Bupleurum Beverage from *The Complete Works of Jing-yue* (景岳全书, Jǐng Yuè Quán Shū): Chái Hú (Radix Bupleuri) 6g, Fáng Fēng (Radix Saposhnikoviae) 3g, Chén Pí (Pericarpium Citri Reticulatae) 4.5g, Sháo Yào (Radix Paeoniae) 6g, Gān Cǎo (Radix et Rhizoma Glycyrrhizae) 3g, and Shēng Jiāng (Rhizoma Zingiberis Recens) three pieces; decoct in water for oral administration to treat exterior wind-cold pattern with symptoms of fever, aversion to cold, headache, and body pain.

3. 柴胡疏肝饮 — Chái Hú Shū Gān Yǐn — Bupleurum Liver-Soothing Beverage from *Doctor's Records* (医医偶录, Yī Yī ǒu Lù): Chái Hú (Radix Bupleuri) 3.6g, Chén Pí (Pericarpium Citri Reticulatae) 3.6g, Chì Sháo (Radix Paeoniae Rubra) 3g, Zhǐ Qiào (Fructus Aurantii) 3g, Xiāng Fù (Rhizoma Cyperi) (stir-fried with vinegar) 3g, and Zhì Gān Cǎo (Radix et Rhizoma Glycyrrhizae Praeparata cum Melle) 1.5g; decoct in water for oral administration to treat rib-side pain, chest oppression, and frequent sighing due to binding constraint of liver qi.

[Precautions] Chái Hú (Radix Bupleuri) is contraindicated in cases of either yin deficiency due to its dispersing property and propensity of damaging yin-fluid or ascendant hyperactivity of liver yang because of its action of uplifting.

Daily practices

1. What are the similarities of Niú Bàng Zǐ (Fructus Arctii), Jú Huā (Flos Chrysanthemi), Chán Tuì (Periostracum Cicadae), and Bò He (Herba Menthae) in terms of releasing the exterior? What are the differences in other actions?
2. What are the similarities and differences between Gé Gēn (Radix Pucrariac Lobatae) and Chái Hú (Radix Bupleuri) in terms of actions and indications?
3. What are the differences between medicinals that release the exterior with acrid and warmth and medicinals that release the exterior with acrid and coolness in terms of actions and indications?

Third Week

1
MEDICINALS THAT CLEAR HEAT

Heat pattern refers to problems attributed to hyperactivity of yang qi that present with heat signs such as fever, thirst, red face, yellow urine, red tongue with yellow coating, and rapid pulse. Treatment of heat patterns should employ cold and cool medicinals. Heat can be found in either the exterior or the interior, the herbs described in this chapter are used for treating interior heat (known as heat-clearing medicinals), and for a description of herbs used for treating exterior heat, see chapter 2.

Internal heat are subdivided into heat in the five *zang* organs, heat in the six *fu* organs, heat in the qi level, heat in the blood level, excess heat, and deficiency heat. Medicinals that clear heat are subdivided by actions into four categories:

1. Herbs that drain heat and fire
   This it refers to medicinals that drain fire downward or attack fire-heat pathogens. Most of these heat-clearing herbs have bitter and cold properties and few of them are pungent cold or sweet cold. They are used for treating higher fever and irritability associated with pathogenic heat exuberance in the interior and the exterior in warm febrile disease. Included in this group are herbs that dry dampness and primarily used for treating damp-heat patterns such as damp-warm disorders, dysenteric disorders, jaundice, and eczema.
2. Herbs that clear heat and resolve toxins
   They are primarily used for high fever, irritability, carbuncles, swellings, sores, ulcers, swollen and painful throat, and dysenteric disorders due to exuberant pathogenic toxin in warm febrile disease.

3. Herbs that cool blood.

These medicinals are most commonly used when a febrile disease enters the *ying*-blood level manifested as persistent high fever, macules, bleeding, lose of consciousness, and delirious speech, or in internal miscellaneous diseases when blood becomes hot with reckless movement and causes different types of hemorrhagic disorders. Some of these herbs can also nourish yin due to its sweet cold property and is applicable for heat with accompany yin deficiency.

4. Herbs that clear deficiency heat

They are mainly used for steaming bone fever, tidal fever, night fever abating at dawn, and vexing heat in the chest, palms and soles due to yin fluid consumption in the late stage of febrile disease or in enduring diseases.

Some of the medicinals in this category have multiple actions. Huáng Lián (Rhizoma Coptidis), for instance, is the medicinal that clear heat and drain fire, and also clear heat and resolve toxins, while Qīng Hāo (Herba Artemisiae Annuae) can clear both deficiency heat and excess heat.

Selection of herbs for clinical use is based on

1. The exterior or interior and deficient or excessive nature of pathogenic heat, and the affected area

2. The secondary pattern

These herbs are often combined with medicinals that open the orifices when accompanied with loss of consciousness and orifice blockage; with medicinals that calm the liver and extinguish wind if accompanied with stirring wind and convulsions; with medicinals that clear qi and ying (or blood) in the cases of both qi and ying (or blood) blazing; and with yin-nourishing medicinals for accompanying symptoms of yin consumption.

3. The etiology of heat

Treatment plan should be designed not only to relieve the heat symptoms but most importantly its root cause. The proper method, for instance, is using purgatives to relieve intestinal excess accumulation for fever caused by *yangming* bowel excess; dissolving food retention to treat fever due to food accumulation; and dispelling static blood to eliminate fever resulting from static blood congestion.

4. Degrees of cold nature of heat-clearing medicinals

Overuse and overdose are not recommended as they may readily injure yang qi of the spleen and stomach. They should be used with caution especially for constitutionally yang qi or yin fluid deficiency as some of these herbs can injure yang qi or transform into dryness to consume yin.

I. Medicinals that Clear Heat and Drain Fire

石膏 **Shí Gāo** *gypsum fibrosum gypsum*

The source is the monoclinic system of gypsum ore, containing hydrous calcium sulfate. Pungent and sweet in flavor and extremely cold in nature.

[Actions] Clear and drain pathogenic heat, quench thirst, and arrest vexation. It is used for high fever, vexation, and thirst in febrile diseases, cough and wheezing due to lung heat, or headache and toothache caused by hyperactivity of stomach fire. Preliminary analysis on natural Shí Gāo (Gypsum Fibrosum) shows its suspension contains silicic acid, calcium sulfate, and aluminium hydroxide; and its solution contains calcium sulfate, ferric sulfate, and magnesium sulfate. Oral administration of its decoction has shown an antipyretic effect against experimental fever of rabbits.

[Quality] Impurities removed, washed clean and dirt removed, and ground with roller into small pieces. Good quality is large, white, and semitransparent with a fibrous vertical section.

[Indications]

1. Lung and stomach excess heat: manifestations include high fever, profuse sweating, intense thirst, and flooding big pulse. Specifically, the high fever is accompanied with aversion to heat (instead of aversion to cold) with moist skin and frequent sweating; the intense thirst is complicated with a desire to drink lots of water or cold water (instead of thirst with little or no desire to drink and a preference of hot beverage); and the pulse is slippery fast, floating big, or flooding big. This

condition is most likely to be found in warm febrile disease, hemorrhagic disorders, metabolic diseases, and sunstroke. Shí Gāo (Gypsum Fibrosum) is often combined with Zhī Mǔ (Rhizoma Anemarrhenae) for high fever and restlessness in the febrile disease; with Zhī Mǔ (Rhizoma Anemarrhenae), Shēng Dì (Radix Rehmanniae), Ē Jiāo (Colla Corii Asini) for subcutaneous bleeding, mouth bleeding, and nosebleed with fever; and with Zhī Mǔ (Rhizoma Anemarrhenae), Rén Shēn (Radix et Rhizoma Ginseng), and Xuán Shēn (Radix Scrophulariae) for intense thirst in diabetes.

2. Cough and wheezing due to lung heat: Shí Gāo (Gypsum Fibrosum) is commonly prescribed together with Má Huáng (Herba Ephedrae) to relieve cough and wheezing caused by lung heat, wheezing with sweating, vexation and agitation with absence of sweating, or sweating with swelling all over the body.

[Mnemonics] Shí Gāo (Gypsum Fibrosum, Gypsum): pungent and cold; good at relieving vexation and thirst with surging big pulse and high fever.

[Simple and Effective Formulas]

1. 玉泉散 Yù Quán Sǎn Jade Spring Powder from *Effective Use of Established Formulas* (成方切用, Chéng Fāng Qiè Yòng): Shí Gāo (Gypsum Fibrosum) 20 g and Gān Cǎo (Radix et Rhizoma Glycyrrhizae) 3 g; decoct in water for oral administration to treat patient with vexation, thirst, fever with sweating, headache, asthma with phlegm, and big pulse. Also used in the treatment of febrile diseases, metabolic disorders, sunstroke, and dermatosis with manifestation listed above.

2. 白虎汤 Bái Hǔ Tāng White Tiger Decoction from *Treatise on Cold Damage* (伤寒论, Shāng Hán Lùn): Shí Gāo (Gypsum Fibrosum) 15–30 g, Zhī Mǔ (Rhizoma Anemarrhenae) 10–20 g, Gān Cǎo (Radix et Rhizoma Glycyrrhizae) 3 g, and Jīng Mǐ (Oryza Sativa L.) 20 g; decoct in water for oral administration to treat patient with high fever, profuse sweating, intense thirst, vexation, agitation, and flooding slippery big pulse. Also applicable for type B encephalitis, epidemic hemorrhagic fever, influenza, pneumonia, epidemic cerebrospinal

meningitis, leptospirosis, high fever of unknown origins, and dermatosis with above-mentioned manifestations.

3. 白虎加人参汤 Bái Hǔ Jiā Rén Shēn Tāng — White Tiger Decoction with Ginseng from *Treatise on Cold Damage* (伤寒论, Shāng Hán Lùn): Shí Gāo (Gypsum Fibrosum) 15–30 g, Zhī Mǔ (Rhizoma Anemarrhenae) 10–20 g, Gān Cǎo (Radix et Rhizoma Glycyrrhizae) 3 g, Rén Shēn (Radix et Rhizoma Ginseng) 10 g or Běi Shā Shēn (Radix Glehniae) 15 g, and Jīng Mǐ (Oryza Sativa L.) 20 g; decoct in water for oral administration to treat patient with intense thirst, dry mouth, and flooding big pulse. Also applicable for diabetes and various types of febrile diseases with the above-manifestations.

4. 苍术白虎汤 Cāng Zhú Bái Hǔ Tāng — White Tiger Decoction with Atractylodes Rhizome from *Treatise on Cold Damage* (伤寒论, Shāng Hán Lùn): Shí Gāo (Gypsum Fibrosum) 15–30 g, Zhī Mǔ (Rhizoma Anemarrhenae) 10–20 g, Gān Cǎo (Radix et Rhizoma Glycyrrhizae) 3 g, Cāng Zhú (Rhizoma Atractylodis) 12 g, and Jīng Mǐ (Oryza Sativa L.) 20 g; decoct in water for oral administration to treat patient with aversion of heat, spontaneous sweating, thirst, painful and heavy body, and inhibited urination. Also applicable for rheumatic fever, diabetes, and dermatosis with above- mentioned symptoms.

5. 竹叶石膏汤 Zhú Yè Shí Gāo Tāng — Lophatherum and Gypsum Decoction from *Treatise on Cold Damage* (伤寒论, Shāng Hán Lùn): Shí Gāo (Gypsum Fibrosum) 12–30 g, Rén Shēn (Radix et Rhizoma Ginseng) 10 g, Mài Dōng (Radix Ophiopogonis) 12 g, Gān Cǎo (Radix et Rhizoma Glycyrrhizae) 5 g, Zhú Yè (Folium Phyllostachydis Henonis) 12 g, Bàn Xià (Rhizoma Pinelliae) 10 g, and Jīng Mǐ (Oryza Sativa L.) 20 g; decoct in water for oral administration to treat patient with emaciation, palpitation, agitation, belching, and cough. Also applicable for febrile diseases in recovery phase, sunstroke, diabetes, and mouth sores with the above manifestations.

[Usage and Dosage] Use raw in general for oral administration, 10–30 g in decoction, very effective for clearing heat; when used for sores, ulcers, eczema, and burns, this substance is calcined to engender flesh and close sore.

[Precautions] Shí Gāo (Gypsum Fibrosum) is an important herb of draining pathogenic heat and clinically indicated only for the excess heat in qi stage. It is contraindicated for patients with aversion to cold, absence of sweating, swelling body, or deep and slow pulse.

Daily practices

1. What is heat-clearing medicinal and how many types of it? What precautions should be taken when using it?
2. What are the actions and indications of Shí Gāo (Gypsum Fibrosum)?

知母 Zhī Mǔ *rhizoma anemarrhenae common anemarrhena rhizome*

The source is from the rhizome of herbaceous perennial *Anemarrhena asphodeloides* Bunge, family Liliaceae. Bitter and sweet in flavor and cold in nature.

[Actions] Clear heat and drain fire, enrich yin and generate body fluids, and moisten dryness. It is applicable to externally-contracted febrile diseases with high fever, vexation, thirst, lung-heat induced dry cough, steaming bone fever, tidal fever, internal heat, wasting-thirst, and intestinal dryness-induced constipation. This herb contains rhizoma anemarrhenae glycosides, flavonoid glycoside, profuse phlegmatic, saccharides, saccharides, and niacin, and a small amount of aromaticity material and fatty oil. Experiments demonstrate sedative and antipyretic effects, and regulation of the adrenal pituitary system.

[Quality] Impurity removed, swashed, softened by moistening, cut into slices, and sun-dried. Good quality is large, thick and hard with a yellowish white and moist cross section.

[Indications]

1. Sweating with vexation: it is identified by vexation or even insomnia and simultaneous sweating, no matter spontaneous sweating, night sweating, or yellow sweat. Zhī Mǔ (Rhizoma Anemarrhenae), Dà

Huáng (Radix et Rhizoma Rhei), Huáng Lián (Rhizoma Coptidis) and Zhī Zǐ (Fructus Gardeniae) all are used for treating vexation. Among their differences, Zhī Mǔ (Rhizoma Anemarrhenae) is often used for deficiency-vexation featured by the absence of pain, stuffiness, and tangible pathogens in the intestines and stomach; Dà Huáng (Radix et Rhizoma Rhei) is for the vexation due to accumulation in the abdomen and pain blockage; Huáng Lián (Rhizoma Coptidis) is for the vexation caused by epigastric *pǐ*, pain, and throbbing; and Zhī Zǐ (Fructus Gardeniae) is for stuffiness and blockage in the chest with coating on the tongue. Clinically, combination of herbs is based on different patterns, Zhī Mǔ (Rhizoma Anemarrhenae) is prescribed together with Shí Gāo (Gypsum Fibrosum) and Rén Shēn (Radix et Rhizoma Ginseng) for fever, dry mouth, thirst, and floating big pulse; with Guì Zhī (Ramulus Cinnamomi) and Shí Gāo (Gypsum Fibrosum) for joint pain; with Guì Zhī (Ramulus Cinnamomi), Sháo Yào (Radix Paeoniae), Fù Zǐ (Radix Aconiti Lateralis Praeparata), and Má Huáng (Herba Ephedrae) for extreme emaciation with swollen enlarged feet; with Bǎi Hé(Bulbus Lilii) for vexation and agitation; and with Suān Zǎo Rén (Semen Ziziphi Spinosae) and Gān Cǎo (Radix et Rhizoma Glycyrrhizae) for insomnia due to deficiency-vexation.

2. Deficiency-heat: manifestations include emaciation, tidal fever, float-ing-red complexion, sweating during sleep, cough with dry throat, red tongue with scanty coating, and dry and hard stool. Zhī Mǔ (Rhizoma Anemarrhenae), capable of nourishing kidney (water) to eliminate defi-ciency fire and potent in relieving deficiency-heat pattern, is often combined with Mài Dōng (Radix Ophiopogonis), Shā Shēn (Radix Adenophorae seu Glehniae), Ē Jiāo (Colla Corii Asini), and Xuán Shēn (Radix Scrophulariae).

3. Cough due to lung dryness: Zhī Mǔ (Rhizoma Anemarrhenae) can clear lung heat and nourish lung yin and is therefore applicable for cough due to either lung yin consumption by excessive heat in the lung or lung yin deficiency in chronic diseases. It is frequently combined with Huáng Qín (Radix Scutellariae) and Zhè Bèi Mǔ (Bulbus Fritillariae Thunbergii) for cough due to lung heat; and with Shā Shēn (Radix Adenophorae seu Glehniae), Mài Dōng (Radix Ophiopogonis), and Chuān Bèi Mǔ (Bulbus Fritillariae Cirrhosae) for cough caused by lung yin deficiency.

[Mnemonics] Zhī Mǔ (Rhizoma Anemarrhenae, Common Anemarrhena Rhizome): bitter and cold; stop sweating, relieve restlessness, drain fire, nourish yin, and remove dryness-heat.

[Simple and Effective Formulas]

1. 玉女煎 Yù Nǚ Jiān — Jade Lady Decoction from *The Complete Works of Jing-yue* (景岳全书, Jǐng Yuè Quán Shū): Zhī Mǔ (Rhizoma Anemarrhenae) 12 g, Shí Gāo (Gypsum Fibrosum) 15 g, Mài Dōng (Radix Ophiopogonis) 10 g, Shú Dì Huáng (Radix Rehmanniae Praeparata) 20 g, and Niú Xī (Radix Achyranthis Bidentatae) 15 g; decoct in water for oral administration to treat patient with vexation heat, thirst, headache, toothache, tooth bleeding, and floating big pulse. Also applicable for different types of febrile disorders, hematopathy, diabetes, and periodontal diseases with above-mentioned manifestations.

2. 滋肾丸 Zī Shèn Wán — Kidney Nourishing Pill from *Illumination of Medicine* (医学发明, Yī Xué Fā Míng): Zhī Mǔ (Rhizoma Anemarrhenae) 10 g, Ròu Guì (Cortex Cinnamomi) 5 g, and Huáng Bǎi (Cortex Phellodendri Chinensis) 10 g; decoct in water for oral administration to treat patient with urinary retention or foot and knee swelling and pain, red tongue, and flooding big pulse. Also applicable for urinary system disorders, arthritis, and gout.

3. 知柏地黄丸 Zhī Bǎi Dì Huáng Wán — Anemarrhena, Phellodendron and Rehmannia Pill from *Golden Mirror of the Medical Tradition* (医宗金鉴, Yī Zōng Jīn Jiàn): Zhī Mǔ (Rhizoma Anemarrhenae) 10 g, Huáng Bǎi (Cortex Phellodendri Chinensis) 10 g, Shú Dì Huáng (Radix Rehmanniae Praeparata) 15 g, Shān Yào (Rhizoma Dioscoreae) 15 g, Shān Zhū Yú (Fructus Corni) 10 g, Zé Xiè (Rhizoma Alismatis) 10 g, Fú Líng (Poria) 12 g, and Mǔ Dān Pí (Cortex Moutan) 6 g; decoct in water for oral administration to treat patient with tidal fever, night sweating, vexation heat, and floating pulse. Also applicable for tuberculosis, urinary system disorders, dysfunction of autonomic nervous system, and chronic infectious diseases with symptoms mentioned above.

4. 二母散 Èr Mǔ Sǎn — Common Anemarrhena Rhizome and Fritillary Bulb Powder from *Effective Use of Established Formulas* (成方切用, Chéng Fāng Qiè Yòng): Zhī Mǔ (Rhizoma Anemarrhenae) 12 g and Bèi Mǔ (Bulbus Fritillaria) 10 g; decoct in water grind into powder (divide

into four equal doses, take one dose/time, twice a day) for oral administration or to treat patient with cough, fever, and sweating during sleep.

[Precautions] Zhī Mǔ (Rhizoma Anemarrhenae), cold and slippery in
nature, is contraindicated in cases of loose stool or diarrhea due to deficiency-cold in the spleen and stomach.

栀子 Zhī Zǐ *fructus gardeniae* gardenia

The source is from a fruit of evergreen shrub *Gardenia jasminoides* Ellis,
family Rubiaceae. Alternate names include 山栀子 Shān Zhī Zǐ, 山栀
Shān Zhī, and 支子 Zhī Zǐ. Bitter in flavor and cold in nature.

[Actions] Clear heat and remove toxin, drain fire and relieve vexation,
and cool the blood and dissipate blood stagnation. It is applicable to
febrile diseases fever, deficiency vexation, insomnia, jaundice, strangury,
wasting-thirst, red eyes, sore throat, hematemesis, epistaxis, dysentery
with stool constaining blood, hematuria, sores due to heat-toxin, ulcers,
and sprain with swelling and pain. This herb contains geniposide, tannin,
pectin, D mannitol, crocin, and ursolic acid. Experiments show these
ingredients have antipyretic, sedative, choleretic, antihypertensive, and
hypolipidemic effects.

[Quality] Sifted to remove dust, impurities removed, ground with roller
into pieces, sifted or cut both ends. Good quality is dry, even fruit, thin-
skinned, full, round, and reddish yellow, and the herb produced in
Zhejiang is the best.

[Indications]

1. Vexing heat and suffocated sensation in the chest: vexing heat refers to
   vexation, irritability, restlessness, fever and sweating; while suffocated
   sensation in the chest means stifling stuffiness or burning sensation in
   the center of the chest and feeling of softness instead of hardness and
   fullness in gastric area upon pressure. In the clinic, patients with vexing
   heat and suffocated sensation in the chest are more susceptible to sore
   throat, red eyes, epistaxis, difficult and painful urination with scanty
   and yellow urine, and red tongue. Physicians need more observation

and inquiry. Zhī Zǐ (Fructus Gardeniae) is often combined with Dàn Dòu Chǐ (Semen Sojae Praeparatum) for this condition, which is most likely to be found in acute febrile diseases, infectious diseases, upper digestive system diseases, and neuropsychiatric disorders. Zhī Zǐ (Fructus Gardeniae) and Zhī Mǔ (Rhizoma Anemarrhenae) both are used in the treatment of vexation, but the former is for vexation and agitation with yellow thin tongue coating caused by fire-heat in or above the chest and diaphragm and the latter is to relieve deficiency-vexation marked by intangible pathogenic influence in the chest, intestines, and stomach and thin tongue coating.

2. Jaundice and strangury: jaundice refers to the yellow colored skin, urine, and whites of the eyes. The jaundice treated by Zhī Zǐ (Fructus Gardeniae) is marked by orange yellow color with accompanying vexing heat, chest oppression, and yellow greasy tongue coating attributed to internal accumulation of damp-heat. In this case, this herb is combined with Dà Huáng (Radix et Rhizoma Rhei), Yīn Chén (Herba Artemisiae Scopariae), and Huáng Bǎi (Cortex Phellodendri Chinensis).

3. Bleeding due to blood-heat: heat in the blood will make blood flow out of the vessel and cause various kinds of hemorrhagic disorders, such as hematemesis, epistaxis, and hematuria. Zhī Zǐ (Fructus Gardeniae) is combined with Lián Qiào (Fructus Forsythiae), Shēng Dì (Radix Rehmanniae), Cè Bǎi Yè (Cacumen Platycladi), and Mǔ Dān Pí (Cortex Moutan) when the bleeding is accompanied with sore throat, red eyes, vexation and agitation, and red tongue. Oral administration of its powder can arrest stomach bleeding.

4. Heat-toxin sores and swelling: Zhī Zǐ (Fructus Gardeniae), capable of clearing heat and resolving toxin, is often combined with Huáng Lián (Rhizoma Coptidis), Huáng Qín (Radix Scutellariae), and Huáng Bǎi (Cortex Phellodendri Chinensis) for abscesses and swelling, erysipelas, sores and ulcers, and burns associated with heat-toxins.

Mixing its powder with vinegar or wine and applying externally can treat sprains and contusions; and mixing its powder with wine or egg white and applying externally can relieve traumatic swelling and pain and erysipelas.

[Mnemonics] Zhī Zǐ (Fructus Gardeniae, Gardenia): bitter and cold; clear heat, resolve restlessness, stuffiness and oppression in the chest, cure hematemesis and epistaxis, and relieve jaundice.

[Simple and Effective Formulas]

1. 栀子豉汤 Zhī Zǐ Chǐ Tāng — Gardenia and Prepared Soybean Decoction from *Treatise on Cold Damage* (伤寒论, Shāng Hán Lùn): Zhī Zǐ (Fructus Gardeniae) 12 g and Dòu Chǐ (Semen Sojae Praeparatum) 12 g; decoct in water for oral administration to treat patients with fever, chest stuffiness and pain, vexation, insomnia due to deficiency-vexation, and yellow thin tongue coating. Also applicable for acute febrile diseases, esophagitis, gastritis, and neuropsychiatric disorders with the above symptoms.

2. 栀子柏皮汤 Zhī Zǐ Bǎi Pí Tāng — Gardenia and Amur Cork-tree Bark Decoction from *Treatise on Cold Damage* (伤寒论, Shāng Hán Lùn): Zhī Zǐ (Fructus Gardeniae) 10 g, Bǎi Pí (Cortex Phellodendri Chinensis) 10 g, and Gān Cǎo (Radix et Rhizoma Glycyrrhizae) 3 g; decoct in water for oral administration to treat patients with fever, jaundice, vexation, and inhibited urination with yellow scanty urine. Also applicable for hepatitis, biliary tract infection with jaundice, or dermatosis of damp-heat pattern.

3. 栀子大黄汤 Zhī Zǐ Dà Huáng Tāng — Gardenia and Rhubarb Decoction from *Essentials from the Golden Cabinet* (金匮要略, Jīn Guì Yào Lüè): Zhī Zǐ (Fructus Gardeniae) 10 g, Dà Huáng (Radix et Rhizoma Rhei) 10 g, Zhǐ Shí (Fructus Aurantii Immaturus) 10 g, and Dòu Chǐ (Semen Sojae Praeparatum) 12 g; decoct in water for oral administration to treat patients with fever, jaundice, chest stuffiness, inhibited urination, and constipation. Also applicable for biliary tract infection, biliary tract stone, and hepatitis with above-mentioned manifestations.

4. 栀子厚朴汤 Zhī Zǐ Hòu Pò Tāng — Gardenia and Officinal Magnolia Bark Decoction from *Treatise on Cold Damage* (伤寒论, Shāng Hán Lùn): Zhī Zǐ (Fructus Gardeniae) 10 g, Hòu Pò (Cortex Magnoliae Officinalis) 10 g, and Zhǐ Shí (Fructus Aurantii Immaturus) 10 g; decoct in water for oral administration to treat patients with vexing heat and abdominal fullness and pain. Also applicable for various digestive tract diseases and febrile diseases.

[Usage and Dosage]

The raw herb is more effective in clearing heat and draining fire; its peel clears external heat, while its kernel clears internal heat; frying with ginger juice to increase its ability of relieving vexation and vomiting, and scorch-frying to strengthen its powder of arresting bleeding. Use 5–12 g in decoction.

[Precautions] Zhī Zǐ (Fructus Gardeniae), bitter and cold in nature, tends to damage the spleen and stomach qi when applied inappropriately and therefore should be used with cautions in cases of loose stool due to deficiency-cold of the spleen and stomach.

Daily practices

1. What are the similarities and differences between Zhī Mǔ (Rhizoma Anemarrhenae) and Zhī Zǐ (Fructus Gardeniae) in terms of actions and indications?
2. What are the similarities and differences among Shí Gāo (Gypsum Fibrosum), Zhī Mǔ (Rhizoma Anemarrhenae), and Zhī Zǐ (Fructus Gardeniae) in terms of nature, flavor, and actions?

黄连 Huáng Lián *rhizoma coptidis coptis rhizome*

The source is from the rhizome of herbaceous perennial *Coptis chinensis Franch. C. deltoidea C. Y. Cheng et Hsiao*, and *Coptis teetoides C. Y. Cheng*, family Ranunculaceae. Alternate names include 川连 Chuān Lián and 雅连 Yǎ Lián. Bitter in flavor and cold in nature.

[Actions] Clear heat and dry dampness, drain fire and relieve vexation, and kill parasites. It is applicable to heat-toxin exuberance, high fever, loss of consciousness, vomiting, diarrhea and dysentery, jaundice, vexation, insomnia, blood heat hematemesis, epistaxis, red, swollen and painful eyes, toothache, wasting-thirst, sores, carbuncles, furuncles, and ulcers. It can be used externally in the treatment of eczema and suppuration from the auditory meatus. This herb contains a variety of alkaloid such as berberine and worenine that exert significant antibacterial effects on shigella dysenteriae, typhoid bacillus, escherichia coli, pseudomonas aeruginosa, staphylococcus, and hemolytic streptococcus. Intravenous injection has an antihypertensive effect and can stimulate gastrointestinal tract and bronchial smooth muscle. Its ingredient berberine has a moderate choleretic, hypolipidemic, and anti-inflammatory effect.

[Quality] Impurity removed, washed clean, moistened thoroughly, cut into slices, and dried under shade. 川连 Chuān Lián produced in eastern Sichuan is of the best quality, its rhizomes are with many interconnections and look like chicken claw, and therefore it is also known as *Jī* 鸡爪连 Zhuǎ Lián. 云连 Yún Lián produced in Deqin, Weixi and Tengchong of Yunnan is of an inferior quality.

[Indications]

1. Vexing heat: symptoms and signs include vexation and agitation, anxiety, nervousness, lack of concentration, hot sensation all over the body, chest stuffiness and oppression, palpitation, rapid pulse or difficult to fall asleep, dreaminess, early-morning awakening insomnia, epigastric discomfort or pain, greasy and yellow tongue coating. This pattern can be seen in acute and chronic infectious diseases, neuropsychiatric disorders, cardiovascular and cerebrovascular diseases, and hypertension. Owning to its effect of clearing heart fire and relieving vexation and agitation, Huáng Lián (Rhizoma Coptidis) is widely used to relieve the manifestations above and usually in a combination with Huáng Qín (Radix Scutellariae), Zhī Zǐ (Fructus Gardeniae), and Gān Cǎo (Radix et Rhizoma Glycyrrhizae).
2. *Pǐ* pattern: manifestations include discomfort, dull pain, and distending pain or burning pain in gastric area with accompanying bitter taste in the mouth, belching, nausea, and vomiting. Pressing, mild, and diffuse pain would occur in the upper abdomen when pressing. It is most commonly found in gastritis, gastric neurosis, and cholecystitis. In this case, Huáng Lián (Rhizoma Coptidis) is often prescribed together with Rén Shēn (Radix et Rhizoma Ginseng), Guì Zhī (Ramulus Cinnamomi), Bàn Xià (Rhizoma Pinelliae), Huáng Qín (Radix Scutellariae), Gān Jiāng (Rhizoma Zingiberis), and Gān Cǎo (Radix et Rhizoma Glycyrrhizae).

3. Dysentery and heat diarrhea: it is often accompanied by abdominal pain, hot sensation in the body, sweating, sticky and smelly stool, and yellow greasy tongue coating. Those symptoms and signs are caused by damp-heat accumulation in the intestines and commonly seen in bacillary dysentery and acute grastroenteritis. Huáng Lián (Rhizoma Coptidis) is usually combined with Huáng Qín (Radix Scutellariae), Mù Xiāng (Radix Aucklandiae), and Hòu Pò (Cortex Magnoliae Officinalis).

4. Wasting-thirst: manifestations include thirst, vexation and agitation, hot sensation all over the body, epigastric *pǐ*, and yellow greasy tongue coating. It can be seen in either acute febrile diseases but also diabetes. Huáng Lián (Rhizoma Coptidis) is frequently used together with Tiān Huā Fěn (Radix Trichosanthis), Shēng Dì (Radix Rehmanniae), and Zhī Mǔ (Rhizoma Anemarrhenae).

5. Heat-toxin patterns: Huáng Lián (Rhizoma Coptidis), potent in clearing heat and resolving toxins, is used as a principal herb for sores and ulcers caused by heat-toxin and hemorrhage, macules, and papules due to heat-toxin resulting from pathogenic heat exuberance in febrile diseases. It is often combined with Huáng Qín (Radix Scutellariae) and Zhī Zǐ (Fructus Gardeniae).

6. Vomiting: Huáng Lián (Rhizoma Coptidis), effective in arresting vomiting, is particularly suitable for vomiting caused by excessive stomach heat and gall bladder heat. It is used in a combination with Zǐ Sū Yè (Folium Perillae) for morning sickness and vomiting during pregnancy.

It is also applicable for restless fetus due to fetal heat, exuberance of liver fire, and damp-heat in the gallbladder channel.

[Usage and Dosage] Use raw in general. Raw herb is more effective in clearing fire and resolving toxins; wine-processed to clear fire in the head and eye; ginger juice-fry to arrest vomiting; and Wú Zhū Yú (Fructus Evodiae)-fried to relieve vomiting due to liver and gallbladder fire exuberance attacking the stomach. Use 3–6 g in decoction, 0.5–2 g in pill and powder. Do not cook overtime as the evaporation of its active ingredients is fast at high temperatures. When used for treating vexation and insomnia, the herb should not be prepared into decoction, but pill and powder, because its sedative ingredients have a low solubility in water.

[Mnemonics] *Huáng Lián* (Rhizoma Coptidis, Coptis Rhizome): clear the heart, relieve *pǐ* pattern and restlessness, drain fire, resolve toxins, arrest dysentery, and calm the fetus.

[Simple and Effective Formulas]

1. 黄连汤 Huáng Lián Tāng — Coptis Decoction from *Treatise on Cold Damage* (伤寒论, Shāng Hán Lùn): Huáng Lián (Rhizoma Coptidis) 5 g, Gān Cǎo (Radix et Rhizoma Glycyrrhizae) 3 g, Gān Jiāng (Rhizoma Zingiberis) 6 g, Guì Zhī (Ramulus Cinnamomi) 6 g, Bàn Xià (Rhizoma Pinelliae) 10 g, Rén Shēn (Radix et Rhizoma Ginseng) 6 g or Dǎng Shēn (Radix Codonopsis) 12 g, and Dà Zǎo (Fructus Jujubae) six pieces; decoct in water for oral administration to treat patient with abdominal pain, nausea, vomiting, epigastric *pǐ*, and palpitation with vexation. Also applicable for digestive system diseases and cardiovascular diseases with above-mentioned manifestations.

2. 半夏泻心汤 Bàn Xià Xiè Xīn Tang — Pinellia and Officinal Magnolia Bark Decoction from *Treatise on Cold Damage* (伤寒论, Shāng Hán Lùn): Huáng Lián (Rhizoma Coptidis) 5 g, Huáng Qín (Radix Scutellariae) 6 g, Gān Jiāng (Rhizoma Zingiberis) 6 g, Gān Cǎo (Radix et Rhizoma Glycyrrhizae) 3 g, Bàn Xià (Rhizoma Pinelliae) 10 g, Rén Shēn (Radix et Rhizoma Ginseng) 6 g or Dǎng Shēn (Radix Codonopsis) 12 g, and Dà Zǎo (Fructus Jujubae) six pieces; decoct in water for oral administration to treat patient with epigastric *pǐ*, nausea, vexing heat, and red tongue with yellow greasy coating. Also applicable for various types of gastrointestinal disorders with symptoms and signs mentioned above.

3. 黄连阿胶汤 Huáng Lián Ē Jiāo Tāng — Coptis and Donkey-Hide Gelatin Decoction from *Treatise on Cold Damage* (伤寒论, Shāng Hán Lùn): Huáng Lián (Rhizoma Coptidis) 5 g, Huáng Qín (Radix Scutellariae) 10 g, Ē Jiāo (Colla Corii Asini) 12 g, Sháo Yào (Radix Paeoniae) 12 g, and one Jī Zǐ Huáng (egg yolk); decoct in water for oral administration to treat patient with vexation, restless sleep, abdominal pain, and stool with pus and blood. Also applicable for insomnia and dysentery caused by exuberance of heart-fire.

4. 黄连解毒汤 Huáng Lián Jiě Dú Tāng — Coptis Toxin-Resolving Decoction from *Arcane Essentials from the Imperial Library* (外台秘要, Wài Tái Mì Yào): Huáng Lián (Rhizoma Coptidis) 6 g, Huáng Qín

(Radix Scutellariae) 12 g, Huáng Bǎi (Cortex Phellodendri Chinensis) 10 g, and Shān Zhī (Fructus Gardeniae)10 g; decoct in water for oral administration to treat patient with vexation and agitation, mania, dry mouth and throat, belching, groan, paraphasia, restless sleep, hematemesis, epistaxis, and macules. Also applicable for infectious diseases, acute communicable diseases, and hemorrhagic diseases due to heat-toxin exuberance.

5. 连苏饮 Lián Sū Yǐn — Coptis and Perilla Leaf Decoction from *Treatise on Damp-heat Induced Diseases* (湿热病篇, Shī Rè Bìng Piān): Huáng Lián (Rhizoma Coptidis) 3 g and Zǐ Sū Yè (Folium Perillae) 6 g; decoct in water for oral administration to treat chest vexation and vomiting. Also applicable for vomiting caused by gastroenteritis and pregnancy.

6. 泻心汤 Xiè Xīn Tāng — Heart-Draining Decoction from *Essentials from the Golden Cabinet* (金匮要略, Jīn Guì Yào Lüè): Huáng Lián (Rhizoma Coptidis) 3 g, Huáng Qín (Radix Scutellariae) 10 g, and Dà Huáng (Radix et Rhizoma Rhei) 10 g; decoct in water for oral administration to treat patient with hematemesis, epistaxis, fever, jaundice, red, swollen and painful eyes, ulcers in the mouth and tongue, sores, and ulcers with accompanying vexing heat in the heart, discomfort and fullness in the chest, constipation, and red tongue with yellow and greasy coating. Also applicable for hemorrhagic diseases, infectious diseases, and digestive tract diseases.

7. 小陷胸汤 Xiǎo Xiàn Xiōng Tāng — Minor Chest Draining Decoction from *Treatise on Cold Damage* (伤寒论, Shāng Hán Lùn): Huáng Lián (Rhizoma Coptidis) 5 g, Bàn Xià (Rhizoma Pinelliae) 12 g, and Guā Lóu (Fructus Trichosanthis) 15 g; decoct in water for oral administration to treat patient with chest oppression and pain, epigastric *pǐ* and pain, cough with sticky sputum, nausea, and constipation. Also applicable for digestive tract disease, respiratory diseases, and cardiovascular diseases with above manifestations.

[Precautions] Huáng Lián (Rhizoma Coptidis), owning to its bitter and cold in nature, tends to damage stomach qi and is therefore contraindicated in cases of vomiting and diarrhea caused by deficiency cold of the spleen and stomach. It is appropriate for vexation and fullness with accompanying hard, tough, dark and reddish tongue, yellow greasy thick tongue coating, and lusterless tongue margin, whereas it should be used with caution when patients present reddish, enlarged and tender tongue with white and thin coating, or sometimes no coating at all. This herb assists dryness and damage yin, and thus should not be taken over a long period of term. Deaths from intravenous injection of berberine have been reported recently.

黄芩 Huáng Qín *radix scutellariae scutellaria root*

The source is from the root of herbaceous perennial *Scutellariae baicalensis* Georgi, family Labiatae. Bitter in flavor and cold in nature.

[Actions] Clear heat and dry dampness, drain fire and resolve toxins, stanch bleeding, and calm the fetus. It is applicable for treating jaundice, diarrhea, dysentery, heat strangury, carbuncle, and sores caused by damp-heat or heat-toxin and such acute febrile diseases as wind-warmth and damp-warmth with the manifestations of high fever, vexation, and thirst. This herb contains baicalin, wogonoside, baicalein, wogonin, and neobaicalein. Baicalin has shown antihypertensive, antipyretic, diuretic, sedative, and antibacterial effects.

[Quality] Impurities removed, residue stem removed, moistened with cool boiled water or soaked in boiled water for a while, obtained and moistened thoroughly, cut into slices, and dried under sunshine. Good quality is long, solid, brownish yellow, and with an intact cross section. The yellow and solid new root is called 子芩, Zi Qín while darkish-brown old root with a hollow center is called 枯芩, Kū Qín.

[Indications]

1. Vexing heat: Huáng Qín (Radix Scutellariae) and Huáng Lián (Rhizoma Coptidis) both can treat vexation, but the former is more impotent in relieving vexation heat in the palms and soles and stuffiness heat in the chest. Huáng Qín (Radix Scutellariae) is often combined with Chái Hú (Radix Bupleuri) and Bàn Xià (Rhizoma Pinelliae) when vexing heat is accompanied with restlessness and retching; with Huáng Lián (Rhizoma Coptidis) for the vexing heat and epigastric *pǐ* and fullness; and with Bái Sháo (Radix Paeoniae Alba) for the vexing heat with abdominal pain and diarrhea.

2. Internal accumulation of heat toxin: Huáng Qín (Radix Scutellariae) is applicable for cough due to exuberance of lung fire; restlessness and unconsciousness caused by exuberance of heart fire; headache, vertigo, and red painful eyes attributed to exuberance of liver fire; jaundice resulting from exuberance of gallblader fire; and alternating chills and fever in *shaoyang* disease.

3. Bleeding due to heat exuberance: manifestations are hematemesis, epistaxis, blood dysentery, profuse menstruation, and restless fetus with accompanying epigastric pǐ. In this case if patients present with strong and tight muscle, red complexion, darkish lips, tough tongue, slippery fast pulse, and sticky and purplish red bleeding, Huáng Qín (Radix Scutellariae) is combined with Huáng Lián (Rhizoma Coptidis) and Zhī Zǐ (Fructus Gardeniae).

4. Internal accumulation of damp-heat: Huáng Qín (Radix Scutellariae), capable of clearing heat and drying dampness, is applicable for jaundice and strangury caused by damp-heat or in cases of unresolved dampness pathogen in damp-warm disease. It is usually combined with Huáng Lián (Rhizoma Coptidis), Tōng Cǎo (Medulla Tetrapanacis), and Huá Shí (Talcum).

5. Restless fetus: Huáng Qín (Radix Scutellariae) is capable of calming the restless fetus caused by fetal heat and is usually in a combination with Bái Zhú (Rhizoma Atractylodis Macrocephalae).

[Usage and Dosage] Use raw in general; wine-fry to clear heat in the upper *Jiao*, and stir-fry until charred to stanch bleeding; 条芩 Tiáo Qín is considered more potent in clearing large intestine fire, and 枯芩 Kū Qín is more effective in relieving lung fire. Use 5–12 g in decoction.

[Mnemonics] Huáng Qín (Radix Scutellariae, Scutellaria Root): drain fire, similar to Huáng Lián (Rhizoma Coptidis), and especially good at arresting bleeding and calming the fetus.

[Simple and Effective Formulas]

1. 黄芩汤 Huáng Qín Tāng — Scutellaria Decoction from *Treatise on Cold Damage* (伤寒论, Shāng Hán Lùn): Huáng Qín (Radix Scutellariae) 10 g, Sháo Yào (Radix Paeoniae) 12 g, Gān Cǎo (Radix et Rhizoma Glycyrrhizae) 3 g, and six Dà Zǎo (Fructus Jujubae); decoct in water for

oral administration to treat patient with fever, vexation, abdominal pain, diarrhea and dysentery with sticky stool containing pus and blood, or epistaxis. Also applicable for damp-heat dysentery and hemorrhagic diseases with blood heat syndrome.

2. 蒿芩清胆汤 Hāo Qín Qīng Dǎn Tāng — Sweet Wormwood and Scutellaria Gallbladder-Clearing Decoction from *Popular Guide to the 'Treatise on Cold Damage'* (通俗伤寒论, Tōng Sú Shāng Hán Lùn): Huáng Qín (Radix Scutellariae) 10 g, Qīng Hāo (Herba Artemisiae Annuae) 10 g, Bàn Xià (Rhizoma Pinelliae) 10 g, Zhǐ Qiào (Fructus Aurantii) 10 g, Fú Líng(Poria) 12 g, Chén Pí (Pericarpium Citri Reticulatae) 5 g, Zhú Rú (Caulis Bambusae in Taenia) 6 g, and Bì Yù Sǎn (Jasper Jade Powder)(decocted while wrapped) 10 g; decoct in water for oral administration to treat patient with alternating chills and fever, chest oppression, nausea, and red tongue with yellow greasy coating. Also applicable for febrile diseases, biliary tract infection and gastritis with above-mentioned manifestations.

[Precautions] Huáng Qín (Radix Scutellariae), bitter and cold in nature, tends to damage yang qi and thus should be used cautiously in patient with constitutional aversion to cold and pale tongue.

Daily practices

1. What are the similarities and differences between Huáng Lián (Rhizoma Coptidis) and Huáng Qín (Radix Scutellariae) in terms of actions and indications?
2. What are the similarities and differences among Huáng Lián (Rhizoma Coptidis), Huáng Qín (Radix Scutellariae), and Shí Gāo (Gypsum Fibrosum) in terms of nature, flavor, and actions?

黄柏 Huáng Bǎi *cortex phellodendri chinensis amur cork-tree bark*

The source is from the cortex of deciduous arbor *Phellodendron Chinense Schneid*, or *Amur Corktree Bark* getting rid of cork, family Rutaceae. Alternate names include 黄檗 Huáng Bò and 檗皮 Bò Pí. Bitter in flavor and cold in nature.

[Actions] Clear heat and dry dampness, and drain fire and resolve toxins. It is used to treat damp-heat diarrhea and dysentery, jaundice, abnormal vaginal discharge, heat strangury, leg qi (edema in the feet), atrophy and weakness in the lower extremities, bone steaming and exhaustion fever, night sweating, seminal emission, sores, ulcers, swelling, pain, eczema and itching. This substance contains berberin, obakunone, and obaculactone. Oral administration of its decoction has shown a significant antibacterial effect, and can protect platelet, decrease blood pressure, and reduce blood sugar.

[Quality] Coarse layer of bark coarse layer of bark scraped and removed, washed in water and moistened thoroughly, cut into slices or slivers, and dried under sunshine. The herb produced in Sichuan and Guizhou, thick and fresh yellow, is with good quality and considered as a genuine regional medicinal.

[Indications]

1. Damp-heat patterns: damp-heat induced jaundice is manifested as yellow body skin, fever, inhibited urination with yellow and scanty urine. Jaundice is divided into two types: yin jaundice is featured by gloomy and smoked yellow, aversion to cold, cold body, and pale tongue with white greasy coating; and yang jaundice is marked by fresh orange yellow, hot body, sweating, and red tongue with yellow greasy coating. Huáng Bǎi (Cortex Phellodendri Chinensis) is indicated for the latter. In the clinic, some patients present with yellow sweat instead of jaundice with accompanying inhibited urination, scantly yellow or even red brown urine, edema in the lower extremities, and yellow greasy tongue coating. Hot body refers to aversion to heat, profuse sweating, red, swollen and painful skin with hot sensation; and inhibited urination often occurs together with thirst and edema. Huáng Bǎi (Cortex Phellodendri Chinensis) is commonly used for impotence, seminal emission, strangury with turbid discharge, abnormal vaginal discharge, prolonged scanty uterine bleeding of variable intervals, atrophy, *bì*, stool containing blood, diarrhea and dysentery, hemorrhoids, fistula, scrotum eczema, and erysipelas of the shank due to damp-heat accumulation in the lower of the body.

2. Dysentery: Huáng Bǎi (Cortex Phellodendri Chinensis) is often combined with Huáng Lián (Rhizoma Coptidis), Qín Pí (Cortex Fraxini),

and Bái Tóu Wēng (Radix Pulsatillae) for tenesmus, stool with pus and blood, fever, vexation, agitation, difficult urination, and yellow urine due to damp-heat dysentery.

3. Heat-toxin sores and ulcers: Huáng Bǎi (Cortex Phellodendri Chinensis) is effective in clearing heat and resolving toxins and therefore widely used for sores, ulcers, abscesses, swelling, erysipelas, and furuncles due to heat-toxin. It can be applied alone externally or used together with Huáng Lián (Rhizoma Coptidis) and Zhī Zǐ (Fructus Gardeniae) for oral administration.

Huáng Lián (Rhizoma Coptidis), Huáng Qín (Radix Scutellariae) and Huáng Bǎi (Cortex Phellodendri Chinensis) have similar properties and are all bitter and cold in nature. Among them, Huáng Lián (Rhizoma Coptidis) is believed best at clearing the fire of heart and stomach to relieve vexation, Huáng Qín (Radix Scutellariae) is most effective in clearing lung fire, stanching bleeding and calming the fetus, and Huáng Bǎi (Cortex Phellodendri Chinensis) is most potent in clearing kidney fire and damp-heat of the lower *jiao*. Meanwhile, Huáng Qín (Radix Scutellariae) is considered most effective in clearing fire in the upper *jiao*, Huáng Lián (Rhizoma Coptidis) the middle *jiao*, and Huáng Bǎi (Cortex Phellodendri Chinensis) the lower *jiao*. This herb is often combined with Zhī Mǔ (Rhizoma Anemarrhenae) to treat kidney fire in the lower *jiao*.

[Usage and Dosage] The raw medicinal is potent for clearing heat and draining fire; stir-frying with wine to relieve fire and heat in the upper part of body, and salt-fry to deficiency fire of the kidney. Use 5–12 g in decoction.

[Mnemonics] Huáng Bǎi (Cortex Phellodendri Chinensis, Amur Cork-tree Bark): dry dampness, relieve swollen feet, and resolve yellow urine, strangury, vaginal discharge, sore, and toxin.

[Simple and Effective Formulas]

1. 二妙散 Èr Miào Sǎn — Two Mysterious Powder from *Teachings of Dan-xi* (丹溪心法, Dān Xī Xīn Fǎ): Huáng Bǎi (Cortex Phellodendri Chinensis)(stir-fried) and Cāng Zhú (Rhizoma Atractylodis)(soaked in rice-washed water, stir-fried) in equal dosage; prepare into fine powder

and take 3–5 g/time and two drops of ginger juice with boiled water for oral administration to treat patient with pain in the sinew and bone due to damp-heat migration, or inhibited yellow urination and weak, red, and swollen foot and knee caused by damp-heat pouring downward, or abnormal vaginal discharge resulting from damp-heat in the lower *jiao*, or eczema in the lower part of the body. Also applicable for different types of infectious diseases, arthritis, dermatosis, and gout.

2. 白头翁汤 Bái Tóu Wēng Tāng — Anemone Decoction from *Treatise on Cold Damage* (伤寒论, Shāng Hán Lùn): Huáng Bǎi (Cortex Phellodendri Chinensis) 10 g, Huáng Lián (Rhizoma Coptidis) 5 g, Bái Tóu Wēng (Radix Pulsatillae) 10 g, and Qín Pí (Cortex Fraxini) 12 g; decoct in water for oral administration to treat patient with heat dysentery, stool containing blood, and vexation with desire to drink. Also applicable for damp-heat dysentery and enteritis.

3. 滋肾丸 Zī Shèn Wán — Kidney Nourishing Pill from *Secrets from the Orchid Chamber* (兰室秘藏, Lán Shì Mì Cáng): Huáng Bǎi (Cortex Phellodendri Chinensis) 10 g, Zhī Mǔ (Rhizoma Anemarrhenae) 10 g, and Ròu Guì (Cortex Cinnamomi) 5 g; grind into fine powder, prepare into pill, and take 5 g/time for oral administration to treat patient with urinary retention, fever, sweating, and thirst with desire to drink. Also applicable for urological diseases and arthritis.

[Precautions] Owning to its bitter and cold nature, Huáng Bǎi (Cortex Phellodendri Chinensis) tends to damage yang qi of the spleen and stomach and should be used with cautions by patients with constitutional aversion to cold and pale tongue. Recent reports show that taking its fine powder with boiled water may cause medical-induced allergic rashes.

苦参 Kǔ Shēn *radix sophorae flavescentis light yellow sophora root*

The source is from the root of sub-shrub *Sophorae flavescentis* Ait., family Leguminosae. Bitter in flavor and cold in nature. It is so named for its extremely bitter flavor.

[Actions] Clear heat and dry dampness, dispel wind and kill parasites, and promote urination. It is applicable to such diseases as skin itching, urticaria, impetigo, and leprosy, as well as damp-heat pattern manifested as jaundice, diarrhea, dysentery, abnormal vaginal discharge, vaginal itching, and difficult urination with burning pain. This herb contains eulexine and sophocarpidine and has antiallergic, antitrichomonal, and diuretic effects. Its preparation has shown an inhibitory effect against a variety of experimental arrhythmia and dermatophyte.

[Quality] Impurity removed, residue stem removed, washed and dirt removed, soaked in water and moistened thoroughly, cut into slices, and dried under sunshine. Good quality is even root, without root tip, and has thin and tender skin; when cut into slices, the tidy slices in yellowish white indicates good quality.

[Indications]

1. Vaginal itching and abnormal vaginal discharge: manifestations include severe itching of pudendum accompanying with yellowish and turbid vaginal discharge, vexation, and difficult urination. This is usually seen in dermatosis, vaginitis, and diabetes. Kǔ Shēn (Radix Sophorae Flavescentis) is often combined with Huáng Bǎi (Cortex Phellodendri Chinensis), Dì Huáng (Radix Rehmanniae), Dì Fū Zǐ (Fructus Kochiae), and Bái Xiān Pí (Cortex Dictamni).
2. Vexation and palpitation: it refers to vexing heat in the heart or palpitations with accompanying reddish complexion, red tongue, and rapid or irregular pulse. Kǔ Shēn (Radix Sophorae Flavescentis) has recently been prepared into injection or tablet for ventricular premature beat.
3. Eczema and intractable tinea: Kǔ Shēn (Radix Sophorae Flavescentis) is often combined with Bái Xiān Pí (Cortex Dictamni), Shé Chuáng Zǐ (Fructus Cnidii), Huáng Bǎi (Cortex Phellodendri Chinensis), Míng Fán (Alumen), Chì Sháo (Radix Paeoniae Rubra), and Dì Huáng (Radix Rehmanniae) for eczema, itching, yellow effusion, and thickened skin.
4. Damp-heat edema: Kǔ Shēn (Radix Sophorae Flavescentis) can promote urination and is often used together with Chē Qián Zǐ (Semen Plantaginis), Zé Xiè (Rhizoma Alismatis), and Mù Tōng (Caulis Akebiae) for edema and difficult urination caused by damp-heat.

In recent years it has been successfully used for treating bacillary dysentery and virus hepatitis, and preventing and treating leukopenia due to different reasons.

[Usage and Dosage] Use raw in general, 3–10 g in decoction for oral administration, also prepared into injection to treat virus hepatitis.

[Mnemonics] Kǔ Shēn (Radix Sophorae Flavescentis, Light Yellow Sophora Root): stop itching, especially for stubborn tinea, promote urination to relieve edema, and relieve restlessness and palpitation.

[Simple and Effective Formulas]

1. 治痢散 Zhì Lì Sàn — Treating Dysentery Powder from *Medical Revelations* (医学心悟, Yī Xué Xīn Wù): Kǔ Shēn (Radix Sophorae Flavescentis) 10 g, Gé Gēn (Radix Puerariae Lobatae) 15 g, Chì Sháo (Radix Paeoniae Rubra) 12 g, Shān Zhā (Fructus Crataegi) 10 g, Chén Pí (Pericarpium Citri Reticulatae) 3 g, and Mài Yá (Fructus Hordei Germinatus) 12 g; decoct in water for oral administration to treat vexation, fever, diarrhea, and dysentery. Also applicable for dysentery, enteritis, cardiovascular and cerebrovascular diseases, and diabetes.
2. 止痒煎 Zhǐ Yǎng Jiān-Arrest Itching Decoction from *Empirical Formulas* (经验方, Jīng Yàn Fāng): Kǔ Shēn (Radix Sophorae Flavescentis) 10 g, Dān Shēn (Radix et Rhizoma Salviae Miltiorrhizae) 10 g, and Shé Chuáng Zǐ (Fructus Cnidii) 12 g; decoct in water for oral administration and meanwhile wash affected area with hot dregs to treat skin itching. Also applicable for various types of eczema and dermatitis.

[Precautions] Kǔ Shēn (Radix Sophorae Flavescentis), extremely bitter in flavor, tends to injure stomach qi or cause vomiting if applied appropriately. It should therefore not be taken on an empty stomach and should rub the tongue with Shēng Jiāng (Rhizoma Zingiberis Recens) prior to taking it. Use with caution in patients with constitutionally aversion to cold, body coldness, and pale tongue. Overdose is discouraged as it will lead to poisoning. Incompatible with Lí Lú (Radix et Rhizoma Veratri Nigri) according to "eighteen antagonisms".

Daily practices

1. What are the similarities and differences between Huáng Bǎi (Cortex Phellodendri Chinensis) and Kǔ Shēn (Radix Sophorae Flavescentis) in terms of actions and indications?
2. What are the similarities and differences among Huáng Lián (Rhizoma Coptidis), Huáng Qín (Radix Scutellariae), and Huáng Bǎi (Cortex Phellodendri Chinensis) in terms of actions and indications?

龙胆草 Lóng Dǎn Cǎo *radix et rhizoma gentianae chinese gentian*

The source is from the rhizome and root of herbaceous perennial *Gentian scabra* Bge, or its varieties, family Gentianaceae. Bitter in flavor and cold in nature.

[Actions] Clear heat-toxin, drain liver fire, and remove damp-heat. It is applicable to damp-heat jaundice, swollen pudendum, vaginal itching, abnormal vaginal discharge, eczema, red eyes, deafness, rib-side pain, bitter taste in the mouth, and infantile convulsion. This herb contains gentiamarin, gentianose, and erythricine. Its preparation has a pronounced *in vitro* inhibitory effect against bacteria and has an inhibitory effect on central nervous system. It also has shown liver cell-protecting, bile secretion-promoting, diuretic, antihypertensive, and antiallergic effects.

[Quality] Impurity removed, residue stem removed, washed clean and moistened thoroughly, cut into segments, and dried under sunshine. Good quality is thick and long, yellow, and with less stems.

[Indications]

1. Headache and red eyes: Lóng Dǎn Cǎo (Radix et Rhizoma Gentianae) is often combined with Huáng Lián (Rhizoma Coptidis), Huáng Qín (Radix Scutellariae), Zhī Zǐ (Fructus Gardeniae), and Gān Cǎo (Radix et Rhizoma Glycyrrhizae) for eyelid erosion, eye with nebula, headache, red eyes, or profuse eye discharge caused by excess fire in the liver and gallbladder .
2. Scrotum swelling and pain: Lóng Dǎn Cǎo (Radix et Rhizoma Gentianae) is frequently prescribed together with Chái Hú (Radix

Bupleuri), Shān Zhī Zǐ (Fructus Gardeniae), Huáng Qín (Radix Scutellariae), and Huáng Bǎi (Cortex Phellodendri Chinensis) for damp-heat pouring downward pattern manifested as localized redness, swelling, itching, or erosion, chest oppression, rib-side pain, and yellow or turbid urine.

3. Heat-toxin transforming into fire: owning to its potent effect on clearing heat and resolving toxins, Lóng Dǎn Cǎo (Radix et Rhizoma Gentianae) is effective in relieving exuberant heat and toxin in febrile diseases. It is combined with Gōu Téng (Ramulus Uncariae Cum Uncis), Shēng Dì (Radix Rehmanniae), and Niú Huáng (Calculus Bovis) to treat convulsion caused by excessive liver heat with internal stirring of liver wind through clearing heat and extinguishing wind; and with Dà Qīng Yè (Folium Isatidis), Bǎn Lán Gēn (Radix Isatidis), and Zhú Rú (Caulis Bambusae in Taenia) for severe headache or with vomiting due to internal exuberance of fire heat.

It is also commonly used for damp-heat induced jaundice and has been recently used in the treatment of cholecystitis.

[Usage and Dosage] Use raw in general, ginger juice-soaking or wine-frying to reduce its bitter-cold nature and potential damage on stomach qi. Use 3–10 g in decoction.

[Mnemonics] Lóng Dǎn Cǎo (Radix et Rhizoma Gentianae, Chinese Gentian): drain fire, relieve red eyes and turbid urine, and use a small amount as it is extremely bitter and cold.

[Simple and Effective Formulas]

1. 龙胆泻肝汤 Lóng Dǎn Xiè Gān Tāng — Gentian Liver Draining Decoction from *Formulas from the Imperial Pharmacy* (局方, Jú Fāng): Lóng Dǎn Cǎo (Radix et Rhizoma Gentianae) 5 g, Huáng Qín (Radix Scutellariae) 10 g, Zhī Zǐ (Fructus Gardeniae) 6 g, Dāng Guī (Radix Angelicae Sinensis) 10 g, Dì Huáng (Radix Rehmanniae) 12 g, Zé Xiè (Rhizoma Alismatis) 10 g, Mù Tōng (Caulis Akebiae) 5 g, Chái Hú (Radix Bupleuri) 6 g, Chē Qián Zǐ (Semen Plantaginis) 10 g, and Gān Cǎo (Radix et Rhizoma Glycyrrhizae) 3 g; decoct in water for oral

administration to treat patients with rib-side pain, bitter taste in the mouth, deafness, swollen ear, strangury, turbid urine, scrotum swelling and pain, headache, vexation, agitation, and jaundice. Also applicable for urological and reproductive disorders, liver and gall bladder diseases, and psychoneuroses with the above manifestations.

2. 龙归散 Lóng Guī Săn — Gentian and Chinese Angelica Powder from *Fei Hong Collection* (飞鸿集, Fēi Hóng Jí): Lóng Dăn Căo (Radix et Rhizoma Gentianae) and Dāng Guī (Radix Angelicae Sinensis) in equal dosage; grind into powder and take 6 g/time for oral administration with warm water to treat pus in the eyes.

[Precautions] Large amount and long-term use are not recommend as Lóng Dăn Căo (Radix et Rhizoma Gentianae) is extremely bitter. It has been used as gastrotonica, however recent reports suggest that ingesting large-dose may cause such side effects as digestive hypofunction, headache, flushing in the face, and vertigo. It should be used with caution in patients with constitutional aversion to cold, cold body, and pale tongue.

夏枯草 Xià Kū *Căo spica prunellae common self-heal fruit-spike*

The source is from the flower and cluster of herbaceous perennial *Prunella vulgaris* L., family Labiatae. Alternate names include 夏枯花 Xià Kū Huā and 棒槌草 Bàng Chuí Căo. Bitter and pungent in flavor and cold in nature.

[Actions] Clear liver fire, relieve stagnation, and dissipate masses. It is applicable to red, swollen, and painful eyes, eyeball pain at night, headache, vertigo, dizziness, scrofula, goiter, tumor, and swollen and painful acute mastitis. From the perspective of experiments, this herb contains volatile oil, ursolic acid, and anthocyanin. Animal experiments reveal it has antihypertensive and diuretic effect. Its preparation has shown an *in vitro* inhibitory effect on a variety of pathogenic bacteria.

[Quality] Good quality is long, short petiole, and brownish red; the herb produced in Nanjing is of the best quality. It is reported that the stem, leaf and whole plant of this herb are superior to the cluster in lowering blood pressure, therefore using the whole plant is recommended for a better effect.

[Indications]

1. Fire-heat in the liver channel: Xià Kū Cǎo (Spica Prunellae) is combined with medicinals that calm the liver and clear heat such as Jú Huā (Flos Chrysanthemi), Mǔ Lì (Concha Ostreae), Shí Jué Míng (Concha Haliotidis), and Bái Sháo (Radix Paeoniae Alba) for headache, dizziness, tinnitus, and blurred vision due to either internal exuberance of liver fire or ascendant hyperactivity of liver yang; and with those that clear heat and improve vision such as Gǔ Jīng Cǎo (Flos Eriocauli), Jú Huā (Flos Chrysanthemi), and Qīng Xiāng Zǐ (Semen Celosiae) for red eyes, photophobia, frequent tearing, and eyeball pain at night caused by fire-heat of the liver channel attacking the upper part of the body.

2. Binding constraint of phlegm fire: binding constraint of phlegm-fire obstruction in the channels and collaterals may cause different kinds of masses, such as scrofula and goiter. Xià Kū Cǎo (Spica Prunellae) is effective in clearing liver fire and dissipating masses, either alone or in combination with Mǔ Lì (Concha Ostreae), Zhè Bèi Mǔ (Bulbus Fritillariae Thunbergii), Xuán Shēn (Radix Scrophulariae), and Kūn Bù (Thallus Laminariae). It is also potent in dissipating masses and therefore combined with Pú Gōng Yīng (Herba Taraxaci) and Qīng Pí (Pericarpium Citri Reticulatae Viride) in the treatment of acute mastitis.

[Usage and Dosage] Use raw in general, 15–30 g in decoction.

[Mnemonics] Xià Kū Cǎo (Spica Prunellae, Common Self-heal Fruit-spike): cold; good at clearing the liver and capable of curing eye problems and dispersing stagnation and accumulation.

[Simple and Effective Formulas]

1. 夏枯草汤 Xià Kū Cǎo Tāng — Common Self-heal Fruit-spike Decoction from *Numerous Miraculous Prescriptions for Health Cultivation* (摄生众妙方, Shè Shēng Zhòng Miào Fāng): Xià Kū Cǎo (Spica Prunellae) 180 g; decoct in water for oral administration to treat

scrofula (no matter ruptured or not, with fistula or not) or prepare into thick soft extracts for oral administration and external application in case of severe deficiency. Also applicable for different types of lymphatic tuberculosis.

2. 补肝散 Bǔ Gān Sàn-Tonifying Liver Powder from *Simple and Essential Prescriptions for Benifiting People* (简要济众方, Jiǎn Yào Jì Zhòng Fāng): Xià Kū Cǎo (Spica Prunellae) 15 g and Xiāng Fù (Rhizoma Cyperi) 12 g; make into powder and take 3 g/time when necessary for liver deficiency induced eyeball pain, uncontrollable cold tears, and photophobia.

[Precautions] Xià Kū Cǎo (Spica Prunellae), bitter and cold in nature, tends to injure the stomach qi and should be used with caution in patients with spleen deficiency. It should be combined with stomachics when long-term use is prescribed.

玄参 Xuán Shēn *radix scrophulariae figwort root*

The source is from the root of herbaceous perennial *Scrophularia ning-poensis* Hemsl, family Scrophulariaceae. Alternate names include 元参 Yuán Shēn and 黑参 Hēi Cān. Bitter, sweet and salty in flavor and cold in nature.

[Actions] Clear heat and enrich yin, drain fire and resolve toxin, and cool blood. It is applicable for vexation with thirst with crimson tongue due to yin consumption in febrile disease, macules due to warm-toxin, constipation caused by fluid consumption, steaming bone fever, tidal fever, red eyes, sore throat, scrofula, carbuncles, swellings, sores, and toxins. This herb contains botanical sterol, scrophularin, alkaloid, asparagine, volatile oil, fatty acid, and vitamin A substances. It has a strong inhibitory effect against pseudomonas aeruginosa and its lixivium and liquid extracts have shown antihypertensive, hypoglycemic, vasodilator, and cardiotonic effects.

[Quality] Impurities removed, the residue of rhizome from root removed, washed clean and moistened thoroughly, cut into slices, and dried in the air; or washed clean and soaked slightly, steamed thoroughly in steamer tub, medium-dried in the air, softened in a sealed container until both the inner and outer side turn into black, and cut into slices. Good quality is moist, solid, heavy, big, and moist with thin skin and bright black color.

[Indications]

1. Enlarged lymph nodes (scrofula): Xuán Shēn (Radix Scrophulariae) is combined with Shēng Dì (Radix Rehmanniae) for enlargement of lymph nodes with accompanying hot sensation all over the body, vexation and agitation, bleeding, and macules caused by heat-toxin accumulation; and with Mǔ Lì (Concha Ostreae) and Lián Qiào (Fructus Forsythiae) for enlargement of lymph nodes with accompanying night sweating, dry and painful throat, dry and hard stool, and red tongue.

2. Throat swelling and pain: Xuán Shēn (Radix Scrophulariae) is prescribed together with Niú Bàng Zǐ (Fructus Arctii), Shè Gān (Rhizoma Belamcandae), Bò He (Herba Menthae), and Bái Jiāng Cán (Bombyx Batryticatus) for swollen and painful throat resulting from externally-contracted wind-heat, or exuberant heat in the lung channel; and with Mài Dōng (Radix Ophiopogonis), Shēng Dì (Radix Rehmanniae), Jié Gěng (Radix Platycodonis), and Gān Cǎo (Radix et Rhizoma Glycyrrhizae) for dry throat and nonproductive cough without sputum attributed to yin-deficiency pharyngitis.

3. Heat-toxin exuberance patterns: owning to its ability to clear heat, resolve toxins, and dissipate masses, Xuán Shēn (Radix Scrophulariae) is effective for different patterns of heat-toxin accumulation. It is combined with Jīn Yín Huā (Flos Lonicerae Japonicae) and Lián Qiào (Fructus Forsythiae) for carbuncles, swelling, sores and ulcers; with Jīn Yín Huā (Flos Lonicerae Japonicae), Dāng Guī (Radix Angelicae Sinensis), Shí Hú (Caulis Dendrobii), and Gān Cǎo (Radix et Rhizoma Glycyrrhizae) for gangrene of finger or toe (thromboangiitis obliterans); and with Shēng Dì (Radix Rehmanniae), Shuǐ Niú Jiǎo (Cornu Bubali), and Dà Qīng Yè (Folium Isatidis) for macules, high fever and crimson tongue caused by exuberant heat-toxin deeply entering into *ying*-blood in febrile disease.

4. Constipation: Xuán Shēn (Radix Scrophulariae), moistening in nature, is applicable for constipation due to insufficiency of intestinal fluids

and often used together with Shēng Dì (Radix Rehmanniae) and Mài Dōng (Radix Ophiopogonis).

[Usage and Dosage] Use steamed slices in general, use raw in some cases, 10–20 g in decoction, and up to 15–30 g for treating constipation due to yin deficiency.

[Mnemonics] Xuán Shēn (Radix Scrophulariae, Figwort Root): bitter and salty; relieve toxin, dissipate accumulation, and relieve scrofula and throat pain.

[Simple and Effective Formulas]

1. 玄麦甘桔汤 Xuán Mài Gān Jié Tāng — Figwort Root, Dwarf Lilyturf Tuber, Licorice Root, and Platycodon Root Decoction from *Empirical Formulas* (经验方, Jīng Yàn Fāng): Xuán Shēn (Radix Scrophulariae) 12 g, Mài Dōng (Radix Ophiopogonis) 10 g, Jié Gěng (Radix Platycodonis) 6 g, and Gān Cǎo (Radix et Rhizoma Glycyrrhizae) 3 g; decoct in water for oral administration to treat throat swelling and pain. Also applicable for chronic pharyngitis and diphtheria.

2. 四妙勇安汤 Sì Miào Yǒng Ān Tāng — Four Wonderfully Effective Heroes Decoction from *New Compilation of Proven Formulas* (验方新编, Yàn Fāng Xīn Biān): Xuán Shēn (Radix Scrophulariae) 30 g, Dāng Guī (Radix Angelicae Sinensis) 20 g, Jīn Yín Huā (Flos Lonicerae Japonicae) 30 g, and Gān Cǎo (Radix et Rhizoma Glycyrrhizae) 10 g; decoct in water for oral administration to treat thromboangitis obliterans.

3. 消瘰丸 Xiāo Luǒ Wán — Dissipating Nodules Pill from *Medical Revelations* (医学心悟, Yī Xué Xīn Wù): Xuán Shēn (Radix Scrophulariae) 20 g, Mǔ Lì (Concha Ostreae) 20 g, and Bèi Mǔ (Bulbus Fritillaria) 10 g; prepare into pill and take 6 g/time for oral administration, twice a day to treat scrofula in early stage.

[Precautions] Xuán Shēn (Radix Scrophulariae), potent in clearing heat and moistening the intestine, should be used with caution in patients with aversion to cold, loose stool, and abdominal distention.

Daily practices

1. What are the similarities and differences among Lóng Dǎn Cǎo (Radix et Rhizoma Gentianae), Xià Kū Cǎo (Spica Prunellae), and Xuán Shēn (Radix Scrophulariae) in terms of actions and indications?
2. Summarize the nature, flavor, actions and indications of heat-clearing and fire-draining medicinals?

II. Medicinals that Clear Heat and Resolve Toxins

金银花 **Jīn Yín Huā** *flos lonicerae japonicae honeysuckle flower*

[Addendum:忍冬藤 Rěn Dōng Téng Caulis Lonicerae Japonicae Honeysuckle Stem]

The source is from the flower bud of semi-evergreen voluble shrub *Lonicera japonica*, *Lonicera hypoglauca Miq*, and other congeneric species, family Caprifoliaceae. Alternate names include 忍冬花 Rěn Dōng Huā, 双花 Shuāng Huā, 二花 Èr Huā, and 银花 Yín Huā. Sweet in flavor and cold in nature.

[Actions] Clear heat and resolve toxin, and cool and dispel wind-heat. It is applicable to treat carbuncles, swellings, boils, furuncles, pharyngitis, erysipelas, toxin dysentery, and fever in warm disease. This herb contains chlorogenic acid, isochlorogenic acid, cyclohexanhexol, luteolin, lonicerin, and tannin. Its thick decoction has shown an antibacterial effect against typhoid bacillus, cholera vibrio, and hemolytic streptococcus, and inhibitory effect against shigella dysenteriae, pneumonia, diplococcus, corynebacterium diphtheriae, and human type tubercle bacillus. This medicinal has significant anti-inflammatory and immunity-regulatory effects. Experiments reveal that it can interact with the cholesterol to reduce intestinal cholesterol absorption.

[Quality] Dirt excluded, impurities removed, and dried under shade. Good quality has many big, soft, pale yellow, unopened or just-opened flowers and is aromatic without branches and leaves. The herb produced in Henan is of good quality.

[Indications]

1. Sores, carbuncles, swelling and toxins: Jīn Yín Huā (Flos Lonicerae Japonicae), potent in clearing heat and resolving toxin, is a commonly used medicinal in TCM external medicines and applicable for all sores and toxins of yang patterns marked by sudden onset with localized redness, swelling, hot sensation and pain. It is often combined with Zǐ Huā Dì Dīng (Herba Violae), Lián Qiào (Fructus Forsythiae), Mǔ Dān Pí (Cortex Moutan), and Chì Sháo (Radix Paeoniae Rubra).
2. Throat swelling and pain: it is usually seen in acute infection of upper respiratory tract, or acute pharyngitis, and tonsillitis. Jīn Yín Huā (Flos Lonicerae Japonicae) is often combined with Lián Qiào (Fructus Forsythiae), Bò He (Herba Menthae), Jié Gěng (Radix Platycodonis), and Gān Cǎo (Radix et Rhizoma Glycyrrhizae) for swollen and painful throat with accompanying enlargement of lymph node in neck and fever.
3. Heat dysentery with stool containing blood: heat dysentery is caused by damp-heat accumulation in the intestines and featured by sudden onset with stool containing mucous and blood and accompanying fever and red tongue with yellow greasy coating. Jīn Yín Huā (Flos Lonicerae Japonicae) is prescribed together with Huáng Lián (Rhizoma Coptidis), Huáng Qín (Radix Scutellariae), and Bái Sháo (Radix Paeoniae Alba).
4. Wind-heat type of common cold and warm febrile disease: owning to its properties of clearing heat, resolving toxins, and scattering wind-heat, Jīn Yín Huā (Flos Lonicerae Japonicae) is combined with Lián Qiào (Fructus Forsythiae), Bò He (Herba Menthae), and Niú Bàng Zǐ (Fructus Arctii) for pathogens entering in the lung-*wei* level in the initial stage of warm disease. It is also applicable when pathogenic heat transmits inwards to the interior in warm febrile disease. It, for instance, is used together with Shí Gāo (Gypsum Fibrosum) and Zhī Mǔ (Rhizoma Anemarrhenae) for pathogenic heat in *qi* level, and with Shēng Dì (Radix Rehmanniae) and Mǔ Dān Pí (Cortex Moutan) for pathogenic heat in blood level. Also used in the summerheat-heat pattern due to its fragrant flavor and effects of clearing heat and resolving summerheat.

[Usage and Dosage] Use raw in general, dry-fry until charred to treat bloody dysentery. Use 3–12 g in decoction, and up to 30–60 g to clear heat and relieve toxin.

[Mnemonics] Jīn Yín Huā (Flos Lonicerae Japonicae, Honeysuckle Flower): sweet and cold; capable of dispersing wind-heat, clearing heat, relieving toxins, and curing sores and dysentery.

[Simple and Effective Formulas]

1. 银翘散 Yín Qiào Sǎn — Lonicera and Forsythia Powder from *Systematic Differentiation of Warm Diseases* (温病条辨, Wēn Bìng Tiáo Biàn): Jīn Yín Huā (Flos Lonicerae Japonicae) 15 g, Lián Qiào (Fructus Forsythiae) 12 g, Jié Gěng (Radix Platycodonis) 5 g, Gān Cǎo (Radix et Rhizoma Glycyrrhizae) 3 g, Jīng Jiè (Herba Schizonepetae) 10 g, Niú Bàng Zǐ (Fructus Arctii) 10 g, Bò He (Herba Menthae) 5 g, Zhú Yè (Folium Phyllostachydis Henonis) 10 g, and Lú Gēn (Rhizoma Phragmitis) 12 g; decoct in water for oral administration to treat externally-contracted wind-heat pattern with fever, sweating, slight aversion to wind, throat pain, and rapid pulse. Also applicable for acute infection of the upper respiratory tract, common cold, pharyngitis, and pneumonia.
2. 回疮金银花散 — Huí Chuāng Jīn Yín Huā Sǎn — Honeysuckle Flower Powder for Curing Sores from *Essentials for Health* (Huó Fǎ Jī Yào, 活法机要): Jīn Yín Huā (Flos Lonicerae Japonicae) 60 g, Huáng Qí (Radix Astragali) 30 g, and Gān Cǎo (Radix et Rhizoma Glycyrrhizae) 10 g; decoct in water for oral administration to treat sores and ulcers in purplish black color and with severe pain.
3. 治乳痈方 Zhì Rě Yōng Fāng — Healing Acute Mastitis Formula from *Empirical Formulas* (经验方, Jīng Yàn Fāng): Jīn Yín Huā (Flos Lonicerae Japonicae) 30 g, Lián Qiào (Fructus Forsythiae) 20 g, Pú Gōng Yīng (Herba Taraxaci) 20 g, Qīng Pí (Pericarpium Citri Reticulatae Viride) 5 g, Chén Pí (Pericarpium Citri Reticulatae) 10 g, and Gān Cǎo (Radix et Rhizoma Glycyrrhizae) 3 g; decoct in water for oral administration to treat acute mastitis.

[Precautions] The infusion of Jīn Yín Huā (Flos Lonicerae Japonicae) is superior to its decoction in terms of antibacterial effect, and therefore it should not be decocted for a long time. In experiment, Jīn Yín Huā (Flos Lonicerae Japonicae) and Lián Qiào (Fructus Forsythiae) are complementary to each other in terms of antibacterial action.

[Addendum] 忍冬藤 Rĕn Dōng Téng *caulis lonicerae japonicae honeysuckle stem*

The source is from the stem and leaf of *Lonicera japonica*, also called 银花藤 Yín Huā Téng. Rĕn Dōng Téng (Caulis Lonicerae Japonicae) and Jīn Yín Huā (Flos Lonicerae Japonicae) have similar flavors and actions. The former is often used to resolve heat-toxin abscesses, swelling, sores, and ulcers, and considered more effective than Jīn Yín Huā (Flos Lonicerae Japonicae) decoction in antibacteria. Rĕn Dōng Téng (Caulis Lonicerae Japonicae) also can clear damp-heat in the channels and collaterals and thus is applicable to wind-heat-damp *bì* syndrome with red, swelling and painful joints. Use 10–20 g in general.

连翘 Lián Qiào *fructus forsythiae weeping forsythia capsule*

The source is from the fruit of deciduous undershrub *Forsythiae suspense* (Thunb.) Vahl, family Oleaceae. Alternate names include 连轺 Lián Yáo. Bitter in flavor and slightly cold in nature.

[Actions] Clear heat and resolve toxins, clear the heart, and alleviate abscesses and dissipate masses. It is applicable for externally-contracted wind-heat or warm disease in early stage manifested as fever, headache, and thirst, or sores, ulcers, carbuncles, and swellings due to heat-toxin accumulation, or scrofula and tuberculosis. This herb contains forsythol, oleanolic acid, forsythoside, vitamin P, and volatile oil. It has shown a significantly inhibitory effect against staphylococcus aureus, shigella dysenteriae, hemolytic streptococcus, pneumonia, coccus, and typhoid bacillus. It can inhibit virus and tubercle bacillus. Its ingredient oleanolic acid has cardiotonic and diuretic effect, and vitamin P can increase capillary resistance. Experiments also show this substance has antipyretic, antemetic, diuretic, and antihypertensive effects.

[Quality] Impurities removed, kneaded off, and branches and peduncles excluded. "Green" 青翹 Qīng Qiào is collected when the fruit has just begun to ripen, good quality is dry, green-brown, and complete without branches or stems. "Old" 老翹 Lǎo Qiào is collected when the fruit already ripened, the fruit should be dry, yellow with a pig petal and thick shell and without branches or stems.

[Indications]

1. Scrofula: Lián Qiào (Fructus Forsythiae) is prescribed together with Xià Kū Cǎo (Spica Prunellae), Mǔ Lì (Concha Ostreae), Bèi Mǔ (Bulbus Fritillaria), Xuán Shēn (Radix Scrophulariae), Chái Hú (Radix Bupleuri), Guǐ Jiàn Yǔ (Ramulus Euonymi), and Gān Cǎo (Radix et Rhizoma Glycyrrhizae) for enlargement of lymph nodes and especially scrofula with accompanying body heat and sweating during sleep.
2. Carbuncles, swelling, sores and toxins: owning to its effect of clearing heat and resolving toxins, Lián Qiào (Fructus Forsythiae) is combined with Chì Sháo (Radix Paeoniae Rubra), Mǔ Dān Pí (Cortex Moutan), and Jīn Yín Huā (Flos Lonicerae Japonicae) for carbuncles, swelling, sores and toxins with localized redness, swelling, hot sensation, pain and before pus formation; and with Pú Gōng Yīng (Herba Taraxaci) and Chuān Bèi Mǔ (Bulbus Fritillariae Cirrhosae) for mastitis and breast nodules. It can also be used topically in the form of fine powder in a combination with other medicinals that clear heat and resolve toxins.
3. Wind-heat pattern: Lián Qiào (Fructus Forsythiae) is combined with Jīn Yín Huā (Flos Lonicerae Japonicae), Zhī Zǐ (Fructus Gardeniae), and Bò He (Herba Menthae) for wind-warm at the initial stage with fever, sweating, throat pain, dizziness, vexation, and cough.
4. Heart fire patterns: Lián Qiào (Fructus Forsythiae) is potent in clearing heart fire and frequently combined with other medicinals that clear the heart such as Mài Dōng (Radix Ophiopogonis), Zhú Yè Xīn (Folium Pleioblasti), and Lián Xīn (Plumula Nelumbinis) for vexation, agitation, unconsciousness, and delirious speech associated with inward

invasion of epidemic warm diseases heat into pericardium; with Shēng Dì (Radix Rehmanniae), Zhú Yè (Folium Phyllostachydis Henonis), Mù Tōng (Caulis Akebiae), and Gān Cǎo (Radix et Rhizoma Glycyrrhizae) for ulcer in the mouth and tongue caused by hyperactivity of heart fire. It is also effective in treating heat strangury and difficult and painful urination due to heart heat transmitting to the small intestine.

[Usage and Dosage] Use raw in general, and its kernel is better at relieving heart fire. Use 10–20 g in decoction.

[Mnemonics] Lián Qiào (Fructus Forsythiae, Weeping Forsythia Capsule): bitter and cold; clear heat, resolve toxins, especially good at clearing the heart, and dissipate sore and accumulation.

[Simple and Effective Formulas]

1. 连翘饮 Lián Qiào Yǐn — Forsythia Beverage from *Book to Safeguard Life Arranged by Categorized Patterns* (类证活人书, Lèi Zhèng Huó Rén Shū): Lián Qiào (Fructus Forsythiae) 12 g, Fáng Fēng (Radix Saposhnikoviae) 10 g, Gān Cǎo (Radix et Rhizoma Glycyrrhizae) 3 g, and Zhī Zǐ (Fructus Gardeniae) 10 g; decoct in water for oral administration to treat pediatric heat patterns with symptoms and signs of fever, night sweating, sores, nosebleed, sore throat, vexation, and agitation.
2. 连翘汤 Lián Qiào Tāng — Forsythia Decoction from Empirical Formulas (经验方, Jīng Yàn Fāng): Lián Qiào (Fructus Forsythiae) 12 g, Xuán Shēn (Radix Scrophulariae) 12 g, Huáng Qín (Radix Scutellariae) 10 g, Chái Hú (Radix Bupleuri) 10 g, and Gān Cǎo (Radix et Rhizoma Glycyrrhizae) 3 g; decoct in water for oral administration to treat enlargement of lymph node in the neck and armpit.

[Precautions] Lián Qiào (Fructus Forsythiae), bitter and cold in nature, should be used with caution in cases of pale tongue, cold body, and loose stool due to deficiency-cold of the spleen and stomach. It is contraindicated in cases of deficiency pattern when carbuncle is ruptured with clean, thin, and light-colored pus.

Daily practices

1. What are the similarities and differences between Jīn Yín Huā (Flos Lonicerae Japonicae) and Lián Qiào (Fructus Forsythiae) in terms of actions and indications?

2. What are the similarities and differences between such heat-clearing and toxin-relieving medicinals as Jīn Yín Huā (Flos Lonicerae Japonicae) and Lián Qiào (Fructus Forsythiae) and these heat-clearing and fire-draining medicinals in terms of indications ?

Fourth Week

1

蒲公英 **Pú Gōng Yīng** *herba taraxaci dandelion*

The source is from the herb of herbaceous perennia *Taraxacum mongolicum* Hand.-Mazz. and other congeneric species, family Compositae. Alternate names include 婆婆丁 Pó Po Dīng and 黄花地丁 Huáng Huā Dì Dīng. Cold and bitter in flavor, and cold in nature.

[Actions] Clear heat and resolve toxins, clear damp-heat, alleviate swelling and dissipate masses, and soothe the liver. It is applicable for boil, carbuncle, swelling, toxin, acute mastitis, scrofula, red eyes, sore throat, lung abscess, intestinal abscess, jaundice, and heat strangury. This herb contains dandelion sterol, cholin, synanthrin, and pectin. Its water extract has shown an inhibitory effect against such bacterials as staphylococcus aureus and hemolytic streptococcus, and its ethanol extractive has a choleretic effect.

[Quality] Impurity removed, washed clean and dirt excluded, cut into segments, and sun-dried. Good quality is dry stem with many green leaves and complete root.

[Indications]

1. Carbuncles, swellings, sores and ulcers: Pú Gōng Yīng (Herba Taraxaci) is considered more effective in clearing heat and resolving toxins and capable of dissipating masses. It can be used for red, swollen, and painful abscesses and sores with hot sensation, either as a decoction for oral administration or by pounding the fresh one for external application. It is often used together with Jīn Yín Huā

(Flos Lonicerae Japonicae) and Lián Qiào (Fructus Forsythiae) for mastitis; and with Yú Xīng Cǎo (Herba Houttuyniae), Yì Yǐ Rén (Semen Coicis), and Táo Rén (Semen Persicae) for internal abscesses such as lung and intestinal abscesses.

2. Damp-heat jaundice: Pú Gōng Yīng (Herba Taraxaci) is often combined with Chái Hú (Radix Bupleuri), Yīn Chén (Herba Artemisiae Scopariae), Huáng Qín (Radix Scutellariae), and Zhī Zǐ (Fructus Gardeniae) for jaundice caused by virus hepatitis and biliary tract infection with accompanying fever and rib-side pain. It is also used to treat chronic hepatitis via soothing the liver and resolving toxins.

3. Liver-stomach qi pain: Pú Gōng Yīng (Herba Taraxaci) is prescribed together with Chái Hú (Radix Bupleuri), Bái Sháo (Radix Paeoniae Alba), Yán Hú Suǒ (Rhizoma Corydalis), and Chén Pí (Pericarpium Citri Reticulatae) for constraint liver qi invading the stomach with manifestations of gastric pain and distention; with Chái Hú (Radix Bupleuri), Qīng Pí (Pericarpium Citri Reticulatae Viride), Zhǐ Qiào (Fructus Aurantii), Jú Hé (Semen Citri Reticulatae), and Zào Jiǎo Cì (Spina Gleditsiae) for premenstrual breast distention with masses resulting from liver constraint and qi stagnation.

[Usage and Dosage] Use raw in general, 15–30 g in decoction, and double the dosage if use fresh.

[Mnemonics] Pú Gōng Yīng (Herba Taraxaci, Dandelion): cold; dissipate heat-toxin, clear and sooth the liver, and remove jaundice.

[Simple and Effective Formulas]
五味消毒饮 Wǔ Wèi Xiāo Dú Yǐn Five Ingredients Toxin-Removing Beverage from *Golden Mirror of the Medical Tradition* (医宗金鉴 Yī Zōng Jīn Jiàn,): Pú Gōng Yīng (Herba Taraxaci) 50 g, De Dīng Cǎo (Herba Corydalis Bungeanae) 30 g, Yě Jú Huā (Flos Chrysanthemi Indici) 20 g, Jīn Yín Huā (Flos Lonicerae Japonicae) 20 g, and Zǐ Bèi Tiān Kuí (Herba Semiaquilegiae) 20 g; decoct in water for oral administration to treat boils, carbuncles, swellings, and toxins.

[Precautions] Pú Gōng Yīng (Herba Taraxaci) is mild in nature and rarely has rare side effect. Gastric hot sensation caused by taking Pú Gōng Yīng (Herba Taraxaci) tablet has been reported. Its injection should be used with caution as it may lead to shivering, pale complexion and psychiatric symptoms.

大青叶 Dà Qīng Yè *folium isatidis woad root*

[Addendum] 板蓝根 Bǎn Lán Gēn Radix Isatidis Isatis Root

青黛 Qīng Dài *indigo naturalis natural indigo*

The source is from the leaf of herbaceous biennial *Isatis tinctoria* L., family Cruciferae, or deciduous shrub *Geum aleppicum*, family Verbenaceae, or herbaceous annual *Polygonum tinctorium* Lour, family Polygonaceae, or shrubby herbaceous perennial *Baphicacanthus cusia* Bremek, family Acanthaceae. Alternate names include 大青 Dà Qīng. Bitter and salty in flavor and cold in nature.

[Actions] Clear heat and resolve toxins, and cool the blood and relieve macules. It is applicable for inward invasion of epidemic warm diseases heat into *ying*-blood manifested as high fever, macules and papules, and crimson or purplish crimson tongue, and such diseases as jaundice, heat dysentery, mumps, erysipelas, and carbuncle. Experiments reveal that *Polygonum tinctorium* Lour has antipyretic, anti-inflammatory, capillary permeability-reducing, and leukocyte phagocytosis-increasing effects. *Geum aleppicum* has shown certain inhibitory effects against staphylococcus aureus, streptococcus, and meningococcus. Indican contained by different types of Dà Qīng Yè (Folium Isatidis) has shown certain antiviral activity, antipyretic, anti-inflammatory, and immunity-regulatory effects.

[Quality] Collected and dried under sunshine. Good quality is complete and grayish-green leaves without impurities.

[Indications]

1. Warm febrile diseases: Dà Qīng Yè (Folium Isatidis) is potent in clearing heat and resolving toxins and therefore widely used for externally-contracted warm febrile diseases with heat-toxin symptoms and signs. For instance, it is often combined with acrid-cool exterior-releasing medicinals such as Jīn Yín Huā (Flos Lonicerae Japonicae), Lián Qiào

(Fructus Forsythiae), and Niú Bàng Zǐ (Fructus Arctii) for warm disease in the initial stage; and with heat-clearing and blood-cooling medicinals such as Shuǐ Niú Jiǎo (Cornu Bubali), Shēng Dì (Radix Rehmanniae), and Mǔ Dān Pí (Cortex Moutan) for pathogenic heat entering *ying*-blood.

2. Heat-toxin swellings and sores: Dà Qīng Yè (Folium Isatidis) is suitable for heat-toxin swelling and sores that affect any part of the body, such as erysipelas, mumps, aphtha, and painful and swelling throat. It can be used alone or in a combination with other medicinals that clear heat and resolve toxin, or for topical application when pounded.

3. Damp-heat jaundice and dysentery: Dà Qīng Yè (Folium Isatidis) is also commonly used for damp-heat diseases with vigorous heat-toxin, such as damp-heat induced jaundice (including virus hepatitis, cholecystitis, and acute cholangitis) and damp-heat induced dysentery with stool containing pus and blood.

From the perspective of modern biomedicine, both Dà Qīng Yè (Folium Isatidis) and Bǎn Lán Gēn (Radix Isatidis) are effective in treating virus infections, epidemic encephalitis B, influenza, leptospirosis, chronic bronchitis, bacillary dysentery, and virus hepatitis. The preparation of the former is especially potent for virus infections such as flat warts.

[Usage and Dosage] Use raw in general, usually prepared into decoction, 10–15 g in decoction, up to 30–60 g when used alone or fresh. It has been recently prepared into granule, tablet and injection for the convenience of application.

[Mnemonics] Dà Qīng Yè (Folium Isatidis, Woad Root) and Bǎn Lán Gēn (Radix Isatidis, Isatis Root): clear heat, relieve toxin, resolve sore, and cure dysentery.

[Simple and Effective Formulas]

1. 大青汤 Dà Qīng Tāng — Woad Root Decoction from *Teachings on the Treatment of Pox* (痘疹心法 Dòu Zhěn Xīn Fǎ,): Dà Qīng Yè (Folium Isatidis), Xuán Shēn (Radix Scrophulariae), Shēng Dì (Radix Rehmanniae), Shí Gāo (Gypsum Fibrosum), Zhī Mǔ (Rhizoma Anemarrhenae), Mù Tōng (Caulis Akebiae), Dì Gǔ Pí (Cortex Lycii),

Jīng Jiè (Herba Schizonepetae), Gān Cǎo (Radix et Rhizoma Glycyrrhizae), and Dàn Zhú Yè (Herba Lophatheri); decoct in water for oral administration to treat red or purplish measles or with excessive rupture due to exuberant heat-toxin.

2. 大青汤 Dà Qīng Tāng — Woad Root Decoction from *Comprehensive Recording of Divine Assistance* (圣济总录, Shèng Jì Zǒng Lù): Dà Qīng Yè (Folium Isatidis) 60 g, Shēng Má (Rhizoma Cimicifugae) 60 g, Dà Huáng (Radix et Rhizoma Rhei) (filed, stir-fried) 60 g, and Shēng Dì (Radix Rehmanniae) (cut, baked) 90 g; grind into fine powder and decoct 6 g/dose in water for oral administration to treat swollen throat and lips, erosion in the mouth and tongue, bitter taste in the mouth, and hot sensation in the face.

3. 大青丸 Dà Qīng Wán — Woad Root Pill from *Comprehensive Recording of Divine Assistance* (圣济总录, Shèng Jì Zǒng Lù): Dà Qīng Yè (Folium Isatidis) 30 g, Dà Huáng (Radix et Rhizoma Rhei) (filed, stir-fried) 30 g, Zhī Zǐ (Fructus Gardeniae) (peel removed) 30 g, Huáng Qí (Radix Astragali) (processed) 30 g, Shēng Má (Rhizoma Cimicifugae) 30 g, Huáng Lián (Rhizoma Coptidis) (fibrous root removed) 30 g, and Pò Xiāo (Mirabilitum) 60 g; grind into fine powder, prepare into phoenix tree seed-sized pill with honey, and take 30 pills/ dose with warm water for oral administration to treat deafness with hot sensation in the head. Also applicable for different types of infectious diseases with internally excessive heat-toxin.

[Precautions] Dà Qīng Yè (Folium Isatidis) has extremely low toxicity, few side effects have been reported. A few patients, however, experience gastrointestinal discomfort such as nausea and vomiting after taking the medicinal.

[Addendum]

板蓝根 Bǎn Lán Gēn *radix isatidis isatis root*

The source is from the root of *Isatis tinctoria* L., or *Baphicacanthus cusia* (Nees) Bremek. It is similar to Dà Qīng Yè (Folium Isatidis) in flavors, natures and actions and commonly used for high fever in warm febrile disease, macules and papules due to heat entering *ying*-blood, or hematemesis, epistaxis, hematuria, and stool with blood caused by exuberant heat stirring blood. It is also applicable for mumps, abscesses, swelling, and ulcers. Use 10–15 g in decoction.

青黛 Qīng Dài *indigo naturalis natural indigo*

The source is from a blue powdery or cloddy substances extracted from the leaf and stem leaf of *Isatis tinctoria* L., *Baphicacanthus cusia* (Nees) Bremek, *Polygonum tinctorium* Lour, and *Ficus hookeriana*, family Leguminosae. With salty flavor and cold nature, it is similar to Dà Qīng Yè (Folium Isatidis) in actions and indications. Recently, it catches the attentions of medical community because its ingredient indirubin exerts better therapeutic effects on chronic granulocytic leukemia.

蚤休 Zǎo Xiū *rhizoma paridis bistorta rhizome*

The source is from the rhizome of herbaceous perennial *Paris polyphylla* Smith or *Paris polyphylla* Smith var. yunnanensis Hand.-Mazz, and other congeneric species, family Liliaceae. Bitter in flavor and slightly cold in nature with slight toxicity. Alternate names include 七叶一枝花 Qī Yè Yī Zhī Huā, 重楼 Chóng Lóu, 重台 Zhòng Tái, and 草河车 Cǎo Hé Chē.

[Actions] Clear heat and resolve toxins, and cool the liver and suppress fright. It is applicable for heat-toxin carbuncles and swellings, viper bite, and spasm due to exuberant heat in the liver channel stirring wind. This herb contains saponin and can inhibit a variety of pathogenic bacteria. It also has shown sedative, antalgic, and antihistaminic effect.

[Quality] Good quality is dry without muddy rootlets.

[Indications]

1. Heat-toxin abscesses and swellings: Zǎo Xiū (Rhizoma Paridis) can clear heat and resolve toxins and is potent in treating various heat-toxins patterns such as carbuncles, boils, swellings, furuncles, swollen and painful throat, and innominate swellings and toxins manifested as redness, pain, and hot sensation. In recent years, it is also used in the treatment of virus hepatitis and other infectious diseases, either alone or

in combination with medicinals that clear heat and resolve toxin such as Pú Gōng Yīng (Herba Taraxaci), Zǐ Huā Dì Dīng (Herba Violae), Jīn Yín Huā (Flos Lonicerae Japonicae), and Lián Qiào (Fructus Forsythiae).

2. Poisonous snake bites: Zǎo Xiū (Rhizoma Paridis), potent in resolving snake venom, can be used alone either for oral administration or external application in mild cases of poisonous snake bites. It is usually combined with Dà Huáng (Radix et Rhizoma Rhei) and Zǐ Huā Dì Dīng (Herba Violae) when fire-heat is exuberant.

3. Liver-heat convulsion: Zǎo Xiū (Rhizoma Paridis) is effective in clearing liver-heat to alleviate convulsions and therefore applicable for febrile diseases with high fever and convulsion. It is often used in a combination with Gōu Téng (Ramulus Uncariae Cum Uncis), Lóng Dǎn Cǎo (Radix et Rhizoma Gentianae), and Dì Lóng (Pheretima) to clear heat and calm liver wind.

[Usage and Dosage] Use raw in general for oral administration, grind into powder for external application. Use 5–15 g in decoction, and decrease the dosage in pill and powder.

[Mnemonics] Zǎo Xiū (Rhizoma Paridis, Bistorta Rhizome): bitter and cold; clear and dissipate heat-toxin, relieve snake venom, extinguish wind, and cool the liver.

[Simple and Effective Formulas]

1. 重台草散 Chóng Tái Cǎo Sǎn — Bistorta Rhizome Powder from *Formulas from Benevolent Sages* (圣惠方, Shèng Huì Fāng): Zǎo Xiū (Rhizoma Paridis) 30 g, Mù Biē Zǐ (Semen Momordicae) (shuck removed) 30 g, and Bàn Xià (Rhizoma Pinelliae) 30 g; grind into fine powder, mix with strong vinegar, and then apply externally to the affected areas to treat sudden onset of localized redness and swelling.

2. 治脱肛方 Zhì Tuō Gāng Fāng — Healing Proctoptosis Formula from *Empirical Formulas* (经验方　Jīng Yàn Fāng): Zǎo Xiū (Rhizoma Paridis); grind into juice with vinegar, apply externally to the affected areas, and conduct the reduction of prolapsed anus with gauze, twice or three times a day to treat proctoptosis.

[Precautions] Bitter and cold in nature, Zǎo Xiū (Rhizoma Paridis) tends to damage yang qi and therefore should be used with caution in patients with original qi deficiency. It is contraindicated in cases haematemesis and epistaxis due to heat damaging *ying* blood.

Daily practices

1. What are the actions and indications of Pú Gōng Yīng (Herba Taraxaci)?
2. What are the actions and indications of Dà Qīng Yè (Folium Isatidis) and what are the similarities and differences between Dà Qīng Yè (Folium Isatidis) and Pú Gōng Yīng (Herba Taraxaci)?
3. What are the similarities and differences among Zǎo Xiū (Rhizoma Paridis), Dà Qīng Yè (Folium Isatidis) and Pú Gōng Yīng (Herba Taraxaci) in terms of actions and indications?

虎杖 **Hǔ Zhàng** *rhizoma polygoni cuspidati giant knotweed rhizome*

The source is from the rhizome of herbaceous perennial *Polygonum cuspidatum* Sieb. et Zucc., family Polygonaceae. Alternate names include 阴阳莲 Yīn Yáng Lián, 大叶蛇总管 Dà Yè Shé Zǒng Guǎn, 花斑竹 Huā Bān Zhú, and 活血丹 Huó Xuè Dān. Bitter in flavor and slightly cold in nature.

[Actions] Clear heat and resolve toxins, invigorate blood and relieve pain, dispel wind and drain dampness, and relieve cough and dissolve phlegm. It is applicable for carbuncles, swellings, sores, toxins, joint *bì* pain, damp-heat induced jaundice, amenorrhea, dysmenorrhea, injuries from falls, fractures, contusions and strains, cough, profuse sputum, and scalding. Its ingredient hellebore phenol-3-heteroside can decrease blood lipid, reduce blood pressure, and dilute coronary artery. Experiments have shown that it has an *in vitro* inhibitory effect against a variety of pathogenic bacteria. It is capable of stanching bleeding and consolidating when applied externally.

[Quality] Good quality is thick and solid with a yellow cross-section.

[Indications]

1. Heat-toxin: Hŭ Zhàng (Rhizoma Polygoni Cuspidati) is applicable for lung-heat cough due to heat-toxin, scalding, burning, abscesses, sores, swellings, and venomous snake bites. It is combined with Sāng Bái Pí (Cortex Mori), Huáng Qín (Radix Scutellariae), and Zhè Bèi Mŭ (Bulbus Fritillariae Thunbergii) for lung-heat cough; and mixed with sesame oil in its dense decoction or fine powder form for external application to cure scalding and burning. Its decoction can be used for oral administration to relieve venomous snake bites, and its fresh plant can be pounded and applied externally as well.
2. Blood stasis with pain: Hŭ Zhàng (Rhizoma Polygoni Cuspidati), effective in invigorating blood and dissolving stasis, is often used together with other medicinals that promote blood flow and eliminate stasis such as Dāng Guī (Radix Angelicae Sinensis), Dān Shēn (Radix et Rhizoma Salviae Miltiorrhizae), Hóng Huā (Flos Carthami), and Táo Rén (Semen Persicae) to relieve amenorrhea, dysmenorrhea, injuries from falls, fractures, contusions, and strains associated with blood stasis.
3. Wind-damp *bì* pain: Hŭ Zhàng (Rhizoma Polygoni Cuspidati) can be decocted alone in wine or combined with Qiāng Huó (Rhizoma et Radix Notopterygii), Fáng Fēng (Radix Saposhnikoviae), and Sāng Jì Shēng (Herba Taxilli) for wind-damp *bì* pain.
4. Damp-heat patterns: Hŭ Zhàng (Rhizoma Polygoni Cuspidati), potent in clearing heat and removing dampness, can be used alone or together with Zhī Zĭ (Fructus Gardeniae), Huáng Băi (Cortex Phellodendri Chinensis), and Bì Xiè (Rhizoma Dioscoreae Hypoglaucae) for damp-heat induced jaundice, strangury, turbid urine, and abnormal vaginal discharge. Nowadays, it is commonly used in the treatment of gallbladder stone, cholecystitis, acute and chronic hepatitis, and urinaty tract stone through not only clearing damp-heat, unblocking collaterals to arrest pain, but also invigorating blood and dissolving masses.

[Usage and Dosage] Use raw in general, 10–30 g in decoction.

[Mnemonics] Hŭ Zhàn (Rhizoma Polygoni Cuspidati, Giant Knotweed Rhizome): bitter and cold; clear heat, invigorate blood, relieve jaundice, strangury and turbid leucorrhea, and cure pain due to blood stasis.

[Simple and Effective Formulas]

1. 治淋散 Zhì Lín Sàn — Healing Strangury Powder from *Yao Seng Tan's Proven Formulas* (姚僧坦集验方, Yáo Sēng Tǎn Jí Yàn Fāng): Hǔ Zhàng (Rhizoma Polygoni Cuspidati); grind into powder and take 6 g/dose with rice soup for oral administration to treat different types of stranguary, such as heat strangury, blood strangury, stony strangury, and chylous strangury.

2. 虎杖散 Hǔ Zhàng Sǎn — Giant Knotweed Rhizome Powder from *The Grand Compendium of Materia Medica* (本草纲目, Běn Cǎo Gāng Mù): Hǔ Zhàng Gēn (Rhizoma Polygoni Cuspidati); grind into powder and take with wine for oral administration to treat postpartum abdominal pain with blood stasis and unconsciousness caused by traumatic injury from falls.

[Precautions] Hǔ Zhàng (Rhizoma Polygoni Cuspidati) is contraindicated during pregnancy because of its blood-invigorating effect.

鱼腥草 Yú Xīng Cǎo *herba houttuyniae heartleaf houttuynia*

The source is from the herb of herbaceous perennial *Houttrynia cordata* Thunb, family Saururaceae. Pungent in flavor and cold in nature. It is called as 鱼腥草 Yú Xīng Cǎo for its strong fishy smell and alternate names include 蕺菜 Jí Cài.

[Actions] Clear heat and resolve toxins, alleviate abscesses and expel pus, promote urination, and relieve strangury. It is applicable for lung abscess with purulent sputum, cough and wheezing, heat dysentery, heat strangury, carbuncles, swellings, sores, and toxins. Houttuynine sodium bisulfite (decanoylacetaldehyde), the major constitutent in its volatile oil, has shown a relative inhibitory effect against a variety of pathogenic bacteria and leptospira, and can increase leukocytotic phagocytosis. Its ingredient quercitrin has a diuretic effect and its decoction has shown an antibechic effect on experimental animal.

[Quality] Washed clean and dried under sunshine. Good quality has many well-shaped leaves and buds with a fishy smell.

[Indications]

1. Lung-heat cough and lung abscess: Yú Xīng Cǎo (Herba Houttuyniae) is good at clearing the lung and thus applicable to cough with yellow sputum caused by phlegm-heat obstruction in the lung. It is also a principal herb for lung abscess and commonly combined with Jié Gěng (Radix Platycodonis), Sāng Bái Pí (Cortex Mori), Zhè Bèi Mǔ (Bulbus Fritillariae Thunbergii), Huáng Qín (Radix Scutellariae), and Lú Gēn (Rhizoma Phragmitis). Its injection has been widely used for different types of pneumonia and the fresh herb can be pounded into juice for oral administration to cure lung abscess.

2. Heat-toxin sores and damp-heat transforming into toxin patterns: Yú Xīng Cǎo (Herba Houttuyniae) is used for abscesses and hemorrhoids due to heat-toxin, as well as snake and insect bites. It is also commonly applied for excessive damp-heat pattern manifested as eczema, itching, vaginal itching, and anus swelling, pain and itching by three approaches, namely decoction for oral administration, pounding fresh herb for external application, and decoction for external wash.

3. Water-damp retention: Yú Xīng Cǎo (Herba Houttuyniae), owning to its urination-promoting property, is suitable for edema and strangury. It can also clear heat and therefore is particularly appropriate for binding of pathogenic heat and water-damp in a combination with Chē Qián Zǐ (Semen Plantaginis), Zhū Líng (Polyporus), and Mù Tōng (Caulis Akebiae).

[Usage and Dosage] Use raw in general, 10–30 g in decoction, double the dosage when used alone or fresh, and do not overcook as its main ingredient is volatile oil.

[Mnemonics] Yú Xīng Cǎo (Herba Houttuyniae, Heartleaf Houttuynia): pungent; principal herb for lung abscess, clear heat-toxin, and cure sore.

[Simple and Effective Formulas]

1. 治肺痈方 Zhì Fèi Yōng Fāng — Healing Lung Abscess Formula from *Materia Medica of South Yunnan* (滇南本草, Diān Nán Běn Cǎo): Yú Xīng Cǎo (Herba Houttuyniae), Cè Bǎi Yè (Cacumen Platycladi), and Tiān Huā Fěn (Radix Trichosanthis) in equal dosage; decoct in water

and take small amounts at frequent intervals for oral administration to treat lung abscess vomiting blood and pus.

2. 清肺散 Qīng Fèi Sàn — Lung Clearing Powder from *Jiang Xi Herbal Medicine* (江西草药, Jiāng Xi Cǎo Yào): Yú Xīng Cǎo (Herba Houttuyniae) 9 g, Hòu Pò (Cortex Magnoliae Officinalis) 9 g, and Lián Qiào (Fructus Forsythiae) 9 g; grind into powder and take 6 g/time with decoction of Sāng Zhī (Ramulus Mori) 30 g for oral administration to treat virus pneumonia, common cold and bronchitis.

[Precautions] Yú Xīng Cǎo (Herba Houttuyniae) is contraindicated to deficiency pattern. Allergic shock, drug-induced dermatitis and peripheral neuritis from its injection have been reported.

射干 Shè Gān *rhizoma belamcandae blackberry lily rhizome*

The source is from the rhizome of herbaceous perennial *Belamcanda chinensis* (L.) DC., family Iridaceae, Bitter in flavor and cold in nature. Alternate names include 乌扇 Wū Shàn and 扁竹 Biǎn Zhú.

[Actions] Clear heat and resolve toxins, and dispel phlegm and alleviate sore throat. It is applicable for swollen and painful throat with exuberant heat phlegm or cough and wheezing due to phlegm exuberance. This herb contains tectoridin, tectorigenin glycoside, and tectorigenin and has an anti-inflammatory effect. Its decoction or infusion has shown *in vitro* inhibitory effect against dermatophyte, adenovirus, and ECHO11 virus.

[Quality] Good quality is dry, thick, big and yellow without rootlets.

[Indications]

1. Pain and swelling of throat: Shè Gān (Rhizoma Belamcandae), good at clearing lung heat and alleviating sore throat, is regarded as a principal medicinal for relieving painful and swollen throat, particularly when patient also present profuse phlegm-drool as it can dispel phlegm-drool. It can be used alone or in a combination with Jié Gěng (Radix Platycodonis), Gān Cǎo (Radix et Rhizoma Glycyrrhizae), and

Bèi Mŭ (Bulbus Fritillaria). Its powder can be blown into the throat to eliminate pain and swelling.

2. Lung-heat cough and wheezing: Shè Gān (Rhizoma Belamcandae), capable of clearing the lung and dispelling phlegm, is usually combined with Sāng Bái Pí (Cortex Mori), Mǎ Dōu Líng (Fructus Aristolochiae), Jié Gĕng (Radix Platycodonis), and Huáng Qín (Radix Scutellariae) for lung-heat induced cough and wheezing with profuse phlegm and phlegm rale in the throat; and with Má Huáng (Herba Ephedrae), Xì Xīn (Radix et Rhizoma Asari), and Bàn Xià (Rhizoma Pinelliae) for cough and asthma due to cold-phlegm obstruction in the lung.

Also used in the treatment of mumps, scrofula and breast abscess in early stage.

[Usage and Dosage] Use raw in general, 5–10 g in decoction.

[Mnemonics] Shè Gān (Rhizoma Belamcandae, Blackberry Lily Rhizome): bitter and cold; good at benefiting the throat and arresting cough and wheezing with phlegm sound.

[Simple and Effective Formulas]
射干麻黄汤 Shè Gān Má Huáng Tāng — Belamcanda and Ephedra Decoction from *Essentials from the Golden Cabinet* (金匮要略, Jīn Guì Yào Lüè): Shè Gān (Rhizoma Belamcandae) 9 g, Má Huáng (Herba Ephedrae) 6 g, Shēng Jiāng (Rhizoma Zingiberis Recens) 6 g, Xì Xīn (Radix et Rhizoma Asari) 4 g, Zǐ Wǎn (Radix et Rhizoma Asteris) 4 g, Kuǎn Dōng Huā (Flos Farfarae) 4 g, Wǔ Wèi Zǐ (Fructus Schisandrae Chinensis) 3 g, Dà Zǎo (Fructus Jujubae) 5 pieces, and Bàn Xià (Rhizoma Pinelliae) 8 g; decoct in water for oral administration to treat cough and wheezing with gurgling frog sound in throat due to qi counterflow. Also applicable for bronchitis and bronchial asthma with profuse sputum.

[Precautions] Shè Gān (Rhizoma Belamcandae), cold and bitter in nature with the action of subduing excess fire and promoting defecation, is contraindicated in cases of cough and wheezing of deficiency pattern. It is not recommended for the pregnant and should be used cautiously in patients with weak stomach and spleen.

白头翁 **Bái Tóu Wēng** *radix pulsatillae chinese anemone root*

The source is from the root of herbaceous perennial *Pulsatilla chinensis* (Bge.) Regel, family Ranunculaceae. Bitter in flavor and cold in nature. It is called "hoary-headed geezer" because the head of the root is white and hairy.

[Actions] Clear heat and resolve toxins, cool the blood and relieve dysentery, and kill intestinal parasites. It is applicable for heat-toxin bloody dysentery, vaginal itching, and abnormal vaginal discharge. This herb contains buttercup glycosides, anemonin, and triterpenoid saponin. Its decoction and ingredient of buttercup glycosides have shown *in vitro* and *in vivo* inhibitory effects against growth of amebic protozoa. Its ingredient of protoanemonin has a strong *in vitro* inhibitory effect against a variety of bacteria.

[Quality] Harvested in spring and autumn, leaf, scape and fibrous root removed, root tip with white fluff included, washed clean, and dried under sunshine. Good quality is solid and brittle with white and hairy head of the root and without impurities.

[Indications]

1. Heat-toxin dysentery: Bái Tóu Wēng (Radix Pulsatillae), potent in clearing damp-heat and toxins in the large intestine, is commonly used for dysentery resulting from excessive damp-heat in the intestine. It is effective in treating bacillary dysentery and amebic dysentery in combination with Huáng Lián (Rhizoma Coptidis), and Huáng Bǎi (Cortex Phellodendri Chinensis).
2. Scrofula, carbuncles and swelling: Bái Tóu Wēng (Radix Pulsatillae) is considered more potent in clearing heat and resolving toxins, and is therefore widely used for heat-induced scrofula and abscesses, either alone or together with other heat-clearing and toxin-resolving medicinals. It can be pounded and applied topically for swollen and painful hemorrhoid and ruptured scrofula.
3. Parasites: Bái Tóu Wēng (Radix Pulsatillae) is capable of killing parasites and thus applicable for white leucorrhea and vaginal itching due to trichomonas vaginalis, as well as tinea favosa. Usually, herb decoction is recommended for external wash.

[Usage and Dosage] Use raw in general, 9–15 g in decoction, use pounded for external application, or apply decoction for external wash.

[Mnemonics] Bái Tóu Wēng (Radix Pulsatillae Chinese, Anemone Root): bitter; cure heat dysentery, kill parasites, stop itching, and remove scrofula.

[Simple and Effective Formulas]

1. 白头翁汤 Bái Tóu Wēng Tāng — Anemone Decoction from *Essentials from the Golden Cabinet* (金匮要略, Jīn Guì Yào Lüè): Bái Tóu Wēng (Radix Pulsatillae) 12 g, Huáng Lián (Rhizoma Coptidis) 9 g, Huáng Bǎi (Cortex Phellodendri Chinensis) 9 g, and Qín Pí (Cortex Fraxini) 9 g; decoct in water for oral administration to treat heat dysentery with severe bloody and purulent stool and tenesmus.

2. 白头翁散 Bái Tóu Wēng Sǎn — Anemone Powder from *Formulas from Benevolent Sages* (圣惠方, Shèng Huì Fāng): Bái Tóu Wēng (Radix Pulsatillae) 15 g, Huáng Lián (Rhizoma Coptidis) 75 g, and Shí Liú Pí (Pericarpium Granati) 30 g; grind into crude powder, decoct 3 g/dose in water, and take for oral administration when necessary to treat pediatric heat-toxin dysentery with stool like a fish brain.

[Precautions] Bái Tóu Wēng (Radix Pulsatillae), cold in nature, is not suitable for cold-damp dysentery or chronic dysentery of deficiency cold. Fresh medicinal is contraindicated in all cases as it contains poisonous protoanemonin that irritates the skin and cause poisoning when used in a big dosage. It should be dried and stored for a long duration to polymezie the protoanemonin into anemonin, which is significantly lower in toxicity and has fewer side effects.

Daily practices

1. What are the similarities and differences in terms of actions and indications among the following heat-clearing and toxin-resolving medicinals, Hǔ Zhàng (Rhizoma Polygoni Cuspidati), Yú Xīng Cǎo (Herba Houttuyniae), Shè Gān (Rhizoma Belamcandae), and Bái Tóu Wēng (Radix Pulsatillae)?

2. Summarize the nature, flavor, and actions of these medicinals that relieve dysentery.

I. Medicinals that Clear Heat and Cool Blood

生地 **Shēng Dì** *radix rehmanniae rehmannia root*

The source is from the underground tuber of herbaceous perennial *Rehmannia glutinosa* (Gaertn.) Libosch., family Scrophulariaceae. Alternate names include Xì Shēng Dì 细生地. Sweet and bitter in flavor and cold in nature.

[Actions] Clear heat and cool the blood, and moisten dryness and promote body fluid. It is applicable for yin consumption in febrile diseases manifested as crimson tongue, vexation, and thirst, bone-steaming fever and taxation fever due to internal miscellaneous diseases, wasting-thirst induced by internal heat, hematemesis, epistaxis, macules, and rashes. This herb contains mannitol, polysaccharide, amino acid, rehmannin, and alkaloid. Its ethanol extractives have antihypertensive effects on anesthetized animal and can promote blood coagulation in rabbits. Some reports state it has a hypoglycemic effect.

[Quality] It is called Xiān Shēng Dì 鲜生地 when used in fresh form, and called Gān Dì Huáng (Radix Rehmanniae Recens) when bake-dried. Good quality is heavy, soft, and slight sweet with a black, oily and moist cross-section.

[Indications]

1. Heat entering *ying*-blood in warm disease: Shēng Dì (Radix Rehmanniae) can clear blood heat and is usually combined with medicinals that cool blood and nourish yin, such as Chì Sháo (Radix Paeoniae Rubra), Mǔ Dān Pí (Cortex Moutan), Shuǐ Niú Jiǎo (Cornu Bubali), Xuán Shēn (Radix Scrophulariae), and Mài Dōng (Radix Ophiopogonis) for fever aggravated at night, vexation and agitation, delirious speech, macules and papules, and crimson tongue.
2. Bleeding due to blood heat: Shēng Dì (Radix Rehmanniae), capable of both cooling blood and stanching bleeding, is applicable for

hematemesis, epistaxis, stool with blood, hematuria, profuse uterine bleeding, prolonged scanty uterine bleeding of variable intervals caused by frenetic movement of hot blood. This substance can be decocted alone or the fresh one can be pounded into juice to be taken directly.

3. Yīn deficiency patterns: owning to its potency of nourishing yin and engendering fluid, Shēng Dì (Radix Rehmanniae) is applicable for both yin deficiency with internal heat and yin consumption in febrile disease. It is combined with Mài Dōng (Radix Ophiopogonis), Běi Shā Shēn (Radix Glehniae), and Yù Zhú (Rhizoma Polygonati Odorati) for lung and stomach yin deficiency; with Xuán Shēn (Radix Scrophulariae) and Mài Dōng (Radix Ophiopogonis) for yin deficiency of the intestines; with Mài Dōng (Radix Ophiopogonis), Ē Jiāo (Colla Corii Asini), and Bái Sháo (Radix Paeoniae Alba) for liver and kidney yin deficiency; and with Dì Gǔ Pí (Cortex Lycii), Biē Jiǎ (Carapax Trionycis), Qīng Hāo (Herba Artemisiae Annuae), and Bái Wēi (Radix et Rhizoma Cynanchi Atrati) for yin deficiency with internal heat.

[Usage and Dosage] Use raw to clear heat, cool blood, nourish yin and promote fluid production; use fresh to better cool the blood and nourish yin; processing with ginger juice to decrease its greasy property; processing with wine to eliminate its side effect on the stomach. Use 10–15 g in decoction, pounding fresh herb to get its juice, and up to above 50 g for treating arthralgia and constipation due to fluid insufficiency of the large intestine.

[Mnemonics] Shēng Dì (Radix Rehmanniae, Rehmannia Root): sweet and cool; good at promoting fluid production, clear heat, cool the blood, and strong at arresting bleeding.

[Simple and Effective Formulas]

1. 增液汤 Zēng Yè Tāng — Humor Increasing Decoction from *Systematic Differentiation of Warm Diseases* (温病条辨, Wēn Bìng Tiáo Biàn): Shēng Dì (Radix Rehmanniae) 24 g, Xuán Shēn (Radix Scrophulariae) 30 g, and Mài Dōng (Radix Ophiopogonis) 24 g; decoct in water for oral administration to treat yin deficiency induced constipation in the late stage of warm disease.

2. 地黄散 Dì Huáng Sǎn — Rehmannia Powder from *Formulas from Benevolent Sages* (圣惠方, Shèng Huì Fāng): Gān Dì Huáng (Radix Rehmanniae Recens) 30 g, Huáng Qín (Radix Scutellariae) 30 g, Bái Sháo (Radix Paeoniae Alba) 30 g, Dāng Guī (Radix Angelicae Sinensis) 30 g, stir-fried Ē Jiāo (Colla Corii Asini) 60 g, and Fú Lóng Gān (Terra Flava Usta) 60 g; grind into fine powder and take 6 g/dose with glutinous rice soup for oral administration to treat deficiency-consumption with hematemesis.

[Precautions] Shēng Dì (Radix Rehmanniae), cold and cloying in nature, should be used with cautions or is even contraindicated in cases of diarrhea due to spleen deficiency, poor appetite due to stomach deficiency, and stagnation of phlegm-dampness.

水牛角 Shuǐ Niú Jiǎo *cornu bubali buffalo horn*

The source is from the horn of water buffalo, *Budalus bubalis* L., family Bovidae. Salty in flavor and cold in nature.

[Actions] Clear heat and cool the blood, and resolve toxins and suppress fright. It can replace Xī Jiǎo (Cornu Rhinocerotis), known as the traditional principal medicinal that cool blood and clear heat. This medicinal is applicable for high fever, vexation, thirst and macules caused by pathogenic heat entering *ying*-blood levels in different types of febrile diseases, hematemesis, epistaxis, stool with blood, hematuria, unconsciousness, convulsive syncope, and pain, and obstruction of the throat. Modern researches suggest this herb has cardiotonic, platelet-increasing, coagulation-promoting, and sedative effects, and its pharmacological effect is similar to that of Xī Jiǎo (Cornu Rhinocerotis).

[Quality] Splitted, soaked in hot water, cut into extremely thin slices with a special knife called *pang dao*, and sun-dried. Good quality is translucent without impurities.

[Indications]

1. Heat entering *ying*-blood: to clear heat and cool blood, Shuǐ Niú Jiǎo (Cornu Bubali) is combined with Shēng Dì (Radix Rehmanniae), Mǔ

Dān Pí (Cortex Moutan), and Chì Sháo (Radix Paeoniae Rubra) for excess heat manifestations caused by pathogenic heat entering into *ying*-blood in warm febrile disease.

2. Unconsciousness and convulsive syncope due to extreme heat: Shuǐ Niú Jiǎo (Cornu Bubali), capable of unblocking heart spirit, opening heart orifice, and arresting convulsive syncope, is often combined with other orifice-opening and fright-suppressing medicinals when above-mentioned symptoms occur in warm febrile disease. It is also commonly used in Chinese patent medicines of opening orifice and suppressing fright.

3. Bleeding due to heat exuberance: Shuǐ Niú Jiǎo (Cornu Bubali) is combined with other medicinals that cool blood and stanch bleeding for frenetic movement of hot blood, manifested either as erupted macules and papules, hematemesis, nosebleed, hemoptysis, hematuria, and stool containing blood in cases of heat entering *ying*-blood in warm febrile disease, or thrombocytopenic purpura in internal miscellaneous diseases.

[Usage and Dosage] Use raw in most cases. Use 10–30 g in decoction, decoct first, increase to large dosage when used in severe case, file into powder, and take with water or medical liquor for oral administration.

[Mnemonics] Shuǐ Niú Jiǎo (Cornu Bubali, Buffalo Horn): similar to Xī Jiǎo (Cornu Rhinocerotis), cool the blood, cure hematemesis and epistaxis, relieve toxin, and stop spasm.

[Simple and Effective Formulas]

1. 牛角地黄汤 Niú Jiǎo Dì Huáng Tāng — Rhinoceros Horn and Rehmannia Decoction (orginally Xī Jiǎo Dì Huáng Tāng) from *Important Formulas Worth a Thousand Gold Pieces* (千金要方, Qiān Jīn Yào Fāng): Shuǐ Niú Jiǎo (Cornu Bubali) (decocted first) 30 g, Shēng Dì (Radix Rehmanniae) 30 g, Sháo Yào (Radix Paeoniae) 12 g, and Mǔ Dān Pí (Cortex Moutan) 9 g; decoct in water for oral administration to treat heat entering into the blood level and frenetic movement of hot blood with manifestations of hematemesis, epistaxis, stool with blood, hematuria, macules and papules purplish dark in color, crimson purplish tongue, or vexation, agitation, and mania.

2. 治淋方 Zhì Lín Fāng — Healing Strangury Formula from *Comprehensive Recording of Divine Assistance* (圣济总录, Shèng Jì Zŏng Lù): Shuĭ Niú Jiǎo (Cornu Bubali) (burnt into ashes, sifted); take 3 g/dose with wine for oral administration to treat stony strangury and hematuria.

[Precautions] Shuĭ Niú Jiǎo (Cornu Bubali), cold and cloying in nature, is contraindicated in the absence of heat in blood level.

牡丹皮 Mŭ Dān Pí *cortex moutan tree peony bark*

The source is from the dry cortex of deciduous undershrub *Paeonia suf-fruticosa* Andr., family Ranunculaceae. Alternate names include 丹皮 Dān Pí. Bitter and acrid in flavor and slightly cold in nature.

[Actions] Clear heat and cool the blood, and invigorate the blood and remove stasis. It is applicable for warm toxin macules, frenetic movement of hot blood, hematemesis, epistaxis, night fever abating at dawn, absence of sweating, steaming bone fever, amenorrhea, dysmenorrhea, carbuncles, swellings, sores, and toxins, and traumatic injury and pain. This herb contains phenol original peony glycosides, peonol, peonoside, peoniflorin, and volatile oil. Experimental researches show it can hinder coagulation through inhibiting platelet aggregation and has a significant inhibitory effect on fibrinolysin. It also has sedative, spasmolytic, analgesic, antihypertensive, and uterus-stimulant effects, and can dilate coronary artery and artery of the lower extremities.

[Quality] Impurity removed, the woody core of root excluded, moistened thoroughly, cut into slices, and dried in the air. Good quality is thick, long and powdery. 凤丹皮 Fèng Dān Pí from Mount Phoenix of Tongling city in Anhui province is of the best quality and has been regarded as a genuine regional medicinal.

[Indications]

1. Lesser abdominal pain with bleeding: manifestations include pain in the lateral aspects of the lower abdomen with hardness feeling upon pressure, and bleeding in the lower part of body in most cases such as stool

and urine containing blood, profuse uterine bleeding, and prolonged scanty uterine bleeding of variable intervals. The bleeding and pain in the lateral aspects of the lower abdomen are intercorrelated. For bleeding without pain in the lateral aspects of the lower abdomen, formulas such as Huáng Tǔ Tāng (Yellow Earth Decoction) and Jiāo Ài Tāng (Donkey-Hide Gelatin and Mugwort Decoction) and medicinals including Ē Jiāo (Colla Corii Asini) and Dì Huáng (Radix Rehmanniae) are commonly used; whereas for pain in the lateral aspects of the lower abdomen without bleeding, medicinals such as Sháo Yào (Radix Paeoniae), Zhǐ Shí (Fructus Aurantii Immaturus), and Dāng Guī (Radix Angelicae Sinensis) are preferred. Mǔ Dān Pí (Cortex Moutan) is suitable for cases of pain in the lateral aspects of the lower abdomen with bleeding, which is most commonly found in colonic disease, irregular menstruation, pelvic infection, adnexitis, gynecologic tumor, and prostate disease. Clinic experiences have shown that Mǔ Dān Pí (Cortex Moutan) and its formulae are suitable for emaciated patients with dark red skin and frequent pain in the lateral aspects of the lower abdomen, or for females who suffer from irregular menstruation with clots, pain in the lateral aspects of the lower abdomen, and darkish red rough tongue.

2. Sores, abscesses, swelling and toxins: Mǔ Dān Pí (Cortex Moutan) is applicable for sores, abscesses, swelling, and toxins when pus has not formed yet with darkish red color, fever every now and then, and abdominal hardness or pain upon pressing. It is combined with Dà Huáng (Radix et Rhizoma Rhei), Táo Rén (Semen Persicae), and Máng Xiāo (Natrii Sulfas) for intestinal abscess; with Lián Qiào (Fructus Forsythiae), Jīn Yín Huā (Flos Lonicerae Japonicae), Bái Zhǐ (Radix Angelicae Dahuricae), Chì Sháo (Radix Paeoniae Rubra), and Zhī Zǐ (Fructus Gardeniae) for sore toxins; and with Chái Hú (Radix Bupleuri), Zhī Zǐ (Fructus Gardeniae), Dāng Guī (Radix Angelicae Sinensis), Sháo Yào (Radix Paeoniae), and Bò He (Herba Menthae) for facial sores.

[Mnemonics] Mǔ Dān Pí (Cortex Moutan, Tree Peony Bark): bitter and pungent; clear blood heat, relieve sores and toxins, invigorate blood, and unblock the channels.

[Simple and Effective Formulas]

1. 大黄牡丹皮汤 Dà Huáng Mǔ Dān Pí Tāng — Rhubar Peony Decoction from *Essentials from the Golden Cabinet* (金匮要略, Jīn Guì Yào Lüè): Mǔ Dān Pí (Cortex Moutan) 10 g, Dà Huáng (Radix et Rhizoma Rhei) 10 g, Táo Rén (Semen Persicae) 15 g, Dōng Guā Zǐ (Semen Benincasae) 30 g, and Máng Xiāo (Natrii Sulfas)10 g; decoct in water for oral administration to treat intestinal abscess. Also applicable for appendicitis and other suppurative diseases of abdominal cavity.

2. 桂枝茯苓丸 Guì Zhī Fú Líng Wán — Cinnamon Twig and Poria Pill from *Essentials from the Golden Cabinet* (金匮要略, Jīn Guì Yào Lüè): Mǔ Dān Pí (Cortex Moutan) 10 g, Táo Rén (Semen Persicae) 15 g, Guì Zhī (Ramulus Cinnamomi) 10 g, Fú Líng (Poria) 12 g, and Sháo Yào (Radix Paeoniae) 12 g; decoct in water for oral administration to treat patient with pain or even masses in lateral aspect of the lower abdomen, headache, vertigo, insomnia, vexation and agitation, palpitations, and dry and scaly skin. Also applicable for menstrual irregularities, dysmenorrhea, hysteritis, annexitis, hysteromyoma, infertility, habitual miscarriage, prostatic hyperplasia, and appendicitis.

[Precautions] Mǔ Dān Pí (Cortex Moutan) has a special aroma, ingesting the decoction of this herb can easily induce vomiting, and it should be used cautiously by patients with stomach qi deficiency and poor appetite.

赤芍 Chì Sháo *radix paeoniae rubra red peony root*

The source is from the root of herbaceous perennial *Preonia lactiflora* Pall, *P. obovata* Maxim, or *P. veitchii* Lynch, family Ranunculaceae. Alternate names include 赤芍药 Chì Sháo Yào. Sour and bitter in flavor and slightly cold in nature.

[Actions] Clear heat and cool the blood, and invigorate the blood and relieve pain. It is applicable for macules and papules, fever, and crimson tongue resulting from warm pathogens entering into *ying*-blood; hematemesis, epistaxis, amenorrhea, and dysmenorrheal due to blood heat; or red, swollen, and painful eyes caused by ascendant hyperactivity of liver fire. This herb contains paeonalin A, B, benzoic acid, paeonol, paeoni-florin, and palmitic acid, and has shown sedative and antalgic effects, especially for abdominal pain caused by intestinal spasm. It can promote body's absorption on inflammatory substances to reduce swelling of and localize the affected area. This substance has also shown an *in vitro* inhibitory effect against a variety of pathogenic bacteria.

[Quality] Impurities removed, washed and soaked in water, obtained and dried in the air until moistened thoroughly, cut into slices, and dried under sunshine. Good quality is long, thick and powdery with a white cross-section, and has an outer cortex that is easily peeled and with deep and coarse wrinkles.

[Indications]

1. Bloody dysentery and abdominal pain: Chì Sháo (Radix Paeoniae Rubra) is combined with Huáng Lián (Rhizoma Coptidis) and Huáng Bǎi (Cortex Phellodendri Chinensis) for purplish black stool containing blood, and unbearable abdominal pain.
2. Static blood obstructing the callaterals: Chì Sháo (Radix Paeoniae Rubra) is combined with Huáng Qí (Radix Astragali), Gé Gēn (Radix Puerariae Lobatae), Hóng Huā (Flos Carthami), and Chuān Xiōng (Rhizoma Chuanxiong) for post-stroke hemiplegia; and with Gān Cǎo (Radix et Rhizoma Glycyrrhizae) and Niú Xī (Radix Achyranthis Bidentatae) for spasm and pain of the lower extremities. The objective indications of blood stasis are dark purple tongue body and rough skin. It is also used for hepatic fibrosis and has been recently used in high dose for liver cirrhosis.
3. Ascendant hyperactivity of liver fire: Chì Sháo (Radix Paeoniae Rubra) is applicable for red, swollen, and painful eyes and headache caused by ascendant hyperactivity of liver fire and is combined with medicinals that clear the liver such as Xià Kū Cǎo (Spica Prunellae) and Lóng Dǎn Cǎo (Radix et Rhizoma Gentianae).

[Usage and Dosage] Use raw in general, dry-fry to reduce its cold nature; when used to treat menstruation disorders, it is fried with vinegar to improve its ability of draining the liver and invigorating blood. Use 6–15 g in decoction, and up to above 60 g when necessary.

[Mnemonics] Chì Sháo (Radix Paeoniae Rubra, Red Peony Root): bitter and sour; specialized in cooling blood, dissolve blood stasis, and disperse liver fire.

[Simple and Effective Formulas]

1. 赤芍药散 Chì Sháo Yào Sǎn — Paeoniae Rubra Powder from *Formulas from Benevolent Sages* (圣惠方, Shèng Huì Fāng): Chì Sháo (Radix Paeoniae Rubra) 15 g and Huáng Bǎi (Cortex Phellodendri Chinensis) 10 g; decoct in water for oral administration to treat bloody dysentery with unbearable abdominal pain.

2. 补阳还五汤 Bǔ Yáng Huán Wǔ Tāng — Yang-Supplementing and Five-Returning Decoction from *Correction of Errors in Medical Works* (医林改错, Yī Lín Gǎi Cuò): Huáng Qí (Radix Astragali) 100 g, Dāng Guī (Radix Angelicae Sinensis) 10 g, Chì Sháo (Radix Paeoniae Rubra) 15 g, Dì Lóng (Pheretima) 10 g, Chuān Xiōng (Rhizoma Chuanxiong) 10 g, Táo Rén (Semen Persicae) 10 g, and Hóng Huā (Flos Carthami) 10 g; decoct in water for oral administration to treat post-stroke hemiplegia.

3. 活血止晕方 Huó Xuè Zhǐ Yūn Fāng — Blood-invigorating and Dizziness-arresting Formula from *Empirical Formulas* (经验方, Jīng Yàn Fāng): Chì Sháo (Radix Paeoniae Rubra) 20 g, Gé Gēn (Radix Puerariae Lobatae) 20 g, Bái Zhú (Rhizoma Atractylodis Macrocephalae) 12 g, and Chuān Xiōng (Rhizoma Chuanxiong) 10 g; decoct in water for oral administration to treat vertigo and stiffness and pain in the nape and back. Also applicable for vertigo resulting from insufficient blood supply to the brain, cerebral arteriosclerosis, cervical spondylosis, and hypertension.

[Precautions] Chì Sháo (Radix Paeoniae Rubra) should be used cautiously in the absence of blood stasis and for patients with pale tongue body and soft muscles.

Daily practices

1. What are the similarities and differences between Shēng Dì (Radix Rehmanniae) and Shuǐ Niú Jiǎo (Cornu Bubali) in terms of actions and indications?

2. What are the other actions of Mǔ Dān Pí (Cortex Moutan) and Chì Sháo (Radix Paeoniae Rubra) apart from cooling blood and what are the similarities and differences among Mǔ Dān Pí (Cortex Moutan), Chì Sháo (Radix Paeoniae Rubra), Shēng Dì (Radix Rehmanniae), and Shuǐ Niú Jiǎo (Cornu Bubali) in terms of actions and indications?

II. Medicinals that Clear Deficiency-Heat

青蒿 Qīng Hāo *herba artemisiae annuae sweet wormwood*

The source is from the acrial part of herbaceous annual *Artemisia annua* L., or *A. apiacea* or and other congeneric species, family Compositae. Bitter and slightly acrid in flavor and cold in nature. Alternate names include 草蒿 Cǎo Hāo.

[Actions] Clear heat and resolve summerheat, resist malaria, and clear deficiency-heat. It is applicable for summerheat fever and yin deficiency fever with manifestations as alternating chills and fever, or night fever abating at dawn, steaming bone fever, hectic fever, and damp-heat induced jaundice. This herb contains volatile oil that has artemisia ketone, isoarte-misia ketone, D-camphor ketone, thujone, cineole, caryophel-lene and other hemiterpene derivatives. Artemisnin, sesquiterpene lactone with peroxide group, is the major ingredient of antimalaria. Its infusion (leach liquor) has shown an inhibitory effect against certain dermatophytes.

[Quality] Impurity removed, washed clean and moistened in water, cut into segments, and dried under sunshine. Good quality is tender, green and fragrant with many leaves.

[Indications]

1. Deficiency-heat patterns: Qīng Hāo (Herba Artemisiae Annuae) is good at clearing deficiency-heat and therefore is applicable for night fever and morning coolness with an absence of sweating caused by unre-solved deficiency-heat in late state of externally-contracted warm febrile disease and steaming bone fever, hectic fever, and afternoon tidal fever due to yin deficiency with vigorous fire in internal

miscellaneous diseases. It can be used alone or in combination with Dì Gŭ Pí (Cortex Lycii), Zhī Mŭ (Rhizoma Anemarrhenae), and Shēng Dì (Radix Rehmanniae).

2. Summerheat and damp-heat patterns: owning to its heat-clearing and dampness-removing properties, the aromatic Qīng Hāo (Herba Artemisiae Annuae) is applicable for both summerheat and damp-heat pattern. It is combined with Xī Guā Cuì Yī (Mesocarpium citrulli) and Jīn Yín Huā (Flos Lonicerae Japonicae) for fever and sweating caused by summerheat or pediatric patient with fever in the summer; and with Huò Xiāng (Herba Agastachis), Pèi Lán (Herba Eupatorii), and Huá Shí (Talcum) for fever induced by damp-heat.

3. Alternating chills and fever: from the perspective of traditional Chinese medicine, this type of fever is caused by pathogen in *shaoyang* and most likely to be found in certain warm febrile diseases and malaria. Qīng Hāo (Herba Artemisiae Annuae) is usually combined with Huáng Qín (Radix Scutellariae), Bàn Xià (Rhizoma Pinelliae), Zhú Rú (Caulis Bambusae in Taenia), and Huò Xiāng (Herba Agastachis). In recent years, artemisinin, an extractive of Qīng Hāo (Herba Artemisiae Annuae), has shown a unique therapeutic effect on malignant malaria.

Also used for skin problems such as pruritus and eczema, either for oral administration or external wash.

[Usage and Dosage] Use raw in most cases, 5–12 g in decoction, up to 200 g/day when use fresh to treat malaria, and grinding into juice for oral administration to prevent the loss of anti-malarial ingredient during decocting.

[Mnemonics] Qīng Hāo (Herba Artemisiae Annuae, Sweet Wormwood): relieve fever, cure malaria as its priority, especially when alternating chills and fever occurs.

[Simple and Effective Formulas]

1. 青蒿鳖甲汤 Qīng Hāo Biē Jiǎ Tāng — Sweet Wormwood and Turtle Shell Decoction form *Systematic Differentiation of Warm Diseases* (温病条辨, Wēn Bìng Tiáo Biàn): Qīng Hāo (Herba Artemisiae Annuae) 12 g, Zhī Mŭ (Rhizoma Anemarrhenae) 10 g, Biē Jiǎ (Carapax Trionycis)

15 g, Shēng Dì (Radix Rehmanniae) 15 g, and Mǔ Dān Pí (Cortex Moutan) 5 g; decoct in water for oral administration to treat malaria or night fever abating at dawn due to yin damage and residual heat hiding internally in later stage of warm febrile disease.

2. 蒿芩清胆汤 Hāo Qín Qīng Dǎn Tāng — Sweet Wormwood and Scutellaria Gallbladder-Clearing Decoction from *Popular Guide to the 'Treatise on Cold Damage'* (通俗伤寒论, Tōng Sú Shāng Hán Lùn): Qīng Hāo (Herba Artemisiae Annuae) 12 g, Huáng Qín (Radix Scutellariae) 10 g, Chén Pí (Pericarpium Citri Reticulatae) 5 g, Bàn Xià (Rhizoma Pinelliae) 10 g, Zhǐ Qiào (Fructus Aurantii) 5 g, Zhú Rú (Caulis Bambusae in Taenia) 6 g, Fú Líng (Poria) 12 g, and Bì Yù Sǎn (Jasper Jade Powder) 15 g; decoct in water for oral administration to treat patients with unremitting fever, slight aversion to cold with fever, sweating but without any improvement of the condition, heaviness of the head, lack of strength of the limbs, and chest oppression and fullness. Also applicable for biliary tract infection, urinary tract infection and common cold in summer.

地骨皮 Dì Gǔ Pí *cortex lycii Chinese wolfberry root-bark*

The source is from the cortex of deciduous shrub *Lycium chinense* Mill, or *L. barbarum L.*, family Solanaceae. Sweet in flavor and cold in nature. Alternate names include 枸杞根皮 Gǒu Qǐ Gēn Pí.

[Actions] Clear heat and cool the blood, clear deficiency heat, and clear the lung and subdue fire. It is applicable for fever due to yin deficiency, steaming bone fever, tidal fever, tidal fever, night sweating, cough caused by lung heat, hemoptysis, epistaxis, and wasting-thirst due to internal heat. This herb contains melissic acid, linoleic acid, β-sitosterin, and betaine. Its preparation has a hypoglycemic effect on rabbits, mild antihypertensive, and angiectatic effects. Its water and ethanol extractive have shown an antipyretic effects. It has shown anti-allergic and anti-inflammatory effects.

[Quality] Impurity and the woody core of root removed, slightly washed, sun-dried, and cut into segments. Good quality is large, thick, and without heartwood.

[Indications]

1. Hemoptysis: Dì Gǔ Pí (Cortex Lycii) is suitable for cough and hemoptysis due to lung heat or fire exuberance due to lung yin deficiency with accompanying cough, wheezing, unremitting low grade fever, and night sweating. It is combined with Sāng Bái Pí (Cortex Mori), Huáng Qín (Radix Scutellariae), Mài Dōng (Radix Ophiopogonis), Bǎi Hé (Bulbus Lilii), and Yù Zhú (Rhizoma Polygonati Odorati) in accordance with the condition of deficiency or excess.
2. Fever due to yin deficiency: see the manifestations in the section of Qīng Hāo (Herba Artemisiae Annuae). However, Dì Gǔ Pí (Cortex Lycii) is particularly suitable for deficiency fever with accompanying sweating during sleep, and often combined with Qīng Hāo (Herba Artemisiae Annuae), Yín Chái Hú (Radix Stellariae), and Hú Huáng Lián (Rhizoma Picrorhizae).
3. Internal heat and wasting-thirst: manifestations include thirst, polydipsia, and emaciation. It is commonly seen in diabetes and internal miscellaneous diseases. Dì Gǔ Pí (Cortex Lycii) is often combined with Tiān Huā Fěn (Radix Trichosanthis), Mài Dōng (Radix Ophiopogonis), Shí Gāo (Gypsum Fibrosum), and Shēng Dì (Radix Rehmanniae). It has also been reported recently that its decoction is used for treating hypertension. It is combined with Xú Cháng Qīng (Radix et Rhizoma Cynanchi Paniculati) in the treatment of chronic urticaria, drug eruption, anapylactoid purpura, and contact dermatitis.

[Usage and Dosage] Use raw in general, 10–15 g in decoction.

[Mnemonics] Dì Gǔ Pí (Cortex Lycii, Chinese Wolfberry Root-bark): sweet; good at clearing deficiency-heat, and can arrest thirst, restlessness, and night sweating.

[Simple Formulas]

1. 泻白散 Xiè Bái Sǎn — White Draining Powder from *Key to Diagnosis and Treatment of Children's Diseases* (小儿药证直诀, Xiǎo Ér Yào Zhèng Zhí Jué): Dì Gǔ Pí (Cortex Lycii) 12 g, Sāng Bái Pí (Cortex

Mori) 12 g, and Gān Cǎo (Radix et Rhizoma Glycyrrhizae) 3 g; decoct in water for oral administration to treat pediatric lung heat, dyspnea, cough, and sputum containing blood. Also applicable for bronchitis and severe cough with scanty phlegm.

2. 地骨皮饮 Dì Gǔ Pí Yǐn — Lycii Decoction from *Comprehensive Recording of Divine Assistance* (圣济总录, Shèng Jì Zǒng Lù): Dì Gǔ Pí (Cortex Lycii) 12 g, Tiān Huā Fěn (Radix Trichosanthis) 15 g, Mài Dōng (Radix Ophiopogonis) 12 g, Lú Gēn (Rhizoma Phragmitis) 15 g, and Dà Zǎo (Fructus Jujubae) seven pieces; decoct in water for oral administration to treat wasting-thirst drinking water all the time. Also applicable for diabetes.

[Precautions] Dì Gǔ Pí (Cortex Lycii) is cold in nature and should be used with caution in cases of deficiency cold in the spleen and stomach manifested as pale tongue, body cold, and loose stool. Its injection may cause dangerous side effects when it is injected too quickly into the vein and blood pressure suddenly drops too low.

Daily practices

1. What are the similarities and differences between Qīng Hāo (Herba Artemisiae Annuae) and Dì Gǔ Pí (Cortex Lycii) in terms of actions and indications?
2. What are the differences between medicinals that clear deficient heat and those clear excessive heat in terms of curing fever?

PURGATIVES

Purgative medicinals are those that either cause diarrhea or lubricate the intestinal tract to facilitate defecation.

Defecation, as a normal physiological function of human, is the act of by which organisms eliminate waste feces from the intestinal tract. Physically, people have bowel movements at fairly regular intervals; in the course of disease, more wastes have been held within the body and defecation is one of the most important ways to discharge. Feces, indigestive food retention in the intestinal tract, water retention or blood stasis accumulation can be expelled in defecation-promoting way with purgatives.

Because the actions and indications of downward-draining herbs are dissimilar, they are divided into three major categories, namely.

1. Purgatives.

   Most of these herbs are bitter and cold in nature, while few acrid and hot with rather strong defecation-promoting effect with accompanying heat-clearing and fire-draining properties.

2. Moist laxatives.

   They are often oily substances, sweet in flavor and moistening in nature. These substances are mild in nature and lubricate the intestines to promote defecation.

3. Harsh expellants (cathartics).

   These are very strong drugs that induce pronounced watery diarrhea with abdominal pain. Most of these herbs are bitter and cold with toxicity. Some of these herbs are also diuretics and useful in the treatment of ascites, hydrothorax, and severe edema.

When using purgatives, the following precautions should be taken: 1) for healthy qi insufficiency or those debilitated by chronic diseases since most laxatives have violent effects; and for women during menstruation, pregnancy and postpartum as some laxatives can also activate blood circulation. 2) constipation caused by yang qi and intestinal fluid insufficiency, especially for the elderly or patient in the recovery phase. The disease should be managed according to its etiology and abuse of purgatives is discouraged. 3) the herbs of draining downward are often combined with other medicinals in prescriptions according to the state of illness. They, for instance, are used together with medicinals that clear heat and drain fire for constipation due to heat accumulation; with medicinals that warm the interior for constipation due to cold accumulation; with medicinals that clear and relieve damp-heat for constipation due to damp-heat accumulation in the intestinal tract; with medicinals that invigorate blood and dissolve stasis when accompanied with blood stasis and heat-blood stagnation; with tonics if accompanied with healthy qi insufficiency; and with medicinals that move qi as smooth qi movement will facilitate smooth bowel movement.

From the perspective of traditional Chinese medicine, the method of draining downward is an important therapy with an instantaneous effect. However, a practitioner needs to be more experienced to prevent the side effects and beginners should be more cautious.

大黄 **Dà Huáng** *radix et rhizoma rhei rhubarb root and rhizome*

The source is from the radix and rhizome of herbaceous perennial *Rheum palmatum L.*, *R. tanguticum Maxim ex Balf*, or *Rheum officinale* Baill, family Polygonaceae. Bitter in flavor and cold in nature. It is so-called as its cross-section is yellowish brown and taking it turns urine bright yellow. Alternate names include 将军 Jiāng Jūn (for its vigorous action of dispelling pathogens) and 川军 Chuān Jūn (mainly from Sichuan).

[Actions] Purge accumulations and remove stagnation, drain fire and promote defecation, and clear heat and invigorate the blood. It is applicable for constipation due to excess heat, accumulation in the intestine, abdominal pain, incomplete defecation, damp-heat jaundice, blood heat hemorrhage, red eyes, sore throat, intestinal abscess, carbuncle, swellings, sores, ulcers, amenorrhea and dysmenorrhea caused by static blood, injuries from falls, fractures, contusions and strains with blood stagnation, and scalding and heat-toxin carbuncle and swelling when applied externally. Its major active ingredients are tannin and anthraquinone derivatives including chrysophanol, aloe-emodin, rhein, rheum emodin, and physcion. This herb can stimulate large intestine, increase peristalsis, and promote defecation. It has shown potent antibacterial and inhibitory effects against virus and fungus. It has spasmolytic, choleretic, hypolipidemic, antihypertensive, bleeding-stanching, and antitumor effects.

[Quality] Washed clean in water, obtained and covered by stupe until moistened thoroughly, cut into slices, and dried under sunshine. Sichuan has the largest output of 南大黄 Nán Dà Huáng, also known as 川大黄 Chuān Dà Huáng, and is regarded as the commonly used quality goods. While 西宁大黄 Xi Níng Dà Huáng produced in Qinghai is recommended as a genuine regional medicinal marked by yellowish and brownish red outer surface, visible whitish rhombic and reticular veins formed by grayish white parenchymatous tissues interlacing with brownish red rays, and aligned stripes inside like brocade. For this reason, it is also known as 锦

纹大黄 Jǐn Wén Dà Huáng. It is the best with optimal curative effects and without side effects.

[Indications]

1. Constipation due to heat accumulation: Dà Huáng (Radix et Rhizoma Rhei), cold in nature, is capable of washing away intestinal accumulations and suitable for excess heat constipation. Clinical manifestations are constipation with abdominal fullness and pain, or stinking water stool with severe abdominal pain, fullness and resistance feeling while pressing, unpleasant, pressing and distending pain in the abdomen upon heavier pressure. In most cases, patients present vexing fever, or red face and eyes, or rave and talkativeness with loud voice, or hot sensation in the body with profuse sweating, or feeling of lightweight body and activeness. This is interior excess heat pattern and Dà Huáng (Radix et Rhizoma Rhei) must be used to purge heat accumulation and unblocking downwards. Other medicinals should be used together according to accompanying symptoms. For instance, Dà Huáng (Radix et Rhizoma Rhei) should be combined with Zhǐ Shí (Fructus Aurantii Immaturus) and Hòu Pò (Cortex Magnoliae Officinalis) for abdominal distention, fullness and pain as if being covered by tiles with feeling of hardness upon pressure; with Máng Xiāo (Natrii Sulfas) for hot body with sweating, constipation lasting for five or six days, hardness and fullness of the abdomen as if clusters of pebbles when pressing, and dry mouth and tongue; with Gān Suì (Radix Kansui) for hardness, fullness and pain from the heart to lateral aspect of the lower abdomen that refuses pressure; with Zhī Zǐ (Fructus Gardeniae) and Yīn Chén (Herba Artemisiae Scopariae) for hot body, dry and greasy mouth, general jaundice, and slight fullness of abdomen; with Máng Xiāo (Natrii Sulfas) and Táo Rén (Semen Persicae) for sudden pain in lateral aspect of the lower abdomen and manic; and with Huáng Lián (Rhizoma Coptidis) and Huáng Qín (Radix Scutellariae) for epigastric *pǐ*, hematemesis, and epistaxis.

For healthy qi deficiency with heat accumulation, Dà Huáng (Radix et Rhizoma Rhei) should be prescribed together with medicinals that reinforce healthy qi in order to avoid injuring healthy qi while dispelling pathogens. For instance, it is used together with Shēng Dì (Radix Rehmanniae), Xuán Shēn (Radix Scrophulariae), and Mài Dōng (Radix Ophiopogonis) for yin fluid insufficiency of the intestines; with Rén Shēn (Radix et Rhizoma Ginseng) and Dāng Guī (Radix Angelicae Sinensis) for qi and blood insufficiency; and with yang-warming medicinals such as Fù Zǐ (Radix Aconiti Lateralis Praeparata) and Gān Jiāng (Rhizoma Zingiberis) for cold accumulation-induced constipation with accompanying spleen yang deficiency.

2. Fire-heat exuberance patterns: owning to potency in clearing heat and resolving toxins, Dà Huáng (Radix et Rhizoma Rhei) is particularly suitable for diseases and patterns of fire-heat flaming upwards, such as headache, red eyes, swollen and painful throat, swollen and painful gum, and ulcers in the mouth and tongue, especially when accompanied with constipation. It can be used alone or together with other medicinals that clear heat and resolve toxin. This substance is combined with Lóng Dǎn Cǎo (Radix et Rhizoma Gentianae), Shēng Dì (Radix Rehmanniae), Zhī Zǐ (Fructus Gardeniae) and Xià Kū Cǎo (Spica Prunellae) for liver and gallbladder exuberant fire; and with Shí Gāo (Gypsum Fibrosum), Sāng Bái Pí (Cortex Mori) and Yú Xīng Cǎo (Herba Houttuyniae) for vigorous fire in the lungs. It is also significantly effective in the treatment of scalding, burns, and heat-toxin induced carbuncles, swellings, ulcers, and sores.

3. Damp-heat patterns: Dà Huáng (Radix et Rhizoma Rhei) is capable of clearing and removing damp-heat and therefore applicable for jaundice, strangury and dysentery caused by damp-heat. It is combined with Zhī Zǐ (Fructus Gardeniae), Yīn Chén (Herba Artemisiae Scopariae), and Huáng Bǎi (Cortex Phellodendri Chinensis) for jaundice; and with Mù Tōng (Caulis Akebiae), Chē Qián Zǐ (Semen Plantaginis), Qú Mài (Herba Dianthi), and Gān Cǎo (Radix et Rhizoma Glycyrrhizae) for strangury. This substance is also used in the treatment of dysentery, either alone or together with other medicinals that clear and drain damp-heat.

4. Internal accumulation of blood stasis: Dà Huáng (Radix et Rhizoma Rhei) is potent in invigorating blood and dissolving stasis and thus has been widely used to treat different diseases and patterns of static blood, such as abdominal pain due to postpartum blood stasis, or abdominal

fullness and pain caused by inhibited menstruation, or traumatic injury resulting in blood stasis blockage in the channels and collaterals manifested as abdominal and lower back pain, hardness and pain in lateral aspect of the lower abdomen when pressing, and restlessness, or irritability, or paraphasia, or restless sleep in most cases. In this case, Dà Huáng (Radix et Rhizoma Rhei) is combined with medicinals that invigorate blood and remove stasis, such as Táo Rén (Semen Persicae), Mǔ Dān Pí (Cortex Moutan), Chì Sháo (Radix Paeoniae Rubra), and Hóng Huā (Flos Carthami) to break up blood and move stasis.

5. Frenetic movement of hot blood: owning to its ability to clear blood heat and stanch bleeding, Dà Huáng (Radix et Rhizoma Rhei) is quite suitable for different types of hemorrhagic disorders caused by blood heat. It can also invigorate blood and remove stasis, thus it can stanch bleeding without retaining blood stasis. This substance can be used alone or in a combination with other medicinals that cool blood and stanch bleeding. Recently, it has been effectively used in a powder form for upper gastrointestinal hemorrhage.

To sum up, this herb is applicable to a wide range of diseases in the clinic and its actions of purgation, clearing heat, invigorating blood and stanching bleeding are interconnected.

[Usage and Dosage] Different preparation methods exert different influences on this herb, namely using raw as a purgative; applying the processed to clear heat, invigorate blood, and remove blood stasis; treating with wine when used to clear fire-heat in the head and face; and using charred one to strengthen its bleeding-arresting action. Use 5–10 g in decoction, increase the dosage for heat-toxin or in severe case of heat accumulation, and 2–3 g as in pill and powder. For decocting, this medicinal can be added later, decocted first, or cooked together with other herbs. When used as a purgative, it should be added at the end since prolonged cooking will reduce its purgative effect. While for clearing heat, it should be cooked together with other herbs. In recent years, it has been prepared into injection to alleviate discomfort in the stomach induced by oral administration and eliminate the purgative effect. Other preparation forms such as tablet and syrup are also available. The dosage of Dà Huáng

(Radix et Rhizoma Rhei) should be prescribed in line with different processing methods, usages, indications and compatibilities. For instance, give 3–15 g for decoction, and up to 15–30 g when used to expel heat accumulation in the intestines by purgation; decrease the dosage when taken with water or powder as 1 g/time can even cause loose and frequent stool; decrease its dosage when added later due to its potent purgative effect; increase the dosage when using processed Dà Huáng (Radix et Rhizoma Rhei) as it is inferior to the raw one in purgation. Taking 1 g in decoction or less than 0.3 g in powder each time would not cause diarrhea. The charred herb is a minor purgative, but more potent for bleeding and dysentery-arresting, usually prescribed 5–10 g.

[Mnemonics] Dà Huáng (*R*adix et Rhizoma Rhei, Rhubarb Root and Rhizome): bitter and cold; expel heat-accumulation by purgation, invigorate blood, arrest bleeding, and relieve jaundice and dysentery.

[Simple and Effective Formulas]

1. 大黄甘草汤 Dà Huáng Gān Cǎo Tāng — Rhubarb and Licorice Decoction from *Essentials from the Golden Cabinet* (金匮要略, Jīn Guì Yào Lüè): Dà Huáng (Radix et Rhizoma Rhei) 6–12 g and Gān Cǎo (Radix et Rhizoma Glycyrrhizae) 3 g; decoct in water for oral administration to treat patient with hardness in the abdomen with constipation. Also applicable for habitual constipation.
2. 小承气汤 Xiǎo Chéng Qì Tāng — Minor Purgative Decoction from *Treatise on Cold Damage* (伤寒论, Shāng Hán Lùn): Dà Huáng (Radix et Rhizoma Rhei) 10 g, Zhǐ Shí (Fructus Aurantii Immaturus) 10 g, and Hòu Pò (Cortex Magnoliae Officinalis) 10 g; decoct in water for oral administration to treat patient suffering from fever with sweating, delirious speech, abdominal pain, distention and fullness, constipation, yellow greasy thick tongue coating, and slippery fast powerful pulse. Also applicable for virus hepatitis, biliary tract infection, flatulence after gastrointestinal surgery, intractable hiccup, and intestinal obstruction with manifestation of heat accumulation in the large intestine.
3. 大柴胡汤 Dà Chái Hú Tāng — Major Bupleurum Decoction from *Treatise on Cold Damage* (伤寒论, Shāng Hán Lùn): Dà Huáng (Radix et Rhizoma Rhei) 10 g, Chái Hú (Radix Bupleuri) 10 g, Zhǐ Shí (Fructus

Aurantii Immaturus) 10 g, Sháo Yào (Radix Paeoniae) 12 g, Huáng Qín (Radix Scutellariae) 10 g, Bàn Xià (Rhizoma Pinelliae) 10 g, Shēng Jiāng (Rhizoma Zingiberis Recens) three pieces, and six Dà Zǎo (Fructus Jujubae); decoct in water for oral administration to treat patient with alternating chills and fever, vomiting with epigastric vexation, epigastric fullness and pain upon pressure, and difficult defecation. Also applicable for acute cholecystitis and acute pancreatitis.

4. 桂枝加大黄汤 Guì Zhī Jiā Dà Huáng Tāng — Cinnamon Twig Decoction plus Rhubar from *Treatise on Cold Damage* (伤寒论, Shāng Hán Lùn): Dà Huáng (Radix et Rhizoma Rhei) 6–10 g, Guì Zhī (Ramulus Cinnamomi) 10 g, Sháo Yào (Radix Paeoniae) 15 g, Gān Cǎo (Radix et Rhizoma Glycyrrhizae) 3 g, Shēng Jiāng (Rhizoma Zingiberis Recens) three pieces, and eight Dà Zǎo (Fructus Jujubae); decoct in water for oral administration to treat patient with abdominal pain, constipation, spontaneous sweating, and feeling of qi rushing up to the chest. Also applicable for dysentery and intractable urticaria.

5. 泻心汤 Xiè Xīn Tāng — Draining Heart Decoction from *Essentials from the Golden Cabinet* (金匮要略, Jīn Guì Yào Lüè): Dà Huáng (Radix et Rhizoma Rhei) 6 g, Huáng Lián (Rhizoma Coptidis) 3 g, and Huáng Qín (Radix Scutellariae) 6 g; decoct in water for oral administration to treat patient with vexing heat, epigastric *pǐ* and pain, hematemesis, epistaxis, and red tongue with yellow coating. Also applicable for acute infectious diseases, upper gastrointestinal hemorrhage, pneumorrhagia, epistaxis, hypertension, cerebral hemorrhage, cerebral thrombosis, hyperlipemia, psoriasis vulgaris, neonatal jaundice, acute inflammation of ear, nose and throat, sores, ulcers, swellings, and toxins.

[Precautious] Dà Huáng (Radix et Rhizoma Rhei) is suitable when patients present with abdominal fullness and pain that refuse pressure, dry mouth, red and tough tongue with red spots and yellow (brownish yellow, burned black) greasy and dry coating, and either slippery powerful, slippery rapid, slow slippery, or deep tight pulse, and diarrhea and dysentery with slippery pulse. Whereas, it should be used with caution in cases of abdominal pain with preference to pressure, constipation for several days but without discomforts and with soft abdomen, or abdomen that feels like a drum, tight on the surface but hollow in the center; listlessness, heavy body, edema, no desire to talk, somnolence, aversion to cold, and absence of sweating; and deep faint pulse, deep slow pulse, deficient floating pulse, or deep weak thin pulse.

Dà Huáng (Radix et Rhizoma Rhei), cold and bitter in nature and potent in purging, may injure yang qi if applied appropriately and therefore should be used cautiously during pregnancy and for the postpartum without stasis blood and people with yang qi deficiency manifested as pale tongue, coldness of body, and loose stool. Long-term consumption of Dà Huáng (Radix et Rhizoma Rhei) is not recommended for patients with chronic constipation, as it may cause more severe constipation after withdrawal.

Daily practices

1. How many types of purgatives and what precautious should be taken when using it?
2. What are the actions and indications of Dà Huáng (Radix et Rhizoma Rhei)?

芒硝 **Máng Xiāo** *natrii sulfas sodium sulphate*

The source is from the refined crystalline sodium sulphate. It is so-called because of its sharp, long, and needle-like precipitate and alternate names include 芒消 Máng Xiāo. Salty and bitter in flavor and cold in nature. It is called 风化硝 Fēng Huà Xiāo when it loses the water of crystallization to form white powder, and alternate names include 玄明粉 Xuán Míng Fěn and 元明粉 Yuán Míng Fěn.

[Actions] Drain heat and promote defection, and soften masses and remove accumulation. It is applicable for excess-heat accumulation, dry stool, sore throat, aphtha, red eyes, sores, and ulcers. This substance contains sodium sulfate and small amount of inorganic salt such as sodium chloride, magnesium chloride, magnesium sulfate, and calcium sulfate. Sodium sulfate is dissoluble in water, however some ionic minerals are not absorbed in the intestines, which may cause hyperosmotic condition in the intestines to hinder intestinal absorption of water. Then severe water retention occurs in the intestines to attenuate intestinal content, enlarge its volume, stimulate intestinal mucosa receptor, cause reflexive hyperfunction of intestinal peristalsis, and eventually result in diarrhea.

[Quality] Good quality is crystalline, prism-shaped, clear, and translucent without impurities.

[Indications]

1. Dry and hard stool: it refers to intestinal dryness and constipation, also known as 燥屎 dry stool. Its manifestations may include constipation for several days, abdomen that feels like clusters of pebbles upon pressing, and thick and dry tongue coating without fluids, stiffness of tongue movement while talking, body heat, red eyes, dry throat, unconsciousness, and delirious speech. It is commonly seen in the elderly, people with constitutionally body fluid insufficiency, febrile diseases, infectious diseases, and consumptive diseases. Dà Huáng (Radix et Rhizoma Rhei) and Gān Căo (Radix et Rhizoma Glycyrrhizae) are often used together with Máng Xiāo (Natrii Sulfas).
2. Fire-heat internal exburance: Máng Xiāo (Natrii Sulfas) is capable of purging and clearing fire-heat pathogen and combined with Dà Huáng (Radix et Rhizoma Rhei), Zhī Zǐ (Fructus Gardeniae), and Zhú Yè (Folium Phyllostachydis Henonis) for high fever, vexation, thirst, cramp, loss of consciousness, and dry and hard stool caused by lung and stomach heat exuberance in externally-contracted warm febrile disease. Its preparation is often applied externally to relieve sore throat, aphtha, and red eyes due to fire-heat through clearing heat and draining fire.
3. Sores and swelling: external application of Máng Xiāo (Natrii Sulfas) has a effect of clearing heat, softening masses, and relieving swelling. It can be wrapped with cloth for external dressing or dissolved into cold water for external wash to treat dermal sores and swelling, red and hot rashes, and mastitis.

[Usage and Dosage] Use raw, 3–12 g in decoction, proper amount when applied topically; slightly stir-fry and add later, or take for oral administration when infused in hot water.

[Mnemonics] Máng Xiāo (Natrii Sulfas, Sodium Sulphate): salty and bitter; drain heat to unblock the bowels, and relieve dry stool when combined with Dà Huáng (Radix et Rhizoma Rhei).

[Simple and Effective Formulas]

1. 调胃承气汤 Tiáo Wèi Chéng Qì Tāng — Stomach Regulating and Purgative Decoction from *Treatise on Cold Damage* (伤寒论, Shāng Hán Lùn): Máng Xiāo (Natrii Sulfas) 10 g, Dà Huáng (Radix et Rhizoma Rhei) 6–10 g, and Gān Cǎo (Radix et Rhizoma Glycyrrhizae) 3 g; decoct in water for oral administration to treat patients presenting fever with sweating, constipation, abdominal pain, and dry yellow thick tongue coating. Also applicable for habitual constipation, intestinal obstruction, and biliary tract diseases.
2. 桃核承气汤 Táo Hé Chéng Qì Tāng — Peach Kernel Qi Guiding Decoction from *Treatise on Cold Damage* (伤寒论, Shāng Hán Lùn): Dà Huáng (Radix et Rhizoma Rhei) 10 g, Táo Rén (Semen Persicae) 12 g, Guì Zhī (Ramulus Cinnamomi) 10 g, Máng Xiāo (Natrii Sulfas) 10 g, and Gān Cǎo (Radix et Rhizoma Glycyrrhizae) 3 g; decoct in water for oral administration to treat patients with spasmodic pain in the lesser abdomen that refuses pressure, uninhibited urination, fever at night, delirious speech, vexation, thirst, mania, amenorrhea due to blood stasis, dysmenorrhea, retention of lochia during postpartum. Also applicable to schizophrenia, epidemic hemorrhagic fever, fulminant bacillary dysentery, diabetes, acute necrotic enteritis, idiopathic hematuresis, chronic nephropyelitis, prostatitis, and crush syndrome.

[Precautious] Máng Xiāo (Natrii Sulfas), owning to its cold and purgative property, should be used with caution by the pregnant and patients with white and slippery tongue coating, coldness of body, and loose stool associated with spleen-stomach deficiency cold.

麻子仁 Má Zǐ Rén *fructus cannabis hemp seed*

The source is from the ripe fruit of herbaceous annual *Cannabis sativa* L., family Moraceae. Alternate names include 火麻仁 Má Zǐ Rén and 大麻仁 Má Zǐ Rén. Sweet in flavor and neutral in nature with mild toxicity.

[Actions] Moisten intestine and promote defecation. It is mainly used for constipation due to intestinal fluid and blood deficiency in the elderly, weak, and parturient.

[Quality] Good quality is dry, full, and grayish-green.

[Indications] Má Zǐ Rén (Fructus Cannabis), moistening and oily in nature, can moisten the intestines and is effective on constipation due to intestinal dryness, especially for the elderly, parturient, weak with constipation resulting from yin and fluid insufficiency. It can be ground into powder and then added into rice congee for oral administration, or used in a combination with other medicinals that promote defecation such as Dà Huáng (Radix et Rhizoma Rhei) and Hòu Pò (Cortex Magnoliae Officinalis) for constipation induced by intestinal dryness.

[Usage and Dosage] Use stir-fried in general to reduce its toxicity, must be grounded before decocting, and 10–15 g in decoction.

[Mnemonics] Má Zǐ Rén (Fructus Cannabis, Hemp Seed): sweet and neutral; moisten the intestines to promote defecation, and applicable and effective for the aged, weak, and puerpera.

[Simple and Effective Formulas]

1. 麻子仁丸 Má Zǐ Rén Wán — Cannabis Fruit Pill from *Treatise on Cold Damage* (伤寒论, Shāng Hán Lùn): Má Zǐ Rén (Fructus Cannabis) 500 g, Sháo Yào (Radix Paeoniae) 250 g, Zhǐ Shí (Fructus Aurantii Immaturus) (roasted) 250 g, Dà Huáng (Radix et Rhizoma Rhei) 500 g, Hòu Pò (Cortex Magnoliae Officinalis) (roasted) 250 g, and Xìng Rén (Semen Armeniacae Amarum) 250 g; grind into fine powder, prepare into pill with honey, and take 9 g/dose with warm water, one or twice a day, or decoct in water for oral administration to treat constipation caused by dryness-heat in the intestines or intestinal dryness with constipation in the elderly or patients in recovery period, or habitual constipation.

2. 麻子粥 Má Zǐ Zhōu — Cannabis Fruit Porridge from *Formulas to Keep Up One's Sleeve* (肘后方, Zhǒu Hòu Fāng): Má Zǐ (Fructus Cannabis); grind, and cook with rice into congee for oral administration to treat constipation.

[Precautions] Má Zǐ Rén (Fructus Cannabis) is contraindicated in cases of constitutionally habitual loose stool and diarrhea. Take once or twice a week is appropriate for chronic constipation. Long-term high dose use is not recommended.

番泻叶 Fān Xiè Yè *folium sennae senna leaf*

The source is from the leaflet of herbaceous undershrub *Cassia angusti-folia* Vahl, or *C. acutifolia* Del., family Leguminosae. Alternate names include 泻叶 Xiè Yè. Sweet and bitter in flavor and cold in nature.

[Actions] Drain heat and remove stagnation, and promote defecation and urination. It is applicable for heat bind and accumulation, constipation with abdominal pain, edema, fullness, and distention. This herb contains sennosides A and B that can be absorbed in the stomach and small intestine and decomposed in the liver. Its hepatic metabolites flowing through the bloodstream stimulate the pelvic ganglion, which leads to contraction of the large intestine and diarrhea.

[Quality] Leaves in fast-growing stage collected on sunny days, and dried under sunshine. Good quality has large, complete, and green leaves with less stems and without soils, sands, and impurities.

[Indications] Owning to its significant purgative effect and convenience for use, Fān Xiè Yè (Folium Sennae) is applicable for heat accumulation and habitual constipation. It is also used nowadays for cleansing the intestinal tract before taking X-ray examination, and in the treatment of acute mechanical ileus, acute pancreatitis, gall-stone, and stomach and duodenum hemorrhage. Using small dosage is effective in reinforcing the stomach.

[Usage and Dosage] Its purgative effect is associated with the dosage and decoction duration, for instance, small dosage causes soft stool or mild diarrhea, large dosage leads to watery diarrhea, and the longer the decoction duration is, the less the purgative effect is. Add at the end of decoction, do not overcook, use 3–9 g when steeped alone as a tea or added later in decoction for the purgative effect, apply less then 2 g in decoction for tonifying the stomach and promoting digestion.

[Mnemonics] Fān Xiè Yè (Folium Sennae, Senna Leaf): bitter and sweet; drain heat and promote defecation.

[Simple and Effective Formulas]

健胃煎 Jiàn Wèi Jiān — Stomach-tonifying Decoction from *Modern Practical Chinese Materia Medica* (现代实用中药, Xiàn Dài Shí Yòng Zhōng Yào): Fān Xiè Yè (Folium Sennae) 3 g, raw Dà Huáng (Radix et Rhizoma Rhei) 1.8 g, Jú Pí (Pericarpium Citri Reticulatae) 3 g, Huáng Lián (Rhizoma Coptidis) 1.5 g, and Dīng Xiāng (Flos Caryophylli) 1.8 g; soak two hours in boiling water, remove dregs, filtrate to get juice, divide into three equal doses, and take one dose/time, three times a day for oral administration to treat constipation due to accumulated heat.

[Precautious] Ingesting large dosage may cause abdominal pain and vomiting. Huò Xiāng (Herba Agastachis) and Chén Pí (Pericarpium Citri Reticulatae) are often added to prescriptions to counteract this effect. It is contraindicated for the pregnant and in cases of spleen-stomach deficiency cold.

Daily practices

1. What are the similarities and differences among Máng Xiāo (Natrii Sulfas), Má Zǐ Rén (Fructus Cannabis) and Fān Xiè Yè (Folium Sennae) in terms of purging actions and indications?
2. Among downward-draining medicinals, which ones are purgatives and which ones are moist laxatives? What are the differences between them in indications?

Fifth Week

1

MEDICINALS THAT DISPEL WIND-DAMP

Exogenous pathogenic wind-cold invasion may cause the exterior pattern when lodged in the superficial layers of the body or lead to joint and muscle pain, spasms of the sinews, joint swelling, and inhibited bending and stretching if invaded the muscle, channels and collaterals, and sinews and bones. Wind-damp dispelling medicinals, acrid to disperse and bitter to dry dampness, primarily treat wind-damp *bì* pattern and dispel wind-damp pathogen from the muscles, sinews, joints, and bones; sooth the sinews, unblock the collaterals, alleviate pain; and strengthen the sinews and bones.

Wind-damp pathopoiesis is further classified into such patterns as wind-cold-damp and wind-damp-heat according to predominance of wind or damp and secondary pathogens of cold or heat. Therefore, the selection and combination of herbs should be based on the state, site, and duration of the disease. For instance, medicinals that dispelling wind should be used for wind-predominant painful obstruction, also known as migratory painful obstruction (行痹 Xíng Bì); medicinals that dispelling wind and relieving the exterior should be combined for the diseases lodged in the exterior or upper part of the body; medicinals that dissipate dampness should be prescribed together with those that dry or drain dampness for damp-predominant painful obstruction, also known as lodged painful obstruction (拙痹 Zhuō Bì) or the disease affected the lower part of the body; medicinals that relieve cold should be used together with medici-nals that warm the channels and collaterals for cold-predominant painful obstruction, also known as afflictive or very painful obstruction (痛痹

Tòng Bì); clear heat-clearing medicinals should be included in the treatment plan for hot painful obstruction, also known as febrile painful obstruction (热痹 Rè Bì); medicinals that invigorate blood and dissolve stasis, or dissolve phlegm, or worm medicinals that search the channels and collaterals to arrest pain should be added for intractable pain or deformative joint due to chronic *bì* pattern with blood stasis and phlegm turbidity; and with herbs that enrich qi and blood or supplement the liver and kidney for enduring disease with qi and blood deficiency or liver and kidney insufficiency.

Because painful *bì* obstruction is often a chronic complaint, these substances are commonly taken in decocted form or as tinctures, pills, and powders. The moving effect of the alcohol used in tinctures is helpful in unblocking the channels and invigorating qi and blood and can provide a better therapeutic effect for wind-damp *bì* pattern.

Most of these substances are aromatic, bitter, warm, and therefore drying in nature. For this reason they may readily injure yin fluid. It should be used with caution in patients with blood or yin deficiency or in a combination with tonics.

独活 Dú Huó *radix angelicae pubescentis double teeth pubescent angelica root*

The source is from the root of herbaceous perennial *Angelica pubescens* Maxim. f. biserrata shan. et Yuan, family Umbelliferae. It is so called due to its self-reliant existing straight stem. Pungent and bitter in flavor and warm in nature. Alternate names include Dú Yáo Cǎo 独摇草.

[Actions] Dissipate wind and relieve dampness, dissipate cold, and unblock *bì* and arrest pain. It is applicable for wind-cold-damp *bì*, pain in the waist and knee, and headache. This herb contains angelol, angelicin, scopoletin, and bergapten. Its decoction or liquid extract have shown antalgic, sedative and anti-inflammatory on animals and can dilate blood vessel, lower blood pressure, and excite respiratory center. Scopoletin has spasmolytic effect on uterus spasm of isolated rats.

[Quality] Impurities removed, moistened thoroughly, cut into slices, and dried under sunshine. Good quality is thick, solid, and aromatic. The source can be found in a variety of plants, but generally, the root of

Angelica pubescens Maxim. f. biserrata shan. et Yuan from Sichuan and Hubei is considered as the quality goods.

[Indications]

1. Wind-cold-damp *bì*: Dú Huó (Radix Angelicae Pubescentis) is particularly suitable for soreness, heaviness, and pain in the waist, back, and the lower part of the body. It is often combined with Fáng Fēng (Radix Saposhnikoviae), Qín Jiāo (Radix Gentianae Macrophyllae), Wēi Líng Xiān (Radix et Rhizoma Clematidis), and Fáng Jǐ (Radix Stephaniae Tetrandrae) when accompanied with muscle contracture and reduced mobility of the leg joints; and with medicinals that supplement the liver and kidney such as Chuān Xù Duàn (Radix Dipsaci), Dù Zhòng (Cortex Eucommiae), and Sāng Jì Shēng (Herba Taxilli) if accompanied with liver and kidney insufficiency.
2. Wind-cold-damp exterior pattern: Dú Huó (Radix Angelicae Pubescentis) is capable of dispersing wind-cold and relieving dampness and combined with Fáng Jǐ (Radix Stephaniae Tetrandrae), Fáng Fēng (Radix Saposhnikoviae), and Qiāng Huó (Rhizoma et Radix Notopterygii) for aversion to cold, fever, headache, heaviness of the head, and soreness and pain of the body with absence of sweating caused by externally-contracted wind-cold-damp.

Qiāng Huó (Rhizoma et Radix Notopterygii) and Dú Huó (Radix Angelicae Pubescentis) both can relieve wind-damp and dissipate cold. The former, however, is considered more potent in dispersing and more commonly used for exterior wind-cold pattern and wind-damp *bì* pain involving the upper part of the body, and the latter is less effective in dispersing but more powerful in relieving dampness and mainly applied to wind-damp in the lower part of the body. They are used together for pain throughout the body.

[Usage and Dosage] Use raw in general, 5–10g in decoction.

[Mnemonics] Dú Huó (Radix Angelicae Pubescentis, Double Teeth Pubescent Angelica Root): acrid and bitter; scatter wind, dissipate cold, dispel dampness, remove the exterior, and arrest arthralgia and *bì* pattern.

[Simple and Effective Formulas]

1. 独活寄生汤 Dú Huó Jì Shēng Tāng — Pubescent Angelica and Mistletoe Decoction from *Effective Formulas from Generations of Physicians* (世医得效方, Shì Yī Dé Xiào Fāng): Dú Huó (Radix Angelicae Pubescentis) 75g, Sāng Jì Shēng (Herba Taxilli) 60g, Dù Zhòng (Cortex Eucommiae) (cut, stir-fried till the gummy threads are broken) 60g, Běi Xì Xīn (Radix et Rhizoma Asari) 60g, Bái Sháo (Radix Paeoniae Alba) 60g, Guì Xīn (Cortex Cinnamomi) 60g, Chuān Xiōng (Rhizoma Chuanxiong) 60g, Fáng Fēng (Radix Saposhnikoviae) (the residue of rhizome removed) 60g, Gān Cǎo (Radix et Rhizoma Glycyrrhizae) 60g, Rén Shēn (Radix et Rhizoma Ginseng) 60g, Shú Dì Huáng (Radix Rehmanniae Praeparata) 60g, and Huáng Dāng Guī (Radix Angelicae Sinensis) 60g; file into powder and decoct 12g/dose in water for oral administration to treat pain in the waist and knee, hemiplegia, cold *bì*, and weakness of the foot associated with wind-damp injuring the kidney, or spasm and pain in the waist and foot during postpartum.

2. 独活细辛汤 Dú Huó Xì Xīn Tāng — Pubescent Angelica and Asarum Decoction from *Symptoms, Causes, Pulses, and Treatment* (症因脉治 Zhèng Yīn Mài Zhì): Dú Huó (Radix Angelicae Pubescentis) 6g, Xì Xīn (Radix et Rhizoma Asari) 6g, Chuān Xiōng (Rhizoma Chuanxiong) 6g, Qín Jiāo (Radix Gentianae Macrophyllae) 6g, Shēng Dì (Radix Rehmanniae) 6g, Qiāng Huó (Rhizoma et Radix Notopterygii) 6g, Fáng Fēng (Radix Saposhnikoviae) 6g, and Gān Cǎo (Radix et Rhizoma Glycyrrhizae) 6g; decoct in water for oral administration to treat headache of *shaoyin* pattern. Also applicable for persistent headache that aggravated by cold.

[Precautions] Dú Huó (Radix Angelicae Pubescentis), warm and drying in nature, is contraindicated for yin deficiency with heat signs, body pain due to qi and blood deficiency, and soreness, pain, and weakness in the waist and knee caused by liver and kidney insufficiency. From the perspective of toxicology, long-term use may cause renal and hepatic injury and ingesting large amount at one dose may lead to compulsive and intermittent convulsions, or even paralysis generalis.

秦艽 Qín Jiāo *radix gentianae macrophyllae large leaf gentian root*

The source is from the root of herbaceous perennial *Gentiana macrophylla* Pall. var. macrophylla or *G. straminea* Maxim., *G. crassicaulis* Duthie ex Burk., or *G. tibetica* King., family Gentianaceae. Bitter and pungent in flavor and slightly cold in nature. Alternate names include 左秦艽, Zuǒ Qín Jiāo among which *Gentiana macrophylla* Pall. looks like chicken drumsticks and therefore also known as 鸡腿艽 Jī Tuǐ Jiāo.

[Actions] Dispel wind-damp, arrest *bì* pain, clear deficiency-heat, and reduce jaundice. It is applicable for wind-damp *bì* pain, spasms of sinews, vexing pain in the joints, afternoon fever, and infantile malnutrition with accumulation fever. From the perspective of traditional Chinese medicine, this herb is called "a moistening but wind-dispelling medicinal" as it is capable of dispelling wind without dry and violent nature consuming yin. It contains gentianidine alkaloid A, B and C and volatile oil, and has significantly antalgic, sedative and anti-inflammatory effect. This substance also has a certain anti-allergic shock and antihistaminic effect, and can reduce capillary permeability.

[Quality] It includes many varieties, good quality is firm, large, thick, and brownish yellow.

[Indications]

1. Wind-damp *bì* pain: owning to its effect of dispelling wind-damp to unblock the channels and collaterals, Qín Jiāo (Radix Gentianae Macrophyllae) is applicable for irritable and painful limbs, cramps of the sinews and bones, and limited range of motion of the hands and feet due to externally-contracted wind-damp, no matter cold or hot, acute or chronic. However, this substance is slightly cold in nature and more suitable for patient with accompanying heat signs. It is combined with Qiāng Huó (Rhizoma et Radix Notopterygii), Dú Huó (Radix Angelicae Pubescentis), and Guì Zhī (Ramulus Cinnamomi) for the cold-natured; with Rěn Dōng Téng (Caulis Lonicerae Japonicae), Fáng Jǐ (Radix Stephaniae Tetrandrae), and Luò Shí Téng (Caulis Trachelospermi) for the hot-natured; and with Chuān Shān Jiǎ (Squama Manitis), Niú Xī (Radix Achyranthis Bidentatae), Bái Jiè Zǐ (Semen Sinapis), Dì Lóng

(Pheretima), and Mù Guā (Fructus Chaenomelis) for chronic *bì* entering the collaterals.

2. Yin deficiency fever: Qín Jiāo (Radix Gentianae Macrophyllae), effective in clearing deficiency-heat, is applicable for steaming bone fever, hectic fever, afternoon tidal fever, and infantile malnutritional fever, and usually combined with Dì Gǔ Pí (Cortex Lycii), Biē Jiǎ (Carapax Trionycis), Qīng Hāo (Herba Artemisiae Annuae), and Bái Wēi (Radix et Rhizoma Cynanchi Atrati).

3. Damp-heat jaundice: Qín Jiāo (Radix Gentianae Macrophyllae), capable of clearing the liver to relieve jaundice, is applicable for damp-heat induced jaundice and often combined with Yīn Chén (Herba Artemisiae Scopariae), Zhī Zǐ (Fructus Gardeniae), and Huáng Bǎi (Cortex Phellodendri Chinensis).

Also combined with Dāng Guī (Radix Angelicae Sinensis), Rén Shēn (Radix et Rhizoma Ginseng), Bái Sháo (Radix Paeoniae Alba), and Fáng Fēng (Radix Saposhnikoviae) for stroke hemiplegia or hand and foot muscle contracture.

It has been recently prepared into injection for intramuscular injection to treat meningococal meningitis, joint pain, headache, toothache, and pain in the waist and legs. From the perspective of modern biomedicine, it is very effective in treating inflammation and pain.

[Usage and Dosage] Use raw in general, 5–10g in decoction, increase the dosage when necessary or used alone.

[Mnemonics] Qín Jiāo (Radix Gentianae Macrophyllae, Large Leaf Gentian Root): bitter and pungent; clear deficiency-heat and resolve *bì* pain and jaundice.

[Simple and Effective Formulas]

1. 秦艽天麻汤 Qín Jiāo Tiān Má Tāng — Gentian and Gastrodia Decoction from *Medical Revelations* (医学心悟, Yī Xué Xīn Wù): Qín Jiāo (Radix Gentianae Macrophyllae) 4.5g, Tiān Má (Rhizoma Gastrodiae) 3g, Qiāng Huó (Rhizoma et Radix Notopterygii) 3g, Chén Pí (Pericarpium Citri Reticulatae) 3g, Dāng Guī (Radix Angelicae Sinensis) 3g, Chuān Xiōng (Rhizoma Chuanxiong) 3g, Gān Cǎo (Radix et Rhizoma Glycyrrhizae) (roasted) 1.5g, Shēng Jiāng (Rhizoma

Zingiberis Recens) 3 pieces, and Sāng Zhī (Ramulus Mori) (stir-fried with wine) 9g; decoct in water for oral administration to treat back pain radiating to the chest, joint pain, and headache.

2. 秦艽汤 Qín Jiāo Tāng — Gentian Decoction from *Essentials of Medical Masters* (不知医必要, Bù Zhī Yī Bì Yào): Qiāng Huó (Rhizoma et Radix Notopterygii) 4.5g, Dāng Guī (Radix Angelicae Sinensis) 6g, Chuān Xiōng (Rhizoma Chuanxiong) 3g, Shú Dì Huáng (Radix Rehmanniae Praeparata) 9g, Bái Sháo (Radix Paeoniae Alba) (stir-fried with wine) 4.5g, and Dú Huó (Radix Angelicae Pubescentis) 4.5g; decoct in water for oral administration to treat pain throughout the body due to wind attacking the channels and collaterals.

3. 秦艽汤 Qín Jiāo Tāng-Gentian Decoction from *Comprehensive Recording of Divine Assistance* (圣济总录, Shèng Jì Zǒng Lù): Qín Jiāo (Radix Gentianae Macrophyllae) 30g, Chái Hú (Radix Bupleuri) 30g, Zhī Mǔ (Rhizoma Anemarrhenae) 30g, and Zhì Gān Cǎo (Radix et Rhizoma Glycyrrhizae Praeparata cum Melle) 30g; decoct in water for oral administration to treat deficiency-consumption tidal fever, cough, and persistent night sweating.

[Precautions] Qín Jiāo (Radix Gentianae Macrophyllae), not drying but acrid, slippery and moistening, is contraindicated in cases with frequent urination and loose stool. It should be used with caution by patients who have chronic diseases and weak constitutions.

Daily practices

1. For the clinical application of wind-damp dispelling medicianls, how to combine it with other medicinals? What precautions should be taken?
2. For treating *bì* pattern, what are the differences between Dú Huó (Radix Angelicae Pubescentis) and Qín Jiāo (Radix Gentianae Macrophyllae) in terms of the nature, flavor, actions, and indications?

威灵仙 Wēi Líng Xiān *radix et rhizoma clematidis chinese clematis root*

The source is from the root and rhizome of climber perennial liana *Clematis chinensis* Osbeck. or upright herbaceous C. *hexapetala* Pall., family Ranunculaceae. Pungent in flavor and warm in nature.

[Actions] Dispel wind-dampness, unblock the channels and collaterals, alleviate *bì* pain, and soften and resolve fish bones. It is applicable for wind-damp *bì* pain, numbness of the limbs, spasms of the sinews, inhibited bending and stretching of joint, and bones stuck in the throat. This herb contains protoanemonin, sterol, phenols, amino acid, and a variety of triterpenoid saponin, Experiments reveal its decoction can reinforce esophagus mobility in frequency and range, relax the upper esophagal contracture, and remove bones stuck in the throat. Recent research states it has a good antipyretic and antalgic effect.

[Quality] Collected in autumn, dirt and sand removed, and dried under sunshine. Good quality is even root and rhizome, solid, and white with a black cortex.

[Indications]

1. Wind-damp *bì* pain: Wēi Líng Xiān (Radix et Rhizoma Clematidis) is applicable for joint muscle pain, numbness of the skin, and reduced mobility of the joints caused by externally-contracted wind-damp. Owning to its strong effect of dispelling wind, it is more suitable for migratory pain that moves from joint to joint caused by wind-predominant pathogen. Combination of herb is based on the state of illness, it is combined with Qiāng Huó (Rhizoma et Radix Notopterygii) and Guì Zhī (Ramulus Cinnamomi) for pain in the upper part of the body; with Chuān Niú Xī (Radix Cyathulae) and Dú Huó (Radix Angelicae Pubescentis) for pain in the lower part; with Fáng Fēng (Radix Saposhnikoviae) for wind-predominant *bì*; with Cāng Zhú (Rhizoma Atractylodis) for damp-predominant *bì*; with Guì Zhī (Ramulus Cinnamomi) for cold-predominant *bì*; with Huáng Bǎi (Cortex Phellodendri Chinensis) and Fáng Jǐ (Radix Stephaniae Tetrandrae) when accompanied with hot pathogen; with Huáng Qí (Radix Astragali), Dāng Guī (Radix Angelicae Sinensis), Mù Guā (Fructus Chaenomelis), and Jī Xuè Téng (Caulis Spatholobi) for qi and blood deficiency caused by enduring disease.
   Mucus of the fresh herb may cause irritation signs and can be used as vesicant and applied externally on the acupuncture point to vesiculate and treat joint, muscle pain, and cirrhosis ascites.

2. Bones stuck in the throat: swallowing slowly the thick decoction of Wēi Líng Xiān (Radix et Rhizoma Clematidis) is effective in treating bones stuck in the throat. If it is too severe, patient needs to go to hospital.

Its preparation has been recently used in the treatment of stomach cold pain, diabetes insipidus, and cholecystitis.

[Usage and Dosage] Use raw in general, 5–10g in decoction, and up to 30g when used alone.

[Mnemonics] Wēi Líng Xiān (Radix et Rhizoma Clematidis, Chinese Clematis Root): warm; good at relieving fish bones stuck in the throat, and wind-cold-damp *bì* pattern.

[Simple and Effective Formulas]

1. 威灵仙散 Wēi Líng Xiān Sǎn — Rhizoma Clematidis Powder from *Formulas from Benevolent Sages* (圣惠方 Shèng Huì Fāng): Wēi Líng Xiān (Radix et Rhizoma Clematidis); grind into fine powder and take 3g/time with warm wine before meal for oral administration to treat patient with persistent pain in the waist and leg.
2. 痹痛丸 Bì Tòng Wán — Painful Obstruction Resolving Pill from *Formulas for Universal Relief* (普济方, Pǔ Jì Fāng): Wēi Líng Xiān (Radix et Rhizoma Clematidis) (stir-fried) 15g, raw Chuān Wū Tóu (Radix Aconiti), and Wǔ Líng Zhī (Faeces Trogopterori) 12g; grind into powder, prepare into phoenix tree seed-sized pill with vinegar paste, and take 7 pills/time with salt solution for oral administration to treat patient with numbness and pain in the hands and feet.

[Precautions] Wēi Líng Xiān (Radix et Rhizoma Clematidis), pungent and warm, may damage qi and blood when misused and therefore contraindicated for pain in the joint and muscle due to qi and blood deficiency. It contains toxic protoanemonin and ingesting large amounts may cause such oral mucosal irritating symptoms such as burning sensation, swelling and erosion, vomiting, abdominal pain, diarrhea, stool with blood, or even spasm of the tongue, decreased heart beat, and difficult breathing.

防己 Fáng Jǐ *radix stephaniae tetrandrae four stamen stephania root*

The source is from the root of perennial woody liana *Stephania tetrandra* S. Moore, family Menispermaceae, or perennial intertwining herbaceous *Aristolochia fangchi* Wu, family Aristolochiaceae. The former is called 汉防己 Hàn Fáng Jǐ or 粉防己 Fěn Fáng Jǐ (as it is firm, heavy, and powdery), and the latter is called 广防己 Guǎng Fáng Jǐ (Radix Aristolochiae Fangchi) or 木防己 *Mù Fáng* Jǐ (as it is mainly produced in Guangxi and Guangdong, woody lightweight). Bitter and pungent in flavor and cold in nature.

[Actions] Promote urination and reduce edema (either facial or systemic), dispel wind and relieve dampness, and arrest *bì* pain. It is applicable for wind-damp *bì* pain, edema, ascites, and leg qi. 汉防己 Hàn Fáng Jǐ (Radix Stephaniae Tetrandrae) is considered more effective in promoting urination and relieving dampness, while 木防己 Mù Fáng Jǐ (Radix Cocculi Trilobi) in dispelling wind and draining dampness. This herb contains a variety of alkaloid such as tetrandrine, hanfangichin, flavonoid glycoside, phenols, and volatile oil. It has antalgic, antihypertensive, antipyretic, anti-inflammatory, diuretic, and coronary flow-increasing effects.

[Quality] Washed clean, obtained and moistened thoroughly, cut into slices, and dried under sunshine. Good quality is firm and powdery without cortex. 汉防己 Hàn Fáng Jǐ is now mainly produced in Anhui, Zhejiang, Jiangxi, and Hubei, but back to ancient times, it was produced in Hankou and therefore named as 汉防己 Hàn Fáng Jǐ.

[Indications]

1. Water-dampness retention patterns: manifestations include edema and ascites, especially edema in the lower limbs with accompanying lumbago, heaviness of the waist, reduced mobility of the knee joints, inhibited urination, body heaviness, abdominal fullness, and panting. Fáng Jǐ (Radix Stephaniae Tetrandrae) can promote urination and reduce swelling, and is usually prescribed together with medicinals that fortify the spleen and promote water circulation such as Huáng Qí (Radix Astragali), Tíng Lì Zǐ (Semen Lepidii), Jiāo Mù (Semen Zanthoxyli), Bái Zhú (Rhizoma Atractylodis Macrocephalae), and Fú Líng (Poria).

2. Wind-damp *bì* pain: Fáng Jǐ (Radix Stephaniae Tetrandrae) is capable of dispelling dampness, unblocking the collaterals, and relieving pain, and applicable for hand and foot cramp and pain, joint swelling and pain, and edema in the lower limbs due to wind-damp *bì* pain. Combination of herbs is often based on the nature of disease. It is prescribed together with Huá Shí (Talcum), Yì Yǐ Rén (Semen Coicis), Cán Shā (Faeces Bombycis) for damp-heat predominance; and with Wū Tóu (Aconite Main Tuber), Fáng Fēng (Radix Saposhnikoviae), and Guì Zhī (Ramulus Cinnamomi) for cold-damp predominance.

In recent reports, oral administration or injection of tetrandrine, the extractive of Hàn Fáng Jǐ 汉防己, has been used for treating hypertension, coronary heart disease, lumbosacral ramitis, prosopalgia, and amoebae dysentery. Using it together with small-dose radiation therapy is of certain effect on late-stage lung cancer. Applying tetrandrine for treating chronic hepatitis and hepatic fibrosis has also been reported.

[Usage and Dosage] Use raw in general, 6–12g in decoction.

[Mnemonics] Fáng Jǐ (Radix Stephaniae Tetrandrae, Four Stamen Stephania Root): cold, bitter, and pungent; promote urination, dispel wind-damp, and cure *bì* pain.

[Simple and Effective Formulas]

1. 防己黄芪汤 Fáng Jǐ Huáng Qí Tāng — Stephania Root and Astragalus Decoction from *Essentials from the Golden Cabinet* (金匮要略, Jīn Guì Yào Lüè): Fáng Jǐ (Radix Stephaniae Tetrandrae) 12g, Huáng Qí (Radix Astragali) 12g, Bái Zhú (Rhizoma Atractylodis Macrocephalae) 10g, and Gān Cǎo (Radix et Rhizoma Glycyrrhizae) 3g; decoct in water for oral administration to treat sweating with swelling and jaundice. Also applicable for hypertension, cerebrovascular diseases, edema, and nephropathy.

2. 四妙丸 Sì Miào Wán — Wonderfully Effective Four Pill from *National Prescription Collection of Chinese Patent Medicine* (全国中药成药处方集, Quán Guó Zhōng Yào Chéng Yào Chǔ Fāng Jí): Fáng Jǐ (Radix Stephaniae Tetrandrae) 12g, Huáng Bǎi (Cortex Phellodendri Chinensis) 6g, Cāng Zhú (Rhizoma Atractylodis) 10g, and Niú Xī (Radix Achyranthis Bidentatae) 12g; prepare into pill and take 4–6 pills/time

to treat patients with edema and numbness in both feet, atrophy and weakness of the lower extremities, fever with yellow sweating, difficult urination with yellow and scanty urine. Also applicable for pain caused by different types of arthritis and skin problems and urinary and reproductive system disorders due to damp-heat.

[Precautions] Fáng Jǐ (Radix Stephaniae Tetrandrae), cold in nature, is suitable for wind-damp-heat *bì* pattern, but can not be used alone for wind-cold *bì* pattern. It should be used with caution in cases of yin deficiency with accompanying emaciation, hot sensation of the body, night sweating, and red tongue without coating. Tetrandrine may cause liver dysfunction.

豨薟草 Xī Xiān Cǎo *herba siegesbeckiae siegesbeckia*

The source is from the aerial part of herbaceous annual *Siegesbeckiae orientalis* L. and other congeneric species, family Compositae. Alternate names include 豨薟 Xī Xiān. Bitter in flavor and cold in nature.

[Actions] Dispel wind-dampness, unblock the channels and collaterals, and strengthen the sinews and bones. It is applicable for wind-damp *bì* pattern, pain in the joint, numbness of the limbs, weakness of the legs, post-stroke paralysis of the limbs, carbuncles, swellings, sores, toxins, eczema, and itching. Clinically, it is often used together with Chòu Wú Tóng (Clerodendri Trichotomi) to generate synergistic effect. This herb contains bitter glycosides and has an anti-inflammatory effect. Its water solution can lower blood pressure.

[Quality] Collected before blossom in summer and dried under sunshine. Good quality is dry and green with many leaves and tender stems.

[Indications]

1. Wind-damp *bì* pain: Xī Xiān Cǎo (Herba Siegesbeckiae), capable of dispersing wind-damp, is used together with Chòu Wú Tóng (Clerodendri Trichotomi) for pain in the sinews and bones and muscle contracture in the limbs caused by wind-damp. Owning to its cold nature, it is considered

more suitable for damp-heat predominance. However, it can also be used for treating the cold-damp natured when combined with Qiāng Huó (Rhizoma et Radix Notopterygii), Dú Huó (Radix Angelicae Pubescentis), and Guì Zhī (Ramulus Cinnamomi).

2. Atrophy and weakness of the limbs: Xī Xiān Cǎo (Herba Siegesbeckiae), capable of strengthening the sinews and bones, is applicable not only for reduced mobility of the sinews and bones caused by wind-damp but also post-stroke hemiplegia, atrophy, weakness, or numbness of the limbs in a combination with medicinals that strengthen the sinews and bones such as Sāng Jì Shēng (Herba Taxilli), Chuān Xù Duàn (Radix Dipsaci), and Gǒu Jǐ (Rhizoma Cibotii).

3. Hypertension: Xī Xiān Cǎo (Herba Siegesbeckiae) is capable of lowering blood pressure and particularly suitable for hypertension patient with numbness of the limbs and soreness and weakness of the waist and knee, either by decocting the single herb or in a combination with Chòu Wú Tóng (Clerodendri Trichotomi).

4. Wind-damp itching: it can be prepared into decoction for external wash to treat unremitting skin itching of rubella and eczema.

[Usage and Dosage] Use raw for dispelling wind-dampness, and treat with yellow wine and steam it until it is cooked for strengthening the sinew and bone. Use 10–15g in decoction.

[Mnemonics] Xī Xiān Cǎo (Herba Siegesbeckiae, Siegesbeckia): cold; cure *bì* and lower blood pressure when combined with Chòu Wú Tóng (Folium Clerodendri), and relieve itching.

[Simple and Effective Formulas]

1. 豨桐丸 Xī Tóng Wán — Siegesbeckia and Firmianae Pill from *Experience Compilations of Health Cultivation* (养生经验合集, Yǎng Shēng Jīng Yàn Hé Jí): Chòu Wú Tóng (Folium Clerodendri) 500g and Xī Xiān Cǎo (Herba Siegesbeckiae) 240g; grind into powder, prepare into phoenix tree seed-sized pill with honey, and take 12 pills/time with boiled water, twice a day, morning and evening for oral administration to treat weakness, soreness and pain in feet failing to walk or muscle contracture in both hands failing to raising up caused by externally-contracted wind-damp pathogen

with internally-generated dampness affecting the channels and collaterals in the limbs. Also applicable for different types of joint pain, weakness of the lower limbs, and hypertension.

2. 豨莶丸 Xī Xiān Wán-Siegesbeckia Pill from *Fang's Orthodox Lineage of Pulses* (方脉正宗, Fāng Mài Zhèng Zōng): Xī Xiān Cǎo (Herba Siegesbeckiae) (steamed with wine, exposed under sunshine 9 times) 1500g, two Qí Shé (Agkistrodon), Rén Shēn (Radix et Rhizoma Ginseng) 240g, Huáng Qí (Radix Astragali) 240g, Gǒu Qǐ Zǐ (Fructus Lycii) 240g, Bì Xiè (Rhizoma Dioscoreae Hypoglaucae) 240g, Bái Zhú (Rhizoma Atractylodis Macrocephalae) 240g, body of Dāng Guī (Radix Angelicae Sinensis) 240g, Cāng ěr Zǐ (Fructus Xanthii) 120g, Chuān Xiōng (Rhizoma Chuanxiong) 120g, Wēi Líng Xiān (Radix et Rhizoma Clematidis) 120g, Bàn Xià Qū (Rhizoma Pinelliae Fermentata) 120g, and Chén Xiāng (Lignum Aquilariae Resinatum) 60g; grind into fine powder, prepare into phoenix tree seed-sized pill with honey, and take 9g/dose with boiled water for oral administration, twice a day, morning and evening to treat post-stroke deviated mouth and eyes, paralysis of the limbs, sluggish speech, slobbering, and weakness in the waist and legs.

[Precautions] Treat Xī Xiān Cǎo (Herba Siegesbeckiae) with wine to improve its ability of strengthen the sinews and bones.

Daily practices

1. What are the indications of Wēi Líng Xiān (Radix et Rhizoma Clematidis), Fáng Jǐ (Radix Stephaniae Tetrandrae), and Xī Xiān Cǎo (Herba Siegesbeckiae) besides relieving *bì* pattern?
2. What precautions should be taken when using Dú Huó (Radix Angelicae Pubescentis) and Wēi Líng Xiān (Radix et Rhizoma Clematidis)?

木瓜 Mù Guā *fructus chaenomelis chinese quince fruit*

The source is from the ripe fruit of deciduous shrub *Chaenomeles lagenaria* (Loisel.) Koidz., *C. sinensis* (Thouin) Koehne or *Chaenomeles speciosa* (Sweet), family Rosaceae. Sour in flavor and warm in nature. Alternate names include 木瓜实 Mù Guā Shí.

[Actions] Dispel wind and eliminate dampness, relax the sinews and unblock the collaterals, and harmonize the stomach and remove phlegm. It is applicable for spasm due to damp *bì*, soreness, heaviness, and pain in the waist and knee joint, vomiting and diarrhea with spasm, and leg qi with edema. This herb contains saponin, malic acid, tartaric acid, citric acid, vitamin C, tannin and flavonoid glycoside. Its decoction has shown a significant anti-inflammatory and swelling-reducing effect on egg albumin-induced arthritis of mice.

[Quality] Washed clean, soaked slightly and moistened thoroughly, steamed in the steamer tub until well-done, cut into slices while it is hot, and exposed to the air day and night until the red color turns into purplish black. Good quality is thick, sour, and firm with wrinkled peel and a purplish red color. The herb produced in Xuancheng of Anhui is even-sized, solid, and thick with best quality and has, therefore, been regarded as a genuine regional medicinal.

[Indications]

1. Vomiting, diarrhea, abdominal pain, and spasm: cholera patients suffer from severe vomiting and diarrhea with accompanying abdominal pain, and muscle contracture, especially in the crural muscle. The combination of herbs is based on the nature of the disorder, Mù Guā (Fructus Chaenomelis) is combined with Wú Zhū Yú (Fructus Evodiae), Zǐ Sū Yè (Folium Perillae), and Shēng Jiāng (Rhizoma Zingiberis Recens) for the cold-natured disorder through warming the middle *jiao*, removing dampness, and soothing the sinews; with Cán Shā (Faeces Bombycis), Huáng Lián (Rhizoma Coptidis), and Zhī Zǐ (Fructus Gardeniae) for the hot-natured via clearing heat, draining dampness, and soothing the sinews. Also applicable for muscle cramps and convulsions in the leg caused by other reasons.
2. Painful *bì* pattern: owning to its wind-damp dispelling and sinew-soothing properties, Mù Guā (Fructus Chaenomelis) is effective on *bì* pattern caused by wind-damp. It is combined with Niú Xī (Radix Achyranthis Bidentatae), Wǔ Jiā Pí (Cortex Acanthopanacis), and Yì Yǐ

Rén (Semen Coicis) for damp *bì* with spasms; and with medicinals that supplement and boost qi and blood for prolonged *bì* pattern with atrophy and weakness of the sinews and bones.

[Usage and Dosage] Use raw in general, stir-frying to strengthen its ability to soothe the sinew and harmonize the spleen and stomach, 5–9g in decoction, and decrease the dosage in pill and powder.

[Mnemonics] Mù Guā (Fructus Chaenomelis, Chinese Quince Fruit): sour and warm; relieve dampness, relax the sinews, cure *bì* pain, relieve cholera, and eliminate cramp.

[Simple and Effective Formulas]

1. 木瓜汤-Mù Guā Tāng — Pawpaw Decoction from *Treatise on Diseases, Patterns, and Formulas Related to the Unification of the Three Etiologies* (三因方, Sān Yīn Fāng): dried Mù Guā (Fructus Chaenomelis) 30g, Wú Zhū Yú (Fructus Evodiae) 15g, Xiǎo Huí Xiāng (Fructus Foeniculi) 0.3g, and Zhì Gān Cǎo (Radix et Rhizoma Glycyrrhizae Praeparata cum Melle) 3g; grind into fine powder, decoct 12g/dose with Shēng Jiāng (Rhizoma Zingiberis Recens) three pieces and Zǐ Sū Yè (Folium Perillae) 10 pieces in water for oral administration before meals to treat vomiting and diarrhea with spasms.
2. 木瓜丸-Mù Guā Wán — Pawpaw Pill from *Formulas from Royal Institute of Medicine* (Yù Yào Yuàn Fāng, 御药院方): Niú Xī (Radix Achyranthis Bidentatae) (soaked in warm wine, baked, cut into slices) 60g, one Mù Guā (Fructus Chaenomelis) (tip and melon pulp removed, add Ài Yè (Folium Artemisiae Argyi) 30g, steamed until it is well-done), Bā Jǐ Tiān (Radix Morindae Officinalis) 30g, Xiǎo Huí Xiāng (Fructus Foeniculi) 30g, Mù Xiāng (Radix Aucklandiae) 30g, and Guì Xīn Guì Xīn (Cortex Cinnamomi) 15g; grind into powder, make into phoenix tree seed-sized pill with honey, and take 20 pills with specially-prepared salt soup for oral administration to treat lumbago and weakness in the sinews and bones.

[Precautions] Mù Guā (Fructus Chaenomelis), sour and astringent, is contraindicated in cases of accumulation and difficult urination.

桑寄生 Sāng Jì Shēng *herba taxilli chinese taxillus*

The source is from the branch and leaf of evergreen undershrub *Taxillus chinensis* (DC.) *Danser* or *Taxillus sutchuensensis* (Lecomte) *danser*, family Loranthaceae. Bitter in flavor and neutral in nature. Alternate names include 寄生 Jì Shēng.

[Actions] Tonify the liver and kidneys, remove wind-dampness, strengthen the sinews and bones, and calm the fetus. It is applicable for wind-damp *bì* pain, soreness and weakness of the waist and knee, vaginal bleeding during pregnancy, and restless fetus. This herb contains quercetin, avicularin, and flavonoid materials. With antihypertensive, coronary artery-diluting, and diuretic effects, it cannot directly dilate the vessel of *ex vivo* blood vessels of healthy rabbits, but has a pronounced vessel dilator effect on *ex vivo* blood vessels in the ear of cholesterol angiosclerotic rabbits. Mistletoe contains maily oleanolic acid and flavonoids compounds, parmocological experiments reveal that ethanol lixivium of the fresh leaf can lower blood pressure for one hour when given subcutaneously to anesthetized rabbits and dogs.

[Quality] Cut into segments. The quality goods is from *Taxillus chinensis* (DC.) *Danser* on old mulberry trees with branches and leaves, but its output is small and mostly limited to southern China, and the commonly-used on is the branches and leaves of *Taxillus sutchuensensis* (Lecomte) *danser* on a variety of deciduous trees. For *Taxillus chinensis* (DC.) *Danser,* good quality is thin, young, and reddish brown, and has many leaves; while for *Taxillus sutchuensensis* (Lecomte) *danser*, good quality is tender and yellowish green, and has many leaves.

[Indications]

1. Lumbago and knee weakness: it refers lack of strength with numbness, soreness, or pain in the waist and lower extremities, which is commonly occur in the elderly and people with liver-kidney deficiency and often accompanied with hypertension, arteriosclerosis, and edema in the lower limbs. Patients always feel heavy head and light feet and cannot walk for a long period of time. If that is the case, Sāng Jì Shēng (Herba Taxilli) is combined with Niú Xī (Radix Achyranthis Bidentatae) and Dù Zhòng (Cortex Eucommiae).

2. Habitual miscarriage or threatened miscarriage: most cases are accompanied with vaginal bleeding or abdominal pain, Sāng Jì Shēng (Herba Taxilli) is usually combined with Ē Jiāo (Colla Corii Asini), Tù Sī Zǐ (Semen Cuscutae), Chuān Xù Duàn (Radix Dipsaci), and Fú Líng (Poria).

Nowadays, it has been widely used in the treatment of hypertension, especially for patients with vertigo, tinnitus, soreness and weakness of the waist and knee.

[Usage and Dosage] Use raw in general, when used for curing rheumatic diseases and strengthening the sinew and bone, it is fried with wine to strengthen its ability to unblock the collaterals and dispel wind-dampness. Use 12–20g in decoction.

[Mnemonics] Sāng Jì Shēng (Herba Taxilli, Chinese Taxillus): bitter and neutral; tonify the liver and kidneys, strengthen the sinews and bones, and calm the fetus.

[Simple and Effective Formulas]

1. 寿胎丸 Shòu Tāi Wán — Miscarriage Preventing Pill from *Records of Chinese Medicine with Reference to Western Medicine* (医学衷中参西录, Yī Xué Zhōng Zhōng Cān Xī Lù): Sāng Jì Shēng (Herba Taxilli) 15g, Tù Sī Zǐ (Semen Cuscutae) 12g, Chuān Xù Duàn (Radix Dipsaci) 12g, and Ē Jiāo (Colla Corii Asini) 10g; prepare into pill with honey or decoct in water for oral administration to treat habitual miscarriage with abdominal pain and vaginal bleeding.

2. 止痢方-Zhǐ Lì Fāng — Dysentery Arresting Formula from *Yang's Life Saving Formula* (杨氏护命方, Yáng Shì Hù Mìng Fāng): Sāng Jì Shēng (Herba Taxilli) 60g, Fáng Fēng (Radix Saposhnikoviae) 7.5g, Chuān Xiōng (Rhizoma Chuanxiong) 7.5g, androasted Gān Cǎo (Radix et Rhizoma Glycyrrhizae) 9g; grind into fine powder and decoct 6g/time in water for oral administration to treat toxin dysentery with stool containing pus and blood.

[Precautions] Sāng Jì Shēng (Herba Taxilli) should be used with cautions as liver dysfunction of some schizophrenia patients who take its decoction or injection has been reported.

五加皮 Wŭ Jiā Pí *cortex acanthopanacis eleutherococcus root bark*

The source is from the root cortex of deciduous undershrub *Acanthopanax gracilistylis* W. W. Smith, family Araliaceae, or liana *Periploca sepium* Bunge, family Asclepiadaceae. The former is called 南五加皮 Nán Wŭ Jiā Pí, and the latter 北五加皮 Běi Wŭ Jiā Pí or 香加皮 Xiāng Jiā Pí. Pungent and bitter in flavor and warm in nature.

[Actions] Dispel wind-dampness, tonify the liver and kidneys, and strengthen the sinews and bones. It is applicable for wind-damp bì pain, atrophy and weakness of the sinews and bones, retarded walking in children, lack of strength, edema, and leg qi. *Acanthopanax gracilistylis* contains volatile oil and tannin, whereas 香加皮 Xiāng Jiā Pí contains periplocoside, 4-methyl salicyladehyde, α and β amyrin, and acetate, and has shown anti-inflammatory effect on experimental arthritis of rats. Its ingredient periplocoside has a digitalis-like cardiotonic effect.

[Quality] 南五加皮 Nán Wŭ Jiā Pí and 北五加皮 Běi Wŭ Jiā Pí have similar actions of dispelling wind-damp, however, comparatively, 南五加皮 Nán Wŭ Jiā Pí is more potent in dispelling wind-damp and strengthening the sinews and bones, and 北五加皮 Běi Wŭ Jiā Pí is more effective in draining dampness and reducing swelling and has certain toxicity. Good quality is large, thick, and aromatic without a woodycenter.

[Indications]

1. Different types of *bì* pain: wind-damp may cause joint pain, soreness and weakness of the waist and knee, and powerlessness of the lower extremites. Wŭ Jiā Pí (Cortex Acanthopanacis) can be taken as a medical wine or together with medicinals that dispel wind-damp and strengthen the sinews and bones such as Gŏu Jĭ (Rhizoma Cibotii), Sāng Jì Shēng (Herba Taxilli), and Dú Huó (Radix Angelicae Pubescentis) in a decoction.

2. Liver-kidney deficiency: Wŭ Jiā Pí (Cortex Acanthopanacis) can also supplement the liver and kidney. It is combined with medicinals that supplement the liver and kidney and strengthen the sinews and bones such as Dù Zhòng (Cortex Eucommiae), Chuān Xù Duàn (Radix

Dipsaci), and Niú Xī (Radix Achyranthis Bidentatae) for soreness and weakness of the waist and knee and retarded walking in children caused by liver and kidney insufficiency.

3. Edema: Wǔ Jiā Pí (Cortex Acanthopanacis) can uninhibit water and reduce swelling and is combined with Fú Líng Pí (Cutis Poriae), Dà Fù Pí (Pericarpium Arecae), and Shēng Jiāng Pí (Cortex Zingiberis Rhizomatis) for edema due to water-dampness retention.

香五加 Xiāng Wǔ Jiā is used in the treatment of congestive heart-failure as its ingredient periplocoside is cardiotonic.

[Usage and Dosage] Use raw in most cases, 6–15g in decoction, and do not overdose as it is toxic.

[Mnemonics] Nán Běi Wǔ Jiā (Cortex Acanthopanacis, Eleutherococcus Root Bark): relieve *bì* pain, strengthen the sinews and bone, drain dampness, and relieve edema.

[Simple and Effective Formulas]

1. 五加皮丸 Wǔ Jiā Pí Wán — Cortex Acanthopanacis Pill from *Treasured Household Formulas for Health* (卫生家宝方, Wèi Shēng Jiā Bǎo Fāng): Wǔ Jiā Pí (Cortex Acanthopanacis) and Dù Zhòng (Cortex Eucommiae) in equal dosage; grind into powder, prepare into phoenix tree seed-sized pill with wine-paste, and take 30 pills/dose with warm wine for oral administration to treat lumbago.

2. 五加皮散 Wǔ Jiā Pí Sǎn — Cortex Acanthopanacis Powder from *Essentials of Infant Care* (保婴撮要, Bǎo Yīng Cuō Yào): Wǔ Jiā Pí (Cortex Acanthopanacis), Chuān Niú Xī (Radix Cyathulae) (soaked in wine for two days), and Mù Guā (Fructus Chaenomelis) in equal dosage; make into powder, take 6g/dose with rice soup on an empty stomach, twice a day, and take with wine sometimes to improve its therapeutic effect on 4- or 5-year-old children who still cannot walk.

[Precautions] Wǔ Jiā Pí (Cortex Acanthopanacis), especially 北五加皮 Běi Wǔ Jiā Pí, warm and dry in nature, can readily injure yin and stir fire. It is contraindicated in the cases of yin deficiency with internal heat. The poisoning symptoms of 北五加皮 Běi Wǔ Jiā Pí include vomiting, nausea, and diarrhea, which can be alleviated or will disappear when stop using. Overdosing may cause bradycardia, then tremor of the body, and eventually paralysis and death.

Daily practices

1. What are the similarities and differences among Mù Guā (Fructus Chaenomelis), Sāng Jì Shēng (Herba Taxilli), and Wǔ Jiā Pí (Cortex Acanthopanacis) in terms of actions and indications?
2. What are the other indications of wind-damp relieving medicinal apart from curing disorder caused by wind-damp?

蚕砂 Cán Shā *feces bombycis silkworm feces*

The source is from the feces of silkworm larvae, family Bombycidae. Sweet and pungent in flavor and warm in nature. Alternate names include 晚蚕砂 Wǎn Cán Shā, 原蚕砂 Yuán Cán Shā, and 蚕矢 Cán Shǐ.

[Actions] Dispel wind and remove dampness, and harmonize the stomach and transform turbidity. It is applicable for rheumatic disease induced pain, acute vomiting, diarrhea, abdominal pain, and spasm and pain of gastrocnemius muscle.

[Quality] Collected in summer, dried under sunshine, and impurities removed. Good quality is intact, black, firm, dry, and without impurity.

[Indications]

1. Wind-damp *bì* pain: Cán Shā (Feces Bombycis) is good at dispelling dampness and usually used for wind-damp *bì* pattern. It is combined with Qiāng Huó (Rhizoma et Radix Notopterygii), Dú Huó (Radix Angelicae Pubescentis), Wēi Líng Xiān (Radix et Rhizoma Clematidis), and Guì Zhī (Ramulus Cinnamomi) for wind-cold-damp *bì*; with Fáng Jǐ (Radix Stephaniae Tetrandrae), Yì Yǐ Rén (Semen Coicis), Huá Shí (Talcum), and Zhī Zǐ (Fructus Gardeniae) for damp-heat *bì*. It can also be stir-fried until hot and then applied on the painful area.
2. Vomiting, diarrhea, and spasm: Cán Shā (Feces Bombycis), capable of relieving turbidity to harmonize the stomach, is effective in the treatment of vomiting, diarrhea, and spasms of gastrocnemius muscle

following severe vomiting and diarrhea due to externally-contacted damp and turbidity.

Owning to its potency of dispelling dampness, it is also effective in treating eczema and skin itching, either via oral administration or external wash. This medicinal is also used in the treatment of white leukorrhea, amenorrhea, and eye problems.

[Usage and Dosage] Use raw in general for oral administration, 4–10g in decoction, and wrap in cheesecloth before decocting.

[Mnemonics] Cán Shā (Feces Bombycis, Silkworm Feces): sweet and pungent; transform turbidity, raise the clear, and good at curing *bì* pain, vomiting, diarrhea, and cramp.

[Simple and Effective Formulas]

1. 宣痹汤 Xuān Bì Tāng — Painful Obstruction Resolving Decoction from *Systematic Differentiation of Warm Diseases* (温病条辨, Wēn Bìng Tiáo Biàn): Fáng Jǐ (Radix Stephaniae Tetrandrae) 15g, Xìng Rén (Semen Armeniacae Amarum) 15g, Huá Shí (Talcum) 15g, Lián Qiào (Fructus Forsythiae) 9g, Zhī Zǐ (Fructus Gardeniae) 9g, Bàn Xià (Rhizoma Pinelliae) (stir-fried with vinegar) 9g, Cán Shā (Feces Bombycis) 9g, and Chì Xiǎo Dòu Pí (Testa Phaseoli) 9g; decoct in water for oral administration to treat damp-heat accumulating in the channels and collaterals manifested as shivering with high fever, vexing pain in the joints, grayish tongue, and sallow complexion.

2. 蚕砂汤 Cán Shā Tāng — Silkworm Feces Decoction from *Long-mu's Ophthalmology* (眼科龙木论 Yǎn Kē Lóng Mù Lùn): Cán Shā (Feces Bombycis) (stir-fried) 120g, Bā Jǐ Tiān (Radix Morindae Officinalis) 90g, and Mǎ Lìn Huā (Flos Iridis Chinensis) 90g; grind into fine powder and take 6g/dose with wine for oral administration when necessary to treat eye problems and tearing on exposure to wind.

[Precautions] Cán Shā (Feces Bombycis) is contraindicated for pain in the sinews, bones, and joints caused by blood deficiency.

海桐皮 Hǎi Tóng Pí *cortex erythrinae erythrina bark*

The source is from the bark of evergreen arbor *Erythrina indica* Lam., family Leguminosae. Bitter and pungent in flavor and neutral in nature.

[Actions] Dispel wind-dampness, and unblock the channels and collaterals. It is applicable for wind-damp *bì* pain, spasm of the limbs, and pain in the waist and knee pain. This herb can also kill parasites and arrest itching and be applied externally to cure scabies and eczema. This herb contains erythraline, erysodine, amino acid, and organic acid. Its infusion has *in vitro* inhibitory effects on common pathogenic dermatophyte and a variety of bacteria.

[Quality] Good quality is dry, thin, wide, and long with many spikes.

[Indications]

1. Wind-damp *bì* pain: Hǎi Tóng Pí (Cortex Erythrinae) can dispel wind-damp, arrest *bì* pain, and sooth spasm, and therefore is effective on wind-damp induced pain in the muscle, joint, waist and knee. It is combined with Niú Xī (Radix Achyranthis Bidentatae), Yì Yǐ Rén (Semen Coicis), and Wǔ Jiā Pí (Cortex Acanthopanacis) for wind-damp *bì* pain; with Fáng Jǐ (Radix Stephaniae Tetrandrae), Mù Tōng (Caulis Akebiae), and Jīn Yín Huā Téng (Caulis Lonicerae Japonicae) for damp-heat *bì* pain; and with Chuān Xù Duàn (Radix Dipsaci), Shú Dì Huáng (Radix Rehmanniae Praeparata), Sāng Jì Shēng (Herba Taxilli), and Gǒu Jǐ (Rhizoma Cibotii) when accompanied with liver kidney deficiency. It can also be decocted with other medicinals that unblock the collaterals and relieve *bì* for external wash to treat joint swelling and pain and muscle contracture.
2. Skin itching: Hǎi Tóng Pí (Cortex Erythrinae) is potent in dispelling wind to arrest itching and applicable for itching caused by scabies and eczema. Use decoction for external wash or grind into powder for external application.

[Usage and Dosage] Use raw in general for oral administration, 6–12g in decoction.

[Mnemonics] Hǎi Tóng Pí (Cortex Erythrinae, Erythrina Bark): bitter and pungent; good at dispelling wind-damp, remove *bì* pain, and relieve itching skin.

[Simple and Effective Formulas]

1. 海桐皮散 Hǎi Tóng Pí Sǎn — Erythrina Bark Powder from *General Guide to the Therapeutic Methods of Leg Qi* (脚气治法总论, Jiǎo Qì Zhì Fǎ Zǒng Lùn): Hǎi Tóng Pí (Cortex Erythrinae) 30g, Líng Yáng Jiǎo (Cornu Saigae Tataricae) scraps 60g, Yì Yǐ Rén (Semen Coicis) 60g, Fáng Fēng (Radix Saposhnikoviae) 30g, Qiāng Huó (Rhizoma et Radix Notopterygii) 30g, Tǒng Guì (Cortex Cinnamomi) (peel removed) 30g, Chì Fú Ling (Poria Rubra) (peel removed) 30g, Shú Dì Huáng (Radix Rehmanniae Praeparata) 30g, and Huáng Bīng Láng (Semen Arecae) 30g; grind into powder and decoct 9g/dose with Shēng Jiāng (Rhizoma Zingiberis Recens) five pieces in water for oral administration to treat wind-damp induced swollen, painful and heavy legs, and contracture and pain in the joint and muscle.

2. 海桐皮散 Hǎi Tóng Pí Sǎn-Erythrina Bark Powder from *General Guide to Infantile Health* (Xiǎo ér Wèi Shēng 小儿卫生总微论, Zǒng Wēi Lùn): Hǎi Tóng Pí (Cortex Erythrinae) 30g, Dāng Guī (Radix Angelicae Sinensis) 30g, Mǔ Dān Pí (Cortex Moutan) 30g, Shú Dì Huáng (Radix Rehmanniae Praeparata) 30g, Niú Xī (Radix Achyranthis Bidentatae) 30g, Shān Zhū Yú (Fructus Corni) 15g, and Bǔ Gǔ Zhī (Fructus Psoraleae) 15g; grind into fine powder and decoct 3g/dose with Cōng Bái (Bulbus Allii Fistulosi) 2/3 decimeter in water for oral administration to treat leg spasm failing to extend in children.

[Precautions] Hǎi Tóng Pí (Cortex Erythrinae) is contraindicated in cases of blood deficiency but with absence of wind-damp.

白花蛇 Bái Huā Shé *agkistrodon agkistrodon*

The source is from the whole dried body without internal organs of *Agkistrodon acutus* (Gunther), family Viperidae. Sweet and salty in flavor and warm in nature with toxicity. Alternate names include 蕲蛇 Qí Shé and 大白花蛇 Dà Bái Huā Shé.

[Actions] Extinguish wind and activate the collaterals, tranquilize the spasm, and relieve toxicity. It is applicable for wind-damp persistent *bì*, numbness, contracture, post-stroke deviated mouth and eyes, hemiplegia, spasm, convulsion, tetanus, leprosies, and scabies. The poison gland in its head contains large amount of hemotoxin, small amount of neurotoxicant, and micro amount of hemolystic and procoagulant components. It has shown sedative, hypnotic, and antalgic effect on mice, and can directly dilate vessel to decrease blood pressure.

[Quality] Good quality is large, completely intact, and thick with a clear pattern. 金钱白花蛇 Jīn Qián Bái Huā Shé (Bungarus Parvus), also known as 小白花蛇 Xiǎo Bái Huā Shé, is from the whole dried body without internal organs of infant *Bungarus multicinctus*, family Elapidae. Its nature, flavors, and actions are similar to but more potent than these of Bái Huā Shé (Agkistrodon).

[Indications]

1. Wind-damp *bì* pain: Bái Huā Shé (Agkistrodon) is good at scattering and penetrating inward to the *zang-fu* organs and outward to the skin and effective in the treatment of wind-damp *bì* pattern. It is often pre-scribed together with Fáng Fēng (Radix Saposhnikoviae), Qiāng Huó (Rhizoma et Radix Notopterygii), and Dāng Guī (Radix Angelicae Sinensis) for wind-damp intractable *bì* with skin numbness and bone contracture.
2. Sroke hemiplegia: Bái Huā Shé (Agkistrodon) can sooth and unblock the channels and collaterals to promote recovery from post-stroke hemiplegia and is usually used together with Huáng Qí (Radix Astragali), Dāng Guī (Radix Angelicae Sinensis), and Bái Sháo (Radix Paeoniae Alba).
3. Convulsion and tetanus: Bái Huā Shé (Agkistrodon) can dispel external wind and extinguish internal wind with a potency of arresting spasm. It is used in different types of spasm, such as infantile convulsion and

tetanus, in a combination with Wū Shāo Shé (Zaocys), Wú Gōng (Scolopendra), and Gōu Téng (Ramulus Uncariae Cum Uncis).

Owning to its potent wind-damp dispelling and toxins-resolving effect, it is applicable for different types of skin problems such as intractable tinea, prurigo, toxic boils, and leprosies.

[Usage and Dosage] If used in decoction, use 3–6g, decrease the dosage in pill and powder, often used in pill and powder or soaked with wine, owing to the limited medicated resource and necessity of long-term consumption.

[Mnemonics] *Bái Huā Shé* (Agkistrodon, Agkistrodon): warm; dispel wind, unblock the collaterals, cure *bì* pain and paralysis, and arrest convulsion.

[Simple and Effective Formulas]

1. 定命散 Dìng Mìng Sǎn — Life Saving Powder from *Comprehensive Recording of Divine Assistance* (圣济总录, Shèng Jì Zǒng Lù): one Wú Gōng (Scolopendra), Wū Shāo Shé (Zaocys) 2/3 decimeter, and Bái Huā Shé (Agkistrodon) (soaked in wine, bone removed, wine-fried) 2/3 decimeter; grind into fine powder and take 6g/dose after mixing with boiled wine for oral administration to treat tetanus, tight, stiff and hard neck, and body rigidity.

2. 地骨皮散 Dì Gǔ Pí Sǎn — Chinese Wolfberry Root-bark Powder from *Comprehensive Recording of Divine Assistance* (圣济总录, Shèng Jì Zǒng Lù): Dì Gǔ Pí (Cortex Lycii) 0.3g, Bái Huā Shé (Agkistrodon) (soaked in wine, roasted, skin and bone removed) 30g, Tiān Nán Xīng (Rhizoma Arisaematis) (cut, baked) 30g, Jīng Jiè Suì (Spica Schizonepetae) 60g, and Shí Gāo (Gypsum Fibrosum) (ground) 60g; grind into fine powder and take 3g/dose with water for oral administration after meal to treat paroxysmal headache or migraine.

[Precautions] Bái Huā Shé (Agkistrodon), warm and dry in nature, tends to damage yin and stir fire. It is therefore contraindicated in cases of yin and blood deficiency with internal heat and should be use with caution by people with weak constitution and post-stoke deficiency pattern.

Daily practices

1. What are similarities and differences among Cán Shā (Feces Bombycis), Hǎi Tóng Pí (Cortex Erythrinae), and Bái Huā Shé (Agkistrodon) into actions and indications?

2. Among medicinals that dispel wind-damp, which ones are cold and cool in nature and which ones are hot and warm in nature? What are the differences between them in indications?

2

AROMATIC MEDICINALS THAT REMOVE DAMPNESS

Medicinals that dispel damp pathogen are divided into four major classes, namely medicinal that clear heat and dry dampness (see chapter 3), wind-damp dispelling medicinal (see chapter 5), aromatic herbs that transform dampness, and diuresis-promoting medicinals with bland flavor. Among them, aromatic medicinals that remove dampness are named after their fragrance, most of them are acrid, warm, and dry in properties, and can move qi to transform dampness, and boost the spleen to assist transportation. They are primarily used for dampness pathogen obstruction in the middle *jiao*, dampness encumbering the spleen, dampness obstruction and qi stagnation, and spleen and stomach failing to transform and transport. The primarily manifestations are gastric oppression, abdominal distention, nausea, vomiting, lack of appetite, tiredness and heaviness of the extremities, loose stool, sticky feeling and sweet taste in the mouth, and greasy tongue coating. Included in this group are some herbs that can relieve summerheat and turbidity, and used for treating such febrile diseases as damp-warm and summerheat-damp.

These herbs are often used together with herbs that move qi, as traditional Chinese medicine holds that qi movement can help to resolve water retention and dampness in the body. They are also generally combined with bland medicinals that percolate and drain dampness. Frequently, damp complicates other mechanisms, such as cold and heat. When dampness is compatible with warm pathogens, patients may experience preponderance of dampness over heat, then equal prominence of dampness and heat when dampness transforms into heat, preponderance of heat over dampness, and eventually transformation into dryness to generate fire. Herbs that aromatically dispel wind-dampness are selected in accordance with the nature of the disorders. They are combined with medicinals that warm yang to relieving damp for cold dampness pattern; and with herbs that clear heat for damp-heat.

These herbs are warm and dry in nature, and therefore should be used with caution in cases of yin consumption. They are aromatic and rich in volatile oil. For this reason, if used in decoction, they should not be over-cooked to prevent loss of active ingredients.

苍术 Cāng Zhú *rhizoma atractylodis atractylodes rhizome*

The source is from the rhizome of herbaceous perennial *Atractylodes lancea* (Thunb.) DC. or *Atractylodes chinensis* (DC.) koidz., family Compositae. Pungent and bitter in flavor and warm in nature.

[Actions] Tonify the spleen and dry dampness, expel wind and dissipate cold, and improve vision. Its volatile oil contains mainly atractylol and atractylon. At a small dosage, volatile oil induces sedation of frog, whereas higher amount has an inhibitory effect on nervus centralis resulting in respiratory paralysis and eventually death. Its extract has shown an hypoglycemic effect on rats and toad, its large dose can decrease blood pressure and has pronounced effect on the discharge of potassium and sodium, but none of significant diuretic effect has been noted.

[Quality] Impurities removed, soaked in rice-washed water or water until medium thoroughly, obtained and cut into slices, and dried under sunshine. 茅术 Máo Shù produced in Maoshan of Jiangsu is the best with clean aroma. Good quality is large, solid, aromatic, and has a yellowish brown cross-section with scattering oily drops, and collected in autumn or in summer before sprouting.

[Indications]

1. Dampness obstruction: damp physical constitution, exposure to a wet environment for long periods of time, externally-contracted coldness, or drinking too much cold all may cause dampness obstruction in the spleen and stomach with the manifestation of abdominal distention, abdominal

fullness, sallow complexion, vertigo, decreased appetite, heaviness of the limbs, lassitude, edema, thirst without desire to drink, diarrhea, dysentery or constipation, enlarged tongue with teeth marks on the margins and greasy tongue coating. This pattern is most likely to be found in disorder of digestive system, liver, gallbladder, and joint. Cāng Zhú (Rhizoma Atractylodis) is known as the principal medicinal that dry dampness and is often combined with Hòu Pò (Cortex Magnoliae Officinalis), Bàn Xià (Rhizoma Pinelliae), and Fú Líng (Poria).

2. Wind-damp *bì* pattern: Cāng Zhú (Rhizoma Atractylodis), pungent-to-disperse and bitter-to-dry in nature, can dispel and disperse wind-damp and particularly suitable for patients with soreness, heaviness, and pain of the muscle. Combination with other medicinals is bases on the state of illness, it is used together with Fù Zǐ (Radix Aconiti Lateralis Praeparata) and Guì Zhī (Ramulus Cinnamomi) for exuberant cold-damp; with Shí Gāo (Gypsum Fibrosum) and Zhī Mǔ (Rhizoma Anemarrhenae) for intense damp-heat with fever, profuse sweating, and joint soreness and pain; and Má Huáng (Herba Ephedrae) and Gān Cǎo (Radix et Rhizoma Glycyrrhizae) for wind-damp in the fleshy exterior manifested as aversion to cold, absence of sweating, edema, and joint swelling and pain; with Huáng Bǎi (Cortex Phellodendri Chinensis) and Yì Yǐ Rén (Semen Coicis) for lower limb redness, swelling, pain or soreness; and with Huáng Qí (Radix Astragali) and Gé Gēn (Radix Puerariae Lobatae) for thirst, edema, and hyperglycemia.

3. Nyctalopia: Cāng Zhú (Rhizoma Atractylodis) is rich in vitamin A substances and therefore applicable for nyctalopia, keratomalacia and rickets due to vitamin deficiency. It is very often cooked with the liver of animal or prepared into pill for oral administration.

Cāng Zhú (Rhizoma Atractylodis) and Bái Zhú (Rhizoma Atractylodis Macrocephalae) have similar indications, but Cāng Zhú (Rhizoma Atractylodis) tends to be scattering and regarded more effective in relieving abdominal distention, swelling, and fullness, joint swelling and pain, and thick tongue with greasy coating; whereas Bái Zhú (Rhizoma Atractylodis Macrocephalae) prones to be tonifying and more potent in fortifying the spleen and boosting qi with a good therapeutic effect on lassitude, lack of strength, and inhibited urination.

[Usage and Dosage] Use raw in general, stir-fry to counteract its drying property. Use 5–12g in decoction, and decrease the dosage as in pill and powder.

[Mnemonics] Cāng Zhú (Rhizoma Atractylodis, Atractylodes Rhizome): bitter and warm; specialized in damp encumbrance and can eliminate night blindness and wind-damp bì pattern.

[Simple and Effective Formulas]

1. 平胃散 Píng Wèi Sǎn — Stomach-Calming Powder from *the Formulas from the Imperial Pharmacy* (和剂局方, Hé Jì Jú Fāng): Cāng Zhú (Rhizoma Atractylodis) 10g, Hòu Pò (Cortex Magnoliae Officinalis) 6g, Gān Cǎo (Radix et Rhizoma Glycyrrhizae) 3g, and Chén Pí (Pericarpium Citri Reticulatae) 6g; decoct in water for oral administration to treat patients with distention and fullness in the chest and abdomen, poor appetite, vomiting, nausea, greasy feeling but bland taste in the mouth, diarrhea, dysentery, and white and greasy tongue coating. Also applicable for digestive system disorders, metabolic diseases, and skin problems with manifestations above.

2. 麻黄加术汤 Má Huáng Jiā Zhū Tāng — Ephedra plus Atractylodes Macrocephalae Decoction from *Essentials from the Golden Cabinet* (金匮要略, Jīn Guì Yào Lüè): Cāng Zhú (Rhizoma Atractylodis) 12g, Má Huáng (Herba Ephedrae) 6g, Guì Zhī (Ramulus Cinnamomi) 6g, Xìng Rén (Semen Armeniacae Amarum) 10g, and Gān Cǎo (Radix et Rhizoma Glycyrrhizae) 3g; decoct in water for oral administration to treat patients with aversion to cold, absence of sweating, and yellowish puffiness and pain of the joint.

3. 越婢加术汤 Yuè Bì Jiā Zhū Tāng — Maidservant from Yue Decoction plus Atractylodes Macrocephalae from *Essentials from the Golden Cabinet*(金匮要略, Jīn Guì Yào Lüè): Cāng Zhú (Rhizoma Atractylodis) 12g, Má Huáng (Herba Ephedrae) 6g, Shí Gāo (Gypsum Fibrosum) 12g, Gān Cǎo (Radix et Rhizoma Glycyrrhizae) 3g, Shēng Jiāng (Rhizoma Zingiberis Recens) three pieces, and ten Dà Zǎo (Fructus

Jujubae); decoct in water for oral administration to treat patients with edema throughout the body, aversion to wind, joint pain, sweating, and difficult urination. Also applicable for acute nephritis and arthritis.

[Precautions] Cāng Zhú (Rhizoma Atractylodis) is suitable when patients present yellowish puffiness complexion, especially in the morning, edema in the lower limbs with loose and soft muscle, heaviness in the body without desire to move, sweating on exertion, and higher risk of suffering vertigo, dizziness, loose or constipated stool, and body pain. It should be used with caution in cases of emaciation, red complexion, and red tongue with thin or scanty coating caused by yin deficiency with interior heat.

厚朴 Hòu Pò *cortex magnoliae officinalis magnolia bark*

The source is from dried bark of the stem, root, and branch of deciduous arbor *Magnolia officinalis* Rehd. et Wils. or *Magnolia officinalis* Rehd. et Wils. var. biloba Reld. et Wils., family Magnoliaceae. Bitter and pungent in flavor and warm in nature.

[Actions] Dry dampness and remove fullness, move qi to resolve distension, and direct rebelling qi downward to relieve wheezing. It is applicable for dampness accumulation in the middle *jiao*, gastric and abdominal distention and fullness, vomiting, diarrhea, food accumulation, abdominal distention, constipation, and cough and wheezing due to phlegm-rheum. This herb contains magnolol, magnocurarine, and volatile oil. Its decoction can reduce the tension of *ex vivo* intestinal canal of rabbit, mildly improve the rigidity of striated muscle, experiment reveals the mechanism lies on its anesthesia effect on the motor nerve ending of striated muscle and its excitatory effect on bronchus of rabbits. It has also shown certain antiulcer and antibacterial effects.

[Quality] The older the plant is, the thicker the bark is, the better the quality is. 紫油厚朴 Zǐ Yóu Hòu Pǔ produced in Sichuan and Hubei is the best. The herb produced in Sichuan is called 川朴 Chuān Pǔ. Good quality bark is thick, finely textured, oily, and aromatic, with a deep purple inner surface containing many shiny spots.

[Indications]

1. Dampness obstruction and food accumulation: Hòu Pò (Cortex Magnoliae Officinalis), capable of moving qi and drying dampness, is effective in abdominal distention and fullness, food accumulation, and indigestion caused by dampness obstruction in the middle *jiao*. It is combined with Cāng Zhú (Rhizoma Atractylodis) and Chén Pí (Pericarpium Citri Reticulatae) for moving qi and relieving distention; and with Zhǐ Shí (Fructus Aurantii Immaturus), Bīng Láng (Semen Arecae), and Dà Huáng (Radix et Rhizoma Rhei) for relieving food accumulation.
2. Phlegm-rheum cough and wheezing: Hòu Pò (Cortex Magnoliae Officinalis) can arrest wheezing and dissolve phlegm and is applicable for cough and wheezing with profuse sputum resulting from damp-phlegm obstruction in the lung. It is combined with Sū Zǐ (Fructus Perillae), Xìng Rén (Semen Armeniacae Amarum), and Lái Fú Zǐ (Semen Raphani) when accompanied with chest oppression, profuse sputum, and thick and greasy tongue coating.

[Usage and Dosage] Use raw in general, treat with ginger to strengthen its ability to warm the center and eliminate its irritability to the throat. Use 3–9g in decoction, 2–3g/time as in pill and powder.

[Mnemonics] Hòu Pò (Cortex Magnoliae Officinalis, Magnolia Bark): pungent and warm; move qi to relieve fullness, dampness obstruction, food accumulation, and arrest panting.

[Simple and Effective Formulas]

1. 厚朴三物汤 Hòu Pò Sān Wù Tāng — Three Substances Decoction with Official Magnolia Bark from *Treatise on Cold Damage* (伤寒论, Shāng Hán Lùn): Hòu Pò (Cortex Magnoliae Officinalis) 9g, Dà Huáng (Radix et Rhizoma Rhei) 5g, and Zhǐ Shí (Fructus Aurantii Immaturus) 6g; decoct in water for oral administration to treat patient with abdominal fullness and pain and inhibited defecation.

2. 平胃散 Píng Wèi Săn-Stomach — Calming Powder from *Formulas for Aiding the Universal Living* (博济方, Bó Jì Fāng): Hòu Pò (Cortex Magnoliae Officinalis) (coarse layer of bark removed, stir-fried with ginger juice until aromatic) 156g, Chén Pí (Pericarpium Citri Reticulatae) (white inner surface of exocarp removed) 156g, Cāng Zhú (Rhizoma Atractylodis) (coarse layer of bark removed, soaked in rice-washed water for two days) 250g, and Gān Căo (Radix et Rhizoma Glycyrrhizae) 90g; grind into fine powder, decoct 6–9g/time with Shēng Jiāng (Rhizoma Zingiberis Recens) 2 pieces and Dà Zăo (Fructus Jujubae) two pieces in water for oral administration to treat patient with dampness retention in the spleen and stomach manifested as gastric and abdominal distention and fullness, poor appetite, bland taste in the mouth, vomiting, nausea, belching, acid regurgitation, heaviness of the limbs, lassitude, somnolence, and white greasy tongue coating.

[Precautions] Hòu Pò (Cortex Magnoliae Officinalis) is generally used for excess pattern and contraindicated for people with qi and blood deficiency because its warm and drying property may deplete qi and blood. It should be used with caution during pregnancy as it can break stagnant qi and injure the fetus.

Daily practices

1. What is aromatic medicinal that remove dampness and what are the indications?
2. What are the actions and indications of Cāng Zhú (Rhizoma Atractylodis) and Hòu Pò (Cortex Magnoliae Officinalis)?

藿香 Huò Xiāng *herba agastachis agastache*

The source is from stem leaf of herbaceous annual or perennial *Agastache rugosa* (Fisch et Mey.) O. Ktze. or *Pogostemon cabin* (Blanco) Benth., family Labiatae. The former is called 土藿香 Tŭ Huò Xiāng and the latter 广藿香 Guăng Huò Xiāng. Pungent in flavor and slightly warm in nature.

[Actions] Remove dampness and harmonize the middle burner, and dispel summerheat and relieve the exterior. It is applicable for externally-contracted summerheat-damp pathogens, fever, aversion to cold, headache, chest oppression, gastric *pǐ*, vomiting, diarrhea, dysentery, malaria, and bad breath. Tǔ Huò Xiāng (Herba Agastachis) and Guǎng Huò Xiāng (Herba Pogostemonis) both contain volatile oil, the former mainly contains patchoulicalcohol, eugenol, and cinnamaldehyde, while the latter mainly contain methyl chavicol. Huò Xiāng (Herba Agastachis) has shown inhibitory and deactivated effect on rhinovirus, sedative effect on gastrointestinal nerve, and promotive effect on gastric juice secretion. Its lixivium has shown a relatively strong inhibitory effect on common dermatophyte *in vitro*.

[Quality] 土藿香 Tǔ Huò Xiāng produced in Jiangsu, Sichuan, Zhejiang, and Liaoning has a lighter taste when compared with 广藿香 Guǎng Huò Xiāng, good quality has many leaves and intense fragrance. While 广藿香 Guǎng Huò Xiāng is originally produced in southeast Asian countries such as Philippines, it now cultivated in Guangdong and Taiwan. Good quality has many leaves and slight bitter and pungent with a special aroma, in general, it is considered to be of better quality. Its stem can also be used as a medicinal and is considered more potent in arresting vomiting.

[Indications]

1. Summerheat-dampness: manifestations include lassitude, powerlessness, chest and abdominal fullness and oppression, poor appetite, nausea, vomiting, and diarrhea. Aromatic medicinals such as Huò Xiāng (Herba Agastachis) are applicable in this case. It is often combined with Zǐ Sū Yè (Folium Perillae) and Pèi Lán (Herba Eupatorii) for slight aversion to cold, abdominal pain, vomiting, diarrhea, and thin greasy tongue coating (especially for gastria and intestinal type of common cold); and with Huáng Qín (Radix Scutellariae) and Huá Shí (Talcum) for summerheat-dampness with heat predominance.
2. Vomiting due to damp-turbidity: it is common in vomiting during pregnancy. Huò Xiāng (Herba Agastachis) is usually combined with Bàn Xià (Rhizoma Pinelliae), Shēng Jiāng (Rhizoma Zingiberis Recens),

and Shā Rén (Fructus Amomi) when accompanied with chest oppression, nausea, and white and greasy tongue coating.

It is also applicable for halitosis due to its filth-dispelling effect.

[Usage and Dosage] Use raw in general, 6–12g in decoction, and use fresh for a better effect of relieving dampness.

[Mnemonics] Huò Xiāng (Herba Agastachis, Agastache): pungent and warm; aromatically remove summerheat-damp, harmonize the stomach, arrest vomiting, and dispel filthy turbidity.

[Simple and Effective Formulas]

1. 藿香正气散 Huò Xiāng Zhèng Qì Sǎn — Agastache Qi Correcting Powder from *Formulas from the Imperial Pharmacy* (和剂局方, Hé Jì Jú Fāng): Huò Xiāng (Herba Agastachis) 10g, Zǐ Sū Yè (Folium Perillae)10g, Hòu Pò (Cortex Magnoliae Officinalis) 5g, Chén Pí (Pericarpium Citri Reticulatae) 5g, Bàn Xià (Rhizoma Pinelliae) 6g, Gān Cǎo (Radix et Rhizoma Glycyrrhizae) 3g, Bái Zhǐ (Radix Angelicae Dahuricae) 6g, Dà Fù Pí (Pericarpium Arecae) 10g, Jié Gěng (Radix Platycodonis) 6g, and Bái Zhú (Rhizoma Atractylodis Macrocephalae) 10g; decoct in water for oral administration to treat cough and wheezing, aversion to cold, fever, abdominal pain, diarrhea, and vomiting. Also applicable for common cold in summer with vomiting and diarrhea or food poisoning-induced diarrhea.

2. 止吐方-Zhǐ Tǔ Fāng — Vomiting Arresting Formula from *Formulas from Benevolent Sages* (圣惠方 Shèng Huì Fāng): Huò Xiāng (Herba Agastachis) 10g, Xiāng Fù (Rhizoma Cyperi) 5g, and Gān Cǎo (Radix et Rhizoma Glycyrrhizae) 3g; decoct in water for oral administration to treat vomiting during pregnancy.

[Precautions] Huò Xiāng (Herba Agastachis) is aromatic and considered most potent in relieving nausea with greasy tongue coating. Warm in nature, it should be used with caution for internal heat or absence of dampness with dry tongue coating.

佩兰 Pèi Lán *herba eupatorii eupatorium*

The source is from the aerial part of herbaceous perennial *Eupatorium fortunei* Turcz., family Compositae. Alternate names include 省头草 Shěng Tóu Cǎo. Pungent in flavor and neutral in nature.

[Actions] Transform dampness and release summerheat, and aromatically remove turbidity. It is applicable for dampness retention in the middle *jiao* with sweet taste in the mouth, profuse drool, and bad breath, externally-contracted summerheat-damp, or damp-warm in early stage. This herb contains volatile oil, its ingredients musk ether and neryl acetate have shown a direct inhibitory effect on influenza virus.

[Quality] Good quality is dry and strongly aromatic with short stem and many green leaves and without inflorescence.

[Indications]

1. Dampness obstruction in the middle *jiao*: Pèi Lán (Herba Eupatorii) is applicable for gastric and abdominal *pǐ* and oppression, poor appetite, nausea, vomiting, lassitude, and white and greasy tongue coating due to dampness obstruction in the middle *jiao* and usually combined with Huò Xiāng (Herba Agastachis), Bái Dòu Kòu (Fructus Amomi Kravanh), and Hòu Pò (Cortex Magnoliae Officinalis).
2. Damp-heat encumbering the spleen: it is called Pí Dān (脾瘅, pyretic abundance) in traditional Chinese medicine, and its manifestations include sweet taste, greasy and sticky feeling in the mouth, increased salivation, and halitosis. If that is the case, Pèi Lán (Herba Eupatorii) can be decocted alone for oral administration.
3. Summerheat-damp or damp-warm disease in early stage: it is featured by damp-turbidity encumbering the fleshy exterior, spleen, and stomach with the manifestations of fever, head distention, chest oppression, epigastric *pǐ*, and white greasy coating. Pèi Lán (Herba Eupatorii) is prescribed together with Huò Xiāng (Herba Agastachis), Qīng Hāo (Herba Artemisiae Annuae), and Hé Yè (Folium Nelumbinis) for the summerheat-damp; and with Huá Shí (Talcum), Yì Yǐ Rén (Semen Coicis), and Huò Xiāng (Herba Agastachis) for damp-warm disease in early stage.

[Usage and Dosage] Use raw in general, 5–10g in decoction, and double the dosage when used in fresh for a better effect in resolving summerheat.

[Mnemonics] Pèi Lán (Herba Eupatorii, Eupatorium): pungent and neutral; good at removing dampness and clearing sweet taste in the mouth caused by damp encumbrance.

[Simple and Effective Formulas]

1. 五叶芦根汤 Wǔ Yè Lú Gēn Tāng — Five Leaves and Reed Decoction from *Revised and Expanded Treatise on Warm-Heat Diseases* (重订广温热论, Chóng Dìng Guǎng Wēn Rè Lùn): Huò Xiāng (Herba Agastachis) leaf 3g, Bò He (Herba Menthae) leaf 3g, Pèi Lán (Herba Eupatorii) leaf 3g, and Hé Yè (Folium Nelumbinis) 3g; decoct Pí Pá Yè (Folium Eriobotryae) 30g, Lú Gēn (Rhizoma Phragmitis) 30g, and fresh wax gourd 60g first and then cook previous herbs in the decoction for oral administration to treat patient of warm-summerheat in early stage with high fever, slight aversion to cold, then fever without chills, intense thirst, profuse sweating, dry teeth, putrid complexion, and vexation.

2. 芳香化湿法 Fāng Xiāng Huà Shī Fǎ — Aromatically Damp Relieving Method from *Treatise on Seasonal Diseases* (时病论, Shí Bìng Lùn): Huò Xiāng Yè (Folium Agastachis) leaf 3g, Pèi Lán Yè (Folium Eupatorii) 3g, Dà Fù Pí (Pericarpium Arecae) 3g, Chén Pí (Pericarpium Citri Reticulatae) 4.5g, processed Bàn Xià (Rhizoma Pinelliae) 4.5g, Hòu Pò (Cortex Magnoliae Officinalis) 2.4g, and fresh Hé Yè (Folium Nelumbinis) 9g; decoct in water for oral administration to treat fever, vertigo, mental confusion, vomiting, and poor appetite caused by invasion of filthy turbidity.

[Precautions] Contraindicated in the absence of internal dampness.

砂仁 Shā Rén *fructus amomi villous amomum fruit*

The source is from the ripe semen of herbaceous perennial *Amomum villosum* lour, A. longiligulare T.L. Wu, *or A. xanthioides* Wall., family Zingiberaceae. Pungent in flavor and warm in nature.

[Actions] Promote qi flow and arrest pain, transform dampness and strengthen the spleen, and calm the fetus and stop vomiting. It is applicable for abdominal pain and distention, poor appetite, food accumulation, cold diarrhea and dysentery, vomiting during pregnancy, and restless fetus. This semen contains volatile oil and its major ingredients are borneol, bornyl acetate, gum camphor, linalool, and nerolidol. At a rather lower concentration, its decoction has an excitatory effect on *ex vivo* intestinal canal of cavia cobaya, whereas its decoction at a high concentration or its volatile oil has shown an inhibitory effect.

[Quality] 阳春砂仁 Yáng Chūn Shā Rén produced in Chunyang county of Guangdong is big, full, and strongly aromatic and regarded as a genuine regional medicinal. 缩砂仁 Suō Shā Rén produced in Vietnam, Laos, and Thailand is inferior to the former in terms of quality. Good quality is large, full, intact, solid, red-brown and intensely aromatic.

[Indications]

1. Abdominal distention and fullness: Shā Rén (Fructus Amomi), capable of moving qi and relieving distention, is combined with Bàn Xià (Rhizoma Pinelliae) and Shēng Jiāng (Rhizoma Zingiberis Recens) for abdominal distention and fullness with accompanying nausea, vomiting, and decreased appetite.
2. Cold dysentery and diarrhea: it marked by abdominal pain and diarrhea aggravated by coldness and watery stool with accompanying abdominal distention, nausea, vomiting, and decreased appetite. In the clinic, Shā Rén (Fructus Amomi) is often used together with Bái Zhú (Rhizoma Atractylodis Macrocephalae), Fú Líng (Poria), Dǎng Shēn (Radix Codonopsis), and Gān Jiāng (Rhizoma Zingiberis).
3. Vomiting during pregnancy: Shā Rén (Fructus Amomi) is usually prescribed together with Zǐ Sū Yè (Folium Perillae) and Bái Zhú (Rhizoma Atractylodis Macrocephalae) for vomiting during pregnancy accompanied with restless fetus in most cases.

[Usage and Dosage] Use raw in most cases, salt solution-fry for the lower *jiao*. Use 2–5g in decoction, and should be added near the end to avoid the loss of active ingredients.

[Mnemonics] Shā Rén (Fructus Amomi, Villous Amomum Fruit): aromatic, pungent, and warm; relieve distention, arrest diarrhea and vomiting, and calm the fetus.

[Simple and Effective Formulas]

1. 香砂枳术丸 Xiāng Shā Zhǐ Zhū Wán — Aucklandia, Amomum, Immature Bitter Orange, and Atractylodes Macrocephala Pill from *Categorized Patterns with Clear-cut Treatments* (类证治裁, Lèi Zhèng Zhì Cái): Shā Rén (Fructus Amomi) 5g, Mù Xiāng (Radix Aucklandiae) 5g, Zhǐ Shí (Fructus Aurantii Immaturus) 6g, Bái Zhú (Rhizoma Atractylodis Macrocephalae) 10g, Chén Pí (Pericarpium Citri Reticulatae) 5g, and Bàn Xià (Rhizoma Pinelliae) 6g; decoct in water for oral administration or prepare into pill to treat patients with indigestion, abdominal fullness, and poor appetite. Also applicable for gastritis, indigestion, gastroptosis, and gastric neurosis.
2. 香砂养胃汤 Xiāng Shā Yǎng Wèi Tāng — Aucklandia and Amomum Stomach Tonifying Decoction from *Supplemental Restoration of Health from the Myriad Diseases* (增补万病回春, Zēng Bǔ Wàn Bìng Huí Chūn): Shā Rén (Fructus Amomi) 5g, Xiāng Fù (Rhizoma Cyperi) 5g, Cāng Zhú (Rhizoma Atractylodis) 6g, Hòu Pò (Cortex Magnoliae Officinalis) 5g, Chén Pí (Pericarpium Citri Reticulatae) 5g, Fú Líng (Poria) 10g, Rén Shēn (Radix et Rhizoma Ginseng) 5g, Mù Xiāng (Radix Aucklandiae) 5g, Bái Zhú (Rhizoma Atractylodis Macrocephalae) 6g, Bái Dòu Kòu (Fructus Amomi Kravanh) 5g, and Zhì Gān Cǎo (Radix et Rhizoma Glycyrrhizae Praeparata cum Melle) 3g; decoct in water for oral administration to treat patients with poor appetite, bland taste in the mouth, and gastric fullness and discomfort. Also applicable for chronic gastritis, gastroptosis, gastric neurosis, and indigestion.

[Precautions] Shā Rén (Fructus Amomi), pungent, warm, and aromatic, is suitable for internal dampness with white and greasy tongue coating. It should be used with caution for red tongue with no coating, which indicates the absence of internal dampness.

白豆蔻 Bái Dòu Kòu *fructus amomi kravanh round cardamon*

The source is from the fruit of herbaceous perennial *Amomum kravanh* Pierre ex Gagnep., family Zingiberaceae. Pungent in flavor and warm in nature. Alternate names include 白豆蔻 Bái Dòu Kòu and 白蔻仁 Bái Dòu Kòu.

[Actions] Transform dampness and move qi, warm the middle *jiao*, and arrest vomiting. It is applicable for dampness obstruction in the middle *jiao*, qi stagnation of the spleen and stomach, abdominal distention, loose stools, and vomiting. This herb can promote gastric juice secretion, excite intestinal peristalsis, relieve gastrointestinal pneumatosis, and inhibit abnormal fermentation of intestinal content. *In vitro* experiments reveal it has an inhibitory effect on shigella dysenteriae, excitatory effect on intestinal canal of cavia cobaya at lower concentration, and inhibitory effect at higher concentration.

[Quality] Good quality is large, full, intact, thin-skinned, acrid, cool, strong-tasting without damage done by worms, mildew, empty shell and impurities.

[Indications]

1. Dampness obstruction in the middle *jiao*: Bái Dòu Kòu (Fructus Amomi Kravanh) is combined with Cāng Zhú (Rhizoma Atractylodis), Hòu Pò (Cortex Magnoliae Officinalis), and Shā Rén (Fructus Amomi) for gastric and abdominal distention and fullness, decreased appetite, and white greasy tongue coating caused by dampness obstruction in the middle *jiao*.
2. Damp-heat patterns: Bái Dòu Kòu (Fructus Amomi Kravanh) is applied to remove damp-heat turbidity pathogen. It is combined with Huò Xiāng (Herba Agastachis), Yì Yǐ Rén (Semen Coicis), Xìng Rén (Semen Armeniacae Amarum), Huá Shí (Talcum), and Zhú Yè (Folium Phyllostachydis Henonis) for damp-warm in the initial stage predominated by dampness; and with Huáng Qín (Radix Scutellariae) and Huá Shí (Talcum) for dampness gradually turning into heat.

3. Stomach cold patterns: Bái Dòu Kòu (Fructus Amomi Kravanh) is effective in warming the stomach and can relieve stomach-cold induced vomiting, gastric pain, and indigestion, either alone or in a combination with Huò Xiāng (Herba Agastachis), Chén Pí (Pericarpium Citri Reticulatae), and Shēng Jiāng (Rhizoma Zingiberis Recens).

Bái Dòu Kòu (Fructus Amomi Kravanh) and Shā Rén (Fructus Amomi) are similar in nature and flavor. However, the former acts on the upper and middle *jiao*, can treat damp-warm disease in the initial state and vomiting caused by stomach cold, and is good at diffusing lung qi to remove dampness; and the latter acts on the middle and lower *jiao* and can treat gastric and abdominal distention, abdominal pain, diarrhea, and restless fetus. They are often used together in the clinic.

[Usage and Dosage] Use raw, should not be stored overtime to prevent the loss of aroma. Crush or grind before use. Use 3–6g in decoction, add near the end of decocting.

[Mnemonics] Bái Dòu Kòu (Fructus Amomi Kravanh, Round Cardamon): warm the stomach, stop vomiting, and relieve the fullness and distention due to the dampness obstruction in the middle *jiao*.

[Simple and Effective Formulas]

1. 白豆蔻散 Bái Dòu Kòu Sǎn — Round Cardamon Powder from *Black Pearl from Red Waters* (赤水玄珠，Chì Shuǐ Xuán Zhū): Bái Dòu Kòu (Fructus Amomi Kravanh) 9g; grind into powder and take with wine for oral administration to treat vomiting and stomachache caused by stomach cold.
2. 白豆蔻汤 Bái Dòu Kòu Tāng — Round Cardamon Decoction from *Shen's Books on Respecting Life* (沈氏尊生书，Shěn Shì Zūn Shēng Shū): Bái Dòu Kòu (Fructus Amomi Kravanh) 5g, Huò Xiāng (Herba Agastachis) 5g, Bàn Xià (Rhizoma Pinelliae) 6g, Chén Pí (Pericarpium Citri Reticulatae) 5g, and Shēng Jiāng (Rhizoma Zingiberis Recens) 3 pieces; decoct in water for oral administration to treat vomiting due to qi counterflow.

[Precautions] Bái Dòu Kòu (Fructus Amomi Kravanh), warm and drying in nature, is contraindicated in cases of yin deficiency and blood dryness without damp-cold.

Daily practices

1. What are the similarities and differences among Huò Xiāng (Herba Agastachis), Pèi Lán (Herba Eupatorii), Shā Rén (Fructus Amomi), and Bái Dòu Kòu (Fructus Amomi Kravanh) in terms of actions and indications?
2. Some of the aromatic medicinals that remove dampness have special effects beside removing dampness, what are they?

Sixth Week

1

MEDICINALS THAT RELIEVE WATER RETENTION

Fluid retention is a pathological product inside of the body. Physiologically, water and food ingestion will be transformed and transported by the spleen and stomach to nourish *zang-fu* organs and tissues all over the body, whereas the redundance will be discharged as urine, feces, and sweating. The term water-dampness in traditional Chinese medicine has two connotations, the first refers to fluid retention in the body, such as edema, ascites, urine retention, strangury, diarrhea, and pleural rheum (hydrothorax), and the second meaning is phlegm-rheum, *bì* pattern, and eczema. Therefore, relieving water-dampness is one the most important therapies in traditional Chinese medicine. The method of promoting urination to relieve water-dampness retention is an extremely important treatment method, also known as urination-promoting method, or dampness-draining method, or diuresis-promoting method with bland flavor medicinals. The ancients stated that draining dampness is often a matter of increasing the production of urine, for this is the primary means by which the accumulation of fluids or dampness is relieved.

Herbs that relieve fluid retention can be further divided by property and function into several classes: the sweet, bland, neutral but relatively cold herbs that promote diuresis are used for inhibited urination and edema; and the bitter and cold herbs that clear heat and drain dampness (also called relieving strangury medicinals) are used for dripping, difficult, and painful urination caused by warm heat accumulation in the lower *jiao*, jaundice and rib-side pain due to damp-heat, and summerheat-damp.

Herbs that promote urination are combined with other medicinals in accordance with the state of the disorders. For instance, they should be used together with medicinals that release the exterior and diffuse the lung when edema in early stage with accompanying symptoms of exterior pattern; with spleen-supplementing herbs if chronic edema is complicated with spleen deficiency; with herbs that warm and strengthen the spleen and kidney when the disorder progresses into spleen and kidney yang deficiency; and with herbs that cool blood and stanch bleeding for hematuria attributed to damp-heat in the lower *jiao* injuring the blood vessel. These herbs are draining in nature and inappropriate use can readily injure yin fluid. For this reason, they must be used with caution in patients with yin deficiency.

茯苓 **Fú Ling** *poria poria*

The source is from the dry sclerotium of *Poria cocos* (schw) Wolf, family Polyporaceae. Sweet and bland in flavor and neutral in nature.

[Actions] Promote urination and leach out dampness, strengthen the spleen, and quiet the heart and calm the spirit. It is applicable for edema with scanty urine, vertigo and dizziness caused by phlegm-rheum, palpitations, less food intake due to spleen deficiency, loose stool, palpitations due to fright, and insomnia. This herb contains β-pachyman, pachymic acid, ergosterol, cholin, histidine, and sylvite. It can directly relax *ex vivo* intestinal canal of rabbit, prevent gastric ulcer induced by ligating pylorus of rat, and reduce gastric acid. Its ethonal extract has shown a significant diuretic effect when injected intraperitoneally in rabbits; its decoction has sedative effect on mice. Its ingredients pachymaran and water-solube carboxymethyl pachymaran have inhibitory effects on mice sarcoma 180, the latter can pronouncedly increase phagocytic function of mice enterocoelia macrophage, restore decreased phagocytic function of macrophage in tumor-bearing mice, and significantly improve spleen and thymic weight.

[Quality] The white part of dry sclerotium of *Poria cocos* (schw) Wolf parasitized on the root of pine (but not around the root), cut into slices. It is produced in many areas, but 云茯苓 Yún Fú Líng from Yunnan is the best and regarded as a genuine regional medicinal, good quality is solid, heavy, and chewy with a brown outer skin, thin skin wrinkles, and a white and finely textured cross section. After removal of the outer skin, the light red variety is called 赤茯苓 Chì Fú Ling (Poria Rubra) and used in the treatment of damp-heat; and the white variety is called 白茯苓 Bái Fú Ling. The outer layer is called 茯苓皮 Fú Líng Pí and often used as a strong diuretic. The part of the fungus around the root is called 茯神 Fú Shén (Sclerotium Poriae Pararadicis) and is considered to be better for calming the restless heart spirit.

[Indications]

1. Vertigo and throbbing: vertigo refers to the feeling of vertigo and dizziness like sitting in the boat; throbbing refers to throbbing in the epigastrium, throbbing below the navel, and throbbing in the muscle. Patients also present restlessness of the heart spirit, dreaminess easy to be frightened, mind-absence, and forgetfulness. Fú Líng (Poria) is effective in relieving vertigo and throbbing caused by phlegm and water retention and accompanied with mild thirst, scanty fluid in the mouth with a desire to drink but less water intake, inhibited urination, less frequency of urination with scanty urine, or edema. In this case, it is combined with Shí Chāng Pú (Rhizoma Acori Tatarinowii) and Yuǎn Zhì (Radix Polygalae). For the disorder caused by the heart and spleen with accompanying insomnia and lassitude, it is combined with Dǎng Shēn (Radix Codonopsis), Lóng Yǎn Ròu (Arillus Longan), and Suān Zǎo Rén (Semen Ziziphi Spinosae).

2. Water-dampness retention: Fú Líng (Poria) can promote urination and therefore applicable for water-dampness retention disorders, no matter cold or hot nature, deficient or excessive. It is often combined with Zhū Líng (Polyporus), Zé Xiè (Rhizoma Alismatis), Dōng Guā Pí (Exocarpium Benincasae), and Chē Qián Zǐ (Semen Plantaginis) for edema; and with Bái Zhú (Rhizoma Atractylodis Macrocephalae), Guì Zhī (Ramulus Cinnamomi), and Bàn Xià (Rhizoma Pinelliae) for vomiting of clear water and gastric distension due to phlegm-rheum retention in the stomach.

3. Spleen deficiency: Fú Líng (Poria) is capable of fortifying the spleen and applicable for decreased appetite and loose stools caused by spleen deficiency failing to transform and transport. It can fortify the spleen to treat the root and drain dampness to treat the branch.

[Usage and Dosage] Bái Fú Líng (Indian Buead) is more effective for fortifying the spleen and boosting qi, while Chì Fú Líng (Poria Rubra, Indian
bread pink epidermis) is more potent in promoting urination and percolating
dampness. Usually the outer layer called Cortex Poriae is removed, when
using with the outer layer is to fortify the spleen and promote urination. Use
raw in most cases, treated with Zhū Shā (Cinnabaris) is called 朱茯苓 Zhū
Fú Líng and to improve its capacity to calm the spirit. Use 10–20 g in decoction, up to above 30 g for edema and diarrhea due to severe water-dampness
accumulation, decoction to be taken hot, and stir suspension or sediment
when taken cold as it contains therapeutic polysaccharide substance.

[Mnemonics] Fú Ling (Poria, Poria): sweet and bland; good at promoting
urination and can tonify the spleen and cure vertigo and palpitation.

[Simple and Effective Formulas]

1. 五苓散 Wǔ Líng Sǎn — Five Substances Powder with Poria from
   Treatise on Cold Damage (伤寒论, Shāng Hán Lùn): Fú Líng (Poria)
   20 g, Bái Zhú (Rhizoma Atractylodis Macrocephalae) 12 g, Zhū Líng
   (Polyporus) 12 g, Zé Xiè (Rhizoma Alismatis) 12 g, and Guì Zhī
   (Ramulus Cinnamomi) 6 g; decoct in water for oral administration to
   treat patients suffering from sweating with floating pulse, vomiting
   with qi rushing up to the chest, fever, thirst, and difficult urination. Also
   applicable for urinary system diseases, digestive system disorders,
   nervous system diseases, febrile diseases, eye problems, ascites, and
   edema with manifestation of water-damp internal retention.
2. 茯苓桂枝白术甘草汤 Fú Líng Guì Zhī Bái Zhú Gān Cǎo Tāng —
   Poria, Cinnamon Twig, White Atractylodes Rhizome, and Licorice
   Root Decoction from *Treatise on Cold Damage* (伤寒论, Shāng Hán
   Lùn): Fú Líng (Poria) 20 g, Guì Zhī (Ramulus Cinnamomi) 10 g, Bái
   Zhú (Rhizoma Atractylodis Macrocephalae) 12 g, and Gān Cǎo (Radix
   et Rhizoma Glycyrrhizae) 5 g; decoct in water for oral administration
   to treat patients with fullness in the epigastrium, qi rushing up to the
   chest, vertigo, dizziness, palpitations with anxiety, thirst, and difficult
   urination. Also applicable for nervous system diseases, cardiovascular
   dirorders, gastrointestinal diseases, respiratory system disorders, aural
   vertigo, and eye problems.

3. 桂苓甘露饮 Guì Líng Gān Lù Yǐn — Cinnamon and Poria Sweet Dew Beverage from *An Elucidation of Formulas* (宣明论方, Xuān Míng Lùn Fāng): Fú Líng (Poria) 15 g, Zé Xiè (Rhizoma Alismatis) 12 g, Zhū Líng (Polyporus) 15 g, Bái Zhú (Rhizoma Atractylodis Macrocephalae) 12 g, Ròu Guì (Cortex Cinnamomi) 5 g, Huá Shí (Talcum) 12 g, Gān Cǎo (Radix et Rhizoma Glycyrrhizae) 3 g, Shí Gāo (Gypsum Fibrosum) 15 g, and Hán Shuǐ Shí (Glauberitum) 15 g; decoct in water for oral administration to treat patients with headache, vexation, thirst, sweating, difficult urination, and yellow and scanty urine. Also applicable for febrile diseases, common cold in summer, and sunstroke.

4. 小半夏加茯苓汤 Xiǎo Bàn Xià Jiā Fú Líng Tāng — Minor Pinellia plus Poria Decoction from *Essentials from the Golden Cabinet* (金匮要略, Jīn Guì Yào Lüè): Fú Líng (Poria) 20 g, Bàn Xià (Rhizoma Pinelliae) 12 g, and Shēng Jiāng (Rhizoma Zingiberis Recens) three pieces; decoct in water for oral administration to treat patients with watery vomiting, vertigo, palpitation, and thirst. Also applicable for neuropsychiatric disorders, digestive system diseases, and aural vertigo.

[Precautions] Fú Líng (Poria) is effective in percolating dampness and therefore cannot be used alone for deficiency pattern. It is contraindicated in cases of frequent and copious urine due to kidney-qi deficiency, spontaneous seminal emission caused by deficiency-cold, and qi deficiency and sinking.

猪苓 Zhū Ling *polyporus polyporus*

The source is from the dry sclerotium of *Polyporus umbellatus* (Pers.) Fr., family Polyporaceae. Sweet and bland in flavor and neutral in nature.

[Actions] Promote urination and leach out dampness. It is applicable for difficult urination, edema, distention, fullness, leg qi, diarrhea, strangury with turbid discharge, and abnormal vaginal discharge. This herb contains ergosterol, biotin, water-soluble polysaccharide compound polysaccharid, and crude protein. Ingesting a large dose of its decoction has shown a diuretic effect on human and dog, but a small dose is non-effective, its extractives can inhibit intracellular DNA synthesis of nice sarcoma 180 ascites tumor, increase tumor intracellular cAMP content, and improve phagocytic function of reticuloendothelial system in mice. Clinical trial has been conducted in the treatment of such malignant tumors as lung cancer, cervical cancer, esophagus cancer, gastric cancer, liver cancer, and lymphosarcoma, indicating preliminarily it can improve symptoms and stabilize tumor progression, and no adverse reactions have been noted.

[Quality] It is produced in many areas, and experimental cultivation has been tried. The one produced in Shaanxi is of the best quality. Good quality is large, has a black outer skin, and is powdery and white on the inside.

[Indications]

1. Heat strangury: Zhū Líng (Polyporus) is often combined with Huá Shí (Talcum) and Zé Xiè (Rhizoma Alismatis) for heat stranguary with manifestations as fever, thirst, difficult and painful urination or cloudy urine, and abnormal vaginal discharge; and with Ē Jiāo (Colla Corii Asini) for hematuria.
2. Edema: Zhū Líng (Polyporus) is combined with Zé Xiè (Rhizoma Alismatis) and Fú Líng (Poria) for edema with thirst and inhibited urination. It can be used alone in a powder form for oral administration to treat edema and thirst during pregnancy.

This herb and its extractives are now commonly used as an adjuvant therapy for cancer and to counteract the side effects of chemotherapy and radiotherapy.

[Usage and Dosage] Use raw in general, 6–12 g in decoction.

[Mnemonics] Zhū Líng (Polyporus, Polyporus): sweet and neutral; promote urination, unblock strangury, relieve fluid retention and edema, and eliminate cancer.

[Simple and Effective Formulas]

1. 猪苓散 Zhū Líng Sǎn — Polyporus Powder from *Essentials from the Golden Cabinet* (金匮要略, Jīn Guì Yào Lüè): Zhū Líng (Polyporus) 15 g, Fú Líng (Poria) 15 g, and Zé Xiè (Rhizoma Alismatis) 15 g; decoct in water for oral administration to treat patient with thirst and inhibited

urination. Also applicable for urinary tract infection, nephritis, febrile diseases, and edema.

2. 猪苓汤 Zhū Líng Tāng — Polyporus Decoction from *Treatise on Cold Damage* (伤寒论, Shāng Hán Lùn): Zhū Líng (Polyporus) 15 g, Fú Líng (Poria) 15 g, Zé Xiè (Rhizoma Alismatis) 12 g, Huá Shí (Talcum) 15 g, and Ē Jiāo (Colla Corii Asini) 10 g; decoct in water for oral administration to treat people with difficult and painful urination, hematuria, and desire to drink water. Also applicable for urinary system disorders and edema.

[Precautions] Zhū Líng (Polyporus), a potent diuretic, may injure yin fluid when misused and is not recommended in the absence of water-dampness.

泽泻 Zé Xiè *rhizoma alismatis water plantain rhizome*

The source is from the tuber of perennial herbaceous mire plant *Alisma orientale* (Sam) Juzep., family Alismataceae. Sweet and bland in flavor and cold in nature.

[Actions] Promote urination and clear damp-heat. It is applicable for difficult urination, edema with fullness and distention, diarrhea, scanty urine, phlegm-rheum induced vertigo and dizziness, heat strangury with difficult and painful urination, and hyperlipemia. This herb contains triterpenes of alisol and acetate, volatile oil, alkaloid, and asparagine. Experiments show it has a diuretic effect and its fat-soluble compounds have a hypolipidemic effect. This herb has shown a significant cholesterol-decreasing effect and anti-atherosclerosis effect on experimental hyperlipemia rats, and can reduce fatty liver.

[Quality] Good quality is big, yellowish white, lustrous, and powdery.

[Indications]

1. Water-dampness retention: Zé Xiè (Rhizoma Alismatis), potent in promoting urination, is applicable for disorders caused by water-dampness retention, such as inhibited urination, edema, ascites, diarrhea, strangury with turbid discharge, and phlegm-rheum vertigo. It is often used in a

combination with medicinals that promote urination such as Fú Líng (Poria), Zhū Líng (Polyporus), Mù Tōng (Caulis Akebiae), and Huá Shí (Talcum); and with Bái Zhú (Rhizoma Atractylodis Macrocephalae) for phlegm-rheum vertigo.

2. Hyperlipidemia: Zé Xiè (Rhizoma Alismatis) is very often used in Chinese patent medicine or formula of lowering blood lipid to treat hyperlipidemia, fatty liver, and atherosclerosis. It is usually prescribed together with Shān Zhā (Fructus Crataegi) and Dà Huáng (Radix et Rhizoma Rhei).

[Usage and Dosage] Use raw in general, avoid using fresh as it contains irritants that cause gastroenteritis, stir-fry with salt to help it enter the kidney to promote urination. Use 6–12 g in decoction, increase the dosage for vertigo caused by phlegm-rheum, decrease the dosage as in powder.

[Mnemonics] Zé Xiè (Rhizoma Alismatis, Water Plantain Rhizome): sweet and cold; promote urination, remove dampness, lower blood lipid, and relieve vertigo.

[Simple and Effective Formulas]

1. 泽泻汤 Zé Xiè Tāng — Water Plantain Rhizome Decoction from *Essentials from the Golden Cabinet* (金匮要略, Jīn Guì Yào Lüè): Zé Xiè (Rhizoma Alismatis) 15 g and Bái Zhú (Rhizoma Atractylodis Macrocephalae) 15 g; decoct in water for oral administration to treat people with vertigo, dizziness, heaviness of the body, spontaneous sweating, shortness of breath, and difficult urination. Also applicable for hyperlipemia, cardiovascular and cerebralvascular diseases, and aural vertigo.

2. 四苓散 Sì Líng Sǎn — Four Líng Powder from *Teachings of [Zhu] Dan-xi* (丹溪心法, Dān Xī Xīn Fǎ): Zé Xiè (Rhizoma Alismatis) 12 g, Fú Líng (Poria) 12 g, Zhū Líng (Polyporus) 12 g, and Bái Zhú (Rhizoma Atractylodis Macrocephalae) 12 g; decoct in water for oral administration to treat patient thirst, spontaneous sweating, and diarrhea and dysentery with inhibited urination. Also applicable for urinary system disorders, acute diarrhea, and common cold in summer.

[Precautions] Zé Xiè (Rhizoma Alismatis), cold and purgative, cannot be used alone in cases of kidney deficiency.

Daily practices

1. What are the indications of medicinals that disinhibit water and what precautions should be taken when using it?
2. What are the similarities and differences among Fú Líng (Poria), Zhū Líng (Polyporus), and Zé Xiè (Rhizoma Alismatis) in terms of actions and indications?

滑石 Huá Shí *talcum talcum*

It is the cube of silicate mineral talcum. Sweet and bland in flavor and cold in nature.

[Actions] Promote urination and relieve strangury, and clear heat and release summerheat. It is applicable for difficult, painful urination, dripping of urine, vexation and thirst due to summer-heat, damp-warmth induced chest oppression, and damp-heat diarrhea. This substance contains hydrous magnesium silicate (major ingredient) and ferrum, sodium, potassium, calcium, and aluminum. Its powder can adsorb large quantity of chemical irritants or poisonous substance to protect the skin and mucous membrane, and oral administration can arrest vomiting and diarrhea and prevent toxics absorption.

[Quality] Washed clean and broke into soybean-sized pieces (滑石块 Huá Shí Kuài); levigated and ground into powders, water removed after sedimenting, cut into cubes when half dried, and dried under sunshine (known as 飞滑石 Fēi Huá Shí). Good quality is white, lustrous, soft, smooth, cool, and without dust.

[Indications]

1. Heat strangury and stone strangury: heat strangury refers to urinary tract infection in modern biomedicine and marked by difficult and painful urination with yellow and scanty urine, frequent urination with

emergency sensation, or hematuria. Most patients present fever, sweating, vexation, and agitation. Huá Shí (Talcum) can be used alone, as *Comprehensive Recording of Divine Assistance* (圣济总录, Shèng Jì Zǒng Lù) stated Huá Shí (Talcum) is applicable for heat strangury with difficult, painful, and decreased urination with hot sensation; *Formulas with Extensive Benefits* (广利方, Guǎng Lì Fāng) recorded it is applicable for qi congestion induced anuria and vomiting, strangury with emergency sensation, and oppression and pain below the navel; *Proven Formulas of Obstetrics and Lactation* (产乳集验方, Chǎn Rǔ Jí Yàn Fāng) stated its effective in the treatment of urinary retention. It can also be used together with Lián Qiào (Fructus Forsythiae), Shān Zhī (Fructus Gardeniae), Zhū Líng (Polyporus), and Chē Qián Zǐ (Semen Plantaginis). Stone strangury refers to urinary tract stone featured by painful urination with sandy stone in urine and severe pain even involving the waist. If that is the case, Huá Shí (Talcum) is often combined with Hǎi Jīn Shā (Spora Lygodii), Jīn Qián Cǎo (Herba Lysimachiae), and Gān Cǎo (Radix et Rhizoma Glycyrrhizae).

2. Edema: Huá Shí (Talcum) is prescribed together with Fú Líng (Poria), Bái Zhú (Rhizoma Atractylodis Macrocephalae), and Zhū Líng (Polyporus) for edema with thirst and inhibited urination.

3. Summerheat: Huá Shí (Talcum), capable of clearing and relieving summerheat, is applicable for damp-warm and summerheat-damp disorder and usually combined with Gān Cǎo (Radix et Rhizoma Glycyrrhizae). For intense damp-heat, it is often combined with Huáng Qín (Radix Scutellariae) and Tōng Cǎo (Medulla Tetrapanacis).

It can dispel dampness and consolidate when applied externally and therefore commonly used for such dermatosis as eczema and miliaria.

[Usage and Dosage] Use raw in general, crush and decoct it first, and place in a cheesecloth bag when decocting 飞滑石 Fēi Huá Shí. Use 6–15 g in decoction,

[Mnemonics] Huá Shí (Talcum, Talcum): sweet and neutral; effective for all kinds of strangury, promote urination, relieve edema, and clear summerheat.

[Simple and Effective Formulas]

1. 六一散 Liù Yī Sǎn — Six-to-One Powder from *The Causes and Manifestations of Cold Damage* (伤寒标本, Shāng Hán Biāo Běn): Huá Shí (Talcum) 180 g and Zhì Gān Cǎo (Radix et Rhizoma Glycyrrhizae Praeparata cum Melle) 30 g; grind into fine powder and take 9 g/dose with warm water for oral administration, three times a day to treat general fever, vomiting, diarrhea, dysentery, urinary retention, and stony strangury.

2. 滑石散 Huá Shí Sǎn — Talcum Powder from *Comprehensive Recording of Divine Assistance* (圣济总录, Shèng Jì Zǒng Lù): Huá Shí (Talcum) 120 g; grind into fine powder and take 5 g/dose with boiled water for oral administration to treat heat strangury and difficult and painful urination with burning sensation.

[Precautions] Huá Shí (Talcum), purgative in nature, can easily injure yin fluid and therefore should be used with caution in cases of deficiency manifestoes as emaciation and red tongue with scanty coating.

薏苡仁 Yì Yǐ Rén *semen coicis coix seed*

The source is from the semen of *Coix lachryma jobi* L., family Gramineae. Alternate names include 苡仁, Yǐ Rén 苡米, Yǐ Mǐ and 米仁 Mǐ Rén. Sweet and bland in flavor and slightly cold in nature.

[Actions] Promote urination to leach out dampness, strengthen the spleen, smooth the sinews, and expel pus. It is applicable for difficult urination, edema, leg qi, spleen deficiency induced diarrhea, wind-damp bì pain, lung abscess, and intestinal abscess. This herb contains coixendide, coixenolide, triterpenoid, and vitamin B1. Animal experiment reveals that its ethanol extractive has an anticancer effect an and coixendide is an active ingredient of anticancer.

[Quality] Outer skin and yellowish-brown outer bark removed, impurities removed, and dried under sunshine. Good quality is dry, large, full, round, white, and without chipping.

[Indications]

1. Wind-damp *bì* pain: Yì Yǐ Rén (Semen Coicis) is cooked with Jīng Mǐ (Oryza Sativa L.) into congee and taken warm, or decocted with Má Huáng (Herba Ephedrae), Xìng Rén (Semen Armeniacae Amarum), and Gān Cǎo (Radix et Rhizoma Glycyrrhizae) for wind-damp bì pain with muscle pain, body heaviness and tiredness, and edema.

2. Edema in the lower limbs: Yì Yǐ Rén (Semen Coicis) is prescribed together with Cāng Zhú (Rhizoma Atractylodis), Fáng Jǐ (Radix Stephaniae Tetrandrae), and Niú Xī (Radix Achyranthis Bidentatae) for edema in the lower limbs with accompanying pain in the lower extremities or weakness of the lower extremities failing to walk.

3. Lung abscess and intestinal abscess: Up to above 30 g of Yì Yǐ Rén (Semen Coicis) is used for oral administration. *Formulas to Aid the Living* (济生方, Jì Shēng Fāng) stated to pound Yì Yǐ Rén (Semen Coicis) 90 g and decoct in water and wine for lung abscess with hematemesis; *Fan Wang's Formulas* (范汪方, Fàn Wāng Fāng) has a similar recording. In the clinic, it can be combined with Lú Gēn (Rhizoma Phragmitis), Táo Rén (Semen Persicae), and Dōng Guā Rén (Semen Benincasae) for lung abscess; and with Bài Jiàng Cǎo (Herba Patriniae), Mǔ Dān Pí (Cortex Moutan), and Táo Rén (Semen Persicae) for intestinal abscess.

4. Wasting-thirst due to spleen deficiency: Yì Yǐ Rén (Semen Coicis) can be used alone or together with Bái Zhú (Rhizoma Atractylodis Macrocephalae), Fú Líng (Poria), and Dǎng Shēn (Radix Codonopsis) for wasting-thirst with accompanying loose stool and loose muscle. *The Grand Compendium of Materia Medica* (本草纲目, Běn Cǎo Gāng Mù) advises to cook Yì Yǐ Rén (Semen Coicis) into congee to treat wasting-thirst with desire to drink.

It has been recently used in the formula of treating cancer. Its extractives are also applicable for the treatment of cancer.

[Usage and Dosage] Use raw in general, 12–30 g in decoction, up to 60–90 g/day when used alone.

[Mnemonics] Yì Yǐ Rén (Semen Coicis, Coix Seed): sweet and bland; promote urination, strengthen the spleen, relieve internal abscesses and dampness, and remove *bì*.

[Simple and Effective Formulas]

1. 麻杏苡甘汤 Má Xìng Yì Gān Tāng — Ephedra, Apricot Kernel, Coix Seed and Licorice Decoction from *Essentials from the Golden Cabinet* (金匮要略, Jīn Guì Yào Lüè): Má Huáng (Herba Ephedrae) 5 g, Yì Yǐ Rén (Semen Coicis) 20 g, Xìng Rén (Semen Armeniacae Amarum) 10 g, and Gān Cǎo (Radix et Rhizoma Glycyrrhizae) 3 g; decoct in water for oral administration to treat patients with externally-contracted wind-damp, pain and heaviness throughout the body aggravated in the afternoon, fever, slight aversion to cold, and edema in the lower extremities. Also applicable for rheumatic diseases, neuralgia, nephritis, edema during pregnancy, and eczema.

2. 苇茎汤 Wěi Jìng Tāng — Phragmites Stem Decoction from *Essentials from the Golden Cabinet* (金匮要略, Jīn Guì Yào Lüè): Lú Gēn (Rhizoma Phragmitis) 20 g, Yì Yǐ Rén (Semen Coicis) 20 g, Dōng Guā Zǐ (Semen Benincasae) 30 g, and Táo Rén (Semen Persicae) 12 g; decoct in water for oral administration to treat patient suffering from lung abscess with fetid sputum with blood and pus, dry scaly skin, and dull pain in the chest. Also applicable for pulmonary abscess, empyema, and bronchiectasia.

3. 薏苡败酱散 Yì Yǐ Bài Jiàng Sǎn — Coix Seed and Patrinia Powder from *Essentials from the Golden Cabinet* (金匮要略, Jīn Guì Yào Lüè): Yì Yǐ Rén (Semen Coicis) 30 g, Bài Jiàng Cǎo (Herba Patriniae) 15 g, and Fù Zǐ (Radix Aconiti Lateralis Praeparata) 6 g; decoct in water for oral administration to treat patients with intestinal abscess when pus is formed, absence of fever, tense abdominal skin with softness upon pressure, cold limbs, and pale tongue. Also applicable for chronic appendicitis, suppurative appendicitis, localized peritonitis, intestine tuberculosis, and skin problems.

木通 Mù Tōng *caulis akebiae akebia stem*

The source is from the woody stem of perennial twining shrub *Akebia trifoliata* (Thunb.) Koidz. subsp. australis (Diels) T. Shimizu, family Lardizabalaceae, or *Clematis armandii* Franch., family Ranunculaceae. The former is called 白木通 Bái Mù Tōng and the latter 川木通 Chuān Mù Tōng. The dry rattan of *Aristolochia manshuriensis* Kom, family

Aristolochiaceae is also used and known as 关木通 Guān Mù Tōng. Bitter in flavor and cold in nature.

[Actions] Clear heart fire, promote urination, and unblock the channels and promote lactation. It is applicable for ulcers in the tongue and mouth, vexation, yellow urine, edema, heat strangury with difficult and painful urination, white leukorrhea, amenorrhea, lack of breast milk, and damp-heat *bì* pain. Its decoction has shown an excitatory effect on ex vivo intestinal canal of mice and uterus. It has a significant diuretic effect.

[Quality] Good quality has even stems with a yellow interior.

[Indications]

1. Damp-heat pouring downward: Mù Tōng (Caulis Akebiae), capable of promoting urination and relieving stranguary, is often combined with Chē Qián Zǐ (Semen Plantaginis), Tōng Cǎo (Medulla Tetrapanacis), and Qú Mài (Herba Dianthi) for scanty, dripping, difficult and painful urination caused by damp-heat in the lower *jiao*.
2. Heart fire flaming upward: Mù Tōng (Caulis Akebiae) is usually combined with Zhú Yè (Folium Phyllostachydis Henonis), Shēng Dì (Radix Rehmanniae), and Gān Cǎo (Radix et Rhizoma Glycyrrhizae) for vexation, ulcers in the mouth and tongue, yellow urine, and red tongue, or difficult urination with hot sensation in some cases due to heart fire flaming upward.
3. Inhibited lactation: for postpartum inhibited lactation, Mù Tōng (Caulis Akebiae) is combinated with Chuān Shān Jiǎ (Squama Manitis) and Wáng Bù Liú Xíng (Semen Vaccariae) or cooked with pig feet.
4. Wind-damp-heat *bì*: Mù Tōng (Caulis Akebiae) is combined with Qín Jiāo (Radix Gentianae Macrophyllae), Fáng Jǐ (Radix Stephaniae Tetrandrae), and Cán Shā (Faeces Bombycis) for patients with joint redness, swelling, pain with hot sensation, reduced mobility of the joints, and even fever with thirst due to wind-damp-heat *bì*.

[Usage and Dosage] Use raw in general, 3–6 g in decoction.

[Mnemonics] Mù Tōng (Caulis Akebiae, Akebia Stem): bitter and cold; clear heart fire, unblock lactation, eliminate *bì*, promote urination, and relieve strangury.

[Simple and Effective Formulas]

1. 导赤散 Dǎo Chì Sǎn — Red-Guiding Powder from *Key to Diagnosis and Treatment of Children's Diseases* (小儿药证直诀, Xiǎo Ér Yào Zhèng Zhí Jué): Shēng Dì (Radix Rehmanniae), Shēng Gān Cǎo (Radix et Rhizoma Glycyrrhizae), and Mù Tōng (Caulis Akebiae) in equal dosage; grind into fine powder, decoct 9 g/dose with Zhú Yè (Folium Phyllostachydis Henonis), and take warm after meal for oral administration to treat pediatric heart heat, fire in the small intestine, dripping discharge of yellow urine, red complexion, vexation, erosion in the mouth and tongue, teeth grinding, and thirst. Also applicable for urinary tract infection.

2. 木通汤 Mù Tōng Tāng — Clematidis Caulis Decoction from *Comprehensive Recording of Divine Assistance* (圣济总录, Shèng Jì Zǒng Lù): Mù Tōng (Caulis Akebiae) 30 g, Zhōng Rǔ Shí (Stalactitum) 30 g, Lòu Lú (Radix Rhapontici) 60 g, Guā Lóu Gēn (Radix Fructus Trichosanthis) 30 g, and Gān Cǎo (Radix et Rhizoma Glycyrrhizae) 30 g; decoct in water for oral administration to treat postpartum lactation inhibition.

[Precautions] Mù Tōng (Caulis Akebiae), effective in unblocking the channels, is contraindicated during pregnancy. Do not overdose, acute renal failure was reported following a dose of 60 g decoction. Guān Mù Tōng (Caulis Aristolochiae Manshuriensis) is discouraged to use as its aristolochic acid can cause renal toxicity.

Daily practices

1. What are the similarities and differences among Huá Shí (Talcum), Yì Yǐ Rén (Semen Coicis), and Mù Tōng (Caulis Akebiae) in terms of actions and indications?

2. Mù Tōng (Caulis Akebiae) and Fú Líng (Poria) both are medicinals that disinhibit water, what are the similarities and differences between them in terms of actions and indications?

茵陈 Yīn Chén *herba artemisiae scopariae virgate wormwood herb*

The source is from the sprout of herbaceous perennial *Artemisia Capillaris* Thunb., family Compositae. Alternate names include 茵陈蒿 Yīn Chén Hāo and 绵茵陈 Mián Yīn Chén. Bitter and pungent in flavor and cool in nature.

[Actions] Clear heat and drain dampness, and promote gallbladder function and relieve jaundice. It is applicable for jaundice, scanty urine, eczema, and itching. Its decoction can promote bile secretion and protect carbon tetrachloride-induced liver injury in rats, and has antipyretic, diuretic, antihypertensive, and hypolipidemic effects.

[Quality] Sifted, impurities removed, residue root excluded, ground with roller into pieces, sifted with sieve to exclude dirt. Wild herb is commonly found in most gravel areas in China. 西茵陈 Xi Yīn Chén produced in Jiangxi is of high quality. Good quality is tender, soft, gray-green, and aromatic.

[Indications] Yīn Chén (Herba Artemisiae Scopariae) is mainly used to treat different types of jaundice. It is applicable for people with abdominal distention and fullness, loose stool, greasy tongue coating, fresh-yellow jaundice with hot sensation all over the body or gloomy-yellow jaundice with aversion to cold. In the clinic, combination of herb is based on the state of illness, it is combined with Dà Huáng (Radix et Rhizoma Rhei), Zhī Zǐ (Fructus Gardeniae), and Huáng Bǎi (Cortex Phellodendri Chinensis) for fresh-yellow jaundice due to damp-heat; and with Bái Zhú (Rhizoma Atractylodis Macrocephalae), Fù Zǐ (Radix Aconiti Lateralis Praeparata), and Gān Jiāng (Rhizoma Zingiberis) for gloomy-yellow jaundice with abdominal distention and loose stool due to cold-damp.

It is also used in the treatment of different types of hepatitis, biliary tract infection, and hemolysis with jaundice.

[Usage and Dosage] Use raw in general, 10–30 g in decoction.

[Mnemonics] Yīn Chén (Herba Artemisiae Scopariae, Virgate Wormwood Herb): bitter and cold; specialized in relieving jaundice, combining with Zhī Zǐ (Fructus Gardeniae) and Dà Huáng (Radix et Rhizoma Rhei) for yang jaundice, and Fù Zǐ (Radix Aconiti Lateralis Praeparata) and Gān Jiāng (Rhizoma Zingiberis) for yin jaundice.

[Simple and Effective Formulas]

1. 茵陈蒿汤 Yīn Chén Hāo Tāng — Virgate Wormwood Decoction from *Treatise on Cold Damage* (伤寒论, Shāng Hán Lùn): Yīn Chén (Herba Artemisiae Scopariae) 15 g, Zhī Zǐ (Fructus Gardeniae) 10 g, and Dà Huáng (Radix et Rhizoma Rhei) 10 g; decoct in water for oral administration to treat patients with fever, orange-yellow jaundice, yellow and scanty urine, constipated stool, slippery fast pulse, and yellow greasy tongue coating. Also applicable for hepatocellular jaundice, jaundice due to acute general infection, and jaundice caused by acute suppurative cholangitis, cholecystitis, and gallbladder stone.

2. 茵陈四逆汤 Yīn Chén Sì Nì Tāng — Virgate Wormwood Frigid Extremities Decoction from *Detailed Explanation of the Jade Pivot* (玉机微义, Yù Jī Wēi Yì): Yīn Chén (Herba Artemisiae Scopariae) 15 g, Fù Zǐ (Radix Aconiti Lateralis Praeparata) 10 g, Gān Jiāng (Rhizoma Zingiberis) 10 g, and Gān Cǎo (Radix et Rhizoma Glycyrrhizae) 3 g; decoct in water for oral administration to treat patients with gloomy complexion, aversion to cold, listlessness, abdominal distention and fullness, loose stool, deep slow pulse, and white and greasy tongue coating. Also applicable for refractory hepatitis, chronic hepatitis, drug-induced hepatitis, cirrhosis, and obstructive jaundice.

金钱草 Jīn Qián Cǎo *herba lysimachiae lysimachia*

The source is from the whole herb of *Lysimachia christinae* Hance, family Primulaceae. Alternate names include 大金钱草 Dà Jīn Qián Cǎo and 神仙对坐草 Shén Xiān Duì Zuò Cǎo. Bitter and sour in flavor and cool in nature.

[Actions] Clear heat and eliminate dampness, improve gall-bladder function and expel stones, and relieve strangury and relieve edema. It is applicable for heat strangury, sand strangury, difficult and painful urination, jaundice, yellow urine, carbuncles, swellings, boils, sores, poisonous snake bites, and stone in the liver and gallbladder. Experiments reveal it has diuretic and choleretic effects.

[Quality] It includes many varieties. In eastern China, *Glechoma longituba* (Nakai) Kupr., family Labiatae is commonly used, and its alternate names include 连钱草 Lián Qián Cǎo and 江苏金钱草 Jiāng Sū Jīn Qián Cǎo; in Guangdong, *Desmodium styracifolium* (Osbeck.) Merr., family Leguminosae is applied and its alternate names include 广东金钱草 Guǎng Dōng Jīn Qián Cǎo; in Jiangxi, *Hydrocotyle dichondroides* Makino, family Umbelliferae is widely used and its alternate names include 江西金钱草 Jiāng Xi Jīn Qián Cǎo; and in Sichuan, *Dichondra repens* Forst, family Convolvulaceae is often applied and its alternate names include 小金钱草 Xiǎo Jīn Qián Cǎo. These herbal plants have similar actions, but their differences still need further research.

[Indications]

1. Damp-heat internal accumulation patterns: Jīn Qián Cǎo (Herba Lysimachiae) can be used alone or together with other medicinals for painful urination, pain in the liver and gallbladder, or stone in the biliary tract or urinary tract due to damp-heat accumulation in the liver, gallbladder, and urinary tract. It is combined with Mù Tōng (Caulis Akebiae), Chē Qián Zǐ (Semen Plantaginis), Qú Mài (Herba Dianthi), and Huá Shí (Talcum) for heat strangury with inhibited, dripping, difficult, and painful urination; with Jī Nèi Jīn (Endothelium Corneum Gigeriae Galli), Shí Wéi (Folium Pyrrosiae), and Hǎi Jīn Shā (Spora Lygodii) for urinary tract stone; and with Yīn Chén (Herba Artemisiae Scopariae), Dà Huáng (Radix et Rhizoma Rhei), and Hǔ Zhàng (Rhizoma Polygoni Cuspidati) for liver and gallbladder stone.
2. Damp-heat jaundice: Jīn Qián Cǎo (Herba Lysimachiae) is combined with Yīn Chén (Herba Artemisiae Scopariae), Zhī Zǐ (Fructus Gardeniae), and Huáng Bǎi (Cortex Phellodendri Chinensis) for jaundice caused by liver and gallbladder diseases.
3. Heat-toxin patterns: Jīn Qián Cǎo (Herba Lysimachiae), especially the fresh one, capable of resolving toxins and reducing swelling, is applicable for redness, swelling and pain with hot sensation in sores, ulcers, and

carbuncles, and poisonous snake bites. It can be twisted into juice for oral administration, or pounded for external application.

It is also applicable for nephritis edema, cough, white leukorrhea, and eczema.

[Usage and Dosage] Use in decoction, 9–30 g, and up to above 100 g when used alone or fresh.

[Mnemonics] Jīn Qián Cǎo (Herba Lysimachiae, Lysimachia): cool; resolve stone, relieve strangury and jaundice, and remove toxins.

[Simple and Effective Formulas]

1. 化石汤 Huà Shí Tāng — Stone Relieving Decoction from *Folk Herb Medicine in Zhejiang* (浙江民间草药, Zhè Jiāng Mín Jiān Cǎo Yào): Jīn Qián Cǎo (Herba Lysimachiae) 15 g, Lóng Xū Cǎo (Medulla Junci) 15 g, and Chē Qián Cǎo (Herba Plantaginis) 15 g; decoct in water for oral administration to treat bladder stone.

2. 治肾炎方 Zhì Shèn Yán Fāng — Nephriti Curing Formula from *Commonly-used Chinese Herbal Medicine in Shanghai* (上海常用中草药, Shànghǎi Cháng Yòng Zhōng Cǎo Yào): Jīn Qián Cǎo (Herba Lysimachiae) 30 g, Biǎn Xù Cǎo (Herba Polygoni Avicularis) 30 g, and Jì Cài Huā (Flos Capsellae) 15 g; decoct in water for oral administration to treat nephritis edema.

[Precautions] No toxic reaction has been reported to occur. However, when taking 江西金钱草 Jiāng Xi Jīn Qián Cǎo, a few patients can develop leucopenia, which is recoverable after cessation of the herb.

车前子 Chē Qián Zǐ *semen plantaginis plantago seed*

The source is from the ripe semen of herbaceous perennial *Plantago asiatica* L. or *P. depressa* Willa., family Plantaginaceae. Sweet in flavor and cold in nature.

[Actions] Clear heat and promote urination, relieve strangury and arrest diarrhea, and improve vision and relieve phlegm. It is applicable for inhibited urination, stranguria with turbid discharge, white leukorrhea, hematuria, cough with profuse sputum, damp *bì*, red eyes with nebula, and diarrhea and dysentery caused by summerheat-damp. This herb contains plantenolic acid, plantasan, protein, and succinic acid, and has diuretic, expectorant, and antibechic effects.

[Quality] Good quality is large, black, round, and full.

[Indications]

1. Water-dampness retention: Chē Qián Zǐ (Semen Plantaginis) has a significant effect on promoting urination and is applicable for different disorders caused by water-dampness retention. It is combined with Fú Líng (Poria), Mù Tōng (Caulis Akebiae), and Huá Shí (Talcum) for stranguary due to damp-heat in the bladder damp-heat; and with Fú Líng Pí (Cortex Poria), Zé Xiè (Rhizoma Alismatis), and Zhū Líng (Polyporus) for edema caused by water retention in the skin.
2. Summerheat-damp diarrhea: Chē Qián Zǐ (Semen Plantaginis) can be used alone or in a combination with Fú Líng (Poria), Zé Xiè (Rhizoma Alismatis), Tōng Cǎo (Medulla Tetrapanacis), Huá Shí (Talcum), and Gān Cǎo (Radix et Rhizoma Glycyrrhizae) for watery diarrhea due to externally-contracted summerheat-damp pathogen.
3. Red, swollen, and painful eyes: Chē Qián Zǐ (Semen Plantaginis) can clear liver fire and is often combined with Xià Kū Cǎo (Spica Prunellae), Jú Huā (Flos Chrysanthemi), and Jué Míng Zǐ (Semen Cassiae) for red, swollen, and painful eyes attributed to liver fire flaming upward; and with medicinals that supplement the liver and kidney for blurred vision due to liver and kidney yin deficiency.
4. Chē Qián Zǐ (Semen Plantaginis), capable of dispelling phlegm and clearing lung heat, is combined with Xìng Rén (Semen Armeniacae Amarum), Sāng Bái Pí (Cortex Mori), Huáng Qín (Radix Scutellariae), and Qián Hú (Radix Peucedani) for lung heat cough with sputum.

According to ancient medical books, its decoction can be used as external wash for vaginal itching.

[Usage and Dosage] Use raw in general, dry-fry with salt when used to clear heat and promote urination, and easily get those active ingredients. Use 6–12 g in decoction, and wrap in cheesecloth during decoction since it is sticky. Chē Qián Căo (Herba Plantaginis, Plantain) is effective at clearing heat and also relieve strangury.

[Mnemonics] Chē Qián Zĭ (Semen Plantaginis, Plantago Seed): resolve strangury, clear damp-heat, and relieve diarrhea, eyes problems, and cough.

[Simple and Effective Formulas]

1. 车前子散 Chē Qián Zĭ Săn — Plantago Seed Powder from *Secret Formulas of the Yang Family* (杨氏家藏方, Yáng Shì Jiā Cáng Fāng): Chē Qián Zĭ (Semen Plantaginis), Rén Shēn (Radix et Rhizoma Ginseng), Xiāng Rú (Herba Moslae), Fú Líng (Poria), and Zhū Líng (Polyporus) in equal dosage; grind into fine powder and take 3 g/time after mixing with Dēng Xīn Căo (Medulla Junci) decoction for pediatric vomiting, diarrhea and epidemic fever due to latent summer-dampness, vexation, intense thirst, and urinary retention.

2. 八正散 Bā Zhèng Săn — Eight Corrections Powder from *Formulas from the Imperial Pharmacy* (局方, Jú Fāng): Chē Qián Zĭ (Semen Plantaginis), Biăn Xù (Herba Polygoni Avicularis), Qú Mài (Herba Dianthi), Huá Shí (Talcum), Zhī Zĭ (Fructus Gardeniae), Zhì Gān Căo (Radix et Rhizoma Glycyrrhizae Praeparata cum Melle), Mù Tōng (Caulis Akebiae), and Dà Huáng (Radix et Rhizoma Rhei) in equal dosage; decoct 6 g/time with Dēng Xīn Căo (Medulla Junci) in water for oral administration to treat difficult and obstructive urination, heat strangury, and blood strangury. Also applicable for urinary tract infection and stone.

[Precautions] Chē Qián Zĭ (Semen Plantaginis), slippery in nature, cannot be used alone for deficiency patterns to prevent damage of vital qi and should be combined with tonics when necessary.

Daily practices

1. What are the similarities and differences among Yīn Chén (Herba Artemisiae Scopariae), Jīn Qián Căo (Herba Lysimachiae), and Chē Qián Zĭ (Semen Plantaginis) in terms of actions and indications?

2. Among medicinals that disinhibit water, which ones can be used to relieve strangury?
3. Among medicinals that disinhibit water, which ones can be used to arrest diarrhea?

MEDICINALS THAT WARM THE INTERIOR

Cold pattern in traditional Chinese medicine refers not only to excess coldness attributable to invasion of exogenous cold pathogen into the body but also internally-generated deficiency-cold due to yang qi deficiency. In general, interior-warming herbs are used in treating interior cold, either through warming and dispersing internal coldness or warming and tonifying yang qi.

Interior cold pattern is featured by systemic functional weakness and a slowing of the metabolism. Symptoms associated with externally-contracted excess cold pattern include cold limbs, fear of cold, abdominal pain, constipation, wheezing, white greasy coating, and deep hidden or wiry tense powerful pulse, whereas the internally-generated patterns of deficiency-old is often resulting from yang qi deficiency manifested as cold extremities, fear of cold, abdominal pain with a preference for pressing, listlessness, loose stool or with undigested food, clear and copious urine, and weak or deep slow powerless pulse.

These interior-warming herbs are warm and hot in nature and most of them have acrid flavor. They can not only warm the interior to dissipate cold, but also warm and tonify yang qi, and restore yang to rescue from counterflow desertion. Therefore, some herbs that tonify yang (see chapter 14) are also can be categorized into interior-warming medicinals, while some herbs that warm the interior (in this chapter) are related to the herbs that tonify the yang.

Medicinals that warm the interior can be further divided by indications into four types: 1) herbs that warm the spleen and stomach are applicable for the pattern of spleen and stomach cold with such symptoms as gastric and abdominal cold pain, vomiting, clear fluid in the mouth, and diarrhea; 2) herbs that warm yang qi of the spleen and kidney are used for the pattern of spleen and kidney yang deficiency manifested as fear of cold, cold extremities, abdominal cold pain, vomiting of clear and cold fluid, loose stool or with indigested food, clear and copious urine or frequent urination, pale tongue with white coating, and deep thin or minute or deep slow powerless pulse; 3) herbs that restore yang qi are suitable for the pattern of yang collapse with ice-cold extremities and feeble pulse; and 4) herbs that warm and unblock the channels and collaterals to dissipate cold and arrest pain are appropriate for different types of pain caused by cold pathogenic influence obstruction in the channels and collaterals.

The selection of herbs for clinical use is based on the etiology of the cold disorder. Specifically, warm and dispersing medicinals should be used in conditions of externally-contracted cold excess; medicinals that warm and tonify yang qi should be applied for the cold pattern resulting from yang qi deficiency; and medicinals that boost the spleen and reinforce the kidney are prescribed in the cases of spleen and kidney yang deficiency. The combination of herbs is based on the state of illness. For instance, they are often used in conjunction with herbs that move qi when patient also present with qi stagnation; with herbs that transform dampness if there is cold-dampness; and with medicinals that strongly tonify original qi in serious cases of yang collapse.

These herbs are warm, hot, and drying in nature. For this reason, they can easily injure yin and stir bleeding. They must therefore be used with the utmost caution or contraindicated in cases of yin deficiency with internal heat or during pregnancy. More attention should be paid on the dosage as some of them have certain degrees of toxicity.

附子 Fù Zǐ *radix aconiti lateralis praeparata monkshood*

The source is from the lateral tuber of herbaceous perennial *Aconitum carmichaeli* Debx., family Ranunculaceae. Pungent in flavor and extremely hot in nature with toxicity.

[Actions] Warm yang and assist fire, restore yang to rescue from counterflow desertion restore devastated yang, and disperse cold and arrest pain. It is applicable for cold excubrance diseases and patterns, exuberant yin repelling yang, yang collapse with profuse sweating, vomiting and diarrhea, reversal counterflow cold of the limbs, cold pain in the chest and abdomen, cold diarrhea and dysentery, leg qi with edema, wind-cold-dampness *bì*, atrophy and weakness of the lower limbs, spasms and tension of the limbs, yin flat-abscess, sores and fistula, and other chronic diseases. This herb contains alkaloid and its major ingredients include aconitine, mesaconitine, and hypaconitine. It also contains non-alkaloid compounds. It has shown antalgic and cardiotonic effects, can increase heart beat, and has shown a significant anti-inflammatory effect on experimental arthritis.

[Quality] It is mainly produced in Sichuan and Shannxi. The one produced in Sichuan is the best and known as 川附子 Chuān Fù Zǐ. 生附子 Shēng Fù Zǐ (untreated herb) is toxic and usually prepared with salt brine to reduce its toxicity. Its major processed products include 盐附子 Yán Fù Zǐ, 黑附子 Hēi Fù Zǐ, 淡附片 Dàn Fù Piàn, and 炮附子 Pào Fù Zǐ.

[Indications]

1. Reversal counterflow cold of the limbs and yang collapse: reversal counterflow means ice-cold limbs and yang collapse refers to sudden loss of yang with accompanying listlessness, cold body with sweating, faint low voice, and deep feeble pulse. It is shock from the perspective of modern biomedicine and commonly occurs in weak people or in cases of profuse sweating, dramatic purgation, and profuse bleeding. Deep feeble pulse, one of the most important indicators of using Fù Zǐ (Radix Aconiti Lateralis Praeparata) means the shape of pulse is extremely thin, feeble and difficult to feel; hidden so deeply that only be felt on hard pressure; or sudden change of the pulse into floating big soggy one. In this case, Fù Zǐ (Radix Aconiti Lateralis Praeparata) is usually combined with Rén Shēn (Radix et Rhizoma Ginseng) and Gān Jiāng (Rhizoma Zingiberis). For accompanying profuse sweating, it is also combined with Mǔ Lì (Concha Ostreae) and Lóng Gǔ (Os Draconis) to consolidate and arrest sweating.
2. Pain: Fù Zǐ (Radix Aconiti Lateralis Praeparata) is applicable for cold pathogen induced severe pain, for instance serious joint pain, muscle contracture and limited joint movement resulting from profuse diaphoresis, rib-side and abdominal intense pain, or chest pain radiating to the back. Meanwhile, patients also present gloomy complexion or slight edema in the face, dull eyes, faint low voice, ice-cold limbs, somnolence, and body tiredness and heaviness. It is combined with Bái Zhú (Rhizoma Atractylodis Macrocephalae), Guì Zhī (Ramulus Cinnamomi),

and Gān Cǎo (Radix et Rhizoma Glycyrrhizae) for cold-damp *bì* pain; and with Dǎng Shēn (Radix Codonopsis), Bái Zhú (Rhizoma Atractylodis Macrocephalae), and Gān Jiāng (Rhizoma Zingiberis) for stomach pain due to cold congealing and qi stagnation.

3. Spleen and kidney deficiency-cold: Fù Zǐ (Radix Aconiti Lateralis Praeparata) can warm yang qi through out the body and is one of principal medicinals to treat different types of deficiency-cold. Kidney yang deficiency pattern is manifested as frequent urination, impotence, aversion to cold, and cold limbs; while spleen yang deficiency pattern is marked by gastric and abdominal cold pain and loose stool. Fù Zǐ (Radix Aconiti Lateralis Praeparata) is applicable for both conditions in a combination with medicinals that either warm the kidney or fortify the spleen. It is used together with Ròu Guì (Cortex Cinnamomi) and Shú Dì Huáng (Radix Rehmanniae Praeparata) for deficiency-cold caused by kidney yang insufficiency; and with Bái Zhú (Rhizoma Atractylodis Macrocephalae) and Gān Jiāng (Rhizoma Zingiberis) for spleen deficiency-cold due to spleen yang insufficiency.

[Usage and Dosage] Processing before use as a medicinal reduces its toxic properties but retains its therapeutic effects. The untreated herb, with strong toxicity, is often applied externally, but rarely prescribed for oral administration, except for the severe case of cold-dampness. Boiling for 30–60 minutes and above before adding other ingredients reduces its toxic properties as its aconine is further hydrolyzed to yield aconine, but its therapeutic effects are retained. Use 3–10 g in decoction, and less than 1 g/time as in pill and powder.

[Mnemonics] Fù Zǐ (Radix Aconiti Lateralis Praeparata, Monkshood): pungent and hot; restore yang to rescue from counterflow, warm the channels to arrest pain, and use with caution as it is toxic.

[Simple and Effective Formulas]

1. 四逆汤 Sì Nì Tāng — Frigid Extremities Decoction from *Treatise on Cold Damage* (伤寒论, Shāng Hán Lùn): Fù Zǐ (Radix Aconiti Lateralis Praeparata) 10 g, Gān Jiāng (Rhizoma Zingiberis) 10 g, and Gān Cǎo (Radix et Rhizoma Glycyrrhizae) 3 g; decoct in water for oral

administration to treat patients with feeble pulse, digestive tract symptoms, reversal cold of the limbs, and diarrhea with undigested food. Also applicable for shock, digestive system diseases, cardiovascular diseases, and arthritis.

2. 桂枝加附子汤 Guì Zhī Jiā Fù Zǐ Tāng — Cinnamon Twig Decoction plus Aconite from *Treatise on Cold Damage* (伤寒论, Shāng Hán Lùn): Fù Zǐ (Radix Aconiti Lateralis Praeparata) 10 g, Guì Zhī (Ramulus Cinnamomi) 10 g, Sháo Yào (Radix Paeoniae) 10 g, Gān Cǎo (Radix et Rhizoma Glycyrrhizae) 3 g, Shēng Jiāng (Rhizoma Zingiberis Recens) 3 pieces, and ten Dà Zǎo (Fructus Jujubae); decoct in water for oral administration to treat patients with aversion to cold, profuse sweating, palpitations, and contracture and pain of the limbs and muscle. Also applicable for common cold, joint pain, allergic rhinitis, and autonomic nerve dysfunction.

3. 芍药甘草附子汤 Sháo Yào Gān Cǎo Fù Zǐ Tāng — Peony Root, Licorice Root, and Aconite Decoction from *Treatise on Cold Damage* (伤寒论, Shāng Hán Lùn): Fù Zǐ (Radix Aconiti Lateralis Praeparata) 10 g, Sháo Yào (Radix Paeoniae) 30 g, and Gān Cǎo (Radix et Rhizoma Glycyrrhizae) 3 g; decoct in water for oral administration to treat patients with aversion to cold and muscle contracture of limbs difficult to bend. Also applicable for sciatica.

4. 附子汤 Fù Zǐ Tāng — Aconite Decoction from *Treatise on Cold Damage* (伤寒论, Shāng Hán Lùn): Fù Zǐ (Radix Aconiti Lateralis Praeparata) 10 g, Bái Zhú (Rhizoma Atractylodis Macrocephalae) 12 g, Sháo Yào (Radix Paeoniae) 12 g, Rén Shēn (Radix et Rhizoma Ginseng) 10 g, and Fú Líng (Poria) 12 g; decoct in water for oral administration to treat patients with aversion to cold in the back, body pain, cold hands and feet, joint pain, and deep pulse. Also applicable for arthritis, lumbar spondylopathy, nephritis with manifestations of cold exuberance or yang qi insufficiency.

5. 大黄附子汤 Dà Huáng Fù Zǐ Tāng — Rhubarb Root and Rhizome and Aconite Decoction from *Essentials from the Golden Cabinet* (金匮要略, Jīn Guì Yào Lüè): Fù Zǐ (Radix Aconiti Lateralis Praeparata) 10 g, Dà Huáng (Radix et Rhizoma Rhei) 6 g, and Xì Xīn (Radix et Rhizoma Asari) 5 g; decoct in water for oral administration to treat patients with rib-side and abdominal severe pain, constipation, and white tongue

coating. Also applicable for neuralgia, habitual constipation, biliary tract disease, urinary tract stone, pharyngitis, hernia, and epididymitis.

6. 麻黄附子甘草汤 Má Huáng Fù Zǐ Gān Cǎo Tāng — Ephedra, Aconite, and Licorice Root Decoction from *Treatise on Cold Damage* (伤寒论, Shāng Hán Lùn): Fù Zǐ (Radix Aconiti Lateralis Praeparata) 6 g, Má Huáng (Herba Ephedrae) 6 g, and Gān Cǎo (Radix et Rhizoma Glycyrrhizae) 3 g; decoct in water for oral administration to treat patients with deep pulse, aversion to cold, absence of sweating, and soreness and heaviness of the body.

[Precautions] Fù Zǐ (Radix Aconiti Lateralis Praeparata), extremely pungent and hot, is contraindicated in cases of excess heat, especially heat syncope with illusionary cold and true heat. This substance is tonic and more attention should be paid to its indications, dosage, usage, and compatibility. Symptoms of poisoning include numbness of limbs, vertigo, lack of strength, nausea, vomiting, sweating, increased salivation, or even palpitations, chest oppression, arrhythmia, decreased blood pressure, and eventually convulsion, coma and heart and respiratory arrest. It is contraindicated to cases of atrioventricular block and should be used with caution for patients with cardiomyopathy and hepatosis. According to some ancient materia medica books, this herb should not to be used together with Bèi Mǔ (Bulbus Fritillaria), Bàn Xià (Rhizoma Pinelliae), Guā Lóu (Fructus Trichosanthis), Bái Jí (Rhizoma Bletillae), and Bái Liǎn (adix Ampelopsis)", however nowadays in the clinic Fù Zǐ (Radix Aconiti Lateralis Praeparata) is commonly combined with Bàn Xià (Rhizoma Pinelliae) and shows no adverse reaction.

干姜 Gān Jiāng *rhizoma zingiberis dried ginger rhizome*

The source is from the dried tuber of herbaceous perennial *Zingibor officinale* Rosc, family Zingiberaceae. Pungent in flavor and hot in nature.

[Actions] Warm the middle *jiao* and rescue devastated yang, warm the lungs and relieve fluid retention, and warm the channels and arrest bleeding. It is applicable for spleen and stomach deficiency-cold pattern manifested as gastric and abdominal cold pain, vomiting, and diarrhea, and deficiency-cold induced bleeding. This herb contains ginger oil and cap-saicine, and can cause reflexible excitation of vasomotor center and sympathetic nerve to rinse up blood pressure.

[Quality] Soaked in water, obtained and softened in a sealed container, cut into slices, and dried under sunshine. It is mainly produced in Sichuan and Hunan, however back to ancient times, the one from Junzhou of Hunan is regarded as genuine regional medicinal and therefore called 均姜 Jūn Jiāng. Nowadays, the one produced in Jian Banchang of Sichuan is the best and known as 川干姜 Chuān Gān Jiāng, good quality is large, solid, white, and powdery with a thin skin.

[Indications]

1. Increased salivation and spittle without thirst: manifestations include increased cold salivation that relieved after spitting out; or turbid and greasy saliva with nausea; absence of thirst without desire of drink or thirst but with little water intake; and white thick or greasy, or white slippery tongue coating covered by a layer of mucus, known as an important indicator to use Gān Jiāng (Rhizoma Zingiberis). For increased saliva and spittle and absence of thirst with accompanying gastric and abdominal cold pain, vomiting, and diarrhea, it is often combined with Bàn Xià (Rhizoma Pinelliae) and Bái Zhú (Rhizoma Atractylodis Macrocephalae).
2. Yang collapse: for the treatment of yang collapse, Gān Jiāng (Rhizoma Zingiberis) is usually prescribed together with Fù Zǐ (Radix Aconiti Lateralis Praeparata) to reduce the toxicity of Fù Zǐ (Radix Aconiti Lateralis Praeparata) and also increase the ability of restore yang to rescue from counterflow desertion.
3. Cough and wheezing due to cold water-retention: Gān Jiāng (Rhizoma Zingiberis) can warm the lung and relieve water-retention, and is combined with Má Huáng (Herba Ephedrae), Xì Xīn (Radix et Rhizoma Asari), and Wǔ Wèi Zǐ (Fructus Schisandrae Chinensis) for cough and wheezing with thin and cleat sputum due to cold-rheum accumulation in the lung.
4. Bleeding due to deficiency-cold: Gān Jiāng (Rhizoma Zingiberis) can warm and reinforce spleen yang to recover its function of governing blood and is applicable for deficiency-cold hematemesis, stool with blood, profuse uterine bleeding, and prolonged scanty uterine bleeding

of variable intervals in a combination with medicinals that supplement qi and stanch bleeding.

[Usage and Dosage] Use raw in general, and frying the herb until the surface is slightly blackened (炮干姜, Pào Gān Jiāng) to warm the center to arrest diarrhea or warm the channels to stanch bleeding. Use 2–10 g in decoction, up to above 10 g when used for rescuing devastated yang.

[Mnemonics] Gān Jiāng (Rhizoma Zingiberis, Dried Ginger Rhizome): pungent and hot; warm the middle *jiao* powerfully, rescue devastated yang, warm the lungs, and arrest bleeding.

[Simple and Effective Formulas]

1. 甘草干姜汤 Gān Cǎo Gān Jiāng Tāng — Licorice and Dried Ginger Rhizome Decoction from *Treatise on Cold Damage* (伤寒论, Shāng Hán Lùn): Gān Jiāng (Rhizoma Zingiberis) 10 g and Gān Cǎo (Radix et Rhizoma Glycyrrhizae) 3 g; decoct in water for oral administration to treat patients with vomiting of watery fluid, vomiting, cough, diarrhea, and dysentery. Also applicable for digestive system diseases and respiratory tract disorders.

2. 干姜附子汤 Gān Jiāng Fù Zǐ Tāng — Dried Ginger Rhizome and Aconite Decoction from *Treatise on Cold Damage* (伤寒论, Shāng Hán Lùn): Gān Jiāng (Rhizoma Zingiberis) 10 g and Fù Zǐ (Radix Aconiti Lateralis Praeparata) 10 g; decoct in water for oral administration to treat patients with reversal cold of the extremities and feeble pulse. Also applicable for shock, digestive system diseases, and cardiovascular diseases.

3. 甘姜苓术汤 Gān Jiāng Líng Zhú Tāng — Licorice Root, Dried Ginger Rhizome, Poria, and White Atractylodes Rhizome Decoction from *Essentials from the Golden Cabinet* (金匮要略, Jīn Guì Yào Lüè): Gān Jiāng (Rhizoma Zingiberis) 10 g, Bái Zhú (Rhizoma Atractylodis Macrocephalae) 12 g, Fú Líng (Poria) 12 g, and Gān Cǎo (Radix et Rhizoma Glycyrrhizae) 3 g; decoct in water for oral administration to treat patients with lumbar and abdominal cold pain, aversion to cold, and inhibited urination. Also applicable for joint pain, lumbar spondylopathy, strain of lumbar muscles, abnormal vaginal discharge, and gastroenteritis.

4. 干姜黄芩黄连人参汤 Gān Jiāng Huáng Qín Huáng Lián Rén Shēn Tāng — Dried Ginger Rhizome, Scutellaria, Coptis, and Ginseng Decoction from *Treatise on Cold Damage* (伤寒论, Shāng Hán Lùn): Gān Jiāng (Rhizoma Zingiberis) 10 g, Huáng Qín (Radix Scutellariae) 6 g, Huáng Lián (Rhizoma Coptidis) 5 g, Rén Shēn (Radix et Rhizoma Ginseng) 10 g or Dǎng Shēn (Radix Codonopsis) 12 g; decoct in water for oral administration to treat epigastric *pǐ*, vexation with agitation, abdominal pain, diarrhea and dysentery, and yellow white tongue coating.

5. 理中汤 Lǐ Zhōng Tāng — Center-Regulating Decoction from *Treatise on Cold Damage* (伤寒论, Shāng Hán Lùn): Gān Jiāng (Rhizoma Zingiberis) 10 g, Rén Shēn (Radix et Rhizoma Ginseng) 10 g, Bái Zhú (Rhizoma Atractylodis Macrocephalae) 10 g, and Gān Cǎo (Radix et Rhizoma Glycyrrhizae) 3 g; decoct in water for oral administration to treat patients with abdominal distention, diarrhea, dysentery, cold sensation in the stomach, and white greasy tongue coating. Also applicable for different types of digestive system diseases.

[Precautions] Gān Jiāng (Rhizoma Zingiberis), pungent and hot, should be used with caution in cases of blood heat, yin deficiency with internal heat manifested as red tongue with scanty coating and dry and hard stool, and during pregnancy.

Daily practices

1. What is the medicinal that warm the interior and what are the actions? What precautions should be taken when using it?
2. What are the similarities and differences between Fù Zǐ (Radix Aconiti Lateralis Praeparata) and Gān Jiāng (Rhizoma Zingiberis) in terms of actions and indications?

吴茱萸 Wú Zhū Yú *fructus evodiae medicinal evodia fruit*

The source is from the unripe fruit of deciduous shrub or subarbor *Evodia rutaecarpa* (Juss) Benth or other congeneric species, family Rutaceae. Pungent and bitter in flavor and hot in nature.

[Actions] Warm the middle *jiao* and dissipate cold to arrest pain, smooth the liver, redirect rebellious qi downward to stop vomiting, and warm the middle *jiao* to stop vomiting. It is applicable for vomiting, acid regurgitation, headache, diarrhea, gastric and abdominal pain, leg qi, hernia, aphtha, ulcer, eczema, and impetigo. This herb contains volatile oil and its major ingredients include evoden, obakulactone, evodiamine, and rutaecarpin. Volatile oil is aromatic and can strengthen the stomach and inhibit intestinal abnormal fermentation. Oral administration of this herb can arrest vomiting and decrease blood pressure.

[Quality] It is mainly produced in Guizhou, Guangxi, Hunan, Yunnan, Shaanxi, and Sichuan, good quality is green, full, round, aromatic, bitter, and slightly pungent. To reduce the its toxicity, the raw Wú Zhū Yú (Fructus Evodiae) should be soaked in boiled water or Gān Cǎo (Radix et Rhizoma Glycyrrhizae) decoction, rinsed by running water, and dried under sunshine before using. It is called 制吴萸 Zhì Wú Yú, also known as 淡吴萸 Dàn Wú Yú.

[Indications]

1. Abdominal pain: Wú Zhū Yú (Fructus Evodiae) is applicable for abdominal pain (persistently distending pain, distending stabbing pain, and eliminated by warmth) with accompanying retching, reversal cold, and white thick tongue coating. It is combined with Wū Yào (Radix Linderae), Xiǎo Huí Xiāng (Fructus Foeniculi), and Gān Jiāng (Rhizoma Zingiberis).
2. Headache: Wú Zhū Yú (Fructus Evodiae) is applicable for severe headache involving the whole head or the parietal region with accompanying reversal cold hands and feet and such digestive tract symptoms as retching, vomiting of clear saliva, chest fullness, and abdominal pain. It is often prescribed together with Rén Shēn (Radix et Rhizoma Ginseng) and Shēng Jiāng (Rhizoma Zingiberis Recens).
3. Disharmony between the liver and stomach: Wú Zhū Yú (Fructus Evodiae) is combined with small amount of Huáng Lián (Rhizoma Coptidis) for disharmony between the liver and stomach manifested as acid regurgitation, vomiting, belching, and gastric pain with distention

and fullness caused by either liver qi exuberance or intense liver qi transforming into fire and attacking the stomach.

4. Cold-damp diarrhea: Wú Zhū Yú (Fructus Evodiae) can be used alone or together with Bǔ Gǔ Zhī (Fructus Psoraleae), Ròu Dòu Kòu (Semen Myristicae), and Wǔ Wèi Zǐ (Fructus Schisandrae Chinensis) for diarrhea attributed to either cold-damp or deficiency-cold.

It can also be ground into powder and applied externally to Yǒng Quán (KI 1) to drain fire downward in the treatment of ulcers in the mouth and tongue, increased salivation in children, and hypertension.

[Usage and Dosage] Process it to reduce its drying property, treat with a decoction of Huáng Lián (Rhizoma Coptidis) to increase its ability of arresting vomiting, and stir-fry with salt solution for hernia. Use 1.5–6 g in decoction, decrease the dosage as in pill and powder.

[Mnemonics] Wú Zhū Yú (Fructus Evodiae, Medicinal Evodia Fruit): bitter and pungent; dispel cold, warm the channels, stop vomiting and diarrhea, and arrest headache.

[Simple and Effective Formulas]

1. 吴茱萸汤 Wú Zhū Yú Tāng — Evodia Decoction from *Treatise on Cold Damage* (伤寒论, Shāng Hán Lùn): Wú Zhū Yú (Fructus Evodiae) 5 g, Rén Shēn (Radix et Rhizoma Ginseng) 10 g or Dǎng Shēn (Radix Codonopsis) 15 g, Shēng Jiāng (Rhizoma Zingiberis Recens) three pieces, and Dà Zǎo (Fructus Jujubae) 12 pieces; decoct in water for oral administration to treat patients with abdominal pain, belching, vomiting of saliva, headache, and vomiting and diarrhea with reversal counterflow cold of the limbs. Also applicable for digestive system diseases, neurotic vomiting, and angioneurotic headache.

2. 四神丸 Sì Shén Wán — Four Spirits Pill from *Corrections and Annotations to Effective Formulas for Women* (校注妇人良方, Jiào Zhù Fù Rén Liáng Fāng): Wú Zhū Yú (Fructus Evodiae) 6 g, Bǔ Gǔ Zhī (Fructus Psoraleae) 10 g, Ròu Dòu Kòu (Semen Myristicae) 6 g, and Wǔ Wèi Zǐ (Fructus Schisandrae Chinensis) 10 g; decoct in water for oral administration to treat patients with diarrhea before dawn or chronic diarrhea, poor appetite, abdominal pain, and cold limbs. Also applicable

for chronic enteritis, tuberculosis of intestines, and especially diarrhea before dawn.

3. 吳茱萸散 Wú Zhū Yú Săn — Evodia Powder from *Formulas from Benevolent Sages Compiled during the Taiping Era* (太平圣惠方, Tài Píng Shèng Huì Fāng): Wú Zhū Yú (Fructus Evodiae) 6 g and Hòu Pò (Cortex Magnoliae Officinalis)10 g; decoct in water for oral administration to treat patients with vomiting and diarrhea, distention and fullness in the heart and abdomen, cramp of the legs, and cold hands and feet. Also applicable for various digestive system diseases.

4. 左金丸 Zuǒ Jīn Wán — Left Metal Pill from *Teachings of Dan-xi* (丹溪心法, Dān Xī Xīn Fǎ): Wú Zhū Yú (Fructus Evodiae) 3 g and Huáng Lián (Rhizoma Coptidis) 5 g; decoct in water for oral administration to treat patients with epigastric upset and pain, vomiting, acid regurgitation, bitter taste in the mouth, red tongue, and wiry fast pulse. Also applicable for digestive system diseases with above-mentioned manifestations.

[Precautions] Overdose and long-term use of Wú Zhū Yú (Fructus Evodiae) is discouraged. Overdose may cause the throat to become extremely dry and extreme overdose can result in poisoning manifested as central nervous excitation, or even visual impairment and illusion. This substance, pungent and hot in nature, can easily consume yin and stir fire and therefore should be used with caution in cases of yin deficiency with heat signs such as red tongue with scanty coating.

细辛 Xì Xīn *radix et rhizoma asari manchurian wild ginger*

The source is from the whole herb of herbaceous perennial *Asarum heterotropoides* Fr. Schmidt var. mandshuricum (Maxim) Litag., or A. sieboldii Miq., family Aristolochiaceae. It is so called because of its thin root and pungent flavor. Pungent in flavor and warm in nature.

[Actions] Warm the channels and arrest pain, warm the lungs and relieve fluid retention, disperse cold and release the exterior, and unblock the nasal orifices. It is applicable for common cold of wind-cold type, headache, toothache, nasal congestion and sinusitis. This herb contains volatile oil and higenamine. Its volatile oil has shown hypnotic, antalgic, and sedative effects, and its higenamine has cardiotonic, blood vessel-dilating, smooth muscle-relaxing, lipid metabolism-incresing, and hyperglycemic effects. Its water or ethanol extractives can inhibit allergic reaction.

[Quality] It is divided into 北细辛 Běi Xì Xīn and 南细辛 Nán Xì Xīn. The former is native in Liaoning, Jilin, and Helongjiang and has been considered as commonly-used quality goods. Good quality is dry, aromatic, has a grayish yellow root and green leaves that are acrid and make the tongue slightly numb.

[Indications]

1. Cough and wheezing due to cold fluid-retention: manifestations include aversion to cold, absence of thirst, white and profuse clear and thin sputum and nasal discharge, or nasal congestion, or unremitting cough and wheezing, and white glossy coating. Xì Xīn (Radix et Rhizoma Asari) is capable of warming the lung and relieving fluid-retention and often combined with Gān Jiāng (Rhizoma Zingiberis) and Wǔ Wèi Zǐ (Fructus Schisandrae Chinensis).

2. Pain patterns: manifestations include headache, body pain, abdominal pain, chest and back pain, sore throat, toothache, and eye pain. The pain is aggravated by cold and accompanied with cold limbs, aversion to cold, and absence of thirst. Xì Xīn (Radix et Rhizoma Asari), capable of warming the channels and relieving pain, can be decocted to rinse the mouth or ground with Chuān Wū (Radix Aconiti) and Rǔ Xiāng (Olibanum) into powder for external application to relieve wind-cold toothache. It is combined with Shí Gāo (Gypsum Fibrosum) for wind-fire toothache; and with Fáng Fēng (Radix Saposhnikoviae) and Dú Huó (Radix Angelicae Pubescentis) for wind-damp *bì* pain.

3. Wind-cold exterior pattern: Xì Xīn (Radix et Rhizoma Asari) can release the exterior and disperse cold, and therefore applicable for wind-cold common cold and other diseases caused by exogenous cold pathogen. It is combined with other medicinals that release the exterior with acrid-warm properties such as Qiāng Huó (Rhizoma et Radix Notopterygii), Guì Zhī (Ramulus Cinnamomi), and Zǐ Sū Yè (Folium Perillae) for wind-cold exterior pattern; and with Má Huáng (Herba

Ephedrae) and Fù Zǐ (Radix Aconiti Lateralis Praeparata) for aversion to cold, fever, lassitude, somnolence, deep pulse, and white glossy tongue coating due to yang deficiency with externally-contract cold pathogen, also called cold entering *shaoyin* in traditional Chinese medicine.

4. Sinusitis: Xì Xīn (Radix et Rhizoma Asari), pungent and warm in nature with an effect of diffusing and unblocking the nasal orifices, is combined with Xīn Yí (Flos Magnoliae) and Bái Zhǐ (Radix Angelicae Dahuricae) for sinusitis with clear nasal discharge and nasal congestion.

[Usage and Dosage] Use raw, 1–3 g in decoction. It has been reported that when used for wind-cold headache, increasing the dosage even up to 15 g brings no side effects at all, as its essential oil evaporates in the decocting process. However, decrease the dosage in pill and powder due to its toxicity.

[Mnemonics] Xì Xīn (Radix et Rhizoma Asari, Manchurian Wild Ginger): pungent and warm; warm and dissolve cold-fluid retention, warm the channels, arrest pain, disperse cold, and dispel wind.

[Simple and Effective Formulas]

1. 小青龙汤 Xiǎo Qīng Lóng Tāng — Minor Green Dragon Decoction from *Treatise on Cold Damage* (伤寒论, Shāng Hán Lùn): Xì Xīn (Radix et Rhizoma Asari) 6 g, Gān Jiāng (Rhizoma Zingiberis) 10 g, Wǔ Wèi Zǐ (Fructus Schisandrae Chinensis) 10 g, Má Huáng (Herba Ephedrae) 5 g, Guì Zhī (Ramulus Cinnamomi) 10 g, Sháo Yào (Radix Paeoniae) 10 g, Bàn Xià (Rhizoma Pinelliae) 6 g, and Gān Cǎo (Radix et Rhizoma Glycyrrhizae) 3 g; decoct in water for oral administration to treat patients with aversion to cold, absence of thirst, cough and wheezing, and profuse clean sputum. Also applicable for bronchial asthma, asthmatic tracheitis, and allergic rhinitis.

2. 麻黄附子细辛汤 Má Huáng Fù Zǐ Xì Xīn Tāng — Ephedra, Aconite and Asarum Decoction from *Treatise on Cold Damage* (伤寒论, Shāng Hán Lùn): Xì Xīn (Radix et Rhizoma Asari) 6 g, Fù Zǐ (Radix Aconiti Lateralis Praeparata) 10 g, and Má Huáng (Herba Ephedrae) 6 g; decoct

in water for oral administration to treat patients with absence of sweating, aversion to cold, fever, and deep pulse. Also applicable for common cold, sciatica, joint pain, and cardiovascular diseases.

3. 细辛散 Xì Xīn Sǎn — Asarum Powder from *Formulas for Universal Relief* (普济方, Pǔ Jì Fāng): Xì Xīn (Radix et Rhizoma Asari) 6 g, Chuān Xiōng (Rhizoma Chuanxiong) 10 g, Má Huáng (Herba Ephedrae) 6 g, and Fù Zǐ (Radix Aconiti Lateralis Praeparata) 10 g; decoct in water for oral administration to treat patients with splitting headache, absence of sweating, aversion to cold, and deep tight pulse. Also applicable for neurotic headache.

[Precautions] The most important indicators of using Xì Xīn (Radix et Rhizoma Asari) include aversion to cold with absence of thirst, listlessness, somnolence without desire to speak, cleat and profuse urine, light red tongue, white and slippery tongue coating with a mucus layer or feeling of cold qi in the mouth, and increased clear salivation with a sensation of cold when swallow it. High-dose use is discouraged, traditional resources stated "use of Xì Xīn (Radix et Rhizoma Asari) should be less than 3 g"; and current animal experiments reveal that large doses of its volatile oil may cause excitement, paralysis, decreased voluntary and respiratory movement, areflexia, respiratory paralysis, and eventually death. However, in practical applications, the toxicity varies from powder to decoction, from single use to in combination, and from short to long period of decoction. Therefore, use of large doses in the clinic has been reported. However, to guarantee patient safety, the dosage should be controlled cautiously when used as powder for oral administration; the amount can be increased properly (not limited to less than 3 g, but should not be overdosed) for decoction, especially when combined with Wǔ Wèi Zǐ (Fructus Schisandrae Chinensis), Gān Jiāng (Rhizoma Zingiberis), and Gān Cǎo (Radix et Rhizoma Glycyrrhizae) and should not be used more than one week.

Daily practices

1. What are the similarities and differences between Wú Zhū Yú (Fructus Evodiae) and Xì Xīn (Radix et Rhizoma Asari) in terms of actions and indications?

2. What are the similarities and differences among Fù Zǐ (Radix Aconiti Lateralis Praeparata), Gān Jiāng (Rhizoma Zingiberis), Wú Zhū Yú (Fructus Evodiae), and Xì Xīn (Radix et Rhizoma Asari) in terms of their actions and indications in warm the interior?

花椒 **Huā Jiāo** *pericarpium zanthoxyli pricklyash peel*

The source is from the ripe peel of shrub or subarbor *Zanthoxylum bungeanum* Maxim. or *Z. schinifolium* Sieb. et Zucc., family Rutaceae. Alternate names include 川椒 Chuān Jiāo or 蜀椒, Shǔ Jiāo as the best is from Sichuan province. Pungent in flavor and hot in nature with mild toxicity.

[Actions] Warm the middle *jiao* to disperse cold, remove dampness and alleviate pain, and kill parasites. It is applicable for cold pain in the heart and abdomen, vomiting, cough, wheezing, wind-cold-damp *bì*, diarrhea, dysentery, hernia, toothache, roundworm, pinworm, vaginal itching, and scabies. This herb contains volatile oil and can kill parasites; its decoction has shown an inhibitory effect against a variety of pathogenic bacteria.

[Quality] Good quality is shiny, thin-skinned, bright red without impurities. Pericarp of other congeneric *Zanthoxylum simulans* Hance, *Zanthoxylum Planispinum* Sieb. Et Zucc., and *Zanthoxylum schinifolium* Sieb. Zucc is also used as 土花椒 Tǔ Huā Jiāo and is inferior in quality.

[Indications]

1. Cold obstruction in the middle *jiao*: Huā Jiāo (Pericarpium Zanthoxyli), capable of warming the middle *jiao* to dispel coldness, can be used alone or together with Gān Jiāng (Rhizoma Zingiberis), Rén Shēn (Radix et Rhizoma Ginseng), and Hòu Pò (Cortex Magnoliae Officinalis) for gastric and abdominal cold pain, vomiting, and diarrhea due to cold obstruction in the middle *jiao*.
2. Worms: Huā Jiāo (Pericarpium Zanthoxyli) can be used alone or in a combination with Wū Méi (Fructus Mume), Huáng Lián (Rhizoma

Coptidis), and Gān Jiāng (Rhizoma Zingiberis) for roundworm with abdominal pain. Nowadays, deep-fry Huā Jiāo (Pericarpium Zanthoxyli) 9 g in 120 ml of sesame oil until scorched and take the prepared oil warm for roundworm ileus.

3. Eczema and itching: Huā Jiāo (Pericarpium Zanthoxyli) can be decocted together with Kǔ Shēn (Radix Sophorae Flavescentis), Dì Fū Zǐ (Fructus Kochiae), Míng Fán (Alumen), and Bái Xiān Pí (Cortex Dictamni) for external wash to treat eczema or vaginal itching.

It is also commonly used as flavorings for Chinese cooking to improve appetite, remove fishy smell, and relieve fish and shrimp poison.

[Usage and Dosage] Use raw in general, or stir-fried in some cases, and 2–5 g in decoction.

[Mnemonics] Huā Jiāo (Pericarpium Zanthoxyli, Pricklyash Peel): pungent and hot; warm the middle *jiao* strongly, remove dampness, arrest itching, and kill parasites.

[Simple and Effective Formulas]

1. 川椒丸 Chuān Jiāo Wán — Pricklyash Peel Pill from *An Elucidation of Formulas for Children's Health* (小儿卫生总微论方, Xiǎo' Ér Wèi Shēng Zǒng Wēi Lùn Fāng): stir-fried Huā Jiāo (Pericarpium Zanthoxyli) 30 g and roasted Ròu Dòu Kòu (Semen Myristicae) 15 g; grind into powder, prepare into millet-sized pill with rice, take 10 pills/time with rice soup for dampness and cold damage in summer with persistent diarrhea.

2. 椒茱汤 Jiāo Zhū Tāng — Pricklyash Peel and Cornus Decoction from *Advancement of Medicine* (医级, Yī Jí): Huā Jiāo (Pericarpium Zanthoxyli) 30 g, Wú Zhū Yú (Fructus Evodiae) 30 g, Shé Chuáng Zǐ (Fructus Cnidii) 30 g, Lí Lú (Radix et Rhizoma Veratri Nigri) 15 g, a handful of aged tea leaf, and roasted salt 60 g; decoct in water for external fumigation and wash to treat unbearable vaginal itching.

[Precautions] Huā Jiāo (Pericarpium Zanthoxyli), pungent and hot, is contraindicated in cases of yin deficiency with internal heat.

胡椒 **Hú Jiāo** *fructus piperis pepper fruit*

The source is from the fruit of evergreen liana *Piper nigrum* L., family Piperaceae. Pungent in flavor and hot in nature.

[Actions] Warm the middle *jiao* and redirect rebellious qi downward, relieve phlegm, and arrest pain. It is applicable for cold-damp induced gastric and abdominal cold pain, vomiting of watery fluids, diarrhea, and cold dysentery, and can remove food poisoning. This herb contains piperine, piperyline, 胡椒油碱, and volatile oil. Piperine has shown sedative and anticonvulsant effects.

[Quality] It is divided into Hēi Hú Jiāo (Fructus Piperis) and Bái Hú Jiāo (Fructus Piperis), the former is collected when the fruits start to turn into red and dried under sunshine with black-brown peel, and the latter is collected when the fruits totally turn into red, dipped in water, pericarp scraped, and dried under sunshine with gray peel. Good quality is large, round, full, and solid, and has a strong taste.

[Indications]

1. Gastric and abdominal cold pain: Hú Jiāo (Fructus Piperis), capable of warming the middle *jiao* and dissipating cold, can be used alone or together with Gān Jiāng (Rhizoma Zingiberis) and Huā Jiāo (Pericarpium Zanthoxyli) for gastric and abdominal pain with cold sensation that eliminated upon warmth and caused by coldness in the stomach and intestines.
2. Vomiting and diarrhea due to cold in the middle *jiao*: Hú *Jiāo* (Fructus Piperis) is combined with Shēng Jiāng (Rhizoma Zingiberis Recens) and Bàn Xià (Rhizoma Pinelliae) for vomiting caused by stomach cold; and with Gāo Liáng Jiāng (Rhizoma Alpiniae Officinarum) and Bái Zhú (Rhizoma Atractylodis Macrocephalae) for cold induced diarrhea. Can also be ground into powder and applied externally on the navel area to relieve vomiting and diarrhea due to cold in the middle *jiao*.

It has been recently reported that "抗灵 Kàng Líng" the synthetic piperine derivant, has been successfully used in the treatment of grand mal of epilepsy.

Also commonly used as flavorings, in small amount to improve appetite, to remove fishy smell, and relieve fish and shrimp poison.

[Usage and Dosage] Use raw, 2–3 g in decoction, and 0.5–1 g/time as in pill and powder.

[Mnemonics] Hú Jiāo (Fructus Piperis, Pepper Fruit): pungent and hot; relieve stomach cold and arrest pain, vomiting, and diarrhea; essential for seasoning.

[Simple and Effective Formulas]

止吐方 Zhǐ Tǔ Fāng — Vomiting Arresting *Formulas from Benevolent Sages* (圣惠方, Shèng Huì Fāng): Hú Jiāo (Fructus Piperis) powder 0.9 g and Shēng Jiāng (Rhizoma Zingiberis Recens) 30 g; decoct in water, divide into three equal doses, and take one dose/time for oral administration to treat persistent vomiting.

[Precautions] Hú Jiāo (Fructus Piperis), pungent and hot, is contraindicated for yin deficiency with internal heat.

高良姜 Gāo Liáng Jiāng *rhizoma alpiniae officinarum galangal*

The source is from the rhizome of herbaceous perennial *Alpinia officinarum* Hance, family Zingiberaceae. Alternate names include 良姜 Liáng Jiāng. Pungent in flavor and hot in nature.

[Actions] Warm the middle *jiao* to disperse cold, and move qi and arrest pain. It is applicable for coldness in the spleen and stomach, gastric and abdominal cold pain, vomiting, diarrhea, dysphagia, nausea, food accumulation, and miasmic malaria. Its volatile oil contains cineole, methyl cinnamate, and such flavonoids and galangol as galangin, kaempferide, and quercetin. Volatile oil can strengthen the stomach and inhibit intestinal canal peristalsis, *in vitro* experiments have shown it has an inhibitory effect on a variety of pathogenic bacteria.

[Quality] Good quality is thick, solid, reddish brown, and aromatic.

[Indications]

1. Pain due to stomach cold: Gāo Liáng Jiāng (Rhizoma Alpiniae Officinarum), effective in dispelling cold and relieving pain, can be

used alone or in a combination with Gān Jiāng (Rhizoma Zingiberis) and Xiāng Fù (Rhizoma Cyperi) for stomachache, vomiting of clear saliva, or gastric distention due to coldness in the stomach.

2. Vomiting and diarrhea due to cold in the middle *jiao*: Gāo Liáng Jiāng (Rhizoma Alpiniae Officinarum) is combined with Shēng Jiāng (Rhizoma Zingiberis Recens) and Bàn Xià (Rhizoma Pinelliae) for vomiting due to coldness in the stomach; and with Mù Xiāng (Radix Aucklandiae) and Bái Zhú (Rhizoma Atractylodis Macrocephalae) for abdominal pain and diarrhea triggered by coldness.

Gāo Liáng Jiāng (Rhizoma Alpiniae Officinarum) and Gān Jiāng (Rhizoma Zingiberis) are similar in actions and indications. The former is less effective than the latter in terms of warming and rescuing yang but more potent in relieving pain and warming the stomach and therefore suitable for pain and vomiting caused by coldness in the stomach; whereas the latter is to warm the spleen and more appropriate for abdominal pain and diarrhea due to spleen yang deficiency and debilitation. These two herbs are often used together to bring out the most potent effect in each other.

[Usage and Dosage] Use raw in general, 3–10 g in decoction.

[Mnemonics] Gāo Liáng Jiāng (Rhizoma Alpiniae Officinarum, Galangal): pungent and hot; warm the stomach, disperse cold, relieve vomiting and diarrhea, and cure stomachache.

[Simple and Effective Formulas]

1. 高良姜汤 Gāo Liáng Jiāng Tāng — Galangal Decoction from *Important Formulas Worth a Thousand Gold Pieces* (千金要方, Qiān Jīn Yào Fāng): Gāo Liáng Jiāng (Rhizoma Alpiniae Officinarum) 15 g, Hòu Pò (Cortex Magnoliae Officinalis) 6 g, Dāng Guī (Radix Angelicae Sinensis) 9 g, and Guì Xīn (Cortex Cinnamomi) 9 g; decoct in water for oral administration to treat patient with sudden onset of colicky and stabbing pain in the heart and abdoman, bilateral rib-side fullness, and unbearable vexing stuffiness.

2. 二姜丸 Èr Jiāng Tāng — Galangals and Dried Ginger Rhizome Pill from *Formulas from the Imperial Pharmacy* (局方, Jú Fāng): Gāo Liáng Jiāng (Rhizoma Alpiniae Officinarum) (blast-fried) and Gān Jiāng (Rhizoma Zingiberis) in equal dosage; grind into fine powder,

prepare into phoenix tree seed-sized pill with flour paste, and take 15–20 pills/dose with Chén Pí (Pericarpium Citri Reticulatae) decoction after meal for oral administration to treat cold pain in the heart and abdomen.

[Precautions] Gāo Liáng Jiāng (Rhizoma Alpiniae Officinarum), pungent and heat in nature, is contraindicated in cases of yin deficiency resulting in vigorous fire.

Daily practices

1. What are the actions and indications of Huā Jiāo (Pericarpium Zanthoxyli), Hú Jiāo (Fructus Piperis), and Gāo Liáng Jiāng (Rhizoma Alpiniae Officinarum) and what precautions should be taken when using them?
2. Among the interior-warming medicinals that we learn, which ones have certain toxicity that require to be used with cautions?

CHAPTER 7

Seventh Week

1

MEDICINALS THAT REGULATE QI

Method of regulating qi is to treat qi disorders caused by the stagnation and the reversed flow of qi. Qi stagnation refers to the obstruction of qi movement in certain part or *zang-fu* organs of the body with subsequent visceral or tissue dysfunctions. Qi movement blockage can occur anywhere in the body, common symptoms include distention, fullness, and pain in affected areas (pain is paroxysmal, migrating, and associated with emotion of patients) with accompanying chest oppression, frequent sighing, belching, and fart. The distending pain is eliminated significantly upon belching or fart. However, there are some differentiated symptoms according to the parts and organs that are primarily involved: stagnant stomach qi-major symptoms include gastric distention, fullness and pain; blocked intestinal qi-major symptoms include abdominal distending pain and inhibited or difficult defecation; constrained liver and gallbladder qi- major symptoms include rib-side distending pain; stagnant lung qi-major symptoms include cough and wheezing. Qi counterflow refers to the disorder arising when qi in certain organs moves abnormally upward (instead of physiologically downward) or extremely upward beyond physiological range. For instance, the lung governs descent and purification, controls breathing, and regulates fluid circulation, the counterflow of lung qi may cause wheezing or edema due to water diffusion; stomach qi governs descent, and reversal flow of stomach qi may lead to vomiting and hiccup; the liver governs ascent and dispersion, but liver qi exuberance or yin deficiency with yang hyperactivity may cause excessive ascent and dispersion that result in headache, vertigo, vomiting of blood, and sudden onset of coma.

Herbs that regulate qi are used to unblock stagnant qi. Most herbs are acrid, warm, and aromatic in nature and potent in activating, dispersing, descending or draining. By definition, they also move qi to relieve distention, disperse stagnation to arrest pain, and direct counterflow downward.

The selection of herbs is based on the site of the qi stagnation and the etiology of qi stagnation. Clinically, causes of stagnant qi include climate factor, inappropriate diet, emotional disturbances, such visible pathogens as phlegm and water retention, water-dampness, blood stasis, and cold congealing, and *zang-fu* organ qi depletion failing to promote qi circulation. The herbs in this chapter therefore should be combined with other herbs based upon the specific nature of the disorders.

橘皮 **Jú Pí** *pericarpium citri reticulatae tangerine pericarp*

The source is from the ripe pericarp of *Citrus reticulate* Blanco, family Rutaceae. Alternate names include 陈皮 Chén Pí indicating the longer it has been aged, the purer moderate the nature, the better the quality. Pungent and bitter in flavor and warm in nature.

[Actions] Regulate the qi and improve the stomach, harmonize the stomach to arrest vomiting, and dry dampness and relieve phlegm. It is applied for fullness in the chest and rib-side region, poor appetite, vomiting, diarrhea, and cough with profuse sputum. Form perspective of modern research, its volatile oil has slight expectorant effect and mild excitatory effect on gastrointestine and can promote digestive juice secretion and remove intestinal flatulence. Its decoction can dilate bronchus to anti-asthmatic effect. Its ingredient aurantiamarin has shown anti-inflammatory, anti-ulcer, choleretic, and serum cholesterol-decreasing effect; hesperidin methyl can dilate blood vessel to slowly reduce blood pressure, and hesperetin can increase blood pressure.

[Quality] Use raw in general, but different preparations are adopted when used in the treatment of different diseases. For instance, it is soaked in fresh urine of boy under 12 and dried under sunshine for phlegm-induced cough, stir-fried with ginger juice for ascending counterflow of stomach qi, and stir-fried with salt solution for diseases of the lower *jiao*. Tangor peel with a lower effect is also available at the market, its pericarp is thicker and puffed and should not be used as a substitute.

[Indications] As an important and typical medicinal of relieving qi stagnation in qi-regulating medicinal, this medicinal has certain effect in treating qi movement obstruction in such organs as the spleen, stomach, lung, intestine, liver, and gallbladder. It can also dry dampness, dissolve phlegm, and arrest cough and wheezing. For this reason, it has been widely used in the clinic:

1. Chest, gastric and abdominal distention, fullness and pain: qi stagnation in the spleen, stomach, intestines, lung, liver, and gallbladder may cause chest, gastria, rib-side, and abdominal distention, fullness, and emotion-associated pain which are unfixed, moving, and waned and waxed with accompanying frequent sighing, belching, and fart. Jú Pí (Pericarpium Citri Reticulatae) is one the principal medicinals for those manifestations. In the clinic, combination of herb is based on cause of qi stagnation in the *zang-fu* organs, it is combined with Cāng Zhú (Rhizoma Atractylodis) and Hòu Pò (Cortex Magnoliae Officinalis) for qi stagnation due to dampness internal obstruction through drying dampness, moving qi, and fortifying the spleen; with Shén Qū (Massa Medicata Fermentata), Shān Zhā (Fructus Crataegi), Mài Yá (Fructus Hordei Germinatus) for qi stagnation resulting from food accumulation via relieving food retention and promoting digestion; and with medicinals that supplement qi and fortify the spleen such as Dǎng Shēn (Radix Codonopsis), Bái Zhú (Rhizoma Atractylodis Macrocephalae), and Fú Líng (Poria) for qi stagnation caused by spleen and stomach qi deficiency. Modern research reveal that actions above are related to its effect of promoting gastrointestinal mobility and relieving gastrointestinal smooth muscle spasms. For chest *bì* manifested as a stifling sensation in the chest and shortness of breath due to stagnated qi movement in the chest, it is combined with Shēng Jiāng (Rhizoma Zingiberis Recens) and Zhǐ Shí (Fructus Aurantii Immaturus).

2. Vomiting and hiccup: food accumulation, phlegm-damp retention, cold congealing, heat stagnation, and stomach qi deficiency may cause ascending counterflow of stomach qi with symptoms of vomiting and hiccup. Jú Pí (Pericarpium Citri Reticulatae), capable of regulating qi, harmonizing the stomach, and subduing the counterflow qi, is applicable for different types of vomiting and hiccup. It is often combined with Shēng Jiāng (Rhizoma Zingiberis Recens) and Bàn Xià (Rhizoma

Pinelliae) for the cold natured problem; with Zhú Rú (Caulis Bambusae in Taenia) and Pí Pá Yè (Folium Eriobotryae) for the hot-natured problem; and Dǎng Shēn (Radix Codonopsis) and Bái Zhú (Rhizoma Atractylodis Macrocephalae) for the deficiency.

3. Cough and wheezing with profuse phlegm: Jú Pí (Pericarpium Citri Reticulatae), capable of drying dampness and dissolving phlegm, is therefore commonly used in treating many different types of cough and wheezing with profuse sputum. As a principal medicinal for relieving damp-phlegm, it is combined with Fú Líng (Poria) and Bàn Xià (Rhizoma Pinelliae) to obtain a stronger ability of drying dampness, dissolving phlegm, and arresting cough and wheezing for different types of acute and chronic cough with accompanying profuse white sputum and chest oppression. These actions are attributed to its expectorator and anti-bronchus spastic contraction effects.

It is also widely used in tonic formulas in a bid to prevent cloying tonic herbs from obstructing the stomach and help improve its effect of supplementing and boosting.

Jú Pí (Pericarpium Citri Reticulatae), similar to Rén Shēn (Radix et Rhizoma Ginseng), can restrain the secretion of sebaceous gland and therefore has recently been used as an important medicinal for hair growing and cosmetics.

[Usage and Dosage] Traditionally, the white inner peel of the tangerine, Jú Bái (Exocarpium Citri Reticulatae Album), is better at moving qi and harmonizing the stomach, while the red part of the tangerine peel, Jú Hóng (Exocarpium Citri Rubrum), is more effective at drying dampness and relieving phlegm. However, nowadays, both are in use. Use 3–9 g in decoction, and decrease the dosage as in pill or powder.

[Mnemonics] *Jú Pí* (Pericarpium Citri Reticulatae, Tangerine Pericarp): pungent and warm; specialized in the spleen and lung; rectify qi, relieve phlegm, dry dampness, and harmonize the stomach.

[Simple and Effective Formulas]

1. 橘皮竹茹汤 Jú Pí Zhú Rú Tāng — Tangerine Peel and Bamboo Shavings Decoction from *Essentials from the Golden Cabinet* (金匮要略

Jīn Guì Yào Lüè): Jú Pí (Pericarpium Citri Reticulatae) 6 g, Zhú Rú (Caulis Bambusae in Taenia) 10 g, Dà Zǎo (Fructus Jujubae) 9 pieces, Gān Cǎo (Radix et Rhizoma Glycyrrhizae) 3 g, Shēng Jiāng (Rhizoma Zingiberis Recens) 3 g, and Rén Shēn (Radix et Rhizoma Ginseng) 10 g; decoction for oral administration to treat patients with chronic diseases and weak constitution or cases of vomiting or hiccup, tender red tongue, and deficient fast pulse caused by qi counterflow resulting from deficiency heat in the stomach after taking purgatives. Also applicable for vomiting during pregnancy and vomiting due to phlegm-heat.

2. 二陈汤 Èr Chén Tāng — Two Matured Substances Decoction from *Beneficial Formulas from the Taiping Imperial Pharmacy* (太平惠民和剂局方 Tài Píng Huì Mín Hé Jì Jú Fāng): Jú Hóng (Exocarpium Citri Rubrum) 6 g, Bàn Xià (Rhizoma Pinelliae) 9 g, Fú Líng (Poria) 10 g, Gān Cǎo (Radix et Rhizoma Glycyrrhizae) 3 g, Shēng Jiāng (Rhizoma Zingiberis Recens) 3 pieces, and Wū Méi (Fructus Mume) 10 g; decoction for oral administration to treat patients with phlegm-damp exuberance patterns, such as phlegm-damp obstruction in the lung with symptoms and signs of cough, profuse sputum, distention and fullness in the chest, nausea, vomiting, white greasy tongue coating, and slippery pulse. It is combined with other formulas when used in the treatment of chronic gastritis and chronic bronchitis.

[Precautions] Jú Pí (Pericarpium Citri Reticulatae), scattering and dispersing in nature like other medicinals that regulate qi, can consume qi if applied inappropriately and should be used with caution. For cases of stagnated qi movement in many organs caused by deficiency, the priority should be given to supplement and boost instead of regulating, otherwise qi will be damaged further. It is contraindicated in cases of yin deficiency with internal heat and hematemesis due to its relatively warm nature.

Daily practices

1. What qi stagnation and qi counterflow are and health problems they can cause?
2. What are the actions and indications of Jú Pí (Pericarpium Citri Reticulatae) and what precautions should be taken when using it?

青皮 Qīng Pí *pericarpium citri reticulatae viride green tangerine peel*

The source is from the unripe pericarp or immature fruit of *Citrus reticulate* Blanco, family Rutaceae. Pungent and bitter in flavor and warm in nature.

[Actions] Break up stagnated qi and soothe the liver, and dissipate clumps and resolve stagnation. It is applicable for chest and rib-side distending pain, distending pain of the breasts, hernia, pain, and food accumulation due to binding constraint of liver qi. Modern researches suggest that its decoction has shown inhibitory and spasmolytic effect on *ex vivo* intestinal canal, and can relax gall bladder of experimental animal to increase biliary secretion. It has been recently found that its preparation has prompt and distinctive hypertensive effect when given intravenously.

[Quality] 个青皮 Gè Qīng Pí is the young fruit of *Citrus reticulate* Blanco, good quality has even fruit, greenish black thick skin, and intense fragrance. 四花青皮 Sì Huā Qīng Pí is immature pericarp of *Citrus reticulate* Blanco; good quality is dry, thick-skinned, and greenish gray without mildew.

[Indications] Jú Pí (Pericarpium Citri Reticulatae) and Qīng Pí (Pericarpium Citri Reticulatae Viride) originate from the same plants, but the former is mature fruit, the latter is immature. They have similar indications, between their differences, the former pertains to regulate qi of the spleen and stomach, while the latter, more effective in moving qi even breaking up qi, pertains to regulate qi of the liver and gallbladder and can relieve stagnation.

1. Binding constraint of liver qi: it refers to a disorder that caused by qi stagnation in the liver with manifestations as blue mood, sentimentality, distending pain in the chest and abdomen, frequent belching and sighing, rib-side distending pain, distending pain or masses of the breasts, dragging pain in the lower abdomen or the lateral aspect of lower abdomen, hernia pain, hepatosplenomegaly in chronic case, menstrual irregularities, distending pain of the breasts before menstruation, dysmenorrhea, and amenorrhea. Qīng Pí (Pericarpium Citri Reticulatae Viride) is often combined with Chái Hú (Radix Bupleuri) and Bái Sháo

(Radix Paeoniae Alba) for rib-side pain caused by binding constraint of liver qi; with Yán Hú Suǒ (Rhizoma Corydalis), Xiǎo Huí Xiāng (Fructus Foeniculi), Lì Zhī Hé (Semen Litchi), and Chuān Liàn Zǐ (Fructus Toosendan) for hernia pain; with Xiāng Fù (Rhizoma Cyperi), Jú Yè (Folium Citri Reticulatae), Chái Hú (Radix Bupleuri), and Pú Gōng Yīng (Herba Taraxaci) for distending pain or masses of the breasts before menstruation; and with Sān Léng (Rhizoma Sparganii) and É Zhú (Rhizoma Curcumae) for hepatosplenomegaly.

2. Food accumulation: Qīng Pí (Pericarpium Citri Reticulatae Viride) is combined with medicinals that improve digestion and relieving accumulation such as Shān Zhā (Fructus Crataegi), Mài Yá (Fructus Hordei Germinatus), and Shén Qū (Massa Medicata Fermentata) for drink and food accumulation with gastric distending pain, putrid belching, and incomplete defecation due to over-drinking and eating or spleen and stomach deficiency failing to transform and transport.

3. Acute mastitis: from the perspective of traditional Chinese medicine, acute mastitis is caused by binding constraint of liver qi and stomach heat exuberance and the most important therapy method is to sooth liver qi. For early stage of acute mastitis, Qīng Pí (Pericarpium Citri Reticulatae Viride) is prepared with Chuān Shān Jiǎ (Squama Manitis) pieces, Bái Zhǐ (Radix Angelicae Dahuricae), Gān Cǎo (Radix et Rhizoma Glycyrrhizae), and Tǔ Bèi Mǔ (Rhizoma Bolbostematis) into powder and taken with warm wine.

[Usage and Dosage] Use raw in general, and stir-fry with vinegar when used to move qi and soothe the liver. Use 3–10 g in decoction, up to above 25 g for acute mastitis, decrease the dosage as in pill and powder,

[Mnemonics] Qīng Pí (Pericarpium Citri Reticulatae Viride, Green Tangerine Peel): bitter and pungent; soothe the liver, resolve stagnation, break up stagnated qi, and cure acute mastitis.

[Simple and Effective Formulas]

1. 青皮散 Qīng Pí Sǎn — Green Tangerine Peel Powder from *Fine Formulas of Zhong Fu Tang Gong* (种福堂公选良方 Zhǒng Fú Táng

Gōng Xuǎn Liáng Fāng): Qīng Pí (Pericarpium Citri Reticulatae Viride), Chuān Shān Jiǎ Zhū (Squama Manitis), Bái Zhǐ (Radix Angelicae Dahuricae), and Tǔ Bèi Mǔ (Rhizoma Bolbostematis) in equal dosage; grind into fine powder and take 3–5 g/dose for oral administration to treat acute mastitis in early stage with localized hardness, redness, swelling, and pain.

2. 青皮丸 Qīng Pí Wán — Green Tangerine Peel Pill from *Shen's Books on Respecting Life* (沈氏尊生书 Shěn Shì Zūn Shēng Shū): Qīng Pí (Pericarpium Citri Reticulatae Viride), Shān Zhā (Fructus Crataegi), Shén Qū (Massa Medicata Fermentata), Mài Yá (Fructus Hordei Germinatus), and Cǎo Guǒ (Fructus Tsaoko) in equal dosage; grind into powder, prepare into pill, and take 3 g/dose for oral administration to treat distention, fullness, and stuffiness after meal with putrid belching. Also applicable for indigestion.

[Precautions] Qīng Pí (Pericarpium Citri Reticulatae Viride), potent in moving qi, should be used with caution for patients with weak constitution. It is contraindicated in cases of qi stagnation caused by deficiency, if that is the case, Jú Pí (Pericarpium Citri Reticulatae) is used. In the opinion of the predecessors, it is also discouraged when patients present with sweating (for reference only).

枳实 Zhǐ Shí *fructus aurantii immaturus immature bitter orange*

[Addendum] 枳壳 Zhǐ Qiào Fructus Aurantii Bitter Orange
The source is from the immature fruit of *Citrus aurantium* L., Citrus *wilsonii* Tanaka, or *Poncirus trifoliata* (L.) Rafin., family Rutaceae. *Li Shizhen* (李时珍) named it Zhǐ 枳, because this medicinal is from the fruit of tree (literally Zǐ 子 in Chinese) and Zhǐ 枳 and Zǐ 子 are almost homophonic. Pungent and bitter in flavor and warm in nature.

[Actions] Regulate qi movements, break up stagnant qi and remove distension, and reduce accumulation and dissolve phlegm. It is applicable for distending pain in the chest and rib-side region, food accumulation, abdominal distention and fullness, and prolapse of certain organs. From the perspective of modern researches, this herb can excite gastrointestinal smooth muscle, stimulate a rhythmic increase in contraction, and therefore relieve gastrointestinal and uterine prolapse. In recent years, its ingredients are shown to have blood pressure-rising effect only when given intravenously.

[Quality] It is divided into 川枳实 Chuān Zhǐ Shí and 江枳实 Jiāng Zhǐ Shí, good quality is a thick and solid fruit with strong fragrance and without damage and decay caused by worms.

[Indications] Zhǐ Shí (Fructus Aurantii Immaturus) is a commonly-used medicinal for regulating qi and relieving distention. Qi movement stagnation may cause different types of disorder, such as qi stagnation in the chest and abdomen with distention, fullness, and pain in the chest and abdomen, sinking of qi with prolapse of organs. Therefore, it is mainly used for stagnated qi movement and sinking of qi movement.

1. Chest and abdominal distending pain: it refers to chest, rib-side, and abdominal distention, *pǐ*, fullness, and pain. Distending pain is unfixed, chest and rib-side pain is migratory, and abdominal pain is often accompanied with distention, sound of grunting, or unfixed, amorphous and moving localized gathering in the abdomen. When pressing the area of pain in the abdomen, doctors feel no obvious tenderness but encounter mild resistance or hear sound of grunting. Pain and distention are closely associated with emotion of patients, emotions like anger, depression and rage tend to increase the degree of distending pain, while good mood may help to improve these symptoms. From the perspective of traditional Chinese medicine, it is qi stagnation and Zhǐ Shí (Fructus Aurantii Immaturus) can regulate qi and relieve stagnation to relieve this kind of abdominal distention and pain. It is often combined with Bái Sháo (Radix Paeoniae Alba), Chái Hú (Radix Bupleuri), and Gān Cǎo (Radix et Rhizoma Glycyrrhizae) to form Sì Nì Sǎn (Frigid Extremities Powder) for this kind of disease.

2. Gastroptosis: it is generally diagnosed by X-ray and most likely happen to people with thin and tall body figure. Its manifestations include abdominal distention aggravated after meal and eliminated when lying flat and with accompanying stomachache and belching, and obvious aortic pulsation in the upper abdomen when touched. Traditional

Chinese medicine holds that gastroptosis is caused by of middle *jiao* qi insufficiency and therefore the formula Center-Supplementing and Qi-Boosting Decoction (补中益气汤, Bǔ Zhōng Yì Qì Tāng) that supplement and boost qi in the middle *jiao* should be combined with Zhǐ Shí (Fructus Aurantii Immaturus).

3. Rectal and anus prolapse: it is common in children or the elderly and may occur due to long term dysentery and diarrhea. In mild case, abnormal descent of the rectal mucosa through the anus occur when defecating, easily restored, whereas in severe case, the prolapse happens when walking or coughing, the intestine protrude from the anus and one segment of the intestine folds within another in cyclic annular, spiral or strip manner, difficult to be restored. The occurrence of this disorder is also related to middle *jiao* qi insufficiency, Zhǐ Shí (Fructus Aurantii Immaturus) can be used together with Bǔ Zhōng Yì Qì Tāng (Center-Supplementing and Qi-Boosting Decoction), or with Dǎng Shēn (Radix Codonopsis), Huáng Qí (Radix Astragali), Shēng Má (Rhizoma Cimicifugae), and Gān Cǎo (Radix et Rhizoma Glycyrrhizae) in decoction for oral administration.

4. Uterine prolapse: This condition is more common in women who have had postpartum injury, too many vaginal births, a weak body, and enduring increased abdominal pressure. Manifestations include patient subjective feeling of dropping in the lower abdomen that aggravates if overstrain, falling or sliding of the womb from its normal position into the area below ischial spine or even the vaginal area, and difficult urination or incontinence. The occurrence of this disorder is related to middle *jiao* qi insufficiency and *dai mai* deficiency, Zhǐ Shí (Fructus Aurantii Immaturus) can be used together with Center-Supplementing and Qi-Boosting Decoction (补中益气汤, Bǔ Zhōng Yì Qì Tāng), or with Shēng Má (Rhizoma Cimicifugae) in decoction for oral administration. Decoction of Zhǐ Shí (Fructus Aurantii Immaturus) can be used to topically soak postpartum prolapsed uterus.

From a modern research perspective, the above-mentioned actions excite gastrointestinal and uterine smooth muscle, stimulate a rhythmic increase in motion and contraction, and eventually relieve gastrointestinal and uterine prolapse.

5. Drink and food accumulation: Zhǐ Shí (Fructus Aurantii Immaturus) is combined with Shān Zhā (Fructus Crataegi), Shén Qū (Massa Medicata Fermentata), and Mài Yá (Fructus Hordei Germinatus) for indigestion due to improper diet through promoting digestion and relieving accumulation; and with Bái Zhú (Rhizoma Atractylodis Macrocephalae) for indigestion caused by spleen and stomach dysfunction to transform and transport via fortifying the spleen to relieve food stagnation.

6. Constipation due to heat accumulation: for constipation resulting from excess heat accumulation in the intestine, Zhǐ Shí (Fructus Aurantii Immaturus) is combined with Dà Huáng (Radix et Rhizoma Rhei) and Hòu Pò (Cortex Magnoliae Officinalis) to drain heat, move qi, and promote defecation.

7. Dysentery and diarrhea: for damp-heat binding with accumulation in the intestine resulting in dysentery with blood and pus in stool, abdominal pain, and tenesmus, Zhǐ Shí (Fructus Aurantii Immaturus) is combined with Dà Huáng (Radix et Rhizoma Rhei), Huáng Lián (Rhizoma Coptidis), Huáng Qín (Radix Scutellariae), and Shén Qū (Massa Medicata Fermentata) to clear damp-heat in the intestine and sooth accumulation so as to relieve dysentery. It can also be ground into powder with Gān Cǎo (Radix et Rhizoma Glycyrrhizae) and decocted for oral administration to treat dysentery with abdominal pain. Modern researches demonstrate that Zhǐ Shí (Fructus Aurantii Immaturus) has certain inhibitory effects against intestinal pathogenic microorganism.

8. Binding of phlegm and qi: Zhǐ Shí (Fructus Aurantii Immaturus) is combined with Guā Lóu (Fructus Trichosanthis), Xiè Bái (Bulbus Allii Macrostemi), Guì Zhī (Ramulus Cinnamomi), and Bàn Xià (Rhizoma Pinelliae) for chest *bì* with chest oppression and chest pain radiating to the back caused by *bì* of binding of phlegm and qi. It is also used to treat angina pectoris and stomachache with above-mentioned symptoms.

[Usage and Dosage] Use raw in general, when used to regulate qi, rectify the stomach, relieve food stagnation, and cure dysentery, it is commonly stir-fried with bran to reduce its volatile oil and irritability, and moderate its property. Use 3–9 g in decoction, up to above 20 g for prolapse of the stomach, intestines, and uterus, and 2–3 g/time in powder.

[Mnemonics] Zhǐ Qiào (Fructus Aurantii, Bitter Orange) and Zhǐ Shí (Fructus Aurantii Immaturus, Immature Bitter Orange): both regulate qi movements; the former is more effective in loosening the center, and the latter is more potent in breaking up stagnant qi.

[Simple and Effective Formulas]

1. 枳术丸 Zhǐ Zhū Wán — Atractylodes Macrocephala Pill from *Treatise on the Spleen and Stomach* (脾胃论, Pí Wèi Lùn): Zhǐ Shí (Fructus Aurantii Immaturus) 30 g and Bái Zhú (Rhizoma Atractylodis Macrocephalae) 60 g; prepare into pill and take 6 g/dose for oral administration to treat food stagnation due to weak spleen and stomach manifested as gastric and abdominal pǐ (痞) and fullness and poor appetite.

2. 枳实导滞丸 Zhǐ Shí Dǎo Zhì Wán — Immature Bitter Orange Stagnation-Moving Pill from *Clarifying Doubts about Damage from Internal and External Causes* (内外伤辨惑论, Nèi Wài Shāng Biàn Huò Lùn): Zhǐ Shí (Fructus Aurantii Immaturus) (stir-fried with bran, pulp removed) 15 g, Dà Huáng (Radix et Rhizoma Rhei) 30 g, Shén Qū (Massa Medicata Fermentata) (stir-fried) 9 g, Fú Líng (Poria) (peel removed) 9 g, Huáng Qín (Radix Scutellariae) (erosion removed) 9 g, Huáng Lián (Rhizoma Coptidis) 9 g, Bái Zhú (Rhizoma Atractylodis Macrocephalae) 9 g, and Zé Xiè (Rhizoma Alismatis) 6 g; grind into powder, prepare into phoenix tree seed-sized pill with steamed cake, and take with 50–70 pills with warm water for oral administration to treat food stagnation and damp-heat accumulation with manifestations of pǐ (痞) and fullness in the chest and abdomen, dysentery, diarrhea, tenesmus, or constipated and hard stool, scanty and yellow urine, red tongue with yellow greasy coating, and deep and excess pulse.

[Precautions] Zhǐ Shí (Fructus Aurantii Immaturus) and Zhǐ Qiào (Fructus Aurantii), pungent, dispersing and consuming qi, should be used with caution in cases of spleen and stomach deficiency, liver and kidney insufficiency and during pregnancy.

[Addendum] 枳壳 Zhǐ Qiào Fructus Aurantii Bitter Orange
Zhǐ Qiào (Fructus Aurantii), the ripe fruit of Zhǐ Shí (Fructus Aurantii Immaturus) or *Citrus aurantium* L. Cv. Daidai, family Rutaceae, is bitter

and sour in flavor and slightly cold in nature. This herb is primarily produced in Jiangxi and is called 江枳壳, Jiāng Zhǐ Ké; good quality is a
thick and solid fruit that is green-brown in color and aromatic. Similar to
but milder in action than Zhǐ Shí (Fructus Aurantii Immaturus), it is especially appropriate for mild disease or when the patient is deficient or
weak. It is also applied in tonic formula to alleviate the negative effect of
greasy and cloying medicinals on gastrointestinal digestive function.
It can be used in raw form or stir-fried with bran to moderate its medicinal nature. Use 3–9 g in general, 3 g in tonic formula.

Daily practices

1. What are the similarities and differences between Qīng Pí (Pericarpium
   Citri Reticulatae Viride) and Jú Pí (Pericarpium Citri Reticulatae) in
   terms of actions and indications?
2. What are the actions and indications of Zhǐ Shí (Fructus Aurantii
   Immaturus)?
3. What are the differences between Zhǐ Shí (Fructus Aurantii Immaturus)
   and Zhǐ Qiào (Fructus Aurantii) in terms of actions?
4. What are the similarities and differences between Zhǐ Shí (Fructus
   Aurantii Immaturus) and Jú Pí (Pericarpium Citri Reticulatae) in terms
   of actions?

薤白 Xiè Bái *bulbus allii macrostemi long stamen onion bulb*

The source is from the underground bulb of herbaceous perennial *Allium
maerostemom* Bunge or *A. chinensis* G. Don, family Liliaceae. Alternate
names include 薤白头, Xiè Bái Tóu. Pungent and bitter in flavor and
warm in nature.

[Actions] Promote qi circulation and unblock the yang, and expand the
chest and remove stagnation. Modern researches reveal it contains alliin,
methyl-alliin, and scorodose, and its decoction has shown *in vitro* inhibitory effects against *shigella dysenteriae* and *staphylococcus aureus*.

[Quality] Good quality is large, hard, full, yellowish white, and semitransparent without stems.

[Indications] Xiè Bái (Bulbus Allii Macrostemi) is mainly used for dysentery and chest distention, oppression and pain.

1. Chest *bì*: it refers to a disorder that marked by chest oppression, pain, and discomfort, even chest pain radiating to the back and back pain radiating the heart, shortness of breath, and wheezing disturbing the sleep. From the perspective of modern biomedicine, it refers to coronary heart disease, angina pectoris, and gastric disorders marked by gastric oppression, distention, and pain radiating to the back. Xiè Bái (Bulbus Allii Macrostemi), effective in unblocking yang, moving qi, and relieving pain, is good at warming and unblocking chest yang and therefore is a principal herb for chest *bì* caused by poor chest yang with phlegm congestion and qi stagnation. In the clinic, it is often combined with Guā Lóu (Fructus Trichosanthis), Guì Zhī (Ramulus Cinnamomi), and Bàn Xià (Rhizoma Pinelliae) for chest *bì*; and with medicinals that invigorate blood and dissolve stasis such as Chuān Xiōng (Rhizoma Chuanxiong), Dān Shēn (Radix et Rhizoma Salviae Miltiorrhizae), Chì Sháo (Radix Paeoniae Rubra), and Sān Qī (Radix et Rhizoma Notoginseng) for chest *bì* due to phlegm and blood stagnation binding and accumulation.

2. Dysentery: from the perspective of traditional Chinese medicine, the occurrence of dysentery is associated with food accumulation and damp-heat accumulation in the large intestine failing to transmit and therefore medicinals that move qi and drain accumulation should be used. Xiè Bái (Bulbus Allii Macrostemi), capable of moving qi and draining accumulation, is commonly used for dysentery, especially when accompanied with tenesmus. It can be used alone or together with Bái Sháo (Radix Paeoniae Alba) and Zhǐ Shí (Fructus Aurantii Immaturus). For severe damp-heat dysentery with stool containing blood and mucus, it is combined with Mù Xiāng (Radix Aucklandiae), Huáng Lián (Rhizoma Coptidis), and Bīng Láng (Semen Arecae).

It can also be pounded into juice for external application to relieve sores and boils.

[Usage and Dosage] Use raw, or steamed thoroughly, or boiled thoroughly and dried under sunshine one; use in decoction generally, 5–10 g.

[Mnemonics] Xiè Bái (Bulbus Allii Macrostemi, Long Stamen Onion Bulb): pungent and warm; unblock yang, eliminate phlegm, relieve tenesmus, and good at treating chest *bì*.

[Simple and Effective Formulas]

1. 栝楼薤白半夏汤, Guā Lóu Xiè Bái Bàn Xià Tāng — Trichosanthes, Chinese Chive and Pinellia Decoction from *Essentials from the Golden Cabinet* (金匮要略, Jīn Guì Yào Lüè): one Guā Lóu (Fructus Trichosanthis) (pounded), Xiè Bái Tóu (Bulbus Allii Macrostemi) 15 g, Bàn Xià (Rhizoma Pinelliae) 10 g, and white wine 30 g; take decoction three times a day for oral administration to treat chest *bì*, inability to lie flat, and cardiac pain radiating to the back. Also applicable for coronary heart disease and gastric diseases with above manifestations.
2. 薤白黄柏汤, Xiè Bái Huáng Bǎi Tāng — Chinese Chive and Phellodendron Decoction from *Supplement to 'The Materia Medica'* (本草拾遗, Běn Cǎo Shí Yí): Xiè Bái (Bulbus Allii Macrostemi) 15 g and Huáng Bǎi (Cortex Phellodendri Chinensis) 15 g; decoct in water for oral administration to treat dysentery with stool containing pus and mucus.

[Precautions] Xiè Bái (Bulbus Allii Macrostemi), warm in nature, should be used with caution in cases with fever or yin deficiency with internal heat.

木香 Mù Xiāng *radix aucklandiae common aucklandia root*

The source is from the root of *Auchlandia lappa* Decne., family Compositae. Alternate names include 蜜香 Mì Xiāng, as its wood frangrance smells like honey. Pungent and bitter in flavor and warm in nature. Literally means wood fragrance.

[Actions] Featured by strongly wood fragrance. Regulate qi to arrest pain and warm the middle *jiao* to harmonize the stomach. From the perspective of modern researches, its water extract and ethnol extract, and volatile oil can counteract bronchus and small intestinal smooth muscle spasms induced by histamine and acetylcholine. Bacteriostasis tests indicate it has a certain inhibitory effect on bacteria.

[Quality] It is called 广木香 Guǎng Mù Xiāng as it was origincally produced in India and exported to Guangzhou. Now, it is also produced in
Yunnan (云木香 Yún Mù Xiāng) and Sichuan (川木香 Chuān Mù Xiāng)
with the same quality as the imported one. Good quality is solid, heavy,
aromatic, and slightly oily.

[Indications] Mù Xiāng (Radix Aucklandiae), effective in regulating qi
and relieving pain, is mainly used for chest and gastric distending pain,
food accumulation with indigestion, poor appetite, and dysentery and
diarrhea with tenesmus caused by qi stagnation.

1. Gastric and abdominal distention and pain: owning to its effect of moving qi, relieving distention, and relieving pain, Mù Xiāng (Radix
   Aucklandiae) is applicable for spleen and stomach stagnated qi movement with gastric and abdominal distending pain caused by cold congealing, dampness obstruction, and food accumulation. It is combined
   with Gāo Liáng Jiāng (Rhizoma Alpiniae Officinarum) and Gān Jiāng
   (Rhizoma Zingiberis) for cold ongealing and qi stagnation; with Cāng
   Zhú (Rhizoma Atractylodis) and Hòu Pò (Cortex Magnoliae Officinalis)
   for dampness obstruction and qi stagnation; and with Shān Zhā (Fructus
   Crataegi), Shén Qū (Massa Medicata Fermentata), and Lái Fú Zǐ
   (Semen Raphani) for food accumulation and qi stagnation. This is
   attributed to its effect of relieving gastrointestinal smooth muscle
   spasm. This substance can be prepared with Zào Jiǎo Cì (Spina
   Gleditsiae) into pill for stabbing pain in the chest.
2. Decreased appetite with abdominal distention: for poor appetite and
   gastric distention especially after meal caused by spleen and stomach
   deficiency failing to transform and transport, Mù Xiāng (Radix
   Aucklandiae) is combined with Dǎng Shēn (Radix Codonopsis), Bái
   Zhú (Rhizoma Atractylodis Macrocephalae), and Shā Rén (Fructus
   Amomi) to regulate qi and fortify the spleen to improve digestion. This
   is relative to its dual-direction regulatory effect on gastrointestinal tract
   motion, which is to inhibit hyperfunctional gastrointestinal motility and
   improve hypofunctional gastrointestinal motility to fortify the spleen
   and relieve food accumulation.
3. Dysentery and diarrhea with tenesmus: Mù Xiāng (Radix Aucklandiae)
   is effective in relieving dysentery and diarrhea with tenesmus due to

damp-heat obstruction in the intestine. According to traditional Chinese medicine, tenesmus is a manifestation of obstructed qi movement in the intestine and can be relieved by sooth qi movement of the intestine. In the clinic, Mù Xiāng (Radix Aucklandiae) is combined with Huáng Lián (Rhizoma Coptidis), or with Sháo Yào (Radix Paeoniae), Dāng Guī (Radix Angelicae Sinensis), Dà Huáng (Radix et Rhizoma Rhei), Huáng Qín (Radix Scutellariae), Huáng Lián (Rhizoma Coptidis), and Bīng Láng (Semen Arecae).

It is also applicable for persistent hiccup and bronchia cough and asthma.

Mù Xiāng (Radix Aucklandiae) is often used in the tonic formula to counteract the cloying nature of tonic medicinals.

[Usage and Dosage] Use raw in general, in a bid to remove its oily substances and strengthen its ability to arrest diarrhea, such processing methods as roasting, plain dry-frying, and dry-frying with bran are applied. Use 1.5–6 g in decoction, and should be added at the end of decoction to retain its effective volatile oil. Additionally, it can be ground into powder for oral administration or taken together with vinegar. Also use in pill or powder form.

[Mnemonics] Mù Xiāng (Radix Aucklandiae, Common Aucklandia Root): pungent and warm; regulate qi to arrest pain, relieve abdominal distension, and eliminate dysentery.

[Simple and Effective Formulas]

1. 香连丸 Xiāng Lián Wán — Costus Root and Coptis Pill from *Formula Collections of Ministry of War (in feudal China)* (兵部手集方 Bīng Bù Shǒu Jí Fāng): Mù Xiāng (Radix Aucklandiae) 14.64 g and Huáng Lián (Rhizoma Coptidis) (stir-fried with Wú Zhū Yú-Fructus Evodiae, Wú Zhū Yú-Fructus Evodiae removed) 60 g; grind into fine powder, prepare into phoenix tree seed-sized pill with vinegar, and take 20 pills/time with thick rice soup on an empty stomach, three times a day for damp-heat dysentery, stool with pus and blood, abdominal pain, and tenesmus.

2. 木香槟榔丸 Mù Xiāng Bīng Láng Wán — Costus Root and Areca Pill from *Confucians' Duties to Their Parents* (儒门事亲 Rú Mén Shì

Qín): Mù Xiāng (Radix Aucklandiae) 90 g, Bīng Láng (Semen Arecae) 90 g, Qīng Pí (Pericarpium Citri Reticulatae Viride) 90 g, Chén Pí (Pericarpium Citri Reticulatae) 90 g, É Zhú (Rhizoma Curcumae) (burned) 90 g, Huáng Lián (Rhizoma Coptidis) 90 g, Huáng Bǎi (Cortex Phellodendri Chinensis) 90 g, Dà Huáng (Radix et Rhizoma Rhei) 90 g, Xiāng Fù (Rhizoma Cyperi) 120 g, and Qiān Niú Zǐ (Semen Pharbitidis) 120 g; grind into fine powder, prepare into small bean-sized pill with water, and take 30 pills/time with Shēng Jiāng (Rhizoma Zingiberis Recens) decoction after meal for oral administration to treat food accumulation, gastric and abdominal pǐ, fullness, and distending pain, or dysentery with stool containing blood and mucus, tenesmus, yellow greasy tongue coating, and excess pulse.

3. 香砂枳术丸 Xiāng Shā Zhǐ Zhū Wán — Aucklandia, Amomum, Immature Bitter Orange, and Atractylodes Macrocephala Pill from *Chinese Traditional Patent Medicine* (中成药 Zhōng Chéng Yào): Mù Xiāng (Radix Aucklandiae), Shā Rén (Fructus Amomi), Shén Qū (Massa Medicata Fermentata), Mài Yá (Fructus Hordei Germinatus), Zhǐ Shí (Fructus Aurantii Immaturus), Bái Zhú (Rhizoma Atractylodis Macrocephalae), Jú Pí (Pericarpium Citri Reticulatae), Xiāng Fù (Rhizoma Cyperi), and Shān Zhā (Fructus Crataegi); grind into pill for oral administration to treat decreased intake of food, chest and gastric distention, fullness and pain, and indigestion caused by spleen-stomach disharmony.

[Precautions] Mù Xiāng (Radix Aucklandiae), intensely pungent, dispersing, aromatic, and dry in nature, should not be used overdose (less than 3 g/time according to some traditional resources). It should be used with caution in cases of constitutionally yin fluid insufficiency and unresolved fire-heat pathogen.

Daily practices

1. What are the actions and indications of Xiè Bái (Bulbus Allii Macrostemi) and how to make combination with other medicinals in accordance with state of illness?

2. What are the actions and indications of Mù Xiāng (Radix Aucklandiae)?

沉香 Chén Xiāng *lignum aquilariae resinatum aquilaria wood*

The source is from the dark brown resinous wood of *Aquilaria agallocha* Roxb. or *Aquilaria sinensis* (Lour) Gilg, family Thymelaeaceae. Alternate names include 蜜香 Mì Xiāng and 沉水香 Chén Shuǐ Xiāng. It can be processed into 伽楠香 Jiā Nán Xiāng. Pungent and bitter in flavor and slightly warm in nature.

[Actions] Move qi to alleviate pain, warm the middle *jiao* to arrest vomiting, and direct rebellious qi downward to relieve asthma. Modern researches display that its volatile oil has anesthesia, muscle-relaxing, and analgesic effect.

[Quality] For the herb produced in China, good quality is heavy, brownish black, oily, and very aromatic; for the imported one, good quality is black, firm, oily, and strong and persistently aromatic.

[Indications] Chén Xiāng (Lignum Aquilariae Resinatum) is mainly used for distention, oppression and pain in the chest and abdomen due to obstruction of qi movement; vomiting and hiccup caused by coldness in the spleen and stomach; and reversed flow of qi and wheezing associated with kidney deficiency.

1. Chest and abdominal distending pain: owning to its qi-moving and pain-relieving property, Chén Xiāng (Lignum Aquilariae Resinatum) is effective in relieving chest and abdominal distention, fullness, and migrating pain due to qi stagnation. It is combined with medicinals that move qi and fortify the spleen such as Xiāng Fù (Rhizoma Cyperi), Shā Rén (Fructus Amomi), and Wū Yào (Radix Linderae) for different patterns of qi stagnation; and with Fù Zǐ (Radix Aconiti Lateralis Praeparata), Gān Jiāng (Rhizoma Zingiberis), and Ròu Guì (Cortex Cinnamomi) for gastric and abdominal cold pain, cold extremities, and loose stool caused by intense cold in the spleen and stomach.

2. Vomiting and hiccup: owning to its ability of warming the spleen and stomach and subsuing counterflow qi, Chén Xiāng (Lignum Aquilariae Resinatum) is mainly used for stomach-cold vomiting and hiccup due

to externally-contracted cold pathogen or yang insufficiency in the middle *jiao*. It can be used together with Bàn Xià (Rhizoma Pinelliae), Jú Pí (Pericarpium Citri Reticulatae), Dīng Xiāng (Flos Caryophylli), and Shì Dì (Calyx Kaki).

3. Cough and wheezing due to lung and kidney deficiency and debilitation: Chén Xiāng (Lignum Aquilariae Resinatum) can not only descend lung qi, but also warm and tonify kidney yang to receive qi. Therefore, it is applicable for cough and wheezing of excess pattern, chronic cough and wheezing, lung disease affecting the kidney, and kidney deficiency-cold. It is combined with Rén Shēn (Radix et Rhizoma Ginseng), Shú Dì Huáng (Radix Rehmanniae Praeparata), Gé Jiè (Gecko), Ròu Cōng Róng (Herba Cistanches), and Wǔ Wèi Zǐ (Fructus Schisandrae Chinensis) for deficiency pattern; and with medicinals that dissolve phlegm and direct qi downward such as Sū Zǐ (Fructus Perillae), Jú Pí (Pericarpium Citri Reticulatae), and Bàn Xià (Rhizoma Pinelliae) when accompanied with chest oppression and qi counterflow with phlegm in the throat.

[Usage and Dosage] Should not be decocted; if used in decoctions, should be added near the end of decocting or taken right after boiled to prevent evaporation of active ingredients, refined powder with water or dissolved water in the finished liquid for oral administration. Use 0.5–1.0 g as in powder and 2–5 g in decoction.

[Mnemonics] Chén Xiāng (Lignum Aquilariae Resinatum, Aquilaria Wood): pungent and warm; direct rebellious qi downward, arrest vomiting, hiccup, cough, and wheezing, and relieve distending pain in the chest and abdomen.

[Simple and Effective Formulas]

1. 沉香降气丸 Chén Xiāng Jiàng Qì Wán — Aquilaria Wood Qi Descending Pill from *Formulas from the Imperial Pharmacy* (局方 Jú Fāng): Chén Xiāng (Lignum Aquilariae Resinatum) 18.5 g, Xiāng Fù (Rhizoma Cyperi) (stir-fried, fuzz removed) 400 g, Shā Rén (Fructus Amomi) 48 g, and Gān Cǎo (Radix et Rhizoma Glycyrrhizae) 120 g; grind into fine powder, take 3 g/dose, boil with few salts, and take decoction on an empty stomach to treat chest and diaphragm *pǐ* and

blockage, abdominal distention and fullness in the heart and abdomen, wheezing, shortness of breath, dry retching, restlessness, and fullness. Also applicable for tachypnea caused by different types of chronic cardiac failure and gastric and abdominal flatulence due to gastrointestinal dysfunction.

2. 沉香化痰丸 Chén Xiāng Huà Tán Wán — Aquilaria Wood Phlegm Resolving Pill from *Comprehensive Medicine According to Master Zhang* (张氏医通 Zhāng Shì Yī Tōng): Chén Xiāng (Lignum Aquilariae Resinatum) 60 g, Bàn Xià Qū (Rhizoma Pinelliae Fermentata) (processed with ginger juice and Zhú Lì (Succus Bambusae) 240 g, Huáng Lián (Rhizoma Coptidis) 60 g, and Mù Xiāng (Radix Aucklandiae) 30 g; grind into fine powder, make into pill with Gān Cǎo (Radix et Rhizoma Glycyrrhizae) decoction, and take 6 g/time with Jiāng Zhī (Succus Rhizomatis Zingiberis) on an empty stomach for abiding phlegm in the chest with phlegm-fire harassing the lungs. Also applicable for chronic bronchitis with yellow sputum, thirst, vexation, cough, wheezing, and shortness of breath.

[Precautions] Chén Xiāng (Lignum Aquilariae Resinatum), pungent, warm and descending in property, should be used with caution or is contraindicated in cases of constitutionally yin deficiency with internal heat manifested as vexing heat in the five centers (chest, palms and soles) or prolapse of anus and uterine due to qi deficiency and sinking.

檀香 Tán Xiāng *lignum santali albi sandalwood*

The source is from the heartwood of evergreen arbor *Santalum album* L., family Santalaceae. Alternate names include 白檀香 Bái Tán Xiāng. Pungent in flavor and warm in nature.

[Actions] Regulate the qi movement and disperse cold, and warm the middle *jiao* to arrest pain.

[Quality] Good quality is collected in summer, aromatic, yellow, hard, dense, and oily.

[Indications] Tán Xiāng (Lignum Santali Albi) and Chén Xiāng (Lignum Aquilariae Resinatum), similar in nature, flavor, and actions, both can treat pain caused by cold congealing and qi stagnation, however the former is mainly used for stomachache and chest and abdominal pain caused by cold congealing and qi stagnation, and the latter is for qi counterflow diseases due to its effect of directing counterflow downward.

1. Gastric and abdominal cold pain: Tán Xiāng (Lignum Santali Albi) is commonly used with Wú Zhū Yú (Fructus Evodiae), Wū Yào (Radix Linderae), Gān Jiāng (Rhizoma Zingiberis), and Guì Zhī (Ramulus Cinnamomi) for gastric and abdominal pain with cold sensation which is triggered and aggravated by exposure to cold with accompanying vomiting of watery fluid, decreased appetite, and gastric distention caused by yang insufficiency of the middle *jiao* or exogenous cold attacking the stomach.
2. Chest *bì* oppression pain: Tán Xiāng (Lignum Santali Albi) is commonly combined with Xì Xīn (Radix et Rhizoma Asari), Yán Hú Suǒ (Rhizoma Corydalis), and Bì Bá (Fructus Piperis Longi) for sudden onset of chest and gastric pǐ, oppression or pain triggered by exposure to cold, absence of thirst in the mouth, and white moist tongue coating; and with Dān Shēn (Radix et Rhizoma Salviae Miltiorrhizae), Pú Huáng (Pollen Typhae), and Wǔ Líng Zhī (Feces Trogopterori) for chest oppression and stabbing pain with blood stasis.

[Usage and Dosage] When used in decoctions, it should be added near the end of decocting or taken when boiled to prevent evaporation of active ingredients; taken in powder or dissolved powder in the strained medical liquid for oral administration. Use 2–5 g in decoction and 0.5–1.0 g as in powder.

[Mnemonics] Tán Xiāng (Lignum Santali Albi, Sandalwood): pungent and warm; specialized at arresting pain, and capable of regulating qi movement and dispersing cold to relieve pain and distention.

[Simple and Effective Formulas]

1. 丹参饮 Dān Shēn Yǐn — Salvia Beverage from *Medical Quintessence* (医学金针 Yī Xué Jīn Zhēn): Dān Shēn (Radix et Rhizoma Salviae Miltiorrhizae) 30 g, Tán Xiāng (Lignum Santali Albi) 4.5 g, and Shā Rén (Fructus Amomi) 4.5 g; decoct in water for oral administration to

treat pain in the heart and abdomen due to half-deficiency half-excess pattern.

2. 檀香饮 Tán Xiāng Yǐn — Sandalwood Beverage from *Recordings of Divine Assistance* (圣济录 Shèng Jì Lù): Tán Xiāng (Lignum Santali Albi) 0.3 g, Chén Xiāng (Lignum Aquilariae Resinatum) 0.3 g, and one Bīng Láng (Semen Arecae); levigate, get the juice, filtrate and remove dregs, decoct until boiled, divide into three equal doses, and take one dose/time and warm for oral administration to relieve toxins and swellings. Also applicable for swollen face with red and itchy skin due to allergic diseases.

[Precautions] Tán Xiāng (Lignum Santali Albi), warm in nature, is contraindicated in cases of yin deficiency with internal heat.

Daily practices

1. What are the similarities and differences between Chén Xiāng (Lignum Aquilariae Resinatum) and Tán Xiāng (Lignum Santali Albi) in terms of actions and indications?
2. What are the similarities and differences among Chén Xiāng (Lignum Aquilariae Resinatum), Tán Xiāng (Lignum Santali Albi), and Mù Xiāng (Radix Aucklandiae) in terms of indications?

丁香 Dīng Xiāng *flos caryophylli clove flower*

The source is from the flower bud of evergreen arbor *Eugenia caryophyllata* Thunb., family Myrtaceae. Alternate names include 公丁香 Gōng Dīng Xiāng, as it looks like Chinese character 丁 Dīng. Pungent in flavor and warm in nature.

[Actions] Warm the middle *jiao* and direct rebellious qi downward, and warm the kidney and assist the yang. It contains such volatile ingredients as oil of cloves, has antibacterial and stomachic effects, and can arrest toothache when applied externally.

[Quality] Good quality is full, large, reddish brown, oily, aromatic, and sinking in water. 母丁香 Mǔ Dīng Xiāng is from the ripe fruit of *Eugenia caryophyllata* Thunb., alternate names include 鸡舌香 Jī Shé Xiāng. Its properties and actions are similar to but weaker than those of 公丁香 Gōng Dīng Xiāng.

[Indications] Dīng Xiāng (Flos Caryophylli) is mainly used for qi stagnation or qi counterflow caused by cold. Also used to supplement kidney and assist yang.

1. Cold congealing the spleen and stomach: owning to its pungent, warm, and fragrant properties, Dīng Xiāng (Flos Caryophylli) is good at treating different types of diseases caused by cold attacking or deficiency-cold of the spleen and stomach. It is combined with Chén Pí (Pericarpium Citri Reticulatae) and Bàn Xià (Rhizoma Pinelliae) for vomiting of phlegm-drool caused by spleen deficiency with coldness in the middle *jiao*; with Wú Zhū Yú (Fructus Evodiae) and Ròu Dòu Kòu (Semen Myristicae) for gastric and abdominal cold pain, vomiting and diarrhea due to coldness in the middle *jiao*; and with Ròu Guì (Cortex Cinnamomi) for unremitting stomach cold pain in a powder form (taken with warm wine before meal).
2. Ascending counterflow of stomach qi: the stomach governs descent; with cold pathogen invasion in the stomach or food accumulation in the middle *jiao*, stomach qi fails to descend and cause vomiting and hiccup. Dīng Xiāng (Flos Caryophylli), effective in relieving ascending counterflow of stomach qi due to coldness, is a principal medicinals for hiccup caused by stomach coldness and can be prescribed together with Shì Dì (Calyx Kaki), Bàn Xià (Rhizoma Pinelliae), and Shēng Jiāng (Rhizoma Zingiberis Recens).
3. Kidney yang deficiency and debilitation: Dīng Xiāng (Flos Caryophylli) can supplement yang and be combined with medicinals that warm the kidney and reinforce yang to treat impotence and seminal cold.

Dīng Xiāng (Flos Caryophylli) can also be applied externally, for instance, by putting it on plaster to treat carbuncles and malignant hyperplasia; wrapping its powder with cotton and filling in the nose to relieve nasal polyp; grinding it with Ròu Guì (Cortex Cinnamomi) into powder for external application to umbilical region to cure abdominal pain and diarrhea caused by coldness. Nowadays, it has been prepared into powder, tincture, or decoction for external application to counteract fungoid skin tinea. It is also an important flavoring ingredient in Chinese cooking.

[Usage and Dosage] When used in decoctions, it should be added near the end of decocting, and taken right after the medicinal liquid is boiled to prevent evaporation of active ingredients. Use 2–5 g in decoction, decrease the dosage as in pill and powder, and appropriate amount for external application.

[Mnemonics] Dīng Xiāng (Flos Caryophylli, Clove Flower): warm the middle *jiao*, specialized at directing rebellious qi downward; capable of relieving vomiting and hiccup often in a combination with Shì Dì (Calyx Kaki).

[Simple and Effective Formulas]

1. 丁夏丸 Dīng Xià Wán — Clove Flower and Pinellia Pill from *Selected Formulas* (百一选方 Bǎi Yī Xuǎn Fāng): Dīng Xiāng (Flos Caryophylli) 30 g and Bàn Xià (Rhizoma Pinelliae) 30 g; grind into fine powder, make into green bean-sized pill with Jiāng Zhī (Succus Rhizomatis Zingiberis), and take 20–30 pills/time with Shēng Jiāng (Rhizoma Zingiberis Recens) decoction for oral administration to treat pediatric vomiting due to common cold.

2. 加味丁桂散 Jiā Wèi Dīng Guì Sǎn — Supplemented Clove Flower and Cinnamon Bark Powder from *Empirical Formulas* (经验方 Jīng Yàn Fāng): Dīng Xiāng (Flos Caryophylli), Ròu Guì (Cortex Cinnamomi), Mù Xiāng (Radix Aucklandiae), and Yán Hú Suǒ (Rhizoma Corydalis) in equal dosage; grind into fine powder, put 2 g/time on adhesive plaster, apply topically on Guān Yuán (RN 4) before menstruation or during dysmenorrheal, add bilateral Sān Yīn Jiāo (SP 6) for unremitting pain, change dressing every other day, apply every day for six days every mouth to treat dysmenorrheal.

[Precautions] Dīng Xiāng (Flos Caryophylli), warm in nature, is contraindicated in cases of excess heat and deficiency heat.

香附 Xiāng Fù *rhizoma cyperi cyperus*

The source is from the rhizome of herbaceous perennial *Cyperus rotundus* L., family Cyperaceae. It literally means aromatic appendage, and alternate names include 香附子 Xiāng Fù Zǐ, 香附米 Xiāng Fù Mǐ, and 莎草根 Suō Cǎo Gēn. Pungent, slightly bitter, and slightly sweet in flavor and neutral in nature.

[Actions] Move qi and relieve stagnation, and regulate menstruation and arrest pain. It is applicable for chest, rib-side, gastric and abdominal distending pain, indigestion, chest and gastric *pǐ* and stuffiness, distending pain in the breasts, menstrual irregularities, amenorrhea, dysmenorrhea, and cold hernia with abdominal pain due to liver constraint qi stagnation. From the perspective of modern research, its volatile oil has a mild androgenic effect and its alcohol extractives have shown anti-inflammatory, antipyretic, antalgic, sedative, and smooth muscle-inhibitory effect.

[Quality] Good quality is large, solid, reddish brown, and aromatic.

[Indications]

1. Binding constraint of liver qi: Xiāng Fù (Rhizoma Cyperi), as a principal medicinal for soothing the liver and relieving stagnation, is applicable for chest and rib-side pain, chest and gastric distending pain, and liver and stomach pain caused by binding constraint of liver qi. It is often combined with Chái Hú (Radix Bupleuri), Qīng Pí (Pericarpium Citri Reticulatae Viride), Chén Pí (Pericarpium Citri Reticulatae), Fó Shǒu (Fructus Citri Sarcodactylis), and Zhǐ Qiào (Fructus Aurantii). For liver and stomach qi pain pattern manifested as gastric pain involving rib-sides and chest oppression and discomfort due to liver qi attacking the stomach, this substance is combined with Gāo Liáng Jiāng (Rhizoma Alpiniae Officinarum) for the cold natured; and with Zhī Zǐ (Fructus Gardeniae) for the hot-natured.
2. Gynecological disorders: most of gynecological disorders are related to liver qi stagnation, and Xiāng Fù (Rhizoma Cyperi) is commonly used in the treatment of gynecological problems. It is often prescribed together with Dāng Guī (Radix Angelicae Sinensis), Bái Sháo (Radix

Paeoniae Alba), Sū Gěng (Caulis Perillae), Chái Hú (Radix Bupleuri), Qīng Pí (Pericarpium Citri Reticulatae Viride), and Chuān Xiōng (Rhizoma Chuanxiong) for menstrual irregularities, dysmenorrhea, and especially distending pain of the breasts before menstruation caused by liver constraint and qi stagnation. This substance can be used alone in a stir-fried powder form (taken with rice soup), or together with medicinals that regulate menstruation and qi for profuse uterine bleeding and prolonged scanty uterine bleeding of variable intervals caused by the liver failing to sooth.

It is also usually used for such external disorders as distending pain of or masses in the breasts due to liver qi stagnation; or ground with Chuān Xiōng (Rhizoma Chuanxiong) into powder for migraine and headache; or prescribed together with medicinals that release the exterior for externally-contracted pathogens with qi stagnation.

[Usage and Dosage] Nowadays, use raw in most cases, but traditionally, there are many requirement for processing, as stated by 李时珍 Li Shi-zhen that "the raw medicinal is considered most effective in going upward to the chest and diaphragm and outward to the skin, the prepared is to go downward to the liver and kidney and exteriorly to the waist and foot, frying until it turns into black is to arrest bleeding, frying in urine of boys under twelve enables it to enter blood phase and tonify deficiency, frying in salt solution helps it enter blood phase and moisten dryness, frying with halite is to supplement kidney qi, frying in wine enables it to penetrate to all the channels and collaterals, frying in vinegar increases the ability of this herb to disperse accumulations and masses, and frying with ginger juice is to relieve phlegm and fluid retention." The processed medicinal is better for gynecological problems, charred one is preferred for hemorrhagic disorders, and vinegar-processed herb is potent for relieving pain due to liver-stomach qi stagnation. Use 5–9 g in decoction, and decrease the dosage as in pill and powder.

[Mnemonics] Xiāng Fù (Rhizoma Cyperi, Cyperus): pungent and neutral; soothe the liver to relieve stagnation, regulate menstruation, arrest pain, and indispensable for gynecological problems.

[Simple and Effective Formulas]

1. 快气汤 Kuài Qì Tāng — Qi Promoting Decoction from *Formulas from the Imperial Pharmacy* (局方 Jú Fāng): Xiāng Fù (Rhizoma Cyperi) (stir-fried, hair removed) 32 g, Shā Rén (Fructus Amomi) 8 g, and Gān Cǎo (Radix et Rhizoma Glycyrrhizae) 4 g; grind into fine powder and take 3 g/dose after mixing with salt solution for qi stagnation patterns manifested as chest and diaphragm *pǐ* and oppression, heart and abdominal distending and pain, belching, acid regurgitation, vomiting, and hangover with poor appetite.

2. 醋附丸 Cù Fù Wán-Vinegar cooked Cyperus Pill from *Fine Formulas for Women* (妇人良方 Fù Rén Liáng Fāng): Xiāng Fù (Rhizoma Cyperi) 250 g; decoct in vinegar, dry by roasting, grind into powder, make into phoenix tree seed-sized pill with vinegar, and take 30 or 40 pills/dose with rice soup for menstrual irregularities, deficiency-cold of organs, vertigo, poor appetite, alternating chills and fever, abdominal distress and pain, red and white leukorrhea, chest oppression, and insecurity of fetal qi.

3. 治腰痛方 Zhì Yāo Tòng Fāng — Lumbago Relieving Formula from *Empirical Formulas* (经验方 Jīng Yàn Fāng): Xiāng Fù (Rhizoma Cyperi); grind into powder and take 4 g/time with cool boiled water for oral administration, three times a day to treat different types of lumbago.

[Precautions] Xiāng Fù (Rhizoma Cyperi), bitter and dry in nature, can consume qi and blood when applied inappropriately and is contraindicated in cases of deficiency without stagnation.

Daily practices

1. What are the similarities and differences among Dīng Xiāng (Flos Caryophylli), Mù Xiāng (Radix Aucklandiae), Chén Xiāng (Lignum Aquilariae Resinatum), and Tán Xiāng (Lignum Santali Albi) in terms of actions and indications?
2. What are the actions and indications of Xiāng Fù (Rhizoma Cyperi) and what are the difference between Xiāng Fù (Rhizoma Cyperi) and Mù Xiāng (Radix Aucklandiae) in terms of actions?

川楝子 Chuān Liàn Zǐ *fructus toosendan toosendan fruit*

The source is from the ripe fruit of deciduous arbor *Melia toosendan* Sieb. et Zucc., family Meliaceae. Alternate names include 楝实 Liàn Shí and 金铃子 Jīn Líng Zi. Bitter in flavor and cold in nature with mild toxin.

[Actions] Move qi and smooth the liver to arrest pain, kill parasites, and relieve tinea. It is applicable for pain in the chest and rib-side, abdominal pain due to worm accumulation, and tinea capitis. Its toosendanin is an active ingredient of dispelling roundworm.

[Quality] Good quality is golden outside, large, and thick.

[Indications] Chuān Liàn Zǐ (Fructus Toosendan) is applicable for rib-side, gastric and abdominal pain and hernia pain caused by liver qi stagnation or disharmony between the liver and stomach, as well as disorders due to parasites and mould.

1. Pain due to liver constraint: it refers to pain caused by liver qi stagnation and localized in the area of liver channel running root, such as rib-side, the lateral aspect of lower abdomen, and pudendum. Such common disorders as intercostal neuralgia, hernia, and dysmenorrheal are all relative with liver constraint. Chuān Liàn Zǐ (Fructus Toosendan) is cold in nature and therefore particularly suitable for liver constraint transforming into fire or with accompanying heat manifestations. In the clinic, it is usually combined with medicinals that sooth the liver and regulate qi such as Qīng Pí (Pericarpium Citri Reticulatae Viride), Xiāng Fù (Rhizoma Cyperi), and Yù Jīn (Radix Curcumae). Combination of herb is based on the nature of disease, specifically, this substance is prescribed together with Wú Zhū Yú (Fructus Evodiae), Xiǎo Huí Xiāng (Fructus Foeniculi), and Ròu Guì (Cortex Cinnamomi) for liver constraint and qi stagnation resulting from cold congealing; and with Pú Gōng Yīng (Herba Taraxaci), Mǔ Dān Pí (Cortex Moutan), and Zhī Zǐ (Fructus Gardeniae) when accompanied with heat signs.

2. Liver and stomach qi disorder: it refers to stomachache and vomiting caused by liver constraint transversely attacking the stomach. In this case, Chuān Liàn Zǐ (Fructus Toosendan) is combined with Yán Hú Suǒ

(Rhizoma Corydalis), Chái Hú (Radix Bupleuri), Zhǐ Qiào (Fructus Aurantii), and Bái Sháo (Radix Paeoniae Alba). If the disorder turns into fire with manifestations of dry mouth and red tongue with scanty fluid, it is combined with Shēng Dì (Radix Rehmanniae) and Běi Shā Shēn (Radix Glehniae).

3. Roundworm: Chuān Liàn Zǐ (Fructus Toosendan) has an effect of dispel worms but less than that of kǔ Liàn Pí (Cortex Meliae). It can also relieve pain and therefore more suitable for abdominal pain caused by roundworm.

Chuān Liàn Zǐ (Fructus Toosendan) can also be applied externally, for instance, pound it into pieces, wrap with cotton, and put into the ear to treat aural sores. It has been reported that its powder are mixed with cooked lard stearin or vaseline for external application to relieve tinea capitis. Its powder is also used topically for tinea of the scalp.

[Usage and Dosage] Use in decoction in general, 5–10 g, use raw, dry-frying until yellow to reduce its toxicity and eliminate its bitter and cold property to protect the stomach; dry-frying with salt to direct the medicinals downwards to increase its ability of curing lower abdominal pain and hernia pain.

[Mnemonics] Chuān Liàn Zǐ (Fructus Toosendan, Toosendan Fruit): bitter and cold; specialized at soothing the liver, arresting rib-side pain, resolving hernia, killing parasites, and relieving tinea.

[Simple and Effective Formulas]

1. 金铃子散 Jīn Líng Zǐ Sǎn — Toosendan Powder from *Essentials for Health* (活法机要 Huó Fǎ Jī Yào): Jīn Líng Zi (Fructus Toosendan) 30 g and Yán Hú Suǒ (Rhizoma Corydalis) 30 g; grind into fine powder and take 6–9 g/time with wine or warm water for oral administration to treat heat syncope with persistent paroxysmal cardiac pain. Also applicable for different types of chest pain, angina pectoris, and stomachache.

2. 导气汤 Dǎo Qì Tāng-Qi — promoting Decoction from *Quintessence of Medical Formulas* (医方简义 Yī Fāng Jiǎn Yì): Chuān Liàn Zǐ (Fructus

Toosendan) 9 g, Xiǎo Huí Xiāng (Fructus Foeniculi) 1.5 g, Mù Xiāng (Radix Aucklandiae) 3 g, and Dàn Wú Zhū Yú (Fructus Evodiae) 3 g; decoct in running water for oral administration to treat cold hernia, sagging testicle, and hernia pain.

[Precautions] Chuān Liàn Zǐ (Fructus Toosendan), with mild toxicity, should not be overdosed. Poisoning symptoms associated with overdosage (above 10 pieces/time) of the fruit of include toxic hepatitis, difficult breathing, numbness of the limbs, convulsion or even death. It is cold and bitter and therefore contraindicated in cases of cold from deficiency of the spleen and stomach.

小茴香 Xiǎo Huí Xiāng *fructus foeniculi fennel*

The source is from the ripe fruit of herbaceous perennial *Foeniculum vulgare* Mill., family Umbelliferae. Alternate names include 谷茴香 Gǔ Huí Xiāng, and 瘪谷茴香 Biě Gǔ Huí Xiāng. Pungent in flavor and warm in nature.

[Actions] Expel cold to alleviate pain, and regulate qi and harmonize the stomach. It is applicable for pain due to cold hernia, sagging testicle, vomiting and decreased intake of food due to stomach cold, and gastric and abdominal distending pain. It contains volatile oil and its major ingredients include anisole and fenchone. Fennel oil can promote gastrointestinal motility and secretion, eliminate flatulence, relieve pain, and remove spasm.

[Quality] Good quality is dry, full, yellowish green, and intensely aromatic without impurities. The best quality is found in Inner Mongolia.

[Indications] Xiǎo Huí Xiāng (Fructus Foeniculi) is mainly used for different types of cold hernia, pain in the lateral aspect of lower abdomen, sagging testicle, and vomiting and decreased appetite caused by stomach cold.

1. Abdominal pain due to cold hernia and sagging testicles: from the perspective of Traditional Chinese Medicine, hernia refers different types of disorders and has different interpretations in the literature resources. *Treatise on the Origins and Manifestations of Various*

Diseases (诸病源候论 Zhū Bìng Yuán Hòu Lùn) stated there are 石疝 Shí Shàn, 血疝 Xuè Shàn, 阴疝 Yīn Shàn, 妒疝 Dù Shàn, and 气疝 Qì Shàn; *The Yellow Emperor's Inner Classic: Basic Questions* (黄帝内经素问 • 骨空论 Huáng Dì Nèi Jīng Sù Wèn) recorded seven types of Shàn (hernia), namely 冲疝 Chōng Shàn, 狐疝 Hú Shàn, 疝 Shàn, 厥疝 Jué Shàn, 瘕疝 Jiǎ Shàn, 疝 Shàn, and 癃疝 Lóng Shàn; *Confucians' Duties to Their Parents* (儒门事亲 Rú Mén Shì Qīn) described seven types of Shàn (hernia), specifically 寒疝 Hán Shàn, 水疝 Shuǐ Shàn, 筋疝 Jīn Shàn, 血疝 Xuè Shàn, 气疝 Qì Shàn, 狐疝 Hú Shàn and 疝 Shàn, among which 寒疝 Hán Shàn refers to abdominal pain caused by cold pathogen, abdominal muscle contracture and umbilical pain in most cases with accompanying cold sweating, aversion to cold, cold limbs, numbness in the hands and feet, or scrotum cold pain. From the perspective of modern biomedicine, sagging testicle is inguinal hernia. Owning to its warm nature and potency of dispelling cold qi in the liver channel, Xiǎo Huí Xiāng (Fructus Foeniculi) is commonly used for the above-mentioned diseases and often combined with Lì Zhī Hé (Semen Litchi), Jú Hé (Semen Citri Reticulatae), and Wú Zhū Yú (Fructus Evodiae). It has often been categorized into interior-warming medicinal because of its strong potency in dispelling cold and warming yang and effectiveness in the treatment of lumbago due to kidney yang insufficiency with exuberant interior-coldness.

2. Vomiting and reduced appetite due to stomach coldness: With a property of warming the middle *jiao*, moving qi, harmonizing the middle *jiao*, and improving appetite, Xiǎo Huí Xiāng (Fructus Foeniculi) is widely used for stomachache, vomiting, decreased appetite, and stomach distention after meal caused by stomach coldness. It can also be prescribed together with Gān Jiāng (Rhizoma Zingiberis), Mù Xiāng (Radix Aucklandiae), and Bàn Xià (Rhizoma Pinelliae).

[Usage and Dosage] Use raw in general, 3–6 g in decoction, and decrease the dosage as in pill and powder. Dry frying in salt solution can increase its ability of dispelling cold pathogen in the lower *jiao*, liver, and kidney, as salty flavor enters into the kidney.

[Mnemonics] Xiǎo Huí Xiāng (Fructus Foeniculi, Fennel): pungent and warm; expel cold, warm the liver and stomach, arrest vomiting, and specialized at curing different types of hernia.

[Simple and Effective Formulas]

1. 小茴香丸 Xiǎo Huí Xiāng Wán — Fennel Pill from *Treatise on Diseases, Patterns, and Formulas Related to the Unification of the Three Etiologies* (三因方 Sān Yīn Fāng): Xiǎo Huí Xiāng (Fructus Foeniculi) and Hú Jiāo (Fructus Piperis) in equal dosage; make into fine powder, prepare into phoenix tree seed-sized pill with wine paste, and take 3 g/dose with warm wine on an empty stomach for pain due to hernia or incarcerated hernia.
2. 茴香猪肾方 Huí Xiāng Zhū Shèn Fāng — Fennel with Pig Kidney Formula from *Essential Teachings on Diagnosis and Treatment* (证治要诀 Zhèng Zhì Yào Jué): Xiǎo Huí Xiāng (Fructus Foeniculi); stir-fry until aromatic, grind into powder, split pig kidney, cut into consecutive slices, dust the power on every slice, wrap with paste paper, roast until well-done, chew slowly, and take with wine for oral administration to treat kidney deficiency lumbago failing to turn around on either side, somnolence, and fatigue. Also applicable for different types of chronic lumbago, fear of cold in the waist, and cold limbs.

[Precautions] Xiǎo Huí Xiāng (Fructus Foeniculi), warm in nature, should be used with caution in cases of yin deficiency with internal heat.

Daily practices

1. What are the similarities and differences between Chuān Liàn Zǐ (Fructus Toosendan) and Xiǎo Huí Xiāng (Fructus Foeniculi) in terms of actions and indications?
2. What are the similarities and differences among qi-regulating medicinals that we learn this week in terms of actions and indications?

CHAPTER 8

Eighth Week

1

荔枝核 Lì Zhī Hé *semen litchi lychee seed*

The source is from the fruit kernel of evergreen arbor *Litchi chinensis* Sonn., family Sapindaceae. Alternate names include 离枝 Lí Zhī because poet 白居易 Bai Ju-yi wrote a poem: "the fruit that taken away (离 Lí) from its branch (枝 Zhī) will lose its color in one day and taste in three days", the later generation then called it Lí Zhī 离枝 and eventually named as Lì Zhī 荔枝. Sweet and astringent in flavor and warm in nature.

[Actions] Dissipate cold to arrest pain, and move qi and soothe the liver. It is applicable for gastric pain, hernia pain, and dysmenorrheal.

[Quality] Good quality is dry, large, and full.

[Indications] Lì Zhī Hé (Semen Litchi) is mainly used for hernia pain, testicle swelling and pain, stomachache, and pain in the lateral aspect of lower abdomen.

1. Abdominal pain due to cold hernia: Lì Zhī Hé (Semen Litchi), warm in nature, can dispel cold pathogen, enter the liver channel blood level, and circulate qi stagnation in blood, and thus is suitable for hernia pain caused by cold congealing and qi stagnation. Clinically, it is usually used together with Xiǎo Huí Xiāng (Fructus Foeniculi) especially for pain in the lateral aspect of lower abdomen radiating downwards to the pudendum; with Wú Zhū Yú (Fructus Evodiae) for severe coldness; with Chuān Liàn Zǐ (Fructus Toosendan) when accompanied with heat

277

pathogen; and with Jú Hé (Semen Citri Reticulatae), Qīng Pí (Pericarpium Citri Reticulatae Viride) if accompanied with testicle swelling and pain.

2. Stomachache, lesser abdominal pain, and dysmenorrheal due to cold congealing and qi stagnation: Lì Zhī Hé (Semen Litchi) can disperse cold pathogen in the liver channel, relieve qi stagnation in the liver channel, and open the liver channel blood level, therefore it is applicable for stomachache, pain in the lateral aspects of the lower abdomen, and dysmenorrheal caused by cold congealing, qi stagnation and blood stasis. It has been recently reported that it is effective in diabetes.

[Usage and Dosage] Use raw in general and crush into pieces before using; dry-frying in salt solution can increase its ability of dispelling cold pathogen in the lower *jiao*, liver, and kidney, as salty flavor enters into the kidney. Use 6–12 g in decoction, decrease the dosage as in pill and powder.

[Mnemonics] Lì Zhī Hé (Semen Litchi, Lychee Seed): sweet and acrid; disperse cold, soothe the liver, promote qi movement, arrest pain, and often used to treat hernia.

[Simple and Effective Formulas]

1. 荔香散 — Lì Xiāng Sǎn — Lychee Seed and Costus Root Powder from *The Complete Works of Jing-yue* (景岳全书, Jǐng Yuè Quán Shū,): Lì Zhī Hé (Semen Litchi) 3 g and Mù Xiāng (Radix Aucklandiae) 2.4 g; make into powder and take 3 g/time after mixing with boiled water for oral administration to treat chronic pain with frequent onsets in the heart, stomach cavity, and abdomen.

2. 荔枝散 Lì Zhī Sǎn — Lychee Seed Powder from *Effective Formulas from Generations of Physicians* (世医得效方, Shì Yī Dé Xiào Fāng,): Xiǎo Huí Xiāng (Fructus Foeniculi), Qīng Pí (Pericarpium Citri Reticulatae Viride) (complete), and Lì Zhī Hé (Semen Litchi) in equal dosage; file into powder, stir-fry and grind into fine powder, and take 6 g/time with wine for oral administration, three times a day for severe swollen testicle (hydrocele of tunica vaginalis).

橘核 Jú Hé *semen citri reticulatae tangerine seed*

The source is from the semen of the ripe fruit of evergreen subarbor *Citrus reticulata* Blanco and its cultivated varieties, family Rutaceae. Bitter in flavor and warm in nature.

[Actions] Dissipate cold to arrest pain, and move qi and smooth the liver. It is applicable for hernia, swollen and painful testicle, acute mastitis, and lumbago.

[Quality] Good quality is white, full, and in even size.

[Indications] Jú Hé (Semen Citri Reticulatae) is mainly used for hernia pain, testicle swelling and pain, stomachache, and 少 abdominal pain. Its indication is similar to that of Lì Zhī Hé (Semen Litchi).

[Usage and Dosage] Use raw in general and crush into pieces before using; dry-frying in salt solution can increase its ability of dispelling cold pathogen in the lower *jiao*, liver, and kidney, as salty flavor enters into the kidney. Use 3–10 g in decoction, decrease the dosage as in pill and powder.

[Mnemonics] Jú Hé (Semen Citri Reticulatae, Tangerine Seed): warm and bitter; disperse cold, move qi, soothe the liver, arrest pain, and applicable for hernia.

[Simple and Effective Formulas]
橘核丸 — Jú Hé Wán — Tangerine Seed Pill from *Formulas to Aid the Living* (Jì Shēng Fāng, 济生方): Jú Hé (Semen Citri Reticulatae) (stir-fried) 30 g, Hǎi Zǎo (Sargassum) (washed) 30 g, Kūn Bù (Thallus Laminariae) (washed) 30 g, Hǎi Dài (Seaweed) (washed) 30 g, Chuān Liàn Zǐ (Fructus Toosendan) (flesh removed, stir-fried) 30 g, Táo Rén (Semen Persicae) (stir-fried with bran) 30 g, Hòu Pò (Cortex Magnoliae Officinalis) (peel removed, stir-fried with ginger juice) 15 g, Mù Tōng (Caulis Akebiae) 15 g, Zhǐ Shí (Fructus Aurantii Immaturus) (stir-fried with bran) 15 g, Yán Hú Suǒ (Rhizoma Corydalis) (stir-fried, peel removed) 15 g, Guì Pí (Cortex Cinnamomi) (use of fire prohibited) 15 g, and Mù Xiāng (Radix Aucklandiae) (use of fire prohibited) 15 g; grind into fine powder, make into phoenix tree seed-sized pill with wine paste, and take 70 pills/ time with salt solution or wine on an empty stomach for swollen scrotum;

swollen, distending, sagging or hard as a stone testicle; umbilical colicky pain; or scrotum sores and toxins with yellow effusion or erosion.

[Precautions] Jú Hé (Semen Citri Reticulatae), capable of moving qi and consuming qi, is suitable for excess pattern and contraindicated in deficiency pattern.

Daily practices

1. What are the commonly-used herbs for cold hernia and what are the similarities and differences among them?
2. What are the similarities and differences among Lì Zhī Hé (Semen Litchi), Jú Hé (Semen Citri Reticulatae), Mù Xiāng (Radix Aucklandiae), and Tán Xiāng (Lignum Santali Albi) in terms of actions and indications?
3. What precautions should be taken when using pungent and warm medicinals that regulate qi and why?

MEDICINALS THAT RELIEVE FOOD STAGNATION

Foods are essential to the normal functioning of the body and its absorption and digestion rely on the spleen and stomach. For this reason, these two organs are known as "the foundation of acquired constitution". Food accumulation is often caused by eating too much that hard to digest or dysfunctional spleen and stomach failing to digest and absorb. This can to be found in indigestion due to eating too much at one time, but most likely in cases of dysfunctional spleen and stomach due to poor dietary habits with alternating overeating and fasting. For this reason, it is most common in children and one of the major causes for infantile malnutrition. Food accumulation, as a pathological agent, will further act to cause many other symptoms and exert negative influences on other organs. Hence, one of common approaches of relieving food accumulation is to restore the function of the spleen and stomach.

This disorder is characterized by gastric and abdominal distention and fullness, decreased appetite, belching with fetid odor, nausea, vomiting, and stool with sour and fetid odor and undigested food. If that is the case, medicinals that relieve blood stasis are primarily used.

The actions of this group of herbs are (1) those that directly help digest food stagnation and mainly used for excess pattern of food accumulation caused by overeating; and (2) those that boost the spleen and harmonize the stomach to improve their ability of transform and transport and mainly applicable for deficiency pattern of food accumulation due to spleen and stomach deficiency. Most of these herbs possess both actions.

Selection for herbs and therapeutic method is based on the state of illness. Herbs that move qi are added to the prescription to help move qi, loosen the center, and promote digestion in cases of food stagnation in the gastrointestinal tract with obstruction of qi dynamics manifested as gastric and abdominal distention and fullness; purgatives may also be required to guide out food stagnation and facilitate defecation if food accumulation is accompanied with dry and hard stool; interior-warming herbs are added to the prescription to dissipate cold and activate stagnation when patient also present with cold manifestations; herbs that clear heat are also prescribed to drain heat and guide out stagnation in cases of food accumulation generating heat. Food accumulation is often in conjunction with damp-turbidity, therefore the herbs in this group are usually combined with aromatic medicinals that relieve dampness. This disorder may arise from spleen and stomach deficiency, but also can result in spleen and stomach depletion upon a prolonged course of disease. It is important to remember that the concurrence of food stagnation and spleen and stomach deficiency is not unusual in the clinic, the herbs in this group are often prescribed together with others that supplement the spleen and stomach to conduct the treatment with both dispersion and supplementation.

山楂 Shān Zhā *fructus crataegi chinese hawthorn fruit*

The source is from the ripe fruit of *Crataegus cuneata* Sieb. et Zucc., family Rosaceae. Alternate names include 赤爪子 Chì Zhuǎ Zi. Sour and sweet in flavor and slightly warm in nature.

[Actions] Strengthen the spleen and assist transportation, reduce and guide out food stagnation, and dissipate stagnation and arrest pain. It is applicable for meat accumulation, gastric distending pain, diarrhea and dysentery with abdominal pain, dysmenorrhea, amenorrhea, postpartum blood stasis, hernia pain, and hyperlipemia. Recent researches reveal it has antihypertensive and hypolipidemic effects and can treat atherosclerosis.

[Quality] Divided into "北山楂 Běi Shān Zhā" and 南山楂 Nán Shān Zhā. The former is from the cultivated *Crataegus pinnatifida* Bge. var. major N.E.Br. mainly produced in Shandong, Henan, Hebei, and Liaoning, and good quality is large, red skinned, and thick with few kernels; whereas the latter is wild Crataegus cuneata Sieb. et Zucc. mainly produced in Jiangsu, Zhejiang, Guangdong, Guangxi, and Yunnan, and good quality is indicated by even size, brownish red skinned, and solid feel.

[Indications]

1. Drink and food accumulation: Shān Zhā (Fructus Crataegi) can help improve digestion and relieve food accumulation, especially for greasy meat accumulation and infantile breast-milk accumulation. It can be used alone for meat accumulation or together with medicinals that move qi and relieve food accumulation such as Mù Xiāng (Radix Aucklandiae), Zhǐ Shí (Fructus Aurantii Immaturus), Shén Qū (Massa Medicata Fermentata), and Mài Yá (Fructus Hordei Germinatus) for different types of drink and food accumulations.
2. Blood stasis accumulation: blood stasis is a kind of pathological substance caused by disturbance of blood circulation and may result in different types of disorders. Blood stasis-relieving medicinals can invigorate blood and dissolve stasis, among them Shān Zhā (Fructus Crataegi), neutral in nature, is a medicinal full of potency. It is widely used for treating abdominal pain and persistent flow of lochia caused by postpartum blood stasis and applicable for dysmenorrheal due to stagnation with blood stasis and featured by severe abdominal pain during menstruation with clots and abdominal pain relieved after discharge of clotting. It can also be combined with Dāng Guī (Radix Angelicae Sinensis), Chuān Xiōng (Rhizoma Chuanxiong), and Yì Mǔ Cǎo (Herba Leonuri) for above-mentioned disorders.

Also applicable for tapeworm and dysentery with stool containing blood and mucus. Nowadays, it has been commonly used in the treatment of hypertension, coronary heart disease, and hyperlipemia.

[Usage and Dosage] Use raw for invigorating blood and relieving blood stasis; dry-fried or scorch-fried for dispersing accumulation, resolving food stagnation, and curing diarrhea an dysentery; and charred for hemorrhagic disorders. Use 9–15 g in decoction, up to 250 g when used alone or for killing parasites, and decrease the dosage as in pill or powder.

[Mnemonics] Shān Zhā (Fructus Crataegi, Chinese Hawthorn Fruit): sour and sweet; lower the blood pressure and blood lipid, dissolve stasis, and disperse meat accumulation.

[Simple and Effective Formulas]

1. 山楂饮 Shān Zhā Yǐn — Chinese Hawthorn Fruit Beverage from *Simple and Convenient Single-medicinal Formula* (简便单方, Jiǎn Biàn Dān Fāng,): Shān Zhā (Fructus Crataegi) flesh 120 g; decoct in water, eat Shān Zhā (Fructus Crataegi) flesh and drink the soup for indigestive meat accumulation.
2. 治痢方 Zhì Lì Fāng — Dysentery Arresting Formula from *Medical Recordes Arranged by Category* (医钞类编, Yī Chāo Lèi Biān): Shān Zhā (Fructus Crataegi) flesh; stir-fry and grind into powder, stir and mix 3–6 g/time with honey for stool containing profuse blood, with white sugar for profuse white mucus, infuse in boiled water, and take on an empty stomach for dysentery with stool containing blood and mucus.

[Precautions] Shān Zhā (Fructus Crataegi), although neutral in nature, is an attacking and dispatching medicinal and therefore is contraindicated to cases of spleen and stomach deficiency, especially poor appetite and food accumulation caused by spleen and stomach deficiency.

神曲 Shén Qū *massa medicata fermentata medicated leaven*

It is a preparation of a fermented mixture of wheat flour, and various herbs including Là Liào (Herba Polygoni Hydropiperis), Qīng Hāo (Herba Artemisiae Annuae), and Xìng Rén (Semen Armeniacae Amarum). Alternate names include 六神曲 Liù Shén Qū. Sweet and pungent in flavor and warm in nature.

[Actions] Reduce food stagnation and harmonize the stomach, and improve appetite. It is applicable for food accumulation, gastric and abdominal distention and fullness, poor appetite, diarrhea, and dysentery. Especially for rice and flour food accumulation and liquor accumulation, this substance contains saccharomycetes and is helpful for digestion.

[Quality] Good quality is old and without damage caused by worms.

[Indications]

1. Indigestion: Shén Qū (Massa Medicata Fermentata) is applicable for gastric and abdominal distention and oppression, belching of putrid qi, and aversion to food cuased by drink and food accumulation and stagnation and often combined with other medicinals that relieving food accumulation such as Shān Zhā (Fructus Crataegi) and Mài Yá (Fructus Hordei Germinatus). Stir-fried three herbs are often used together and known as "焦三仙 Jiāo Sān Xiān".
2. Dysentery and diarrhea: Shén Qū (Massa Medicata Fermentata) can be used alone or together with Cāng Zhú (Rhizoma Atractylodis) and Wú Zhū Yú (Fructus Evodiae) for dysentery and diarrhea with incomplete defecation or tenesmus, mucus in stool, and severe abdominal pain attributed to drink and food retention.

[Usage and Dosage] Use dry-fried until yellow or scorched-fried in general, 6–12 g in decoction, decrease the dosage as in pill or powder. Using in pill containing mineral medicinal as excipients to prevent the negative effect of mineral medicinal on digestive system, such as Cí Zhū Wán (Loadstones and Cinnabar Pill).

[Mnemonics] Shén Qū Massa Medicata Fermentata, Medicated Leaven): warm; promote digestion, guide out food stagnation, and relieve dysentery and diarrhea.

[Simple and Effective Formulas]
曲术丸 Qū Zhú Wán — Medicated Leaven and Atractylodes Rhizome Pill from *Formulas from the Imperial Pharmacy* (局方, Jú Fāng): Shén Qū (Massa Medicata Fermentata) (stir-fried) and Cāng Zhú (Rhizoma Atractylodis) (soaked in rice-washed water for one night, baked) in equal dosage; grind into powder, make into phoenix tree seed-sized pill with flour paste, and take 15–20 pills/time with rice soup for oral administration,

twice a day to treat summer fulminant diarrhea and diarrhea due to food accumulation with chest and diaphragm *pǐ* and oppression.

[Precautions] Shén Qū (Massa Medicata Fermentata), warm and dry in nature, is contraindicated in cases with accumulation transforming into heat. It is also contraindicated in cases of constitutionally hyperchlorhydria as its ingestion may cause acid upflow. Use with caution during pregnancy according to some literature resources.

Daily practices

1. What are the causes and manifestations of food accumulation? What are the actions of medicinal that relieve food stagnation?
2. What are the similarities and differences between Shān Zhā (Fructus Crataegi) and Shén Qū (Massa Medicata Fermentata) in terms of actions?

麦芽 Mài Yá *fructus hordei germinatus germinated barley*

The source is from the dried germinant fruit of herbaceous *Hordeum vulgare* L., family Gramineae. Alternate names include 大麦芽 Dà Mài Yá. Sweet in flavor and neutral in nature.

[Actions] Reduce food stagnation and harmonize the middle *jiao*, and inhibit lactation. It is applicable for food accumulation, indigestion, poor appetite, gastric stuffiness, and abdominal distention, especially rice and flour-based food accumulation, and distending pain of the breasts during terminating lactation period and breast milk stagnation.

[Quality] Good quality is yellow, large, full, dry, and fully sprouted.

[Indications]

1. Indigestion and food accumulation: Mài Yá (Fructus Hordei Germinatus), capable of relieving food accumulation and improving appetite, is applicable for poor appetite, gastric oppression, abdominal distention, belching of putrid qi, and acid regurgitation attributed to indigestion with food accumulation. It is often used together with Shén

Qū (Massa Medicata Fermentata), Gǔ Yá (Fructus Setariae Germinatus), and Shān Zhā (Fructus Crataegi). For food accumulation and poor appetite caused by spleen deficiency failing to transform and transport, it is combined with medicinals that supplement qi and fortify the spleen such as Dǎng Shēn (Radix Codonopsis) and Bái Zhú (Rhizoma Atractylodis Macrocephalae).

2. Breast milk accumulation: accumulation of breast milk during postpartum and lactation period may cause breast swelling and pain, even localized redness, masses and abscesses, and eventually acute mastitis. Mài Yá (Fructus Hordei Germinatus) is capable of removing breast mild accumulation and therefore can be used for acute mastitis before the formation of abscess, or combined with medicinals that clear heat, resolve toxins, unblock the collaterals, and reduce swelling when abscess is formed. It can also be used as decoction for terminating lactation due to its breast milk inhibitory effect.

[Usage and Dosage] Traditionally used raw for a stronger stomach-reviving and qi-descending effect, and stir-fried for a better potency of fortifying the spleen to transform. However, modern research indicates that during dry-fried until scorched process, the high temperature will easily destroy amylase that help digestion in this herb and reduce its content to 1/6 of that of the raw one. Therefore, this substance should not be over-scorched if used for helping digestion. Use 10–30 g in decoction, up to 60–90 g for inhibiting lactation. Modern researches suggest the stir-fried form is considered less effective for aiding in digestion, some scholars therefore suggest it is better just to slightly stir-fry the raw herb, grind into powder and take it after mixing with water, decrease the amount when used in powdered form.

[Mnemonics] Mài Yá (Fructus Hordei Germinatus, Germinated Barley): neutral and sweet; reduce food stagnation, improve appetite, and arrest and inhibit lactation even when used alone.

[Simple and Effective Formulas]

1. 消食丸 Xiāo Shí Wán — Digestion Promoting Pill from *The Grand Compendium of Materia Medica* (本草纲目, Běn Cǎo Gāng Mù): Mài

Yá (Fructus Hordei Germinatus) 120 g, Shén Qū (Massa Medicata Fermentata) 60 g, Bái Zhú (Rhizoma Atractylodis Macrocephalae) 30 g, Jú Pí (Pericarpium Citri Reticulatae) 30 g; grind into powder, process them into cakes then steam into phoenix tree seed-sized pill, and take 30 or 50 pills/time with Rén Shēn (Radix et Rhizoma Ginseng) decoction for oral administration to treat different types of food accumulation with poor appetite.

2. 麦芽散-Mài Yá Sǎn — Germinated Barley Powder from *Teachings of Dan-xi* (丹溪心法, Dān Xī Xīn Fǎ): Mài Yá (Fructus Hordei Germinatus) 60 g; stir-fry, grind into fine powder, and take with light soup for oral administration, four times in total to treat postpartum fever, inhibited lactation, distention of the breasts, or nursing mother who wants to terminate lactation.

[Precautions] Mài Yá (Fructus Hordei Germinatus), one of the medicinals that help digestion and remove accumulation, is featured by dispersing without supplementing property and therefore should not be used alone and over a long period of time for spleen and stomach deficiency. It is contraindicated to cases of poor appetite with the absence of accumulation and stagnation.

鸡内金 Jī Nèi Jīn *endothelium corneum gigeriae galli chicken gizzard lining*

The source is from the inside membrane of the gizzard of *Gallus domesticus* Brisson, family Phasianidae. Alternate names include 鸡肫皮 Jī Zhūn Pí. Sweet in flavor and neutral in nature.

[Actions] Strengthen the stomach to remove food accumulation, and secure essence and arrest enuresis and spermatorrhea. It is applicable for food accumulation, diarrhea and dysentery, infantile malnutrition with accumulation, seminal emission, enuresis. It has been recently used for different types of stone disorders via its effect of removing accumulation. It is also used in the treatment of wasting-thirst (diabetes). Modern researches reveal ingestion of this substance can promote gastric juice secretion and significantly improve gastric motor function.

[Quality] Good quality is large, intact, yellow, and clean.

[Indications]

1. Indigestion and food accumulation: Jī Nèi Jīn (Endothelium Corneum Gigeriae Galli) is potent in relieving food accumulation, capable of supplementing spleen and stomach, and therefore applicable for different types of food accumulation in a powder form. It is prescribed with other medicinals that relieve food stagnation such as Shān Zhā (Fructus Crataegi) and Mài Yá (Fructus Hordei Germinatus) for severe gastric abdominal distention and fullness due to food accumulation; with Huò Xiāng (Herba Agastachis), Zǐ Sū Yè (Folium Perillae), Bàn Xià (Rhizoma Pinelliae), and Chén Pí (Pericarpium Citri Reticulatae) for diarrhea and vomiting; and with medicinals that supplement the spleen such as Dǎng Shēn (Radix Codonopsis), Bái Zhú (Rhizoma Atractylodis Macrocephalae), and Shān Yào (Rhizoma Dioscoreae) for food accumulation caused by spleen deficiency failing to transform and transport or infantile malnutrition with food accumulation due to spleen deficiency.

2. Seminal emission, enuresis, and frequent urination: due to its effect of restraining and consolidating, Jī Nèi Jīn (Endothelium Corneum Gigeriae Galli) is commonly used for disorders that caused by kidney deficiency failing to consolidate such as seminal emission, enuresis, and frequent urination and usually combined with medicinals that supplement the kidney and consolidate such as Jīn Yīng Zǐ (Fructus Rosae Laevigatae), Fù Pén Zǐ (Fructus Rubi), Qiàn Shí (Semen Euryales), Tù Sī Zǐ (Semen Cuscutae), Sāng Piāo Xiāo (Oötheca Mantidis), calcined Lóng Gǔ (Os Draconis), and calcined Mǔ Lì (Concha Ostreae).

3. Stone disorders: Jī Nèi Jīn (Endothelium Corneum Gigeriae Galli) is usually prescribed with Jīn Qián Cǎo (Herba Lysimachiae) and Hǔ Zhàng (Rhizoma Polygoni Cuspidati) for such stone disorders as lithangiuria and cholelithiasis.

It can also be applied externally, for instance, grind into powder with Kū Fán (Alumen Dehydratum) and put on the skin for galloping gan of the teeth and gums; or burn into ashes and apply externally for aphtha, and swollen and painful throat.

[Usage and Dosage] Usually use its raw form in northern China and stir-fried form in southern China. According to some scholars, heating will easily destroy its gastric hormones that help digestion and therefore the raw one should be used for improving digestion. Other resources indicate liquid-fried one, neutral in nature, is more appropriate for people with chronic disease and spleen and stomach deficiency and weak digestive function. Use 3–9 g in decoction, or as a pill and powder (considered more effective), capsule or dissolved in the decoction.

[Mnemonics] Jī Nèi Jīn (Endothelium Corneum Gigeriae Galli, Chicken Gizzard Lining): neutral; promote digestion, strengthen the spleen, remove stone, and arrest enuresis and frequent urination.

[Simple and Effective Formulas]

1. 鸡金散 — Jī Jīn Sǎn — Chicken Gizzard Lining Powder from *Important Formulas Worth a Thousand Gold Pieces* (千金要方, Qiān Jīn Yào Fāng): Jī Nèi Jīn (Endothelium Corneum Gigeriae Galli); burn into ashes and take with wine for oral administration to treat nausea, vomiting after meal. In *Seeking Sources in the Materia Medica* (本草求原, Běn Cǎo Qiú Yuán), it is used in the treatment of food accumulation with abdominal fullness. In *The Grand Compendium of Medical Works* (医林集要, Yī Lín Jí Yào), it is applied to relieve urinary tract stone with dripping of urine and unbearable pain.

2. 治遗精方, Zhì Yí Jīng Fāng — Seminal Emission Curing Formula from *Chinese Herbal Medicine in Jilin* (吉林中草药, Jí Lín Zhōng Cǎo Yào,): Jī Nèi Jīn (Endothelium Corneum Gigeriae Galli) 18 g; dry-fry until scorched, grind into powder, divide into six equal doses, infuse one dose/time with half small cup of hot yellow wine, and take twice a day for oral administration, morning and evening, to treat seminal emission.

[Precautions] Jī Nèi Jīn (Endothelium Corneum Gigeriae Galli) is neutral in nature and effective in fortifying the spleen, however should not be used alone in cases of gastric and abdominal distention, indigestion, and poor appetite caused by deficiency.

Daily practices

1. Shān Zhā (Fructus Crataegi), Shén Qū (Massa Medicata Fermentata), Mài Yá (Fructus Hordei Germinatus), and Jī Nèi Jīn (Endothelium Corneum Gigeriae Galli) are all medicinals that relieve food stagnation, what are the differences among them in terms of indications?
2. How to make the combination with other medicinals in accordance with the state of illness when using medicinal that relieve food stagnation?

MEDICINALS THAT EXPEL WORMS

The herbs in this chapter are used primarily for expelling or killing intestinal parasites such as roundworms, pinworms, hookworms, tapeworms, and fasciolopsiasis. Recent research reveals some herbs are also effective on schistosome and plasmodium. Mild parasites cases often have no overt symptoms and may only be identified by testing feces. While patients with severe parasites often experience such symptoms as para-umbilical pain, vomiting of saliva and drool, decreased appetite, swift digestion with rapid hungering, change in appetite or deranged appetite such as pica of soil and paper, and itching in such places as the rectum especially at night in the cases of pinworm. If the condition is prolonged they may suffer from qi and blood exhaustion with sallow complexion, emaciated body, and distended abdomen. Hookworm disease is featured by sallow complexion, edema, and lack of strength.

The selection of herbs, types or dosage, must be matched to the particular parasite and the constitution of the individual patient. They may need to be used in conjunction with other herbs to dispel and kill parasites on the one hand and protect healthy qi of the body on the other hand. The herbs are usually taken on an empty stomach to make their active ingredients directly act on the worms. Most of these herbs have certain degree of toxicity and therefore should be used with utmost caution during pregnancy and for the debilitated and elderly. The dosage therefore should be prescribed with more cautions. On the other hand, patients need to pay more attention on dietetic hygiene to avoid reinfection.

Worm-dispelling herbs are always used in combination with other substances. They are prescribed together with purgatives for patients with strong constitution and constipation to facilitate the discharge of worms; with medicinals that tonify the spleen and stomach in cases of spleen and stomach deficiency to avoid further injury to the spleen and stomach; with medicinals that relieve food stagnation when accompanied with food stagnation; with interior-warming herbs when patients also present with cold congealing; with heat-clearing herbs if accompanied with stagnated heat. For weak patients due to chronic or severe diseases, treatment plan should be simultaneous attack and supplementation or supplementation followed by attack.

使君子 Shǐ Jūn Zǐ *fructus quisqualis rangoon creeper fruit*

The source is from the ripe semen of lianoid shrub *Quisqualis indica* L., family Combretaceae. Alternate names include 五棱子 Wǔ Léng Zi and 留求子 Liú Qiú Zi. Bitter in flavor and warm in nature.

[Actions] Kill parasites and dissolve accumulation. It is applicable for roundworm, pinworm, abdominal pain caused by worm accumulation, and infantile malnutrition with accumulation. Modern research indicate it contains a variety of anthelmintic ingredients.

[Quality] Good quality is large, purplish black, and shiny; the kernels should be full, yellow, fragrant, sweet, and oily.

[Indications] Shǐ Jūn Zǐ (Fructus Quisqualis) can be stir-fired until aromatic and chewed to treat roundworm and pinworm. For severe worm disease, it is combined with medicinals that expel worms such as Kǔ Liàn Pí (Cortex Meliae) and Bīng Láng (Semen Arecae) to increase its ability of dispelling worms. It is prescribed together with medicinals that supplement the spleen and stomach and other medicinals that expel worms such as Dǎng Shēn (Radix Codonopsis), Bái Zhú (Rhizoma Atractylodis Macrocephalae), Jī Nèi Jīn (Endothelium Corneum Gigeriae Galli), and Bīng Láng (Semen Arecae) for sallow complexion, emaciation, poor appetite or deranged appetite such as pica of soil and uncooked rice, abdominal distention, and loose stool caused by infantile malnutrition with accumulation.

It is also applicable for vaginal trichomoniasis. According to ancient recordings, everyday soaking three or five pieces Shĭ Jūn Zĭ (Fructus Quisqualis) in a small amount of sesame oil and slowly chewing the kernel before sleep over a long period of time is useful for relieving facial sores and acnes. This substance can also be applied externally, for instance, using Shĭ Jūn Zĭ (Fructus Quisqualis) decoction to rinse the mouth for decayed tooth with pain; and using Shĭ Jūn Zĭ (Fructus Quisqualis) water infusion to relieve different types of tinea due to fungus infections.

[Usage and Dosage] Stir-frying until aromatic to reduce its side effects (use raw substance can cause many side effects). Long-term storage will cause the loss of active ingredients and therefore the fresh substance that collected and stored in the same year is preferred. Can also be used fresh, or the shell broken into pieces and used in a decoction, use 6–12 g in decoction. The dosage in children is one seed per year of age on an empty stomach, not to exceed 20 per day, two or three days in a row.

[Mnemonics] Shĭ Jūn Zĭ (Fructus Quisqualis, Rangoon Creeper Fruit): kill parasites when dry-fried until aromatic and relieve toothache when decocted to rinse the mouth.

[Simple and Effective Formulas]
使君子散 — Shĭ Jūn Zĭ Săn — Rangoon Creeper Fruit Powder from *Pediatric Standards* (幼科准绳, Yòu Kē Zhǔn Shéng): Shĭ Jūn Zĭ (Fructus Quisqualis) (stir-fried on the tile, prepared into powder) 10 pieces, Gān Căo (Radix et Rhizoma Glycyrrhizae) (soaked in bile for one night) 0.3 g, Wú Yí (Fructus Ulmi Macrocarpae Praeparata) 0.3 g, and five Chuān Liàn Zĭ (Fructus Toosendan) (blast-fried, kernel removed); grind into powder and decoct 3 g/time in water for oral administration to treat pediatric roundworm and infantile malnutrition with accumulation.

[Precautions] Shĭ Jūn Zĭ (Fructus Quisqualis) has a fairly low toxicity compared with other medicinals that expel worms and is safe to use in a defined dose range. Overdoses of this herb lead to hiccups, vertigo, dizziness, or vomiting, abdominal pain, diarrhea, even cold sweating, convulsion, difficult breathing, and decreased blood pressure in serious cases. Hot tea should not be taken before or after oral administration of Shǐ Jūn Zǐ (Fructus Quisqualis) to prevent aggravation of side effects. Frequent ingestion of Dīng Xiāng (Flos Caryophylli) decoction is recommended in mild poisoning cases, and a visit to the hospital is required if the poisoning is severe.

槟榔 Bīng Láng *semen arecae betel nut*

The source is from the ripe semen of evergreen arbor *Areca catechu* L., family Palmae. Alternate names include 大腹子, Dà Fù Zǐ, 海南子, Hǎi Nán Zi, and 槟榔子. Back ancient times in southern China, people used to treat distinguished guests (宾郎 Bīn Láng) with this substance; 槟榔 Bīng Láng and 宾郎 Bīn Láng are mostly homophonic. Bitter and pungent in flavor and warm in nature.

[Actions] Kill parasites, lead stagnation out by mildly draining downward, and move qi and promote urination. It is applicable for tapeworm, roundworm, fasciolopsiasis, abdominal pain due to worm accumulation, dysentery and diarrhea caused by accumulation, leg qi with edema, and malaria. Recent research suggests it has a excitatory effect on M-choline receptor and can increase intestinal peristalsis, promote digestive juice secretion, improve appetite, reinforce cholecyst and choledoch contractile force, and speed up biliary discharge. Therefore, this substance is applicable for invigorating stomach, helping digestion, and expelling gall stones.

[Quality] Good quality is large, firm, and heavy with a fresh-looking cross-section.

[Indications]

1. Intestinal parasites: Bīng Láng (Semen Arecae) can treat tapeworm, roundworm, fasciolopsiasis, and pinworm, especially for tapeworm and fasciolopsiasis as its ingredient arecoline has an anesthetic effect on these worms. It is often combined with Nán Guā Zǐ (Semen Cucurbitae) for tapeworm to get a better therapeutic effect; with Qiān Niú Zǐ (Semen Pharbitidis) for fasciolopsiasis; and with Kǔ Liàn Pí (Cortex Meliae) for roundworm. Its decoction with Bǎi Bù (Radix Stemonae) can be used as retention enema before sleep to kill pinworm.

2. Food accumulation qi stagnation: owning to its effect of dispersing and moving qi with pungency and slight laxative to promote defecation, Bīng Láng (Semen Arecae) is applicable for food accumulation and qi stagnation with abdominal distention and prescribed together with other medicinals that relieve food accumulation and move qi. It is combined with Mù Xiāng (Radix Aucklandiae), Zhǐ Shí (Fructus Aurantii Immaturus), Qīng Pí (Pericarpium Citri Reticulatae Viride), Dà Huáng (Radix et Rhizoma Rhei), and Huáng Lián (Rhizoma Coptidis) for dysentery caused by damp-heat accumulation in the intestine manifested as dysentery with stool containing blood and mucus, tenesmus, and abdominal pain.
3. Different types of edema: Bīng Láng (Semen Arecae), effective in disinhibiting water to reduce swelling, is applicable for edema caused by different reasons, such as nephritis edema, cardiopathic edema, and leg qi with edema, especially for patients with accompanying constipation. It is used together with medicinal that warm yang and drain dampness for edema caused by cold-damp, and with medicinals that clear and drain damp-heat for edema due to damp-heat.

It is also prescribed with medicinals that prevent attack of malaria such as Cháng Shān (Radix Dichroae) and Cǎo Guǒ (Fructus Tsaoko) for malaria; with Jīn Qián Cǎo (Herba Lysimachiae), Chái Hú (Radix Bupleuri), Zhǐ Shí (Fructus Aurantii Immaturus), and Yù Jīn (Radix Curcumae) for gall stone. It can be applied externally, for instance, burning Bīng Láng (Semen Arecae) into ashes, grinding into fine powder, applying topically for sores in the corner of the mouth, or using its decoction as eye droppings for miotic.

[Usage and Dosage] Use raw to kill worms and break up accumulation, especially the fresh one with the strongest potency; stir-frying to moderate its effect and for regulate qi and remove food accumulation, dry-frying until scorched to further moderate its effect and for patient of weak constitution with food accumulation and qi stagnation. Traditionally, this medicinal should be soaked in water for around 30 days before cutting into slices, which may consume half of the active ingredients. Insteadly, nowadays, it is just soaked in water for a few hours or break into granules.

Use 6–15 g in decoction, or 60–90 g when used alone for tapeworms and fasciolopsiasis.

[Mnemonics] Bīng Láng (Semen Arecae, Betel Nut): bitter and pungent; kill parasites, promote urination, relieve edema, and resolve accumulation.

[Simple and Effective Formulas]

1. 槟榔散 — Bīng Láng Sǎn — Betel Nut Powder from *General Treatise on the Diseases of Cold Damage* (伤寒总病论, Shāng Hán Zǒng Bìng Lùn): two Bīng Láng (Semen Arecae) (one use raw, the other roasted); grind into fine powder, decoct in two small cups of wine until only 1 and 2/5 cup left, divide into two equal doses, and take one dose/time for oral administration to treat cold damage resulting from purgation or diaphoresis, chest and gastric *pǐ* and fullness, blocked qi circulation, or syncope due to roundworms, and sever pain in the heart and abdomen (similar to biliary tract roundworm disease).

2. 槟榔散 Bīng Láng Sǎn — Betel Nut Powder from *Formulas for Universal Relief* (普济方, Pǔ Jì Fāng): half of Bīng Láng (Semen Arecae) if using a big one, grind 3 g with Mài Mén Dōng (Radix Ophiopogonis) decoction, stew hot, and take for oral administration to treat inhibited defecation and urination or hematuria with stabbing pain.

[Precautions] Bīng Láng (Semen Arecae), potent in descending qi, is contraindicated in cases of weak constitution without excess pathogen. Overdoses of this herb lead to increased salivation, headache, nausea, vomiting, lethargy, and convulsions.

榧子 Fěi Zǐ *semen torreyae torreya*

The source is from the ripe semen of evergreen arbor *Torreya grandis* Fort., family Taxaceae. Alternate names include 榧实 Fěi Shí. Sweet in flavor and neutral in nature.

[Action] Kill intestinal parasites including roundworm, tapeworm, hookworm, and fasciolopsiasis. It also has a slight laxative effect. Stir-frying can make it fragrant, sweet, more effective, and safe to use. These qualities make it an important anti-parasitc herb for children.

[Quality] Good quality is large with a thin shell, yellowish white kernels, oily, and without cracks.

[Indications] It is applicable for different types of intestinal parasite, by either chewing the stir-fried one or decocting with other medicinals. Fěi Zǐ (Semen Torreyae) (choped into pieces) is combined with Bīng Láng (Semen Arecae) and Nán Guā Zǐ (Semen Cucurbitae) for tapeworm; and with Shǐ Jūn Zǐ (Fructus Quisqualis), Chuān Liàn Zǐ (Fructus Toosendan), and Wū Méi (Fructus Mume) for roundworm.

Application of this substance to treat filariasis has been reported recently, specifically grinding Fěi Zǐ (Semen Torreyae) flesh 150 g and Xuè Yú Tàn (Crinis Carbonisatus) 30 g into powder, prepare into 150 pills with honey, and take two pills/time, three times a day for 4–8 days.

It is also applicable for cough due to lung dryness due to its effect of moistening the lung and arresting cough.

[Usage and Dosage] Break into pieces and use in a decoction, 15–30 g/time; stir-fry until cooked, remove the shell, and chew the semen; or decrease the amount as in a pill and powder for oral administration.

[Mnemonics] Fěi Zǐ (Semen Torreyae, Torreya): sweet and aromatic; specialized in killing parasites; capable of moistening the lungs and arresting cough.

[Simple and Effective Formulas]
驱虫汤 Qū Chóng Tāng — Parasites Dispelling Decoction from *Modern Practical Chinese Medicines* (现代实用中药, Xiàn Dài Shí Yòng Zhōng Yào,): Fěi Zǐ (Semen Torreyae) (choped into pieces) 30 g, Shǐ Jūn Zǐ (Fructus Quisqualis) (chopped up) 30 g, and garlic bulblet (chopped up) 30 g; decoct in water for oral administration to treat hookworm, round-worm, and pinworm.

[Precautions] Fěi Zǐ (Semen Torreyae) (chopped into pieces) is safe to use due to its relatively neutral nature compared with other worm-dispelling medicinals, no damage to the spleen and stomach, and a fairly low toxicity. However, it is contraindicated to loose stool because of its oily and moistening texture.

Besides the above-mentioned medicinals, others that are mainly used for expelling intestinal worms include Kǔ Liàn Pí (Cortex Meliae), Nán Guā Zǐ (Semen Cucurbitae), Hè Cǎo Yá (Herba et Gemma Agrimoniae),

Léi Wán (Omphalia), Hè Shī (Fructus Carpesii), Wú Yí (Fructus Ulmi Macrocarpae Praeparata), and Guàn Zhòng (Rhizoma Cyrtomii). Among which, Kǔ Liàn Pí (Cortex Meliae) has a bigger toxicity, Hè Cǎo Yá (Herba et Gemma Agrimoniae) and Léi Wán (Omphalia) should not be used in decoction but should be given in powder. Guàn Zhòng (Rhizoma Cyrtomii) can also clear heat and resolve toxins, and the charred one can stanch bleeding.

Daily practices

1. What are the common intestinal parasites and what are the major clinic manifestations?
2. What are the major medicinals used for roundworm, tapeworm, hook-worm, pinworm, and fasciolopsiasis, respectively? What precautions should be taken when using it?
3. For above-mentioned worm-expelling medicinals, what other actions do they have beside worm-expelling?

MEDICINALS THAT STANCH BLEEDING

Bleeding-stanching medicinals are used for traumatic or internal hemorrhage.

Hemorrhagic disorders are common in the clinic, such as coughing with blood, vomiting blood, blood in the stool, blood in the urine, teeth bleeding, nosebleed, profuse menstruation, and bleeding associated with trauma. Causes for bleeding include breakage of blood vessel; reckless movement of blood due to exuberant blood heat; enduring non-healing blood vessel due to static blood stagnation; yang qi insufficiency failing to contain blood; or failure of deficient spleen to control blood. Excessive bleeding will cause blood deficiency in the body, and also lead to qi collapse following blood desertion, even death. Therefore, it is important to use hemostatic herbs whether for general cases or first-aid. Modern research reveals that most of the hemostatic herbs can speed up blood clotting or recovery of blood vessel.

Hemostatic herbs are divided into several types and differentiated from each other in the nature of hemorrhagic disorders they treat, namely (1) herbs that cool blood to stanch bleeding are cool or cold in nature and capable of clearing heat in blood to arrest bleeding; (2) herbs that restrain and consolidate to stanch bleeding are astringent and applicable for bleeding without blood stasis; (3) herbs that dissolve stasis to stanch bleeding are effective in invigorating blood and dissolving stasis and suitable for bleeding with blood stasis; and (4) herbs that warm the channels to stanch bleeding are warm and hot in nature and appropriate for bleeding caused by deficiency-cold.

When these hemostatic herbs are needed, it is important to use them together with herbs that treat the underlying condition. Therefore, the selection and combination of herbs for arrest bleeding are based on the underlying reason of the disorder. If the bleeding is due to reckless movement of hot blood, cool and cold herbs that clear heat to cool blood should be used in combination with herbs that clear heat to cool blood and clear heat to drain fire. If the bleeding is due to yin deficiency with ascendant yang and deficiency-fire flaming upward, cool and cold hemostatic herbs should be used in conjunction with herbs that enrich yin to subdue fire. If the persistent bleeding difficult to stop is due to blood stasis, herbs that relieve stasis to arrest bleeding should be prescribed together with herbs that invigorate blood and resolve stasis. If the bleeding is due to deficiency-cold, the herbs that warm the channels and stanch bleeding should be used together with herbs that warm yang, boost qi, and tonify the spleen.

It is important to note that in general when these herbs are needed for hemorrhagic disorders they should not be used alone. It is also essential to follow the rule of "stanch bleeding without restraining blood stasis" and avoid overuse of medicinals that cool blood and stanch bleeding and those that astringe and stanch bleeding as they may cause blood stasis, which is another factor in bleeding. In severe bleeding cases, herbs that strongly tonify original qi to rescue from desertion should be included in the treatment plan.

小薊 Xiǎo Jì *herba cirsii field thistle*

[Addendum:] 大薊 Dà Jì Herba Cirsii Japonici Japanese Thistle
The source is from the aerial part of herbaceous perennial *Cephalanoplos segetum* (Bunge) kitam. or *C. setosum* Kitam, family Compositae. Sweet in flavor and cool in nature.

[Actions] Cool the blood and stanch bleeding, relieve toxins to close sore and relieve carbuncle, and promote urination. It is applicable for hemoptysis, epistaxis, hematemesis, hematuria, profuse uterine bleeding, prolonged scanty uterine bleeding of variable intervals, and heat-toxin carbuncles and swellings associated with frenetic movement of hot blood. Experiments reveal it can shorten the bleeding time and has certain antibacterial effect.

[Quality] Good quality is clean, relatively complete, and without mildew.

[Indications]

1. Hemorrhage due to blood heat: Xiǎo Jì (Herba Cirsii), cold in nature with ability of clearing blood heat to stanch bleeding, is appropriate for hemorrhagic disorders due to frenetic movement of hot blood, such as hematemesis, hemoptysis, and epistaxis. Owning to its potency of promoting urination, it is considered particularly suitable for cases of hematuria caused by heat accumulation in the lower *jiao* and commonly combined with medicinals that cool blood and promote urination such as Pú Huáng (Pollen Typhae), Mù Tōng (Caulis Akebiae), Shēng Dì (Radix Rehmanniae), Huá Shí (Talcum), and Dàn Zhú Yè (Herba Lophatheri). Also applicable for postpartum uterine involution incomplete and profuse uterine bleeding.
2. Heat-toxin carbuncles and swellings: for carbuncles, swellings, sores, and ulcers resulting from heat-toxin accumulation, Xiǎo Jì (Herba Cirsii) is decocted for oral administration or the fresh one is pounded for external application.

Application of its root in the treatment of infectious virus hepatitis has been reported. Its decoction has been used as a wash in casese of vaginal itching.

[Usage and Dosage] Use raw in general, stir-fry until charred to improve its ability of stanching bleeding. Use 10–15 g in decoction, up to 30–60 g in decoction or pounded into juice when used fresh.

[Mnemonics] Xiǎo Jì (Herba Cirsii, Field Thistle): cool; relieve swelling, cure sore, and stop bleeding, especially bloody urine.

[Simple and Effective Formulas]

1. 小蓟饮子 Xiǎo Jì Yǐn Zǐ — Field Thistle Drink from *Teachings of Dan-xi* (丹溪心法, Dān Xī Xīn Fǎ,): Shēng Dì (Radix Rehmanniae) 15 g, Xiǎo Jì (Herba Cirsii) 15 g, Huá Shí (Talcum) 15 g, Tōng Cǎo (Medulla Tetrapanacis) 15 g, stir-fried Pú Huáng (Pollen Typhae) 15 g, Dàn Zhú Yè (Herba Lophatheri) 15 g, ǒu Jié (Nodus Nelumbinis Rhizomatis) 15 g, Dāng Guī (Radix Angelicae Sinensis) 15 g, Zhī Zǐ (Fructus Gardeniae) 15 g, and Gān Cǎo (Radix et Rhizoma Glycyrrhizae) 15 g; decoct in water for oral administration to treat hematuria and blood strangury caused by heat accumulation in the lower *jiao*. Also applicable for bloody urine or difficult and painful urination with blood in urine with heat manifestations as thirst, fever, heat in the center of palms and soles, rapid pulse, and red tongue.

2. 清心散 Qīng Xīn Sǎn — Heart Clearing Powder from *Comprehensive Recording of Divine Assistance* (圣济总录, Shèng Jì Zǒng Lù,): a handful of Xiǎo Jì (Herba Cirsii); smash into juice and take after mixing with a small cup of wine for oral administration to treat persistent bleeding on the tongue.

[Precautions] Xiǎo Jì (Herba Cirsii), neutral in nature without pronounced toxicity, has less side effects. However, it is cold in nature and therefore should be used with caution in cases of deficiency-cold of the spleen and stomach. According to literature, it has an effect of dissolving stasis and should be used cautiously in cases of absence of blood stagnation. Just for reference.

[Addendum] 大蓟 Dà Jì Herba Cirsii Japonici Japanese Thistle
The source is from the aerial part or with root of herbaceous perennial *Cirsium japonicum* DC., family Compositae. It is sweet and bitter in flavor and cool in nature with the actions of cooling blood, stanching bleeding, clearing heat, relieving toxin, dispersing blood stagnation, and eliminating carbuncles. It is applicable for heat-induced bleedings, alone or combined with such blood-cooling and bleeding-arresting herbs as Xiǎo Jì (Herba Cirsii), Shēng Dì (Radix Rehmanniae), and Cè Bǎi Yè (Cacumen Platycladi). For heat-toxin and carbuncle and swollen caused by accumulation of heat and blood stagnation, it can be pounded into juice

for either oral administration or external application, or combined with other herbs of clearing heat, resolving toxins, relieving carbuncle and sores. It has been reported that Dà Jì (Herba Cirsii Japonici) is effective on controlling hypertension due to ascendant hyperactivity of liver yang. Dà Jì (Herba Cirsii Japonici) and Xiǎo Jì (Herba Cirsii) are with the similar actions, but the former is primarily used for sores and swellings, and the latter for hematuria.

地榆 Dì Yú *radix sanguisorbae garden burnet root*

The source is from the root and rhizome of herbaceous perennial *Sanguisorba officinalis* L., family Rosaceae. It is so called because its leaf looks like that of elm (榆树 Yú Shù) and grows on the ground (地 Dì). Bitter and sour in flavor and slightly cold in nature.

[Actions] Cool the blood and stanch bleedings, and relieve toxin and close sores. It is applicable for various hemorrhagic disorders of heat nature, such as hemoptysis, hematemesis, epistaxis, stool with blood, hemorrhoids bleeding, hematuria, profuse uterine bleeding, and prolonged scanty uterine bleeding of variable intervals. It is also used for scalding, eczema, skin erosions, and dysentery. Modern research suggest it has relatively significant anti-scalding, procoagulant and anti-bacteria effect.

[Quality] Good quality is dry, firm, and reddish colored in cross section.

[Indications]

1. Bleeding due to blood heat: Dì Yú (Radix Sanguisorbae), cold in nature and sour in flavor to astringe, can cool blood to stanch bleeding and consolidate to stanch bleeding. It is a commonly-used herb for hemorrhagic disorders, especially for bleeding in the lower part of body such as stool with blood, hemorrhoids bleeding, hematuria, profuse uterine bleeding, and prolonged scanty uterine bleeding of variable intervals. It can be used alone or together with other medicinals. It is combined with Huái Huā (Flos Sophorae), Shēng Dì (Radix Rehmanniae), Huáng Qín (Radix Scutellariae), and Dāng Guī (Radix Angelicae Sinensis) for stool with blood; and with Mǔ Dān Pí (Cortex Moutan), Shēng Dì (Radix Rehmanniae), and Xiān Hè Cǎo (Herba Agrimoniae) for

profuse uterine bleeding and prolonged scanty uterine bleeding of variable intervals.

2. Carbuncles, swollen, sores, ulcers: owning to its potency of clearing heat, resolving toxins, removing dampness, and closing sores, Dì Yú (Radix Sanguisorbae) is applied externally in a variety of external diseases and skin problems. For instance, it can be used alone in a powder form after mixing with sesame oil or together with Dà Huáng (Radix et Rhizoma Rhei) powder to relieve scalding; its decoction can be used for external wash or application to cure eczema, sores, and ulcers. It also can be combined with Duàn Shí Gāo (Gypsum Fibrosum Praeparatum) powder and Kū Fán (Alumen Dehydratum) powder for external application.

3. Damp-heat dysentery: Dì Yú (Radix Sanguisorbae), capable of clearing heat, resolving toxins, and cooling blood to stanch bleeding, is effective in treating dysentery caused by damp-heat in the intestines, especially for dysentery with stool containing blood. It can be prescribed alone or together with Bái Tóu Wēng (Radix Pulsatillae), Huáng Bǎi (Cortex Phellodendri Chinensis), and Huáng Qín (Radix Scutellariae).

It also can be decocted with Tài Zǐ Shēn (Radix Pseudostellariae) and 怀牛膝 Huái Niú Xī in water for oral administration to treat thrombocytopenic purpura.

[Usage and Dosage] Its raw plant is considered more potent in resolving toxins and closing sores. Modern research suggests heating will decrease its antibacterial effect and therefore the stir-fried is more effective for stanching bleeding.

[Mnemonics] Dì Yú (Radix Sanguisorbae, Garden Burnet Root): cool the blood, indispensable for stool with blood, relieve abscesses and dysentery, and cure scalding.

[Simple and Effective Formulas]

1. 地榆汤 — Dì Yú Tāng — Garden Burnet Root Decoction from *Comprehensive Recording of Divine Assistance* (圣济总录, Shèng Jì Zǒng Lù,): Dì Yú (Radix Sanguisorbae) 60 g and Gān Cǎo (Radix et Rhizoma Glycyrrhizae) (roasted, filed) 15 g; grind into fine powder,

decoct 6 g/time in water, remove dregs, and take the liquid three times/ day for oral administration to treat persistent blood dysentery or stool with blood.

2. 地榆煎 — Dì Yú Jiān-Garden Burnet Root Decoction from *Formulas from Benevolent Sages* (圣惠方, Shèng Huì Fāng,): Dì Yú (Radix Sanguisorbae) 60 g (filed); boil in 250 ml vinegar for ten times, remove dregs, and take 100 ml hot before meal for hematemesis and unremitting vaginal bleeding with yellow complexion and emaciation.

[Precautions] Dì Yú (Radix Sanguisorbae), bitter and cold, is contraindicated in cases of deficiency-cold induced bleeding and dysentery. In the opinion of some predecessors, it should not be used in the early stage of dysentery as its sour and astringing property would restrain pathogen, however, nowadays it has been widely used in the treatment of acute damp-heat dysentery with a good therapeutic effect. Although as a commonly-used herb for burning and scalding, it is not suitable for scald covering a large skin area as it contains hydrolyzed tannin that may cause toxic hepatitis when absorbed by the body.

Daily practices

1. What are the differences among the medicinals that cool blood to stanch bleeding, those that astringe to stanch bleeding, those that dissolve stasis to stanch bleeding, and those that warm the channels to stanch bleeding in terms of actions and indications?
2. What precautions should be taken when treating hemorrhagic disorders?
3. What are the similarities and differences between Xiǎo Jì (Herba Cirsii) and Dì Yú (Radix Sanguisorbae) in terms of actions and indications?

槐花 Huái Huā *flos sophorae pagoda tree flower*

The source is from the flower bud of *Sophora japonica* L., family Leguminosae. Alternate names include 槐米 Huái Mǐ and 槐芯 Huái Xīn. Bitter in flavor and slightly cold in nature.

[Actions] Cool the blood and stanch bleeding, and clear the liver and drain fire. It is applicable for blood heat induced stool with blood, hemorrhoids bleeding, blood dysentery, profuse uterine bleeding, prolonged scanty uterine bleeding of variable intervals, hematemesis, and epistaxis. It is also used in the treatment of red eyes, headache, vertigo and dizziness caused by liver heat. Modern experiments indicate its ingredients rutin sophorin and its aglycon quercetin can maintain normal resistance of blood capillary and have anti-inflammatory, anti-spasmic, anti-ulcer, and arteriosclerosis-preventing and treating effects.

[Quality] Good quality is dry, large, tight, and yellowish green. 槐花米 Huái Huā Mǐ is of better quality as its contents of such active ingredients as rutin are higher than that of blooming sophora flower.

[Indications]

1. Bleeding due to blood heat: Huái Huā (Flos Sophorae), bitter and cold in nature, is effective in treating a variety of hemorrhagic disorders due to frenetic movement of hot blood. Similar to Dì Yú (Radix Sanguisorbae), it is considered more potent for the bleeding in the lower part of the body such as stool containing blood, blood dysentery, haemorrhoids bleeding, profuse uterine bleeding, prolonged scanty uterine bleeding of variable intervals, and hematuria. This substance is very often prescribed together with Cè Bǎi Yè (Cacumen Platycladi) and Dì Yú (Radix Sanguisorbae).

2. Liver fire flaming upward: exuberant liver channel fire-heat may cause disorders in the head and face, such as red, swollen, and painful eyes, headache, vertigo, and dizziness. If that is the case, Huái Huā (Flos Sophorae) is applicable with its capability of clearing and draining liver heat. It can be used alone or together with Xià Kū Cǎo (Spica Prunellae), Jué Míng Zǐ (Semen Cassiae), Jú Huā (Flos Chrysanthemi), and Huáng Qín (Radix Scutellariae). It is nowadays commonly used in the treatment for headache and vertigo caused by hypertension.

[Usage and Dosage] Raw form is more effective in draining fire and clearing heat, stir-fry until charred is more potent in stanching bleeding, stir-fry until yellow is a better way to preserve active ingredients. Use 6–12 g in decoction, decrease the dosage as in pill and powder.

[Mnemonics] Huái Huā (Flos Sophorae, Pagoda Tree Flower): bitter and cold; drain fire and clear the liver, use raw to clear fire, and use charred to stop bleeding.

[Simple and Effective Formulas]

1. 槐花散 — Huái Huā Sǎn — Pagoda Tree Flower Powder from *Experienced and Effective Formulas* (经验良方, Jīng Yàn Liáng Fāng,): Huái Huā (Flos Sophorae) (half raw half stir-fried) 30 g and Shān Zhī Zǐ (Fructus Gardeniae) (peel removed, stir-fried) 30 g; make into fine powder and take 6 g/time with water before meal for stool containing blood.
2. 槐花散-Huái Huā Sǎn-Pagoda Tree Flower Powder from *A Compilation of Empirical Formula* (良朋汇集, Liáng Péng Huì Jí,): aged Huái Huā (Flos Sophorae) 30 g and Bǎi Cǎo Shuāng (Palvis Fumi Carbonisatus) 15 g; make into powder and take 9–12 g/time with warm wine for oral administration to treat abnormal vaginal bleeding without signs of blood stasis.

[Precautions] Huái Huā (Flos Sophorae), bitter and cold, is contraindicated in cases of deficiency-cold of the spleen and stomach and bleeding caused by deficiency.

侧柏叶 Cè Bǎi Yè *cacumen platycladi arborvitae*

The source is from the leaf of tender branch of evergreen arbor *Biota orientalis* (L.) endl., family Cupressaceae. Alternate names include 扁柏叶, Biǎn Bǎi Yè, 丛柏叶 Cóng Bǎi Yè, and 柏叶 Bǎi Yè. Bitter and astringent in flavor and slightly cold in nature.

[Actions] Cool the blood and stanch bleeding, and expel phlegm and arrest cough. It is applicable not only for hemorrhagic disorders especially frenetic movement of hot blood but also cough due to lung heat.

Experiments indicate its extractive has shown antibechic, expectorant, and central-nerve-system sedative effects on mice.

[Quality] Good quality is tender, light green, and without fragments.

[Indications]

1. Bleeding due to blood heat: Cè Bǎi Yè (Cacumen Platycladi) can stanch bleeding through cooling blood and consolidation. It is commonly combined with Xiǎo Jì (Herba Cirsii), Dà Jì (Herba Cirsii Japonici), Bái Máo Gēn (Rhizoma Imperatae), Huáng Lián (Rhizoma Coptidis), and Shēng Dì (Radix Rehmanniae) for hemorrhagic disorders caused by blood heat; and with medicinals that warm the channels to stanch bleeding such as Páo Jiāng (Rhizoma Zingiberis Praeparatum) and Ài Yè (Folium Artemisiae Argyi) for hemorrhagic disorders caused by deficiency-cold.
2. Lung heat cough: Cè Bǎi Yè (Cacumen Platycladi) is capable of clearing lung heat and dissolving phlegm and therefore applicable for cough with yellow and thick sputum difficult to expectorate due to lung heat. It is usually combined with medicinals that clear the lung and dissolve phlegm such as Běi Shā Shēn (Radix Glehniae), Bèi Mǔ (Bulbus Fritillaria), and Huáng Qín (Radix Scutellariae).

Mixing its decoction with wine can treat pain in the joint. In recent reports, it has been prepared into tincture to relieve dysentery, decoction for whooping cough, hypertension, and ulcer with bleeding. Also can be applied externally, for instance, external application of 60% ethanol solution of Cè Bǎi Yè (Cacumen Platycladi) for baldness, and mixing its powder with wine for external application can treat deep-localized abscess and epidemic parotitis.

[Usage and Dosage] Raw herb is more effective in dissolving phlegm and arresting cough, use stir-fried to stanch bleeding as modern research suggests that stir-frying can improve its potency of shortening the bleeding and clotting time. Use 10–15 g in decoction, decrease the dosage as in pill and powder.

[Mnemonics] Cè Bǎi Yè (Cacumen Platycladi, Arborvitae): cold and bitter; cool the blood, stop bleeding, and arrest cough due to lung heat.

[Simple and Effective Formulas]

1. 柏叶汤 Bǎi Yè Tāng — Arborvitae Decoction from *Essentials from the Golden Cabinet* (金匮要略, Jīn Guì Yào Lüè,): Cè Bǎi Yè (Cacumen Platycladi) 10 g, Gān Jiāng (Rhizoma Zingiberis) 10 g, and a handful of Ài Yè (Folium Artemisiae Argyi); decoct in water and add urine of boys under 12 years old (originally used 马通汁, Mǎ Tōng Zhī, dissolve horse shit into water and twist the clear juice) for oral administration to treat center qi deficiency-cold with failure of qi to contain blood mani- fested as chronic hematemesis, sallow complexion, and deficient, fast and powerless pulse.

2. 侧柏叶汤 Cè Bǎi Yè Tāng — Arborvitae Decoction from *Essentials of Materia Medica* (本草切要, Běn Cǎo Qiè Yào,): Cè Bǎi Yè (Cacumen Platycladi) 15 g, Mù Tōng (Caulis Akebiae) 6 g, Dāng Guī (Radix Angelicae Sinensis) 6 g, Hóng Huā (Flos Carthami) 6 g, Qiāng Huó (Rhizoma et Radix Notopterygii) 6 g, and Fáng Fēng (Radix Saposhnikoviae); decoct in water for oral administration to treat patient with severe joint pain immigrating the whole body failing to turn around to either sides.

[Precautions] Cè Bǎi Yè (Cacumen Platycladi) is bitter in flavor and cold in nature. Long-term ingestion can damage stomach qi. Vertigo, nausea, gastric discomfort, and decreased appetite from long-term ingestion or a large dose has been reported. It may cause such allergic reaction as edema and dermatitis in few cases.

仙鹤草 Xiān Hè Cǎo *herba agrimoniae hairy vein agrimonia*

The source is from the whole plant of herbaceous *Agrimonia pilosa* ledeb., family Rosaceae. Alternate names include 龙芽草 Lóng Yá Cǎo, 脱力草 Tuō Lì Cǎo, and 黄龙尾, *Huáng Lóng Wěi*. Bitter and astringent in flavor and neutral in nature.

[Actions] Astringent and stanch bleeding, reduce food stagnation and strengthen the stomach, and kill parasites. It is applicable for hemorrhagic disorders such as hemoptysis, hematemesis, hematuria, stool containing blood, profuse uterine bleeding, prolonged scanty uterine bleeding of variable intervals, dysentery, overstrain, carbuncles, swelling, and injuries from falls, fractures, contusions and strains. Modern research indicate it has certain vasoconstrictive and coagulative, antibacterial, pesticidal, and anti-inflammatory effects.

[Quality] Good quality has purplish red stems, tender branches, and well-shaped leaves.

[Indications]

1. Hemorrhagic disorders: owning to its astringing and stanching bleeding effect, Xiān Hè Cǎo (Herba Agrimoniae) is applicable to different types of bleeding only when there is no obvious stagnation. Combination with other herbs is based on the state of illness. It is combined with Shēng Dì (Radix Rehmanniae) and Zhī Zǐ (Fructus Gardeniae) for frenetic movement of hot blood through clearing heat and stanching bleeding; with Dǎng Shēn (Radix Codonopsis), Huáng Qí (Radix Astragali), and Páo Jiāng (Rhizoma Zingiberis Praeparatum) for bleeding caused by deficiency-cold. It has recently been prepared into powder and applied externally to treat different types of bleeding.
2. Food accumulation: Xiān Hè Cǎo (Herba Agrimoniae), effective in supplementing the stomach and promoting digestion, is applicable for food accumulation and infantile malnutrition with accumulation. It can be used alone in decoction form, or together with other medicinals that fortify the spleen and promote digestion. It also can be cooked together with pig liver, drink the soup and eat liver.
3. Chronic diarrhea and dysentery: Xiān Hè Cǎo (Herba Agrimoniae), astringent in flavor and effective in consolidation, is capable of arresting dysentery for chronic diarrhea and dysentery. It can be used alone or together with medicinals that fortify the spleen and arrest dysentery.
4. Lack of strength and overstrain: Xiān Hè Cǎo (Herba Agrimoniae) is decocted with Dà Zǎo (Fructus Jujubae) for listlessness due to qi and blood insufficiency or fatigue and lack of strength due to overwork. For this reason, it is also known as 脱力草 Tuō Lì Cǎo.

5. Parasitic worms: its 200% decoction is locally applied to the vagina for trichomonas vaginitis. Its root is applicable for tapeworm and schistosome. Grinding 9 g of Xiān Hè Cǎo (Herba Agrimoniae) into powder and taking with liquor before the onset of malaria for oral administration can relieve malaria.

Ingesting its decoction can treat neurasthenia, night sweating, aural vertigo, dizziness, allergic purpura, infantile summer non-acclimatization, and acute mastitis.

[Usage and Dosage] Use raw in general and stir-fried to stanch bleeding. Use 10–15 g in decoction, up to 30–60 g when used alone or fresh, decrease the dosage as in pill and powder.

[Mnemonics] *Xiān Hè Cǎo* (Herba Agrimoniae, Hairy Vein Agrimonia): stop bleeding, improve fatigue, and relieve diarrhea and dysentery due to food stagnation.

[Simple and Effective Formulas]

1. 治咯血方-Zhì Kǎ Xiě Fāng — Hemoptysis Relieving Formula from *Commonly Used Folk Medicinals and Formulas in Guizhou* (贵州民间方药集, Guì Zhōu Mín Jiān Fāng Yào Jí,): fresh Xiān Hè Cǎo (Herba Agrimoniae) 30 g (dried one 18 g) and white sugar 30 g; pound Xiān Hè Cǎo (Herba Agrimoniae), add a small bowl of cool boiled water, mix them up, squeeze juice, add white sugar, and drink the juice all at one time to treat lung tuberculosis with hemoptysis.
2. 止血方 Zhǐ Xuè Fāng — Bleeding Arresting Formula from *Sichuan Provincial Records of Chinese Medicinals* (四川中药志 Sìchuān Zhōng Yào Zhì,): Xiān Hè Cǎo (Herba Agrimoniae) 15 g, Pú Huáng (Pollen Typhae) 15 g, Bái Máo Gēn (Rhizoma Imperatae) 15 g, and Dà Jì (Herba Cirsii Japonici) 15 g; decoct in water for oral administration to treat epistaxis and stool containing blood.

[Precautions] Xiān Hè Cǎo (Herba Agrimoniae) is astringent in nature and should be combined with medicinal that invigorate blood and dissolve stasis for bleeding with static blood.

Daily practices

1. What are the similarities and differences among Huái Huā (Flos Sophorae), Cè Băfi Yè (Cacumen Platycladi), and Xiān Hè Căo (Herba Agrimoniae) in terms of actions and indications?
2. Please review the actions and indications of what we learn this week, namely qi-regulating, food accumulation-relieving, worm-dispelling, bleeding-stanching medicinals.

CHAPTER 9

Ninth Week

1

白及 **Bái Jí** *rhizoma bletillae bletilla rhizome*

The source is from the rhizome of herbaceous perennial *Bletilla striata* (Thunb.) Reichb. f., family Orchidaceae. It is so called because its roots are white and interconnected. Bitter, sweet, and acrid in flavor and slightly cold in nature.

[Actions] Restrain and arrest, reduce swelling and generate flesh. It is applicable for different types of hemorrhagic disorders, sores, carbuncles, swellings, toxins, rhagadia of hands and feet, and lung abscess. Experiments show it has favorable effects of topical administration and its mucoid substance can induce erythrocyte agglomeration and promote thrombopoiesis. *In vitro* experiments indicate it has an inhibitory effect against tubercle bacillus and other bacteria.

[Quality] Good quality is dry, large, semi-transparent, and firm.

[Indications]

1. Hemorrhagic disorders: Bái Jí (Rhizoma Bletillae), sticky in texture and astringent in nature, is effective in consolidating and stanching bleeding and applicable for hematemesis, hemoptysis, and hemorrhage caused by traumatic injury. It can be used alone in a powder form or together with medicinals that stanch bleeding. This substance is combined with Pí Pá Yè (Folium Eriobotryae), Shēng Dì (Radix Rehmanniae), and Ē Jiāo (Colla Corii Asini) for hemoptysis; and with Sān Qī (Radix et Rhizoma Notoginseng) for hemoptysis and hematemesis due to traumatic injury of the lung and stomach.

311

2. Skin and mucous membrane breakage: Bái Jí (Rhizoma Bletillae), effective in generating flesh and promoting wound healing, is applicable for skin rhagadia in the hands and feet, anal fissure, or non-healing wound of sores and ulcers by either ground into powder or mixed with sesame oil for external application. The ancients believe it can repair the injury in the lung and therefore it is suitable in the cases of lung tuberculosis no matter with or without hemoptysis. Owning to its flesh-generating property, it can be used alone or ground with Hǎi Piāo Xiāo (Endoconcha Sepiae) into powder to treat gastric and duodenum ulcer, especially when a small amount of bleeding in the digestive tract.

3. Carbuncles and swellings: Bái Jí (Rhizoma Bletillae), capable of reducing swelling, is combined with Jīn Yín Huā (Flos Lonicerae Japonicae), Zào Jiǎo Cì (Spina Gleditsiae), and Tiān Huā Fěn (Radix Trichosanthis) for carbuncles in early stage with redness, swelling, hot sensation, and pain.

Grinding with Wū Tóu (Aconite Main Tuber) into fine powder, wrapping a small amount with gauze, and putting into vagina can treat prolapse of uterus. Its decoction or powder can be applied topically for tuberculous fistula and burning.

[Usage and Dosage] Use raw in general, 3–10 g in decoction (overdose may cause decoction sticky and difficult to swallow), decrease the amount as in pill and powder, and taken after mixing with warm water.

[Mnemonics] Bái Jí (Rhizoma Bletillae, Bletilla Rhizome): sticky in texture; restrain and stanch bleeding; effective for arresting hematemesis and hemoptysis.

[Simple and Effective Formulas]

1. 白及散　Bái Jí Sǎn — Bletilla Rhizome Powder from *Medical Enlightenment* (医学启蒙　Yī Xué Qǐ Méng): Bái Jí (Rhizoma Bletillae), Ē Jiāo (Colla Corii Asini), Kuǎn Dōng Huā (Flos Farfarae), and Zǐ Wǎn (Radix et Rhizoma Asteris) in equal dosage; decoct in water for oral administration to treat lung *wěi* (痿 atrophy) and cough and hemoptysis of pulmonary tuberculosis.

2. 白及丸 Bái Jí Wán — Bletilla Rhizome Pill from *The Great Compendium of External Medicine* (外科大成 Wài Kē Dà Chéng): Bái Jí (Rhizoma Bletillae); grind into fine powder, make into pill with wine paste, and take 9 g/time with yellow wine for oral administration, everyday for 15 days, to treat sinusitis, clear nasal discharge and headache.

[Precautions] Bái Jí (Rhizoma Bletillae), astringent in nature, is contraindicated in early stage of externally-contracted diseases and fire-heat exuberance. According to "eighteen antagonisms", it is incompatible with Wū Tóu (Aconite Main Tuber).

三七 **Sān Qī** (*aka Tián Qī*) *radix et rhizoma notoginseng pseudoginseng root*

The source is from the root of herbaceous perennial *Panax notoginseng* (Burk.) T. H. Chen, family Araliaceae. It is so called because this plant has three leaves on the left side of the main stem and four leaves on the right. In the opinion of some people, it was originally named 山漆 Shān Qī as it can close stab wound like glutinous lacquer and eventually known as 三七 Sān Qī. Alternate names include 山漆 Shān Qī, 参三七 Cān Sān Qī, 田三七 Tián Sān Qī, and 田漆 Tián Qī. Sweet and slight bitter in flavor and warm in nature.

[Actions] Stanch bleeding and disperse blood stagnation, and relieve swelling and arrest pain. It is applicable for different types of hemorrhagic disorders, such as hematemesis, hemoptysis, hemoptysis, epistaxis, stool with blood, hematuria, blood dysentery, profuse uterine bleeding, prolonged scanty uterine bleeding of variable intervals, injuries from falls, fractures, contusions and strains, postpartum inhibited lochia, traumatic bleeding, carbuncles, swellings, tumor, and pain. Experiments indicate it can shorten clotting time of experimental animals, increase blood flow volume of coronary artery, lower blood pressure, strengthen the heart, and reduce blood capillary permeation.

[Quality] Good quality is large, solid, and heavy, has a thin and smooth cortex and a grayish green, yellowish green or brownish black cross-section without cracks.

[Indications]

1. Hemorrhagic disorders: *New Compilation of Materia Medica* (本草新编 Běn Cǎo Xīn Biān) regarded Sān Qī (Radix et Rhizoma Notoginseng) as "panacea of stanching bleeding", indicating it is very effective in stanching bleeding and applicable for different types of hemorrhagic disorders. Owning to its secondary effect of dissolving stasis, it is applicable for hemorrhagic disorders, no matter with or without blood stasis. It can stanch bleeding without retaining blood stasis and can be used alone in a powder form or together with other bleeding-stanching medicinals. It can be ground into powder and applied externally for traumatic bleeding.
2. Swelling and pain due to blood stagnation: Sān Qī (Radix et Rhizoma Notoginseng), effective in invigorating blood and dissolving stasis, is applicable for swelling and pain caused by blood stagnation, such as blood stasis with swelling and pain resulting from injuries from falls, fractures, contusions and strains. It can be ground into powder for oral administration and mixed with wine for external application, or used in the formula that invigorate blood and move qi. This medicinal has been recently used in the treatment of coronary heart disease and angina pectoris due to its effects of invigorating blood, dissolving stasis, and relieving pain. Nowadays, it is ground into powder to treat stomachache, chronic hepatitis, anti-liver fibrosis, acute segmental necrotizing enteritis, and hemorrhagic cerebral stroke.

It is also applied externally to treat a variety of disorders. For instance, it is ground with Lóng Gǔ (Os Draconis), Xiàng Pí (Elephant Hide), Xuè Jié (Sanguis Draconis), and Rǔ Xiāng (Olibanum) into powder and applied externally to treat non-healing stab wound; or ground into juice and applied externally on the rim of the eye to treat red and painful eyes.

[Usage and Dosage] Use as powder or pill in most cases, and decoction in few cases. Use 1–3 g when taken directly as a powder.

[Mnemonics] *Sān Qī* (Radix et Rhizoma Notoginseng, Pseudoginseng Root): sweet and bitter; specialized in stanching bleeding, invigorating blood, arresting pain, and popular with traumatology.

[Simple and Effective Formulas]

1. 化血丹 Huà Xuè Dān — Blood Relieving Elixir from *Records of Chinese Medicine with Reference to Western Medicine* (医学衷中参西录 Yī Xué Zhōng Zhōng Cān Xī Lù): Sān Qī (Radix et Rhizoma Notoginseng) 6 g, Huā Ruǐ Shí (Ophicalcitum) (calcined but medical nature preserved) 9 g, and Xuè Yú Tàn (Crinis Carbonisatus) (calcined but medical nature preserved) 3 g; grind into fine powder, divide into two equal doses, and take one dose/time with boiled water for oral administration to treat hemoptysis, hematemesis, epistaxis and blood in urine and stool.

2. 军门止血方 Jūn Mén Zhǐ Xuè Fāng — Army Blood Arresting Formula from *Saving Life Collection* (回生集 Huí Shēng Jí): Rén Shēn (Radix et Rhizoma Ginseng), Sān Qī (Radix et Rhizoma Notoginseng), Bái Là (Cera Chinensis), Rǔ Xiāng (Olibanum), Jiàng Xiāng (Lignum Dalbergiae Odoriferae), Xuè Jié (Sanguis Draconis), Wǔ Bèi Zǐ (Galla Chinensis), and Mǔ Lì (Concha Ostreae) in equal dosage; grind into powder and apply externally for traumatic bleeding.

[Precautions] Sān Qī (Radix et Rhizoma Notoginseng) is effective in invigorating blood and dissolving stasis and therefore should be used with caution during pregnancy.

Daily practices

1. What are the similarities and differences among Cè Bǎi Yè (Cacumen Platycladi), Xiān Hè Cǎo (Herba Agrimoniae), Bái Jí (Rhizoma Bletillae), and Sān Qī (Radix et Rhizoma Notoginseng) in terms of stanching bleeding?
2. What are the other actions of Bái Jí (Rhizoma Bletillae) and Sān Qī (Radix et Rhizoma Notoginseng) apart from bleeding-stanching?
3. What precautions should be taken when using medicinals that astringe and stanch bleeding?

茜草 **Qiàn Cǎo** *radix et rhizoma rubiae Indian madder root*

The source is from the root and rhizome of herbaceous perennial *Rubia cordifolia* L., family Rubiaceae. Alternate names include 茜根 Qiàn Gēn,

血见愁 Xuè Jiàn Chóu, 活血丹 Huó Xuè Dān, and 过山龙 Guò Shān Lóng. Bitter in flavor and cold in nature.

[Actions] Cool the blood and stanch bleeding, and invigorate blood and dissolve stasis. It is applicable for different types of hemorrhagic disorders due to blood heat, blood stasis caused amenorrhea, injuries from falls, fractures, contusions and strains, pain due to blood stasis and qi stagnation, and *bì* pattern with pain. From the perspective of modern experiment researches, its lixivium can shorten blood clotting time of rabbits, its water extract can excite *ex vivo* uterus of cavia cobaya and stimulate uterus contraction. It has shown antibechic, expectorant, spasmolytic, and certain antibacterial effects.

[Quality] Good quality is dry, coarse, long, reddish-brown outside, deep-red inside, few branches, and without stems, shoots, and rootlets.

[Indications]

1. Hemorrhagic disorders: Qiàn Cǎo (Radix et Rhizoma Rubiae), cold in nature with bleeding-stanching effect, is applicable for hemorrhagic disorders caused by blood heat and often used together with medicinals that cool blood and stanch bleeding for different disorders of blood heat, such as hematemesis, hemoptysis, epistaxis, stool with blood, hematuria, profuse uterine bleeding, and prolonged scanty uterine bleeding of variable intervals. It is particularly suitable for bleeding with blood stasis as it can also dissolve stasis. It should be combined with Huáng Qí (Radix Astragali), Bái Zhú (Rhizoma Atractylodis Macrocephalae), and Hǎi Piāo Xiāo (Endoconcha Sepiae) for bleeding caused by insecurity of the *chong* and *ren* mai or bleeding due to qi deficiency failing to control blood.

2. Amenorrhea with blood stasis: Qiàn Cǎo (Radix et Rhizoma Rubiae), capable of invigorating blood and dissolving stasis, is applicable for amenorrhea due to blood stasis, injuries from falls, fractures, contusions and strains, and *bì* with joint pain. It is used alone as medical wine or often together with medicinals that invigorate blood, dissolve stasis, and unblock channels with Dāng Guī (Radix Angelicae Sinensis), Hóng Huā (Flos Carthami), Táo Rén (Semen Persicae), and Chì Sháo (Radix Paeoniae Rubra). This substance is also used in the

treatment of boils, carbuncles, and urticaria due to its effect of invigorating blood.

It has been recently prepared with Jú Pí (Pericarpium Citri Reticulatae) into tablet for chronic bronchitis. Its extractives have also been prepared into tablet for leukocytopenia and profuse menstruation.

[Usage and Dosage] Use raw or wine-fried for invigorating blood, and charred to stop bleeding. Fresh plant is more potent in cooling the blood and stanching bleeding. Use 10–15 g in decoction, double the dosage when use fresh, and decrease the amount as in pill and powder.

[Mnemonics] Qiàn Cǎo (Radix et Rhizoma Rubiae, Indian Madder Root): cold and bitter; cool the blood, stanch bleeding, dispel blood stasis, and promote menstruation.

[Simple and Effective Formulas]

1. 茜草丸 Qiàn Cǎo Wán — Indian Madder Root Pill from *Comprehensive Recording of Divine Assistance* (圣济总录 Shèng Jì Zǒng Lù): Qiàn Cǎo (Radix et Rhizoma Rubiae) (filed), Xióng Hēi Dòu (Semen Sojae Nigrum) (peel removed), and Gān Cǎo (Radix et Rhizoma Glycyrrhizae) (roasted, filed) in equal dosage; grind into fine powder, make into hoodle-sized pill with water, and take one pill/time with warm water for oral administration to treat asthenic fever, agitation, and thirst after hematemesis. Also applicable for preventing hemorrhage and resolving toxins.

2. 茜梅丸 Qiàn Méi Wán — Indian Madder Root and Mume Pill from *Experiential Formulas for Universal Relief* (普济本事方 Pǔ Jì Běn Shì Fāng): Qiàn Cǎo Gēn (Radix et Rhizoma Rubiae) 30 g, Ài Yè (Folium Artemisiae Argyi) 30 g, and Wū Méi (Fructus Mume) flesh (baked) 15 g; grind into fine powder, make into phoenix tree seed-sized pill with honey, and take 30 pills/time with Wū Méi (Fructus Mume) decoction for oral administration to treat epistaxis at variable interval and chronic and recurrent nosebleed and gum bleeding.

[Precautions] Qiàn Cǎo (Radix et Rhizoma Rubiae), cold in nature, should be used with caution in cases of deficiency-cold of the spleen and stomach or in the absence of blood stagnation.

蒲黄 Pú Huáng *pollen typhae cattail pollen*

The source is from the pollen of aquatic herbaceous *Typha angustifolia* L., or *T. latifolia* Linn., or *T. orientalis* Presl, family Typhaceae. Alternate names include 蒲花 Pú Huā, 蒲厘花粉 Pú Lí Huā Fěn, and 蒲棒花粉 Pú Bàng Huā Fěn. Sweet in flavor and neutral in nature.

[Actions] Stanch bleeding, dispel blood stasis, and relieve strangury. It is applicable for different types of hemorrhagic disorders such as hematemesis, hemoptysis, epistaxis, stool containing blood, hematuria, profuse uterine bleeding, prolonged scanty uterine bleeding of variable intervals, and traumatic bleeding. This herb can also promote urination and dissolve stasis and therefore is especially suitable for hematuria with dripping and difficult urination. It is applicable for stomach, gastric, abdominal pain, and swelling and pain caused by injuries from falls, fractures, contusions and strains. Experiments indicate it can shorten clotting time and increase platelet count and postpartum uterus contraction, and has certain hypolipidemic effects.

[Quality] Good quality is fresh yellow, smooth and glossy, pure, light-weight, creamy when twisted. The herb containing plenty of capillaments and anther is called 草蒲黄 Cǎo Pú Huáng with an inferior quality.

[Indications]

1. Hemorrhagic disorders: Pú Huáng (Pollen Typhae), neutral in nature with stasis-dissolving effect, is applicable for hemorrhagic disorders, no matter cold or hot, with or without stasis. It can be used alone or together with other medicinals that stanch bleeding. For instance, It is combined with Shēng Dì (Radix Rehmanniae), Cè Bǎi Yè (Cacumen Platycladi), Dà Jì (Herba Cirsii Japonici), and Xiǎo Jì (Herba Cirsii) for blood heat bleeding; with Páo Jiāng (Rhizoma Zingiberis Praeparatum) and Ài Yè (Folium Artemisiae Argyi) for deficiency-cold bleeding; and with Huá Shí (Talcum) and Xiǎo Jì (Herba Cirsii) for dripping, difficult and painful urination. It can also be applied externally to stanch bleeding.
2. Pain caused by blood stagnation: owning to its blood-invigorating and stasis-dissolving property, Pú Huáng (Pollen Typhae) can dissolve stasis and relieve pain, and is effective on pain caused by static blood

accumulation. It is commonly used to treat gastric pain, dysmenorrhea, and postpartum abdominal pain in a combination with Wǔ Líng Zhī (Feces Trogopterori).

Its external application can relieve swollen tongue, sublingual swelling with sores, wet and itchy pudendum and pus draining out of the ear. Nowadays, it is commonly used in the treatment of coronary heart disease, hyperlipidemia, and hypertension.

[Usage and Dosage] Use in raw form to dispel blood stasis and relieve pain, stir-fried to stop bleeding. The ancients stated that "use raw to invigorate and move blood, stir-fried until black to stanch bleeding", however modern experiments display that the raw substance is also effective in stanching bleeding, in the opinion of some researchers, it is unnecessary to stir-fry this herb into black. Use 5–10 g in decoction. If decocted, it should be placed in cheesecloth due to its lightweight nature. Decrease the amount as in pill and powder, appropriate amount for external application.

[Mnemonics] Pú Huáng (Pollen Typhae, Cattail Pollen): sweet and neutral; use raw to promote blood circulation, use fried to stanch bleeding, arrest pain, and relieve strangury.

[Simple and Effective Formulas]

1. 蒲黄丸 Pú Huáng Wán — Cattail Pollen Pill from *Comprehensive Recording of Divine Assistance* (圣济总录 Shèng Jì Zǒ ng Lù): Pú Huáng (Pollen Typhae) (slightly stir-fried) 90 g, Lóng Gǔ (Os Draconis) 75 g, and Ài Yè (Folium Artemisiae Argyi) 30 g; grind into fine powder, make into phoenix tree seed-sized pill with honey, and take 20 pills/time with rice soup for oral administration to treat profuse menstruation or dripping of uterine bleeding.

2. 失笑散 Shī Xiào Sǎn — Sudden Smile Powder from *Formulas from the Imperial Pharmacy* (局方 Jú Fāng): Pú Huáng (Pollen Typhae) (stir-fried until aromatic) and Wǔ Líng Zhī (Feces Trogopterori) (ground with wine, panned to remove sand and soil) in equal dosage; grind into fine powder, mix 6 g/time with vinegar, make into decocted extract, then decoct in water, and take warm before meal for severe pain in the heart and

abdomen during postpartum. Also applicable for gastric pain, abdominal pain, and dysmenorrheal associated with static blood obstruction.

[Precautions] Pú Huáng (Pollen Typhae) should be used with cautions during pregnancy as it can induce uterine contraction.

Besides the above-mentioned medicinals, others that commonly used for stanching bleeding include Zhù Má Gēn (Radix Boehmeriae), Bái Máo Gēn (Rhizoma Imperatae), Zōng Lǚ Tàn (Petiolus Trachycarpi Carbonisatus), Xuè Yú Tàn (Crinis Carbonisatus), Ài Yè (Folium Artemisiae Argyi), and Zào Xīn Tǔ (Terra Flava Usta).

Daily practices

1. What are the similarities and differences between Qiàn Cǎo (Radix et Rhizoma Rubiae) and Pú Huáng (Pollen Typhae) in terms of stanching bleeding?
2. What are the other actions of Qiàn Cǎo (Radix et Rhizoma Rubiae) and Pú Huáng (Pollen Typhae) beside stanching bleeding?
3. What are the differences among those medicinals that stanch bleeding in terms of treating hemorrhagic disorders?
4. Summarize the medicinals that stanch bleeding and can also dissolve blood stasis.

MEDICINALS THAT INVIGORATE BLOOD

Blood stasis refers to the condition in which the flow of blood has retarded, become blocked, or is static. It can be caused by disturbance of blood circulation due to exogenous pathogen invasion; disorder of qi movement failing to promote blood circulation; blood stasis caused by traumatic hemorrhage; and phlegm-damp hindering blood flow. Blood stasis are often associated with such pathogenic factors as cold, heat, phlegm, damp, and qi stagnation to form such complicated patterns as cold-blood stasis, heat-blood stasis, phlegm-blood stasis, turbidity-blood stasis, and qi stagnation with blood stasis. This can lead to many types of problems due to different affected areas of static blood. For instance, blood stasis in the organs may cause dysfunction of relative organs; blood stasis in the heart may cause cardiac pain, or mental disturbance, or even heart qi external desertions; blood stasis obstructing the liver may cause rib-side *pĭ*, masses, and pain; blood stasis in the stomach may cause gastric stabbing pain; blood stasis lodged in the uterus may cause amenorrhea or dysmenorrhea; blood stasis in the lower *jiao* may cause pain, hardness, and fullness in the lateral aspects of lower abdomen (blood amassment pattern); and blood stasis in the sinews may cause general pain. Blood stasis is also often involved in the traumatic injury, and pathogenesis of dermatosis, sores, and ulcers.

These herbs can sooth the flow of blood and resolve blood stasis. Once blood stasis is relieved, such symptoms as stagnation, accumulation, pain, swelling, distention, amenorrhea will disappear. Blood stasis is a common pathological state in the clinic, and therefore blood-invigorating herbs are widely used in treating unsmooth flow of blood and blockage of blood stasis. In recent years, herbs that invigorate blood and method that invigorate blood and dissolve stasis has became a highlight of research on treatment methods of traditional Chinese medicine, and many new achievements have been obtained. These herbs have been widely used in the treatment of coronary heart disease, sequelae of cerebral apoplexy, cirrhosis, tumor, ectopic pregnancy, acute abdominal disease, and thromboangitis obliterans. Systematic researches have been conducted on their mechanisms of action.

Clinically, the herbs in this section are often combined in prescriptions with other herbs in accordance with state of illness and demand of treatment. From the perspective of traditional Chinese medicine, qi is the commander of blood, moving qi is beneficial for blood circulation, and therefore blood-invigorating herbs are often used in conjunction with qi-moving herbs to activate qi circulation promoting blood flow. For cold-blood stasis, herbs that warm the interior are also used to warm cold and dissolve blood stagnation. For heat-blood stasis, heat-clearing herbs are also indicated to clear heat and resolve blood stagnation. For phlegm-blood stasis, phlegm-dissolving herbs are added. For damp-turbidity binding with blood stasis, herbs that dispel dampness and relieve turbidity also included in the treatment plan. For *pĭ*, accumulation, and masses, herbs that soften hardness and dissipate masses are also used. For the debilitated patient, tonics are also prescribed.

Blood-invigorating herbs can consume blood and stir bleeding and therefore should be used with cautions during pregnancy or in cases of profuse menstruation or patients susceptible to bleeding.

川芎 Chuān Xiōng *rhizoma chuanxiong sichuan lovage root*

The source is from the rhizome of *Ligusticum chuanxiong* Hort., family Umbelliferae. Alternate names include 芎藭 Xiōn Qióng (as this medicinal is specialized in relieving disorders in the head and brain which is considered as vault 芎藭 Xiōng Qióng) and 西芎 Xi Xiōng. Pungent in flavor and warm in nature.

[Actions] Invigorate blood and move qi, and dispel wind and arrest pain. It is applicable for menstrual irregularities, dysmenorrhea, amenorrhea, chest and rib-side stabbing pain, traumatic swelling and pain, headache, wind-damp *bì* pain, and tumor attributed to blood stasis. Modern researches suggest its active ingredient ligustrazine can dilate blood vessels, increase blood flow volume of coronary artery and myocardial systolic function, improve blood circulation, inhibit platelet aggregation, and reduce thrombopoiesis. Therefore it is effective for treating different types of ischemic disorders. Other ingredients such as alkaloid, volatile oil, and lactones also have certain pharmacological effects.

[Quality] Good quality is large, solid, and oily with a yellowish white cross-section and strong aroma.

[Indications]

1. Blood stasis qi stagnation: owning to its pungent, dispersing, warm and unblocking properties, Chuān Xiōng (Rhizoma Chuanxiong) is capable of invigorating blood and moving qi and suitable for disorder caused by blood stasis and qi stagnation, especially when accompanied with pain such as menstrual irregularities, dysmenorrhea, gastric pain, and *bì* pattern. It is combined with medicinals that invigorate blood, regulate qi, and regulate menstruation such as Hóng Huā (Flos Carthami), Táo Rén (Semen Persicae), Dāng Guī (Radix Angelicae Sinensis), Dān Shēn (Radix et Rhizoma Salviae Miltiorrhizae), Xiāng Fù (Rhizoma

Cyperi), and Yì Mǔ Cǎo (Herba Leonuri) for menstruation disorders; with medicinals that sooth the liver and regulate qi such as Chái Hú (Radix Bupleuri), Bái Sháo (Radix Paeoniae Alba), and Xiāng Fù (Rhizoma Cyperi) for chest and rib-side pain due to liver constraint blood stasis qi stagnation; with Dān Shēn (Radix et Rhizoma Salviae Miltiorrhizae), Yù Jīn (Radix Curcumae), and Jiàng Xiāng (Lignum Dalbergiae Odoriferae) for blood stasis obstruction in the heart vessels; with Wǔ Líng Zhī (Faeces Trogopterori), Yán Hú Suǒ (Rhizoma Corydalis), Chì Sháo (Radix Paeoniae Rubra), and Hóng Huā (Flos Carthami) for *pǐ* and masses with pain; and with Sān Qī (Radix et Rhizoma Notoginseng), Rǔ Xiāng (Olibanum), and Mò Yào (Myrrha) for blood stasis, swellings, and pain attributed to injuries from falls, fractures, contusions and strains.

2. Pain: Chuān Xiōng (Rhizoma Chuanxiong), effective in relieving pain, is applicable for different types of pain, such as headache, muscle and joint pain, wind-damp *bì* in a combination with other medicinals. It is pungent, warm, ascending, and dispersing in nature, and is commonly used in the treatment of different types of headache when prescribed together with different herbs. It is used together with Qiāng Huó (Rhizoma et Radix Notopterygii), Gǎo Běn (Rhizoma Ligustici), and Xì Xīn (Radix et Rhizoma Asari) for wind-cold headache; with Jú Huā (Flos Chrysanthemi), Shí Gāo (Gypsum Fibrosum), and Huáng Qín (Radix Scutellariae) for wind-heat headache; with Qiāng Huó (Rhizoma et Radix Notopterygii), Dú Huó (Radix Angelicae Pubescentis), and Fáng Fēng (Radix Saposhnikoviae) for wind-damp headache; with Dāng Guī (Radix Angelicae Sinensis), Shú Dì Huáng (Radix Rehmanniae Praeparata), and Hé Shǒu Wū (Radix Polygoni Multiflori) for blood deficiency headache; with Chì Sháo (Radix Paeoniae Rubra), Táo Rén (Semen Persicae), Hóng Huā (Flos Carthami), and Rǔ Xiāng (Olibanum) for static blood headache; and with Dú Huó (Radix Angelicae Pubescentis), Guì Zhī (Ramulus Cinnamomi), Xì Xīn (Radix et Rhizoma Asari), and Má Huáng (Herba Ephedrae) for joint and muscle pain caused by wind-cold-dampness.

It has recently been used for hematopoietic dysfunction and cytopenia caused by radioactive rays. This herb is combined with Yì Mǔ Cǎo (Herba

Leonuri) for chronic nephritis and with Hóng Huā (Flos Carthami) for angina pectoris.

[Usage and Dosage] Use raw in general, wine-processed for headache or to invigorate blood and move qi with a better effect in going upward to unblock the blood vessels. Use 3–6 g in decoction, a bigger amount to invigorate blood, and up to 30 g may be used for migraine. However, overdose may cause vomiting and vertigo. Ligustrazine has been recently prepared into tablets for different types of cardiocerebral vascular disorders.

[Mnemonics] Chuān Xiōng (Rhizoma Chuanxiong, Sichuan Lovage Root): pungent and warm; invigorate blood, move qi, arrest pain, and good at regulating menstruation.

[Simple and Effective Formulas]

1. 散偏汤 Sàn Piān Tāng — Migraine Relieving Decoction from *Secret Records in a Stone Room* (石室秘录 Shí Shì Mì Lù): Chuān Xiōng (Rhizoma Chuanxiong) 30 g, Bái Sháo (Radix Paeoniae Alba) 15 g, Yù Lǐ Rén (Semen Pruni) 3 g, Chái Hú (Radix Bupleuri) 3324 g, Xiāng Fù (Rhizoma Cyperi) 6 g, Bái Jiè Zǐ (Semen Sinapis) 9 g, Gān Cǎo (Radix et Rhizoma Glycyrrhizae) 3 g, and Bái Zhǐ (Radix Angelicae Dahuricae) 1.5 g; decoct in water for oral administration to treat migraine.

2. 川芎丸 Chuān Xiōng Wán — Sichuan Lovage Root Pill from *An Elucidation of Formulas* (宣明论方 Xuān Míng Lùn Fāng): Chuān Xiōng (Rhizoma Chuanxiong) 500 g and Tiān Má (Rhizoma Gastrodiae) 120 g; grind into powder, make into pill (3 g each) with honey, chew slowly one pill/time, and take with tea after drinking wine or meal for oral administration to treat head wind with vertigo and dizziness, migraine, headache, body tension, and lassitude.

[Precautions] Chuān Xiōng (Rhizoma Chuanxiong), pungent, warm, and scattering in nature, is contraindicated to cases of excess heat and yin deficiency resulting in vigorous fire. It should be used with caution in patients with weak constitution and different types of hemorrhagic disorders as it can stir and consume blood.

乳香 Rǔ Xiāng *olibanum frankincense*

[Addendum] 没药 Mò Yào Myrrha Myrrh
The source is from the resin of the stem cortex of subarbor *Boswellia carterii* Birdw and other plants of the same genus and species, family Burseraceae. It is so called because the drips of nipple-like resin hanging down from the tree. Alternate names include 熏陆香 Xūn Lù Xiāng, 多伽罗香 Duō Jiā Luō Xiāng, and 马尾香 Mǎ Wěi Xiāng. Bitter and pungent in flavor and warm in nature.

[Actions] Regulate qi and invigorate blood, smooth the sinews and arrest pain, and expel pus and reduce swelling. It is applicable for chest, gastric and abdominal pain, carbuncles, swellings, sores, and toxins, injuries from falls, fractures, contusions and strains, dysmenorrhea, and postpartum abdominal pain attributed to qi stagnation and blood stasis.

[Quality] Good quality is light yellow, granular, semitranslucent, aromatic, and sticky without impurities such as sandy stone and bark.

[Indications]

1. Blood stasis and qi stagnation: Rǔ Xiāng (Olibanum), capable of invigorating blood and moving qi, is applicable for disorders caused by blood stasis and qi stagnation, especially pain. It is combined with Mò Yào (Myrrha), Wǔ Líng Zhī (Faeces Trogopterori), and Xiāng Fù (Rhizoma Cyperi) for stomachache caused by blood stasis; with Mò Yào (Myrrha), Dān Shēn (Radix et Rhizoma Salviae Miltiorrhizae), and Chuān Xiōng (Rhizoma Chuanxiong) for chest *bì*, coronary heart disease, and angina pectoris; with Mò Yào (Myrrha), Xuè Jié (Sanguis Draconis), and Shè Xiāng (Moschus) for blood stasis, swellings, and pain due to injuries from falls, fractures, contusions and strains; and with Qiāng Huó (Rhizoma et Radix Notopterygii), Dú Huó (Radix Angelicae Pubescentis), and Dāng Guī (Radix Angelicae Sinensis) for joint pain and spasms of the limbs attributed to wind-damp *bì* pain.
2. Carbuncles, swellings, sores, and ulcers: Rǔ Xiāng (Olibanum), capable of invigorating blood, reducing swelling, generating muscle, and relieving pain, is a commonly-used medicinals for external diseases. It

is combined with Jīn Yín Huā (Flos Lonicerae Japonicae), Lián Qiào (Fructus Forsythiae), and Tiān Huā Fěn (Radix Trichosanthis) for localized redness, swelling and pain with a hot sensation in the early stage of carbuncles; and Mò Yào (Myrrha), Shè Xiāng (Moschus), and Xióng Huáng (Realgar) for hard carbuncles, scrofula, and phlegm node. Ground into powder for sores, chronic open non-healing ulcers.

It is also applicable for seminal emission and hiccup.

[Usage and Dosage] Use in decoction, but stir-fried or vinegar-processed one is preferred due to its strong and smelly fragrance may readily cause nausea. Frying with vinegar is to enhance its blood-invigorating, pain-relieving, and astringing, and flesh-generating properties. Use 3–9 g in decoction, decrease the dosage in pill and powder.

[Mnemonics] Rǔ Xiāng (Olibanum, Frankincense): pungent and bitter; invigorate blood, reduce sore and swelling, and arrest pain.

[Simple and Effective Formulas]

1. 抽刀散　Chōu Dāo Sǎn — Chou Dao Powder from *Numerous Miraculous Prescriptions for Health Cultivation* (摄生众妙方　Shè Shēng Zhòng Miào Fāng): Rǔ Xiāng (Olibanum) 3 g and Hú Jiāo (Fructus Piperis) 49 pieces; grind into powder and men take with Jiāng Zhī (Succus Rhizomatis Zingiberis) and women take with Dāng Guī (Radix Angelicae Sinensis) decoction for oral administration to treat sudden onset of precordium pain, stomachache, and angina pectoris.
2. 乳香定痛散　Rǔ Xiāng Dìng Tòng Sǎn — Frankincense Pain-resolving Powder from *Elaboration on External Medicine* (外科发挥　Wài Kē Fā Huī): Rǔ Xiāng (Olibanum) 6 g, Mò Yào (Myrrha) 6 g, Hán Shuǐ Shí (Glauberitum) (calcined) 12 g, Huá Shí (Talcum) 12 g, and Bīng Piàn (Borneolum Syntheticum) 0.3 g; make into fine powder and apply externally to the affected areas for sores and ulcers with unbearable pain.

[Precautions] Rǔ Xiāng (Olibanum) is effective in invigorating blood and therefore should be used with caution during pregnancy. Taking large-dose is not recommended for patient with spleen and stomach weakness due to its stimulation effect on the spleen and stomach. It is also contraindicated in cases of ulcerated sores and ulcers or with profuse pus.

[Addendum] 没药 Mò Yào Myrrha Myrrh
The source is from the resin of the stem cortex of *Commiphora myrrha* Engl., family Burseraceae. It is bitter in flavor and neutral in nature. Rǔ Xiāng (Olibanum) and Mò Yào (Myrrha) both can invigorate blood, dissolve stasis and move qi, and are applicable for dispersing blood stasis, arresting pain, reducing swelling, and engendering flesh. However, the former is considered to be more potent in moving qi, while the latter dispersing blood stasis. They are clinically similar in usage and dosage and are usually prescribed together.

Daily practices

1. What are the causes for blood stasis and what problems can it cause?
2. What is the medicinal that invigorates blood and what precautions should be taken when using it?
3. What are the similarities and differences between Chuān Xiōng (Rhizoma Chuanxiong) and Rǔ Xiāng (Olibanum) in terms of actions and indications?

郁金 *Yù Jīn Radix Curcumae Turmeric Root Tuber*

The source is from the tuberous root of herbaceous perennial *Curcuma aromatica* Salisb., *C. zedoaria* (Berg) Rosc., and *C. longa* L., family Zingiberaceae. It is so called because of its effect of relieving stagnation and yellow cross section, and alternate names include 玉金 Yù Jīn. Pungent and bitter in flavor and cold in nature.

[Actions] Invigorate blood and arrest pain, move qi and dissolve phlegm, relieve stagnation, cool the blood and clear the heart, and improve gallbladder function and relieve jaundice. It is applicable for chest, abdominal, rib-side distending pain, hematemesis, epistaxis, depressive psychosis, mania, menstrual irregularities, dysmenorrhea, gallstone, tumor, *pi* and masses associated with liver qi stagnation with internal obstruction of blood stasis. Modern research reveal that this medicinal contains many types of volatile oil and curcumin.

[Quality] There are four major varieties with different production area, species, and names. 黄郁金 Huáng Yù Jīn is from the root tuber of *Curcuma aromatica* Salisb. in Sichuan, alternate names include 黄丝郁金 Huáng Sī Yù Jīn and 广郁金 Guǎng Yù Jīn, and good quality is large and full, has thin wrinkles on the surface and a orange-yellow cross-section. 温郁金 Wēn Yù Jīn is from the root tuber of *Curcuma. zedoaria* (Berg) Rosc. in Zhejiang, alternate names include 黑郁金 Hēi Yù Jīn and 川郁金 Chuān Yù Jīn, and good quality is large and has few thin wrinkles on the surface and a grayish black cross-section. 白丝郁金 Bái Sī Yù Jīn is from the root tuber of *Curcuma aromatica* Salisb. in Sichuan, and good quality is large and thin-skinned and has a solid cross-section. Lǜ Sī Yù Jīn is from the root tuber of *Curcuma longa* L. in Sichuan and poor in quality.

[Indications]

1. Blood stasis and qi stagnation: Yù Jīn (Radix Curcumae), pungent and dispersing in nature, is capable of moving qi and invigorating blood and therefore applicable for chest, rib-side, and abdominal pain caused by blood stasis and qi stagnation. It is combined with Mù Xiāng (Radix Aucklandiae) and Sū Gěng (Caulis Perillae) for the cases predominated by qi stagnation; with Dān Shēn (Radix et Rhizoma Salviae Miltiorrhizae) and Chì Sháo (Radix Paeoniae Rubra) for the cases predominated by blood stasis; and with Xiāng Fù (Rhizoma Cyperi), Dāng Guī (Radix Angelicae Sinensis), and Bái Sháo (Radix Paeoniae Alba) for dysmenorrheal.

2. Phlegm turbidy confounding the pericardium: Yù Jīn (Radix Curcumae), capable of dispersing with pungency, draining with bitterness, and removing stagnation and phlegm turbidity, is commonly used for mental disturbance due to phlegm turbidity confounding the pericardium. It is combined with Shí Chāng Pú (Rhizoma Acori Tatarinowii), Zhī Zǐ (Fructus Gardeniae), and Zhú Lì (Succus Bambusae) for unconsciousness with delirious speech caused by damp-warm, phlegm, and turbidity confounding the pericardium through clearing the heart, dissolving phlegm, and opening the orifices; and with Bái Fán (Alumen) and Dǎn

Nán Xīng (Arisaema cum Bile) for depressive psychosis and mania caused by phlegm confounding the heart orifices.

3. Liver and gallbladder damp-heat: damp-heat accumulation in the liver and gallbladder may cause jaundice or generate stone. Owning to its ability of moving qi, relieving stagnation, soothing the liver and gallbladder, and clearing and draining damp-heat, Yù Jīn (Radix Curcumae) is widely used in cases of liver and gallbladder damp-heat. It is combined with Yīn Chén (Herba Artemisiae Scopariae), Zhī Zǐ (Fructus Gardeniae), Huáng Bǎi (Cortex Phellodendri Chinensis), and Dà Huáng (Radix et Rhizoma Rhei) for damp-heat jaundice; and with Jīn Qián Cǎo (Herba Lysimachiae), Hǔ Zhàng (Rhizoma Polygoni Cuspidati), and Jī Nèi Jīn (Endothelium Corneum Gigeriae Galli) for cases of stone.

4. Bleeding due to blood heat: Yù Jīn (Radix Curcumae), cold in nature, can clear pathogenic heat in blood and is commonly used for hemorrhagic disorders caused by blood heat, especially for hematemesis, epistaxis, and vicarious menstruation due to liver constraint transforming into fire in a combination with Mǔ Dān Pí (Cortex Moutan) and Zhī Zǐ (Fructus Gardeniae). It is combined with Shēng Dì (Radix Rehmanniae), Xiǎo Jì (Herba Cirsii), and Huá Shí (Talcum) for difficult, dripping and painful urination and hematuria due to heat accumulation in the lower *jiao*.

Nowadays, it has been prepared into tablets for premature heart beat or injection for acute and chronic hepatitis. It is also used in t the treatment of liver fibrosis.

[Usage and Dosage] Use raw in most cases, process with alums solution to improve its ability of dispelling phlegm. 广郁金 Guǎng Yù Jīn is considered more effective in moving qi and suitable for blood stasis and qi stagnation pattern with qi stagnation predominance, whereas 川郁金 Chuān Yù Jīn is more potent in invigorating blood and suitable for blood stasis qi and stagnation pattern predominated by static blood. Use 3–9 g in decoction, 2–3 g/dose in pill and powder.

[Mnemonics] Yù Jīn (Radix Curcumae, Turmeric Root Tuber): pungent and cold; relieve stagnation and phlegm, cool the blood, stanch bleeding, open the orifices, and relieve jaundice.

[Simple and Effective Formulas]

1. 郁金散 Yù Jīn Sǎn — Turmeric Root Tuber Powder from *Formulas for Universal Relief* (普济方 Pǔ Jì Fāng): Yù Jīn (Radix Curcumae), Pú Huáng (Pollen Typhae), and Gān Dì Huáng (Radix Rehmanniae Recens) in equal dosage; grind into fine powder and take 3 g/time with Chē Qián Cǎo (Herba Plantaginis) decoction before meal for patient with blood strangury, difficult and painful urination, and hematuria.
2. 白金丸 Bái Jīn Wán — Turmeric Root Tuber and Alum Pill from *Experiential Formulas for Universal Relief* (普济本事方 Pǔ Jì Běn Shì Fāng): Yù Jīn (Radix Curcumae) 210 g and Bái Fán (Alumen) 90 g; grind into fine powder, make into phoenix tree seed-sized pill with rice paste, and take 50 pills/time with boiled water for oral administration to treat mania and depression induced by phlegm-turbidity obstructing the heart orifice.

[Precautions] Yù Jīn (Radix Curcumae), effective in invigorating blood and moving qi, is contraindicated in the absence of either qi stagnation and blood stasis, in the cases of bleeding due to yin deficiency resulting in vigorous fire, and during pregnancy. According to "nineteen incompatibilities", this herb is discouraged to be used together with Dīng Xiāng (Flos Caryophylli).

延胡索 **Yán Hú Suǒ** *rhizoma corydalis corydalis rhizome*

The source is from the tuber of herbaceous perennial *Corydalis Yanhusuo* W. T. Wang, family Papaveraceae. Alternate names include 玄胡索 Xuán Hú Suǒ , 元胡 Yuán Hú, and 元胡索 Yuán Hú Suǒ . Bitter and pungent in flavor and warm in nature.

[Actions] Regulate qi and arrest pain, and invigorate blood and relieve blood stasis. It is applicable for chest, rib-side, gastric and abdominal pain, amenorrhea, dysmenorrhea, static blood during postpartum, and injuries from falls, fractures, contusions and strains attributed to qi stagnation and blood stasis. Modern research has shown that its major antalgic ingredient is and alkaloid, and that the effects of corydalis B, C, and D are superior to that of corydaline. Tetrahydropalmatine has shown significant sedative, hypnotic, sedative, and antipyretic effects.

[Quality] There are several varieties. The one most commonly found in Zhejiang is of good quality featured by large, full, hard, and yellow with the inside being bright yellow; poor quality is small and grayish yellow with white center. The one produced in the northeast of China is 山延胡索 Shān Yán Hú Suǒ and 迷延胡索 Mí Yán Hú Suǒ, and the one produced in Jiangsu is called 苏延胡 Sū Yán Hú with a poor quality.

[Indications]

1. Qi stagnation and blood stasis: Yán Hú Suǒ (Rhizoma Corydalis), effective in dispersing with pungency and unblocking with warmth, can sooth and unblock qi and blood, and therefore is applicable for cases caused by qi stagnation and blood stasis. It is combined with Guā Lóu (Fructus Trichosanthis), Xiè Bái (Bulbus Allii Macrostemi), and Dān Shēn (Radix et Rhizoma Salviae Miltiorrhizae) for chest *bì* pain; with Chái Hú (Radix Bupleuri), Xiāng Fù (Rhizoma Cyperi), Zhǐ Qiào (Fructus Aurantii), and Yù Jīn (Radix Curcumae) for chest, rib-side, and gastric pain caused by the predominance of qi stagnation; with Táo Rén (Semen Persicae), Hóng Huā (Flos Carthami), and Dān Shēn (Radix et Rhizoma Salviae Miltiorrhizae) for the predominance of blood stasis; with Gāo Liáng Jiāng (Rhizoma Alpiniae Officinarum) and Gān Jiāng (Rhizoma Zingiberis) for the cold-natured manifestations; with Chuān Liàn Zǐ (Fructus Toosendan), Zhī Zǐ (Fructus Gardeniae) for the heat-natured manifestations; with Xiǎo Huí Xiāng (Fructus Foeniculi), Lì Zhī Hé (Semen Litchi), and Jú Hé (Semen Citri Reticulatae) for hernia pain; with Dāng Guī (Radix Angelicae Sinensis), Chuān Xiōng (Rhizoma Chuanxiong), and Pú Huáng (Pollen Typhae) for dysmenorrheal and postpartum abdominal pain; and with Rǔ Xiāng (Olibanum), Mò Yào (Myrrha), and Guì Zhī (Ramulus Cinnamomi) for injuries from falls, fractures, contusions and strains, and wind-damp pain.

2. Pain patterns: Yán Hú Suǒ (Rhizoma Corydalis) is effective not only on pain caused by qi stagnation and blood stasis but also pain in many other diseases, such as headache, abdominal pain, joint pain, and

toothache. Treatment plan based on the root cause of pain will relieve pain better.

Its active ingredients have been prepared into tablet or injection to reinforce its ability of arresting pain. It is also applicable for cough and wheezing.

[Usage and Dosage] Use raw to arrest pain and regulate qi, stir-frying or liquid-frying to harmonize blood and regulate menstruation, stir-frying with vinegar is more effective in invigorating blood and arresting pain, while toasting in vinegar enters the liver channel and is more potent in dispelling stagnation and relieving pain. Modern researches suggest that processing in vinegar can enhance the solubility of analgesic active ingredients to improve its analgesic effect. Use 4–9 g in decoction, 2–5 g/dose as in pill and powder.

Toasting or frying in vinegar enhances its blood-invigorating properties. For a stronger effect, it should be used as a powder.

[Mnemonics] Yán Hú Suǒ (Rhizoma Corydalis, Corydalis Rhizome): pungent and bitter; keep qi and blood flow smoothly, and relieve different kinds of pain.

[Simple and Effective Formulas]
三神丸 Sān Shén Wán — Three Spirits Pill from *Formulas to Aid the Living* (济生方 Jì Shēng Fāng): Yán Hú Suǒ (Rhizoma Corydalis) (decocted in vinegar, peel removed) 30 g, Dāng Guī (Radix Angelicae Sinensis) (the residue of rhizome removed, soaked in wine, filed, slightly stir-fried) 30 g, and Jú Hóng (Exocarpium Citri Rubrum) 60 g; grind into fine powder, make into phoenix tree seed-sized pill with wine-treated rice paste, and take 70 pills/time and gradually up to 100 pills/time with Ài Yè (Folium Artemisiae Argyi) decoction or rice soup for oral administration to treat virgin with abdominal stabbing pain, scanty menstruation, and dysmenorrheal.

[Precautions] Yán Hú Suǒ (Rhizoma Corydalis) is capable of invigorating blood and therefore contraindicated in cases of profuse menstruation and early menstruation, and during pregnancy.

丹参 Dān Shēn *radix et rhizoma salviae miltiorrhizae* danshen root

The source is from the root and rhizome of herbaceous perennial *Salvia miltiorrhiza* Bunge, family Labiatae. It is so called because of its purplish red color and ginseng-like shape and alternate names include 紫丹参 Zǐ Dān Shēn and 赤参 Chì Cān. Bitter in flavor and slightly cold in nature.

[Actions] Dispel blood stasis and arrest pain, invigorate blood and unblock the channels, and clear the heart and relieve restlessness. It is applicable for gynecological problems such as menstrual irregularities, dysmenorrhea, and amenorrhea, accumulations, gatherings, *pǐ*, masses, hepatosplenomegaly, insomnia with vexation, chest *bì*, cardiac pain, and swelling and painful sores and ulcers. Many modern studies have been conducted regarding this herb and reveal it contains such active ingredients as salviol I, IIA, and III B that can improve body's anoxia resistance, dilate coronary artery, promote myocardial contractile force, enhance tissue reparation and regeneration, inhibit blood clotting, activate fibrinolysis, induce sedation, and regulate immunological function.

[Quality] Good quality is coarse and purplish black inside with small chrysanthemi-shaped white spots.

[Indications]

1. Static blood: Dān Shēn (Radix et Rhizoma Salviae Miltiorrhizae), effective on invigorating blood and dissolving stasis, is the principal herb that treat blood stasis. It is relatively cold in nature and regarded most suitable for the pattern of heat-blood stagnation. It is combined with Sān Léng (Rhizoma Sparganii), É Zhú (Rhizoma Curcumae), and Zào Jiǎo Cì (Spina Gleditsiae) for abdominal masses caused by blood stasis; with Bīng Láng (Semen Arecae), Qīng Pí (Pericarpium Citri Reticulatae Viride), Jú Pí (Pericarpium Citri Reticulatae), and Xiǎo Huí Xiāng (Fructus Foeniculi) for vulva swelling and pain. It has been recently prepared into injection and tablets to treat coronary heart disease, cerebrovascular accident, and arteriosclerosis with its property of invigorating blood. However, research has indicated that preparation should be

used with caution when given intravenously in cases of coronary heart disease with cerebrovascular circulatory disorder as the herbs improves coronary artery circulation but contracts cerebral vessels. Modern clinic experiences show it is effective in central retinitis, systemic lupus erythematosus, dermatosclerosis, hepatitis, psoriasis, and DIC.

2. Gynecological disorders: Dān Shēn (Radix et Rhizoma Salviae Miltiorrhizae) is a principal medicinal that regulate menstruation, as the ancients stated "powder of Dān Shēn (Radix et Rhizoma Salviae Miltiorrhizae) is as potent as Sì Wù Tāng-Four Substances Decoction". It is prescribed together with medicinals that regulate, clear heat, cool blood, and invigorate blood according to the nature of such diseases as menstrual irregularities, dysmenorrhea, and amenorrhea.

3. Restlessness of heart spirit: Dān Shēn (Radix et Rhizoma Salviae Miltiorrhizae) can also nourish and boost heart blood and therefore is combined with Fú Shén (Sclerotium Poriae Pararadicis), Hé Huān Pí (Cortex Albiziae), Yè Jiāo Téng (Caulis Polygoni Multiflori), and Bǎi Zǐ Rén (Semen Platycladi) for palpitations and insomnia due to heart blood insufficiency through nourishing blood and calming the spirit.

It can also be applied externally, for instance, decocting with Kǔ Shēn (Radix Sophorae Flavescentis) and Shé Chuáng Zǐ (Fructus Cnidii) for external wash to treat skin itching, urticaria, and scabies; or preparing with Bái Sháo (Radix Paeoniae Alba) and Bái Zhǐ (Radix Angelicae Dahuricae), and lard into paste for external application to relieve swelling and pain in female breasts.

[Usage and Dosage] Use raw in general, mixing or stir-frying with Zhū Shā (Cinnabaris) to nourish the heart and calm the mind, processing with wine for cold-natured disorders. Use 5–9 g in decoction, up to 15–30 g when used for severe case of blood stasis, decrease the amount as in pill and powder. It has been recently prepared into injection alone or together with Jiàng Xiāng (Lignum Dalbergiae Odoriferae) (Fù Fāng Dān Shēn Zhù Shè Yè, Compound Salvia Injection) and widely used in the clinic.

[Mnemonics] Dān Shēn (Radix et Rhizoma Salviae Miltiorrhizae, Danshen Root): cold and bitter; specialized in relieving blood stasis, nourishing the heart, arresting pain, and regulating menstruation.

[Simple and Effective Formulas]

丹参饮 Dān Shēn Yǐn — Salvia Beverage from *Medical Quintessence* (Yǐ Xué Jǐn Zhēn, 医学金针): Dān Shēn (Radix et Rhizoma Salviae Miltiorrhizae) 30 g, Bái Tán Xiāng (Lignum Santali Albi) 4.5 g, and Shā Rén (Fructus Amomi) 4.5 g; decoct in water for oral administration to treat chest and abdomen pain due to half-deficiency half-excess pattern. It is capable of moving qi, dissolving stasis, and arresting pain and therefore applicable for such disorders as stomachache, abdominal pain, and angina pectoris.

[Precautions] Dān Shēn (Radix et Rhizoma Salviae Miltiorrhizae), although "as effective as Sì Wù Tāng-Four Substances Decoction", is most potent in invigorating blood and less potent in supplementing the blood. It cannot be used alone in cases of blood deficiency. According to "eighteen antagonisms", it is incompatible with Lí Lú (Radix et Rhizoma Veratri Nigri), but still needs experimental proof. Traditionally, this substance has been commonly used in the treatment of tumor, however, modern research has shown that this substance can aggravate the spread of cancer cells no matter in which way it has been administrated. Thus, more caution should be taken when using it.

Daily practices

1. What are the similarities and differences among Yù Jǐn (Radix Curcumae), Yán Hú Suǒ (Rhizoma Corydalis), and Dān Shēn (Radix et Rhizoma Salviae Miltiorrhizae) in terms of actions?
2. Yù Jǐn (Radix Curcumae), Yán Hú Suǒ (Rhizoma Corydalis), and Dān Shēn (Radix et Rhizoma Salviae Miltiorrhizae) all are capable of invigorating blood, what are their other actions and indications?

益母草 Yì Mǔ Cǎo *herba leonuri motherwort*

The source is from the whole plant of herbaceous annual or biennial *Leonurus heterophyclus* Sweet, family Labiatae. Alternate names include 茺蔚草 Chōng Wèi Cǎo and 坤草 Kūn Cǎo. Bitter and pungent in flavor and slightly cold in nature.

[Actions] Invigorate blood and regulate menstruation, and promote urination and reduce swelling. It is applicable for menstrual irregularities, dysmenorrhea, amenorrhea, persistent flow of lochia, edema with scanty urine, and hypertension. Experiments reveal its decoction and ethonal infusion have an excitatory effect on the uterus and a certain inhibitory effect against thrombus formation, and can dilute blood vessel, increase coronary artery blood flow volume, and regulate immunological function.

[Quality] Good quality is tender and grayish green, and has thin stems and many leaves without impurities. Whereas poor quality is old, withered, and yellow without leaves. Modern researches display its active ingredients are most commonly found in young stems and leaves.

[Indications]

1. Gynecological problems: owning to its feature of "activating blood without hindering generation of new blood", Yì Mǔ Cǎo (Herba Leonuri) is widely used in gynecological disorders during menstruation and childbirth and especially suitable for menstrual irregularities, amenorrhea, dysmenorrhea, postpartum static blood abdominal pain, and persistent flow of lochia. It can be used alone in a decoction or decocted extract form, or together with Dāng Guī (Radix Angelicae Sinensis), Chuān Xiōng (Rhizoma Chuanxiong), and Chì Sháo (Radix Paeoniae Rubra).

   It is also effective for red and white leucorrhea, either alone in a powder form or in a combination with other medicinals.
2. Nephritis edema: Yì Mǔ Cǎo (Herba Leonuri) can promote urination and improve renal blood flow and therefore is effective in the treatment of nephritis edema. It can be used alone or together with Fú Líng (Poria) and Chē Qián Zǐ (Semen Plantaginis). It is also capable of lowering blood pressure and thus more suitable for nephritis edema with hypertension.

According to recent reports, it has been prepared into injection to treat coronary heart disease.

[Usage and Dosage] Use raw, 10–30 g in decoction, up to 60–100 g when used alone or for nephritis, increase the amount when used fresh, and decrease the dosage in pill and powder.

[Mnemonics] Yì Mǔ Cǎo (Herba Leonuri, Motherwort): bitter and pungent; invigorate blood, regulate menstruation, promote urination, and lower blood pressure, especially for the postpartum.

[Simple and Effective Formulas]
治恶露不下方 Zhì È Lù Bù Xià Fāng — Lochia Retention Relieving Formula from *Formulas from Benevolent Sages* (圣惠方, Shèng Huì Fāng): Yì Mǔ Cǎo (Herba Leonuri); grind and make into juice and take a small cup of juice for oral administration to treat postpartum inhibited lochia and abdominal pain. Or prepared into Yì Mǔ Cǎo (Herba Leonuri) decocted extract for menstrual irregularities, dysmenorrhea, and postpartum poor uterine contraction resulting from static blood.

[Precautions] Yì Mǔ Cǎo (Herba Leonuri) is neutral in nature but it still unblocks and invigorates blood. Therefore it is contraindicated in cases of yin and blood insufficiency. Although it is known as "benefiting mother (益母, Yì Mǔ)", it should not be used for deficiency pattern during prepartum and postpartum period.

桃仁 **Táo Rén** *semen persicae peach kernel*

The source is from the dried semen of deciduous subarbor *Prunus persica* (L.) Batsch or *P. davidiana* Franch., family Rosaceae. In ancient literatures, it is called 桃核 Táo Hé. Bitter in flavor and neutral in nature.

[Actions] Invigorate blood and dispel blood stasis, moisten the intestines to unblock the bowels, and arrest coughing. It is applicable for dysmenorrhea, amenorrhea, postpartum abdominal pain, accumulation, gathering, pǐ, masses, and injuries from falls, fractures, contusions and strains associated with blood stasis. This herb is also used for constipation due to intestinal dryness and cough caused by lung yin deficiency. Modern research has shown that contains amygdalin, volatile oils, and fatty acids, and its ethanol extracting solution has antithrombogenic effect, indicating this substance can invigorate blood and dissolve stasis.

[Quality] Good quality is even in size, full, and intact.

[Indications]

1. Static blood patterns: Táo Rén (Semen Persicae), a commonly-used medicinal for static blood, is applicable for masses, pain, and dysfunction of *zang-fu* organs associated with blood stasis. It is combined with Hóng Huā (Flos Carthami), Dān Shēn (Radix et Rhizoma Salviae Miltiorrhizae), Chuān Xiōng (Rhizoma Chuanxiong), and Dāng Guī (Radix Angelicae Sinensis) for menstrual irregularities, dysmenorrhea, and amenorrhea; with Hóng Huā (Flos Carthami), Sū Mù (Lignum Sappan), and Chuān Shān Jiǎ (Squama Manitis) pieces for injuries from falls, fractures, contusions and strains. Their extractive has been successfully used in the treatment of liver fibrosis and cirrhosis in recent years.

   Táo Rén (Semen Persicae) is effective in the treatment of sores, ulcers, and carbuncle because of its property of invigorating blood, dissolving stasis, and reducing swelling. It is combined with Jīn Yín Huā (Flos Lonicerae Japonicae), Lián Qiào (Fructus Forsythiae), and Pú Gōng Yīng (Herba Taraxaci) for heat patterns of sores and ulcers; with Dōng Guā Rén (Semen Benincasae), Lú Gēn (Rhizoma Phragmitis), and Yì Yǐ Rén (Semen Coicis) for pulmonary abscess; and with Bài Jiàng Cǎo (Herba Patriniae), Dà Huáng (Radix et Rhizoma Rhei), and Mǔ Dān Pí (Cortex Moutan) for intestinal abscess (appendicites).
2. Constipation due to intestinal dryness: Oily Táo Rén (Semen Persicae) can moisten the intestines to promote defecation and is commonly combined with Bǎi Zǐ Rén (Semen Platycladi), Xìng Rén (Semen Armeniacae Amarum), and Yù Lǐ Rén (Semen Pruni).
3. Cough and wheezing: Táo Rén (Semen Persicae), capable of moistening the lung to arrest cough, is combined with Xìng Rén (Semen Armeniacae Amarum) for relieving cough and wheezing.

[Usage and Dosage] Use raw to invigorate blood, stir-fried one to moisten the intestines and promote defecation. Use 6–10 g in decoction, decrease the dosage in pill and powder.

[Mnemonics] Táo Rén (Semen Persicae, Peach Kernel): bitter and neutral; essential for dispelling blood stasis, unblock the collaterals, relieve edema, and effective for constipation.

[Simple and Effective Formulas]

1. 桃仁散 Táo Rén Sǎn — Peach Kernel Powder from *Secret Formulas of the Yang Family* (杨氏家藏方, Yáng Shì Jiā Cáng Fāng): Táo Rén (Semen Persicae) (baked), Hóng Huā (Flos Carthami), Dāng Guī (Radix Angelicae Sinensis) (washed, baked), and Dù Niú Xī (Radix Achyranthis Bidentatae) in equal dosage; make into powder and take 9 g/time with warm wine on an empty stomach for amenorrhea and vexing heat in the chest, palms and soles.

2. 桃核承气汤 Táo Hé Chéng Qì Tāng — Peach Kernel Qi-Guiding Decoction from *Treatise on Cold Damage* (伤寒论, Shāng Hán Lùn): Táo Rén 10 pieces (Semen Persicae) (peel and tip removed), Dà Huáng (Radix et Rhizoma Rhei) 10 g, Guì Zhī (Ramulus Cinnamomi) 5 g (peel removed), Gān Cǎo (Radix et Rhizoma Glycyrrhizae) (roasted) 5 g, and Máng Xiāo (Natrii Sulfas) 5 g; decoct in water for oral administration to treat blood amassment in the lower *jiao* manifested as heat accumulation in the bladder, mental agitation, and spasmodic pain in the lateral aspect of lower abdomen.

[Precautions] Táo Rén (Semen Persicae) is the medicinal that invigorate blood and thus contraindicated during pregnancy and in cases of blood deficiency.

红花 **Hóng Huā** *flos carthami safflower*

The source is from the tubular flower without ovary of herbaceous annual *Carthamus tinctorius* L., family Compositae. Alternate names include 草红花 Cǎo Hóng Huā, 杜红花 Dù Hóng Huā, 刺红花 Cì Hóng Huā, and 红蓝花 Hóng Lán Huā. Pungent in flavor and warm in nature.

[Actions] Remove blood stasis, unblock the channels, and arrest pain. It is applicable for dysmenorrhea, amenorrhea, postpartum abdominal pain, gatherings, accumulations, *pǐ*, masses, injuries from falls, fractures, contusions and strains, and swollen and painful sores and ulcers attributed to static blood. Modern research has shown that it contains carthamin, neocarthamin, and carthamone, and can increase coronary artery blood flow volume, lower blood pressure, inhibit platelet aggregation, and reinforce fibrinolysis, and excite the uterus, especially for the uterus during pregnancy.

[Quality] Good quality is dry and soft, and has long, thin, and fresh red petals without branches, leaves, and impurities. Zàng Hóng Huā (Stigma Croci, Tibetan saffron) is the stigma of herbaceous *Crocus sativus* Linn., family Iridaceae, its actions are similar to those of Hóng Huā (Flos Carthami), but much more expensive and need to be imported from other countries.

[Indications]

1. Static blood patterns: Hóng Huā (Flos Carthami), a commonly-used herb for cases of static blood, is applicable for masses, pain, and dysfunction of *zang-fu* organs associated with blood stasis. It is combined with Táo Rén (Semen Persicae), Dān Shēn (Radix et Rhizoma Salviae Miltiorrhizae), Chuān Xiōng (Rhizoma Chuanxiong), and Dāng Guī (Radix Angelicae Sinensis) for menstrual irregularities, dysmenorrhea, and amenorrhea; and with Táo Rén (Semen Persicae), Sū Mù (Lignum Sappan), and Chuān Shān Jiǎ (Squama Manitis) pieces for injuries from falls, fractures, contusions and strains. Táo Rén (Semen Persicae) and Hóng Huā (Flos Carthami) are often used together for the treatment of blood stasis. For the darkish macules and papules due to heat constraint with blood stasis in febrile diseases, Hóng Huā (Flos Carthami) is prescribed together with medicinals that clear heat and cool blood such as Zǐ Cǎo (Radix Arnebiae) and Dà Qīng Yè (Folium Isatidis).

2. Pain due to blood stasis: owing to its effectiveness of invigorating blood and dissolving stasis, Hóng Huā (Flos Carthami) is widely used in the treatment of pain caused by blood stagnation. It is combined with Sū Mù (Lignum Sappan), Chì Sháo (Radix Paeoniae Rubra), Dāng Guī (Radix Angelicae Sinensis), and Rǔ Xiāng (Olibanum) for static blood swellings and pain caused by injuries from falls, fractures, contusions and strains; with Guì Zhī (Ramulus Cinnamomi), Guā Lóu (Fructus Trichosanthis), and Dān Shēn (Radix et Rhizoma Salviae Miltiorrhizae) for chest *bì* with heart pain; and with Bái Jiè Zǐ (Semen Sinapis), Táo Rén (Semen Persicae), and Chuān Shān Jiǎ (Squama Manitis) pieces for enduring painful *bì* pattern with blood stasis.

It is prepared into tincture or oiling agent and applied topically to relieve pain, or external application of plaster to treat bedsores. This substance is also prepared into injection for intramuscular injection or intravenous drip to treat thromboangiitis, coronary heart disease, cerebral thrombosis, and sudden onset of deafness.

[Usage and Dosage] Use 3–9 g in decoction, bigger dosage to invigorate blood, 1–3 g to harmonize and nourish blood, dispel stasis, and create new blood. Therefore the ancients stated "larger dosage for breaking up blood, small dosage for nourishing blood". Adding small amount of Hóng Huā (Flos Carthami) in the formula that enriches blood is helpful for blood circulation, and it can improve the effect of blood-nourishing medicinals.

[Mnemonics] Hóng Huā (Flos Carthami, Safflower): pungent and warm; remove blood stasis, arrest pain, invigorate blood , unblock the channels, and generate the blood when used a small amount.

[Simple and Effective Formulas]
通经方 Tōng Jīng Fāng — Menstration-inducing Formula from *Doctor Zhu's Effective Medical Formulas* (朱氏集验医方, Zhū Shì Jí Yàn Yī Fāng): Hóng Huā (Flos Carthami), Sū Mù (Lignum Sappan) (pounded into pieces), and Dāng Guī (Radix Angelicae Sinensis) in equal dosage; chop up, decoct 30 g/time with Hóng Huā (Flos Carthami) and Sū Mù (Lignum Sappan) in water until boiled, add a small cup of wine and Dāng Guī (Radix Angelicae Sinensis), continue to decoct, and take warm on an empty stomach for amenorrhea.

[Precautions] Hóng Huā (Flos Carthami) is potent in invigorating blood and therefore contraindicated for patients with a tendency of bleeding. It should not be used during pregnancy as it can cause uterine stimulation.

Daily practices

1. What are the similarities and differences among Yì Mǔ Cǎo (Herba Leonuri), Táo Rén (Semen Persicac), and Hóng Huā (Flos Carthami) in terms of actions?

2. Yì Mǔ Cǎo (Herba Leonuri), Táo Rén (Semen Persicae), Hóng Huā (Flos Carthami), Chuān Xiōng (Rhizoma Chuanxiong), Rǔ Xiāng (Olibanum), Yù Jīn (Radix Curcumae), and Yán Hú Suǒ (Rhizoma Corydalis) all can invigorate blood, what are the similarities and differences among them in terms of actions and indications?

牛膝 Niú Xī *radix achyranthis bidentatae two-toothed achyranthes root*

The source is from the root of herbaceous perennial *Achyrantes bidentata* Blume and *C. officinalis* Kuan, family Amaranthaceae. Bitter and sour in flavor and neutral in nature. The herb produced in Henan is called 怀牛膝 Huái Niú Xī, and the herb produced in Sichuan, Guizhou, and Yunnan is called 川牛膝 Chuān Niú Xī.

[Actions] Tonify the liver and kidneys, strengthen the sinews and bones, remove blood stasis and unblock the channels, promote urination and relieve strangury, and induce the downward movement of fire. It is applicable for soreness and pain of the waist and knee, weakness of the sinews and bones, amenorrhea, accumulation and gathering, and ascendant hyperactivity of liver yang. 怀牛膝 Huái Niú Xī is considered more potent in supplementing the liver and kidney and strengthening the sinews and bones, while 川牛膝 Chuān Niú Xī in invigorating blood and dissolving stasis. Modern pharmacological experiments has shown that it has an inhibitory effect on experimental arthritis, a pronounced contractory effect on uterus during pregnancy, and certain antihypertensive and diuretic effects.

[Quality] Good quality is long, thin, and hard with a light yellow color.

[Indications]

1. Blood stagnation: owning to its blood-invigorating and stasis-dissolving property, Niú Xī (Radix Achyranthis Bidentatae) is widely used in disorders caused by static blood obstruction. It is combined with Táo Rén (Semen Persicae), Hóng Huā (Flos Carthami), Dāng Guī (Radix Angelicae Sinensis), and Dān Shēn (Radix et Rhizoma Salviae Miltiorrhizae) for amenorrhea, dysmenorrhea, and postpartum static

blood abdominal pain due to static blood obstruction; and with Dāng Guī (Radix Angelicae Sinensis), Chuān Xiōng (Rhizoma Chuanxiong), and Chuān Xù Duàn (Radix Dipsaci) for static blood, swelling, and pain caused by injuries from falls, fractures, contusions, and strains. It is also applicable for postpartum retention of the placenta.

2. Liver and kidney deficiency: owning to its property of supplementing the liver and kidney and strengthening the sinews and bones, Niú Xī (Radix Achyranthis Bidentatae) is often prescribed together with Shú Dì Huáng (Radix Rehmanniae Praeparata), Dù Zhòng (Cortex Eucommiae), Chuān Xù Duàn (Radix Dipsaci) for liver and kidney deficiency manifested as soreness and pain in the waist and knee, lack of strength in the lower limbs, and vertigo; and with Dú Huó (Radix Angelicae Pubescentis), Sāng Jì Shēng (Herba Taxilli), and Qín Jiāo (Radix Gentianae Macrophyllae) for atrophy and weakness of the sinews and bones resulting from prolonged *bì* pattern.

3. Damp-heat pouring downward: Niú Xī (Radix Achyranthis Bidentatae) is descending in nature and commonly used for damp-heat pouring downward or damp-heat in the lower part of the body. It is combined with Chē Qián Zǐ (Semen Plantaginis), Huáng Bǎi (Cortex Phellodendri Chinensis), and Cāng Zhú (Rhizoma Atractylodis) for foot atrophy and weakness with redness, swelling and pain resulting from damp-heat pouring downward; and with Dōng Kuí Zǐ (Fructus Malvae), Huá Shí (Talcum), Qú Mài (Herba Dianthi), and Zhī Zǐ (Fructus Gardeniae) for strangury and difficult and painful urination with blood or sandy stone in urine caused by damp-heat accumulation in the bladder.

4. Pathogenic fire flaming upward: owning to its descending nature, Niú Xī (Radix Achyranthis Bidentatae) is commonly used for the disorders in the head, face, mouth, and tongue caused by pathogenic fire flaming upward or hemorrhagic disorders in the upper part of the body. It is used together with Dài Zhě Shí (Haematitum), Mǔ Lì (Concha Ostreae), and Bái Sháo (Radix Paeoniae Alba) to relieve headache and vertigo caused by ascendant hyperactivity of liver yang through calming the liver and subduing yang; with Dì Huáng (Radix Rehmanniae), Shí Gāo (Gypsum Fibrosum), and Zhī Mǔ (Rhizoma Anemarrhenae) to treat ulcers in the mouth and tongue and swollen, painful, and bleeding gum due to upward reversal of stomach fire by clearing the stomach and

subduing fire; and with Bái Máo Gēn (Rhizoma Imperatae), Zhī Zǐ (Fructus Gardeniae), and Dài Zhě Shí (Haematitum) to arrest hematemesis and epistaxis attributed to ascending counterflow of qi and fire and frenetic movement of blood via subduing fire and stanching bleeding.

Pounding raw Niú Xī (Radix Achyranthis Bidentatae) and applying externally can relieve pain of traumatic wound and injury.

[Usage and Dosage] Use raw to invigorate blood, dissolve stasis and direct medicinals go downward; wine-processed one to supplement the liver and kidney, harmonize blood, and regulate menstruation. Use 6–10 g in decoction, double the dosage when used alone or for retention of the placenta, and decrease the amount as in pill and powder.

[Mnemonics] Niú Xī (Radix Achyranthis Bidentatae, Two-toothed Achyranthes Root): bitter and sour; invigorate blood; 川牛膝 Chuān Niú Xī is more effective to drain, 怀牛膝 Huái Niú Xī to tonify, but both pertain to induce the downward movement.

[Simple and Effective Formulas]

1. 下胞衣方 Xià Bāo Yī Fāng — Placenta Retention-inducing Formula from *Doctor Mei's Effective Medical Formulas* (梅师集验方, Méi Shī Jí Yàn Fāng): Niú Xī (Radix Achyranthis Bidentatae) 240 g and Dōng Kuí Zǐ (Fructus Malvae) 30 g; decoct into 1500 ml water until only 500 ml left, divide into three equal doses, and take one dose/time for oral administration for postpartum retention of the placenta.
2. 鹤膝风方 Hè Xī Fēng Fāng — Knee Joint Tuberculosis Relieving Formula from *Treasury of Words on the Materia Medica* (本草汇言, Běn Cǎo Huì Yán): Niú Xī (Radix Achyranthis Bidentatae), Mù Guā (Fructus Chaenomelis), Wǔ Jiā Pí (Cortex Acanthopanacis), Gǔ Suì Bǔ (Rhizoma Drynariae), Jīn Yín Huā (Flos Lonicerae Japonicae), Zǐ Huā Dì Dīng (Herba Violae), Huáng Bǎi (Cortex Phellodendri Chinensis), Bì Xiè (Rhizoma Dioscoreae Hypoglaucae), and Gān Jú Gēn (Radix Cancrinia Discoidea); decoct in water for oral administration to treat tuberculosis of knee joint.

[Precautions] Niú Xī (Radix Achyranthis Bidentatae) can supplement the liver and kidney, however, it is descending in nature. It is contraindicated in cases of seminal emission, urinary incontinence and profuse menstruation associated with kidney deficiency, diarrhea, prolapse of anus, prolapse of the uterus, and also during pregnancy due to its hastening of parturition effect.

五灵脂 **Wǔ Líng Zhī** *faeces trogopterori flying squirrel feces*

The source is from the dry feces of *Trogopterus xanthipes* Milne-Edward, family Petauristidae. Alternate names include 寒号虫粪 Hán Hào Chóng Fèn. Bitter and sweet in flavor and warm in nature.

[Actions] Invigorate blood, disperse blood stasis, arrest pain, stop bleeding, and relieve toxin. It is applicable for internal obstruction of static blood manifested as chest, rib-side, gastric and abdominal stabbing pain, dysmenorrhea, amenorrhea, postpartum blood stasis with abdominal pain, and swelling and pain due to injuries from falls, fractures, contusions and strains.

[Quality] It has been devided by shape into 灵脂米 Líng Zhī Mǐ (散灵脂 Sàn Líng Zhī) and 灵脂块 Líng Zhī Kuài (糖灵脂 Táng Líng Zhī). For the former, good quality is coarse, blackish brown outside, yellowish green inside, lightweight, and without impurities; whereas the latter is a chunk of dry feces, good quality is clumped, blackish-brown, shiny, oily, moist, and without impurities. The latter is better than former.

[Indications]

1. Pain caused by blood stagnation: Wǔ Líng Zhī (Faeces Trogopterori), capable of invigorating blood and dissolving stasis, is often combined with other medicinals for pain caused by static blood obstruction. It is always combined with Pú Huáng (Pollen Typhae) for stomachache, chest pain, abdominal pain, and dysmenorrheal caused by static blood; and with Yán Hú Suǒ (Rhizoma Corydalis), Rǔ Xiāng (Olibanum), and Mò Yào (Myrrha) to relieve qi stagnation and blood stasis through moving qi and invigorating blood.

2. Static blood with bleeding: Wǔ Líng Zhī (Faeces Trogopterori) can invigorate blood and also dissolve stasis and stanch bleeding. It is featured by stanching bleeding without retaining blood stasis for hemorrhagic disorders and therefore particularly suitable in the cases of static blood with bleeding. It is usually combined with medicinals that dissolve stasis and stanch bleeding such as Sān Qī (Radix et Rhizoma Notoginseng) and Pú Huáng (Pollen Typhae).

It is prescribed together with Xiǎo Huí Xiāng (Fructus Foeniculi) and Rǔ Xiāng (Olibanum) for external application to relieve pain caused by fracture and injury; or ground with Xióng Huáng (Realgar) into powder for either oral administration or external application to treat poisonous bites of snake, scorpio, and scolopendra.

[Usage and Dosage] Use raw to invigorate blood, dissolve stasis, and arrest pain, stir-fried to stop bleeding. Stir-frying with vinegar is to reduce its gamey smell and enhance its stasis-dissolving and bleeding-stanching properties, and stir-frying with wine is to improve its ability of invigorating blood and arresting pain. Use 4–9 g in decoction, decrease the dosage as in pill and powder.

[Mnemonics] Wǔ Líng Zhī (Faeces Trogopterori, Flying Squirrel Faeces): bitter and sweet; disperse blood stasis, arrest pain and bleeding, and relieve toxin.

[Simple and Effective Formulas]

1. 灵脂散 Líng Zhī Sǎn — Flying Squirrel Faeces Powder from *Yong Lei Qian Formulas* (永类钤方 Yǒng Lèi Qián Fāng): Wǔ Líng Zhī (Faeces Trogopterori) (grind into fine powder, stir-fried until smoked); grind into powder and take 3 g/time with warm wine for oral administration to treat various kinds of pain due to blood stasis, profuse uterine bleeding with pain, and chest, gastric, rid-side, and abdominal pain.

2. 治吐血方 Zhì Tù Xiě Fāng — Hematemesis Arresting Formula from *The Grand Compendium of Materia Medica* (本草纲目 Běn Cǎo Gāng Mù): Wǔ Líng Zhī (Faeces Trogopterori) 30 g and Huáng Qí (Radix

Astragali) 15 g; grind into powder and take with cool boiled water for oral administration to treat persistent hematemesis.

[Precautions] Wǔ Líng Zhī (Faeces Trogopterori) is effective in invigorating blood and therefore contraindicated in cases of blood deficiency and during pregnancy. According to "nineteen incompatibilities", this herb was traditionally considered to be antagonized by Rén Shēn (Radix et Rhizoma Ginseng). But clinically, these two herbs are often combined in prescriptions for qi deficiency and blood stasis and no adverse reactions have been reported.

三棱 Sān Léng *rhizoma sparganii common burr reed tuber*

[Addendum] 莪术 É Zhú Rhizoma Curcumae Curcumae Rhizome
The source is from the tuberous rhizome of herbaceous perennial *Sparganium stoloniferum* Buch. Ham., family Sparganiaceae. It is so called as its leaf has three ridges and alternate names include 京三棱 Jīng Sān Léng and 三棱草 Sān Léng Cǎo. Bitter in flavor and neutral in nature.

[Actions] Break up blood and expel stasis, move qi to alleviate pain, and dissolve accumulation and reduce food stagnation. It is applicable for amenorrhea, abdominal pain, accumulations, gatherings, *pǐ*, masses, and food accumulation attributed to qi stagnation and blood stasis.

[Quality] Good quality is dry, even-sized, heavy, solid, and yellowish white with a light grayish-yellow cross section and without cuticle. 荆三棱 Jīng Sān Léng is from the tuber of herbaceous *Scirpus planiculmis* Fr. Schmidt, family Cyperaceae.

[Indications]

1. Qi stagnation and blood stasis: Sān Léng (Rhizoma Sparganii) is very effective in invigorating blood, also known as blood-breaking up medicinal (破血药, Pò Xiě Yào). It can also move qi and commonly prescribed together with medicinals that dissolve stasis and move qi such as Rǔ Xiāng (Olibanum), Mò Yào (Myrrha), and Yán Hú Suǒ

(Rhizoma Corydalis) for accumulations, gatherings, *pǐ*, masses, chest and abdominal pain, and chest and rib-side distending pain caused by qi stagnation and blood stasis.

2. Food accumulation: Sān Léng (Rhizoma Sparganii) can promote digestion and remove accumulation, and is combined with medicinals that remove food accumulation and move qi such as Shān Zhā (Fructus Crataegi), Mài Yá (Fructus Hordei Germinatus), and Qīng Pí (Pericarpium Citri Reticulatae Viride) for gastric and abdominal distention, oppression, and pain resulting from food accumulation.

[Usage and Dosage] Use raw in most cases, stir-fry with vinegar to enhance its pain-arresting property.

[Mnemonics] Sān Léng (Rhizoma Sparganii, Common Burr Reed Tuber): bitter and neutral; break up blood stasis, move qi, dissolve accumulation, and reduce food stagnation.

[Simple and Effective Formulas]
三棱煎丸 Sān Léng Jiān Wán — Common Burr Reed Tuber Pill from *Formulas to Aid the Living* (济生方, Jì Shēng Fāng): Jīng Sān Léng (Rhizoma Sparganii), Péng É Zhú (Rhizoma Curcumae) 60 g, Yuán Huā (Flos Genkwa) 15 g, Qīng Pí (Pericarpium Citri Reticulatae Viride) (pulp removed) 45 g; file into fine powder, decoct into vinegar 500 ml, bake into fine powder, make into phoenix tree seed-sized pill with vinegar, and take 50 pills/time with light vinegar soup for oral administration to treat amenorrhea and intractable masses located below the navel.

[Precautions] Sān Léng (Rhizoma Sparganii), potent in breaking up blood stagnation and relieving masses, can easily consume healthy qi and therefore should be used with caution for patients with weak constitution. It is contraindicated during pregnancy and in cases of amenorrhea due to blood deficiency.

[Addendum] 莪术 É Zhú Rhizoma Curcumae Curcumae Rhizome
The source is from the rhizome of herbaceous perennial *Curcuma Kwangsinensis* S. G. Lee et C.F. Liang, *C. aromatica* Salisb. and *C. zedoaria* Rosc., family Zingiberaceae. Alternate names include 蓬莪术 Péng É Zhú and 蓬莪茂 Péng É Mào. It, bitter and pungent in flavor and

warm in nature, can move qi, break up blood stasis, resolve accumulation, and arrest pain. It is applicable for accumulations, gatherings, *pǐ*, masses, amenorrhea due to static blood, food accumulation, and abdominal distention. Sān Léng (Rhizoma Sparganii) and É Zhú (Rhizoma Curcumae), both capable of breaking up and removing blood stasis, are similar in terms of actions, indications, usage, dosage, and precautions, and usually prescribed together. There do exist, however, distinctions between the two: the former is more potent in breaking up blood obstruction, the latter is moving qi.

This herb should be yellowish white and slightly granular in cross-section, aromatic, acrid, and slightly bitter; yellowish brown to dark brown with many clear vessels in cross section, very aromatic and bitter and slightly spicy; or grayish yellowish or yellowish brown, shiny, aromatic, slightly bitter and acrid. In all cases good quality is solid, firm and aromatic.

Daily practices

1. What are the similarities and differences among Niú Xī (Radix Achyranthis Bidentatae), Wǔ Líng Zhī (Faeces Trogopterori), and Sān Léng (Rhizoma Sparganii) in terms of actions and indications?
2. What are these medicinal capable of invigorating blood and moving qi, among them which ones are considered more potent in invigorating blood and which are more effective in moving qi ?
3. Among medicinals that stanch bleeding and medicinals that invigorate blood, which ones can not only invigorate blood but also stanch bleeding?

CHAPTER 10

Tenth Week

1

MEDICINALS THAT DISSOLVE PHLEGM

Phlegm-dissolving herbs are primarily used for removing phlegm and turbidity.

In traditional Chinese medicine, the term "phlegm" refers to the pathological accumulation caused by disturbance of water metabolism. It is also important to know that phlegm can turn into a new pathogenic factor to cause diverse set of disorders. Physiologically, production and circulation of body fluid are based on the normal function of such *zang-fu* organs as the lung, spleen, kidney, and *sanjiao*, dysfunction of any organs may cause fluid retention and generate phlegm. However, the term "phlegm" in traditional Chinese medicine is not limited to the presence of sputum but also intangible phlegm that is often implicated in such disorder as vertigo, dizzy vision, palpitations, vomiting, chest and gastric *pǐ* and fullness, disturbance of consciousness, delirious speech, masses, greasy tongue coating, and slippery pulse.

Phlegm disorder is featured by widely-affected sites involving *zang-fu* organs, sinews, bones, skins, and muscles, complicated state of illness, and subsequent pathological changes of *zang-fu* organ and extremities. Phlegm accumulation in the lung may cause coughing and wheezing with profuse sputum; phlegm confounding the heart orifice may cause absence of consciousness; phlegm obstructing the liver may cause vertigo, dizzy vision, or even spasm; phlegm stagnation in the chest may cause chest oppression and labored breathing; phlegm blockage in the channels and collaterals may cause various disorders like numbness of the limbs, hemiplegia, and deviated mouth and eyes; phlegm obstruction in the throat

350

may generate a blocking feeling in the throat that cannot be spit out or swallowed; phlegm gathering subcutaneously may cause nodules and masses; phlegm flowing into the joint may cause pain of the limbs and joint deformation; and phlegm stagnated in the bone and muscle may cause yin-type carbuncle or fistula with pus. Phlegm can be further divided by nature into cold-, heat-, dry-, and damp-type. It is not unusual that phlegm is complicated by other pathogens like static blood and food accumulation, therefore the selection and combination of herbs for phlegm disorder is based on the site and nature of the phlegm and concurrent pathogens.

Clinically, it is important to treat the underlying conditions that generate phlegm and pay more attention to regulate functions of *zang-fu* organs. Smooth qi movement is of great significance to dissolve phlegm. Combination of herbs is based on the state of illness. For instance, herbs that warm yang are also used for cold phlegm; heat-clearing herbs are added for heat-phlegm; herbs that moisten drying are included in the prescription for dry-phlegm; herbs that leech out dampness and disinhibit water are also used for damp-phlegm; herbs that supplement the spleen are also applied for spleen deficiency generating phlegm; herbs that diffuse and descend lung qi are also used for phlegm accumulation in the lung. Phlegm-dissolving herbs should be used in conjunction with stasis-dissolving and food accumulation-removing herbs for the secondary pathogenesis of static blood and food accumulation.

Phlegm-dissolving medicinals act on dispelling pathogens, if applied inappropriately, it can injure healthy qi of human body. For this reason, it should be used with caution. In cases of healthy qi deficiency with accompanying phlegm, treatment plan is based on both reinforcing healthy qi and dispelling pathogens.

半夏 Bàn Xià *rhizoma pinelliae pinellia rhizome*

The source is from the tuber of herbaceous perennial *Pinellia ternata* (Thunb.) Breit, family Araceae. It is so called because it grows in May, the middle (*Bàn,* 半) of summer (*Xià,* 夏). Alternate names include 野芋头 Yě Yù Tou, 蝎子草 Xiē Zǐ Cǎo, and 地文 Dì Wén. Pungent in flavor and warm in nature with toxicity.

[Actions] Dry dampness and dissolve phlegm, direct counterflow downward to relieve vomiting, and disperse *pǐ* and dissipate masses. It is applicable for cough and wheezing with profuse sputum, wind-phlegm vertigo and dizziness, phlegm-obstruction headache, vomiting and nausea, chest and gastric *pǐ* and oppression, plum-pit qi (globus hystericus). It also can reduce swelling and resolve toxins when applied externally. Modern pharmacological experiments reveal it has certain antibechic, glandular secretion-inhibitory, antanacathartic, anti-pregnant, and anti-cancer effects.

[Quality] Good quality is large, white, solid, powdery and without peels. Shēng Bàn Xià (Rhizoma Pinelliae) is heavily toxic, it is then called 清半夏 Qīng Xàn Xià after being prepared with Míng Fán (Alumen), called 姜半夏 Jiāng Bàn Xià after being prepared with Shēng Jiāng (Rhizoma Zingiberis Recens) and Míng Fán (Alumen), and called 法半夏 Fǎ Bàn Xià after being processed with Míng Fán (Alumen), Gān Cǎo (Radix et Rhizoma Glycyrrhizae), and calcarea. 水半夏 Shuǐ Bàn Xià is also available in the market, but it is different from Bàn Xià (Rhizoma Pinelliae) in terms of actions, and can not be used as a substitute.

[Indications]

1. Damp-phlegm patterns: Bàn Xià (Rhizoma Pinelliae), a principal medicinal of dissolving phlegm, is effective on disorders caused by different types of phlegm. It is warm and dry in nature and therefore particularly suitable for patient with damp-phlegm. It is combined with Chén Pí (Pericarpium Citri Reticulatae) and Fú Líng (Poria) for cough and wheezing with profuse thick sputum caused by damp-phlegm accumulation in the lung; and with Bái Zhú (Rhizoma Atractylodis Macrocephalae), Tiān Má (Rhizoma Gastrodiae), Zé Xiè (Rhizoma Alismatis), and Fú Líng (Poria) for vertigo and tinnitus due to damp-phlegm clouding clear yang.

2. Binding of phlegm and qi pattern: stagnated qi movement is one of the major causes for phlegm generation, phlegm will in turn stagnate qi movement further, eventually phlegm and qi bind together. Bàn Xià (Rhizoma Pinelliae), pungent and dispersing, is capable of regulating qi and also dissolving phlegm. It is combined with Gān Jiāng (Rhizoma Zingiberis), Huáng Lián (Rhizoma Coptidis), and Huáng Qín (Radix

Scutellariae) for gastric *pǐ* and fullness associated with phlegm and qi binding below the heart via opening with pungency and descending with bitterness; and with Hòu Pò (Cortex Magnoliae Officinalis), Zǐ Sū Yè (Folium Perillae), and Fú Líng (Poria) for "plum-pit qi (globus hystericus)" defined by the sensation as if something were stuck in the throat, which can neither be spit up or swallowed down due to phlegm and qi obstructing in the throat.

3. Vomiting and nausea: Bàn Xià (Rhizoma Pinelliae), known as a principal medicinal to arrest vomiting, is effective on vomiting due to a variety of causes in a combination with other medicinals. It is prescribed together with Shēng Jiāng (Rhizoma Zingiberis Recens) and Fú Líng (Poria) for vomiting caused by cold or phlegm-damp invading the stomach; with Huáng Lián (Rhizoma Coptidis) and Zhú Rú (Caulis Bambusae in Taenia) for stomach heat vomiting; with Mài Dōng (Radix Ophiopogonis) and Shí Hú (Caulis Dendrobii) for vomiting due to stomach yin insufficiency; with Rén Shēn (Radix et Rhizoma Ginseng) and Bái Mì (Mel) for vomiting attributed to stomach deficiency failing to receive; and with Zǐ Sū Yè (Folium Perillae), Zào Xīn Tǔ (Terra Flava Usta), Zhú Rú (Caulis Bambusae in Taenia) and medicinals that calm the fetus for vomiting during pregnancy.

4. Carbuncles, deep-rooted ulcers, swellings, and toxins: external application of Bàn Xià (Rhizoma Pinelliae) can reduce swelling and resolve toxins, and therefore is applicable for early stage of carbuncles, sores, and ulcers with localized redness, swelling, and pain, and poisonous snake and insect bites. In those cases, the powder of raw Bàn Xià (Rhizoma Pinelliae) or the ground fresh Bàn Xià (Rhizoma Pinelliae) can be applied externally.

[Usage and Dosage] Due to its toxicity, Shēng Bàn Xià (Rhizoma Pinelliae) is rarely used for oral administration and more commonly used as external application. Qīng Bàn Xià (Rhizoma Pinelliae Concisum), less acrid and dry in nature after processing, is applicable for the weak with profuse phlegm; Jiāng Bàn Xià (Rhizoma Pinelliae Praeparatum), low in toxicity, is potent in drying dampness, removing phlegm, unblocking with pungency, and reliving vomiting, and therefore applicable for cases of cold-phlegm and vomiting; and Fǎ Bàn Xià (Rhizoma Pinelliae Praeparatum) is considered more effective in dissolving phlegm and suitable for cases of profuse phlegm. Use 5–10 g in decoction, decrease to less than 1 g when use Shēng Bàn Xià (Rhizoma Pinelliae). Use with caution when special usage is required. Should be decocted for a long time. Reduce the amount in pill and powder.

[Mnemonics] Bàn Xià (Rhizoma Pinelliae, Pinellia Rhizome): pungent and warm; use with caution as it is toxic; specialized in relieving vomiting and resolving phlegm.

[Simple and Effective Formulas]

1. 小半夏汤 Xiǎo Bàn Xià Tāng — Minor Pinellia Rhizome Decoction from *Essentials from the Golden Cabinet* (金匮要略, Jīn Guì Yào Lüè): Bàn Xià (Rhizoma Pinelliae) 10 g and Shēng Jiāng (Rhizoma Zingiberis Recens) 5 g; decoct in water for oral administration to treat thoracic rheum below the heart with vomiting. Also applicable for vomiting caused by different types of gastritis.
2. 半夏散 Bàn Xià Sǎn — Pinellia Rhizome Powder from *Treatise on Cold Damage* (伤寒论, Shāng Hán Lùn): Bàn Xià (Rhizoma Pinelliae) (washed), Guì Zhī (Ramulus Cinnamomi) (peel removed), and Gān Cǎo (Radix et Rhizoma Glycyrrhizae) (roasted) in equal dosage; grind into fine powder and take 4 g/time with boiled water for oral administration to treat *shaoyin* disease with painful throat. Also applicable for swollen and painful throat due to deficiency-heat flaming upward.

[Precautions] Bàn Xià (Rhizoma Pinelliae), warm in nature, may damage yin fluid when misused and therefore should be used cautiously in cases of yin fluid insufficiency. According to traditional literature, it is contraindicated during pregnancy, but no adverse reaction has been reported when used for vomiting during pregnancy. According to "eighteen antagonisms", it is incompatible with Wū Tóu (Aconite Main Tuber), but still needs modern experiment proof.

Taking an overdose of raw Bàn Xià (Rhizoma Pinelliae) can cause poisoning symptoms such as sense of burning, pungency, and numbness of oral and throat mucosa, gastric discomfort, chest compression, even suffocation and numbness of limbs in serious cases.

天南星 Tiān Nán Xīng *rhizoma arisaematis jackinthepulpit tuber*

The source is from the tuber of herbaceous perennial *Arisaema Consanguineum* Schott, *Arisaema amurense* Maxim., or *Arisaema heterophyllum* Bl., family Araceae. Alternate names include 虎掌 Hǔ Zhǎng (its leaf looks like the palms of tiger), and 南星 Nán Xīng (its round and white root looks like the god of longevity living in South Mountain-Nán Shān). Bitter and pungent in flavor and warm in nature with toxicity.

[Actions] Dry dampness and dissolve phlegm, and dispel wind and arrest convulsion. It is applicable for cough due to remnant phlegm, chest and diaphragm distention and oppression, wind-phlegm vertigo, wind-stroke phlegm exuberance, depressive psychosis, and tetanus. External application of 生南星 Shēng Nán Xīng can reduce swelling and relieve pain to treat carbuncles, deep-rooted ulcers, and phlegm node. Modern experiments have indicated this substance and its preparation have certain anticonvulsant, antalgic, analgesic, expectorant, and antitumor effects.

[Quality] Good quality is dry, white, solid, powdery and with lateral sprouts. It is seldom used in raw form and generally prepared with Shēng Jiāng (Rhizoma Zingiberis Recens) and Míng Fán (Alumen), which are then called as 制南星 Zhì Nán Xīng. Also prepared with bile of pig or caw and called 胆南星 Dǎn Nán Xīng.

[Indications]

1. Damp-phlegm patterns: Tiān Nán Xīng (Rhizoma Arisaematis), warm and dry in nature, is commonly used for damp-phlegm obstruction with stagnated qi movement. Its actions are similar to that of Bàn Xià (Rhizoma Pinelliae) and they are usually used together. It is combined with Bàn Xià (Rhizoma Pinelliae), Chén Pí (Pericarpium Citri Reticulatae), and Zhǐ Shí (Fructus Aurantii Immaturus) for cough with profuse sputum caused by damp-phlegm obstruction in the lung; and with medicinals that clear heat such as Dǎn Nán Xīng (Arisaema cum Bile) and Huáng Qín (Radix Scutellariae) for phlegm heat pattern.

2. Wind-phlegm: wind-phlegm is defined by wind pathogen binding with phlegm obstructs in the *zang-fu* organs or the channels and collaterals. Tiān Nán Xīng (Rhizoma Arisaematis) is combined with Bàn Xià (Rhizoma Pinelliae), Tiān Má (Rhizoma Gastrodiae) for most commonly-occurred headache and vertigo caused by wind-phlegm harassing the upper part of the body; with Bàn Xià (Rhizoma Pinelliae), Bái Jiāng Cán (Bombyx Batryticatus), and Bái Fù Zǐ (Rhizoma Typhonii) for numbness of hands and feet, hemiplegia, deviated eyes and mouth resulting from wind-phlegm obstruction in the channels and collaterals; and with Shí Chāng Pú (Rhizoma Acori Tatarinowii), Míng Fán (Alumen), and Shè Xiāng (Moschus) for mental disturbance or epilepsy attributed to wind-phlegm obstructing in the heart orifices.
3. Carbuncles, deep-rooted ulcers, swellings, and toxins: owing to its pungent and dispersing nature and swelling-reducing effect, Tiān Nán Xīng (Rhizoma Arisaematis) can be applied externally to treat carbuncles, deep-rooted ulcers, swellings, and toxins. The raw substance can be ground into powder and mixed with vinegar for external application to treat carbuncles, deep-rooted ulcers, phlegm node, or poisonous snake bites.

In recent years, it has been used to treat tumors with certain therapeutic effects. It has been prepared into tincture, suppository, topical agents, or injection for topical application to cure cervical cancer. Soaking its powder into vinegar and using the medical liquid for external application can treat parotitis.

[Usage and Dosage] The raw substance has a relatively high toxicity, and 制南星 Zhì Nán Xīng is preferred and potent in dispelling wind, dissolving phlegm, unblocking the collaterals, and relieving convulsions. 胆南星 Dǎn Nán Xīng, the least dry and violent and relatively cool in nature, is particularly suitable for cases of phlegm-heat or wind-phlegm. Use 3–6 g in decoction, increase the dosage but less than maximum 15 g when used in the treatment of tumors.

[Mnemonics] Tiān Nán Xīng (Rhizoma Arisaematis, Jackinthepulpit Tuber): pungent and bitter; dissolve phlegm, unblock the collaterals, arrest convulsion, relieve swelling, and applicable externally and internally.

[Simple and Effective Formulas]

1. 三生饮 Sān Shēng Yǐn — Life Saving Beverage from *Formulas from the Imperial Pharmacy* (局方, Jú Fāng): Shēng Nán Xīng (Rhizoma Arisaematis) 30 g, Mù Xiāng (Radix Aucklandiae) 0.3 g, raw Chuān Wū (Radix Aconiti) (peel removed) 3 g, and raw Fù Zǐ (Radix Aconiti Lateralis Praeparata) (peel removed) 15 g; grind into fine powder, decoct 15 g/time with 15 pieces of Shēng Jiāng (Rhizoma Zingiberis Recens) in water for oral administration to treat post-stroke hemiplegia, deviated eyes and mouth, and phlegm accumulation in the throat.
2. 天南星膏 Tiān Nán Xīng Gāo — Jackinthepulpit Tuber Decocted Extract from *Secret Formulas of the Yang Family* (杨氏家藏方, Yáng Shì Jiā Cáng Fāng): Tiān Nán Xīng (Rhizoma Arisaematis); grind into fine powder, mix with Shēng Jiāng (Rhizoma Zingiberis Recens) juice, spread on a piece of paper, and apply externally to the affected areas for deviated eyes and mouth caused by facial nerve paralysis.

[Precautions] Tiān Nán Xīng (Rhizoma Arisaematis), warm and dry in nature, should be used cautiously by patients with yin deficiency. It should also be applied cautiously in clinic for its toxicity, particularly, the raw plant may cause serious irritation manifested as oral mucosa erosion and necrosis. Overdose use will present such poisoning symptoms swollen tongue, mouth, and lips, saliva, mouth and tongue numbness, hoarseness, and difficult in opening mouth. Long-term use is discouraged as this substance is toxic to the liver. It is also contraindicated to patients with liver diseases and during pregnancy.

Daily practices

1. What are the causes for phlegm generation? What are the characteristics of phlegm diseases? What precautions should be taken when treating phlegm diseases?
2. What are the similarities and differences between Bàn Xià (Rhizoma Pinelliae) and Tiān Nán Xīng (Rhizoma Arisaematis) in terms of actions and indications? What precautions should be taken when using them?

白附子 **Bái Fù Zǐ** *rhizoma typhonii typhonium rhizome*

The source is from the tuber of herbaceous perennial *Typhonium giganteum* Engl., family Araceae. It is so called as it is white and looks like Fù Zǐ (Radix Aconiti Lateralis Praeparata) and alternate names include 禹白附 Yǔ Bái Fù and 鸡心白附 Jī Xīn Bái Fù. It is known as 关白附 Guān Bái Fù and 竹节白附 Zhú Jié Bái Fù when the tuberous root of herbaceous perennial *Aconitum coreanum* (Lévl.) Rapaics, family Ranunculaceae. Acrid and sweet in flavor, and warm nature with toxicity.

[Actions] Dry dampness and dissolve phlegm, dispel wind and arrest convulsion, and resolve toxins and dissipate masses. It is applicable for wind-phlegm exuberance, deviated eyes and mouth, tetanus, migraine, scrofula, and venomous snake bites. 禹白附 Yǔ Bái Fù and 关白附 Guān Bái Fù are similar in actions, but the former is more potent in resolving toxins and dispersing masses and thus more suitable for scrofula and venomous snake bite, whereas the latter can arrest pain.

[Quality] Good quality is large, white, firm, and powdery. It is commonly prepared with Míng Fán (Alumen), Shēng Jiāng (Rhizoma Zingiberis Recens), and known as 制白附子 Zhì Bái Fù Zǐ. Bái Fù Zǐ (Rhizoma Typhonii) mainly refers to 关白附 Guān Bái Fù in ancient literatures, but nowadays 禹白附 Yǔ Bái Fù is most commonly used in the clinic.

[Indications]

1. Wind-phlegm in the upper part of the body: manifestations include chronic headache and vertigo, heaviness of the head, and greasy tongue coating. Due to its dry, ascending, and pain-relieving property, Bái Fù Zǐ (Rhizoma Typhonii) is commonly combined with Bàn Xià (Rhizoma Pinelliae), Tiān Nán Xīng (Rhizoma Arisaematis), and Bái Zhǐ (Radix Angelicae Dahuricae).

2. Wind-phlegm convulsive syncope: Bái Fù Zǐ (Rhizoma Typhonii) is often combined with Quán Xiē (Scorpio), Bái Jiāng Cán (Bombyx Batryticatus), and Dì Lóng (Pheretima) for either deviated eyes and mouth and pain throughout the body caused by wind-phlegm obstructing in the channels and collaterals, or convulsive syncope attributed to wind-phlegm entering the liver channel; and with Fáng Fēng (Radix

Saposhnikoviae), Tiān Má (Rhizoma Gastrodiae), and Tiān Nán Xīng (Rhizoma Arisaematis) for tetanus with opisthotonos and locked jaw.

3. Scrofula, carbuncles and deep-rooted ulcers: Bái Fù Zǐ (Rhizoma Typhonii), capable of reducing swelling and dissipating masses, is applicable for carbuncles, deep-rooted ulcer, phlegm node, and scrofula. It can also be applied externally and ground into juice for oral administration to treat poisonous snake bites.

[Usage and Dosage] 生白附子 Shēng Bái Fù Zǐ is often used for external application, while 制白附子 Zhì Bái Fù Zǐ for oral administration. Use 3–5 g in decoction, and 0.1–1 g/time in pill and powder.

[Mnemonics] Bái Fù Zǐ (Rhizoma Typhonii, Typhonium Rhizome): warm and pungent; dissolve phlegm, arrest convulsion, and specialized in relieving pain and dissipating masses.

[Simple and Effective Formulas]

1. 牵正散 Qiān Zhèng Sǎn — Symmetry Correcting Powder from *Secret Formulas of the Yang Family* (杨氏家藏方, Yáng Shì Jiā Cáng Fāng): Bái Fù Zǐ (Rhizoma Typhonii), Bái Jiāng Cán (Bombyx Batryticatus), and Quán Xiē (Scorpio) (detoxicated) in equal dosage; use raw, grind into fine powder, and take 3 g/time with warm wine, three times a day for post-stroke deviated eyes and mouth and hemiplegia.

2. 白附散 Bái Fù Sǎn — Typhonium Rhizome Powder from *An Elucidation of Formulas for Children's Health* (小儿卫生总微论方, Xiǎo' Ér Wèi Shēng Zǒng Wēi Lùn Fāng): Bái Fù Zǐ (Rhizoma Typhonii) and Huò Xiāng (Herba Agastachis) leaf in equal dosage; grind into fine powder and 1.5–3 g/time with rice soup for pediatric vomiting and asthma.

[Precautions] Bái Fù Zǐ (Rhizoma Typhonii), warm and dry in nature, can easily consume qi and blood and therefore is contraindicated in dizziness, headache and convulsion caused by blood deficiency generating wind or excessive heat generating wind. Attentions should be paid to the usage and dosage for it is toxic.

白芥子 Bái Jiè Zǐ *semen sinapis white mustard seed*

It is from the semen of herbaceous annual or biennial *Brassica alba* (L.) Boiss, family Cruciferae. Alternate names include 辣菜子 Là Cài Zǐ. Pungent in flavor and warm in nature.

[Actions] Dissolve phlegm and free qi movement, and alleviate swelling and dissipate masses. It is considered good at dispersing phlegm and effective in treating the phlegm no matter where it lodges. This herb is applicable for cough and wheezing with chest and rib-side pain caused by internal obstruction of phlegm-rheum, masses due to phlegm accumulation in the channels and collaterals, and yin flat-abscess.

[Quality] Good quality is large, round, full, white, and purified.

[Indications]

1. Internal obstruction of phlegm-rheum: Bái Jiè Zǐ (Semen Sinapis), warm in nature and pungent in flavor, is capable of warming, dispersing, unblocking, and moving qi and most appropriate for disorders caused by cold-phlegm. It is combined with Lái Fú Zǐ (Semen Raphani) and Sū Zǐ (Fructus Perillae) for cough and wheezing with profuse sputum, and chest oppression caused by cold-phlegm congestion in the lung; with Gān Suì (Radix Kansui) and Jīng Dà Jǐ (Radix Euphorbiae Pekinensis) for chest and rib-side pain and hydrothorax due to phlegm rheum retention in the chest and rib-side. This substance can be ground with Yán Hú Suǒ (Rhizoma Corydalis), Gān Suì (Radix Kansui), and Xì Xīn (Radix et Rhizoma Asari) into powder, then mixed with small amount of Shè Xiāng (Moschus), and used in topically-applied powders to Fèi Shù (BL 13) and Gāo Huāng (BL 43) in the hot period between early July and early September for chronic and unremitting asthma caused by cold-phlegm encumbering the lung.

2. Phlegm coagulation: Bái Jiè Zǐ (Semen Sinapis) is combined with Mò Yào (Myrrha), Guì Zhī (Ramulus Cinnamomi), and Bàn Xià (Rhizoma Pinelliae) for numbness and pain due to phlegm obstruction in the channels, collaterals, and joints; and with Má Huáng (Herba Ephedrae), Ròu Guì (Cortex Cinnamomi), and Lù Jiǎo Jiāo (Colla Cornus Cervi) for yin type of deep-rooted ulcer with unchanged skin

color and diffuse swelling, and aching pain caused by phlegm coagulation in the muscle.

[Usage and Dosage] Use stir-fried in most cases, 3–6 g in decoction, decrease the dosage as in pill and powder. Grind and then mix with sesame oil or other liquids for external application.

[Mnemonics] Bái Jiè Zǐ (Semen Sinapis, White Mustard Seed): pungent and warm; warm and unblock the channels and effective for deep-rooted abscess, swelling, and pain.

[Simple and Effective Formulas]

1. 三子养亲汤 Sān Zǐ Yǎng Qīn Tāng — Three Seed Filial Devotion Decoction from *Han's Clear View of Medicine* (韩氏医通, Hán Shì Yī Tōng): Zǐ Sū Zǐ (Fructus Perillae), Bái Jiè Zǐ (Semen Sinapis), and Lái Fú Zǐ (Semen Raphani); clean, prescribing dosage of each herb based on the state of illness, i.e. Sū Zǐ (Fructus Perillae) for severe asthma, Lái Fú Zǐ (Semen Raphani) for qi stagnation, and Bái Jiè Zǐ (Semen Sinapis) for profuse phlegm difficult to expectorate; decoct 9 g/time while wrapped with gauze for oral administration to treat the elderly patients with cough, wheezing and profuse phlegm accumulation.

2. 白芥子散 Bái Jiè Zǐ Sǎn — White Mustard Seed Powder from *Fine Formulas for Women* (妇人良方, Fù Rén Liáng Fāng): Bái Jiè Zǐ (Semen Sinapis) 90 g, Mù Biē Zǐ (Semen Momordicae) (stir-fried with bran) 90 g, Mò Yào (Myrrha) (ground) 15 g, Guì Xīn (Cortex Cinnamomi) 15 g, and Mù Xiāng (Radix Aucklandiae) 15 g; grind into powder and take 3 g/time with warm wine for phlegm stagnation in the channels and collaterals with manifestations as paroxysmal pain in the arm radiating to scapular region with limited range of motion, periarthritis of shoulder, and pain in the upper extremities.

[Precautions] Bái Jiè Zǐ (Semen Sinapis) may consume qi and yin, and is therefore contraindicated in patients with vigorous fire due to yin deficiency. Topical application may cause blisters.

桔梗 Jié Gěng *radix platycodonis platycodon root*

The source is from the root of herbaceous perennial *Platycodon grandiflorum* (Jacq.) A. DC., family Campanulaceae. Alternate names include 苦桔梗 Kǔ Jié Gěng, 大药 Dà Yào, and 荠苨 Jì Ní. Bitter and pungent in flavor and neutral in nature.

[Actions] Diffuse lung and dispel phlegm, and benefit throat and discharge pus. It is applicable for cough, profuse sputum, chest oppression, sore throat, hoarseness, lung abscess with spitting of pus, and sores and ulcers with unsmooth discharge of pus. Modern research has shown that reveal it has significant antibechic, expectorant, hypoglycemic, anti-ulcer, and anti-inflammatory effects.

[Quality] Good quality is even, thick, firm, white, and bitter. The good quality is found in eastern China, the herb collected in summer is of higher active ingredients. Traditionally, the skin should be removed before using, but recent researches reveal the skin is rich in active ingredient and should be used.

[Indications]

1. Phlegm-qi congestion in lung: the lung governs diffusion and descending, phlegm qi obstruction in the lung may cause lung qi fail to diffuse and descend with the manifestation of cough and wheezing with expectoration of sputum. Jié Gěng (Radix Platycodonis), bitter and draining in nature, can diffuse and descend lung qi and dissolve phlegm to disinhibit chest and diaphragm and is therefore commonly prescribed together with other medicinals for cough, profuse sputum, nasal congestion, and chest oppression caused by exogenous pathogens invading the lung. It is combined with Xìng Rén (Semen Armeniacae Amarum), Zǐ Sū Yè (Folium Perillae), Fáng Fēng (Radix Saposhnikoviae), and Jīng Jiè (Herba Schizonepetae) for wind-cold; with Jīn Yín Huā (Flos Lonicerae Japonicae), Lián Qiào (Fructus Forsythiae), Jú Huā (Flos Chrysanthemi), and Niú Bàng Zǐ (Fructus Arctii) for wind-heat; and with medicinals that dissolve phlegm and diffuse and descend lung qi such as Bàn Xià (Rhizoma Pinelliae), Má Huáng (Herba Ephedrae),

Chén Pí (Pericarpium Citri Reticulatae), and Fú Líng (Poria) for chronic cough and wheezing.

2. Throat disorders: Jié Gěng (Radix Platycodonis), pungent, dispersing, and ascending in nature, is combined with Bò He (Herba Menthae), Gān Cǎo (Radix et Rhizoma Glycyrrhizae), and Shè Gān (Rhizoma Belamcandae) for swollen and painful throat with loss of voice; with Bǎn Lán Gēn (Radix Isatidis), Mǎ Bó (Lasiosphaera seu Calvatia), and Qīng Guǒ (Fructus Canarii) for severe cases of swollen and painful throat.

3. Unsooth discharge of pus: Jié Gěng (Radix Platycodonis) has an effect of expelling pus and therefore is combined with Gān Cǎo (Radix et Rhizoma Glycyrrhizae), Bài Jiàng Cǎo (Herba Patriniae), and Yì Yǐ Rén (Semen Coicis) for pulmonary abscess with expectoration of purulent sputum; and with Zào Jiǎo Cì (Spina Gleditsiae) for ruptured sores and ulcers with unsmooth evacuation of pus.

Owning to its ascending nature, this herb can be used in the treatment of urinary retention and inhibited defecation to realize "bringing up the pot and opening its cover". But it has to be combined with defecation and urination-promoting medicinals, respectively.

This substance can also be applied externally. For instance, it can be burned and ground into powder with Xiǎo Huí Xiāng (Fructus Foeniculi) and applied topically for ulcerative gingivitis with bad smell and erosion.

[Usage and Dosage] Use raw in general, 3–9 g in decoction, increase the amount when used to expel pus from pulmonary abscess, but overdose is discouraged as it may readily cause nausea.

[Mnemonics] Jié Gěng (Radix Platycodonis, Platycodon Root): bitter and pungent; diffuse lung, dispel phlegm, benefit throat, and discharge pus.

[Simple and Effective Formulas]

1. 桔梗汤 Jié Gěng Tāng — Platycodon Root Decoction from *Treatise on Cold Damage* (伤寒论, Shāng Hán Lùn): Jié Gěng (Radix Platycodonis) 6 g and Gān Cǎo (Radix et Rhizoma Glycyrrhizae) 12 g; decoct in water for oral administration to treat *shaoyin* disease with painful throat.

2. 济生桔梗汤 Jì Shēng Jié Gěng Tāng — Life Saving Platycodon Root Decoction from *Formulas to Aid the Living* (济生方, Jì Shēng Fāng): Jié Gěng (Radix Platycodonis) 30 g, Bèi Mǔ (Bulbus Fritillaria) 30 g, Dāng Guī (Radix Angelicae Sinensis) 30 g, Guā Lóu Rén (Semen Trichosanthis) 30 g, Zhǐ Qiào (Fructus Aurantii) 30 g, Yì Yǐ Rén (Semen Coicis) 30 g, Sāng Bái Pí (Cortex Mori) 30 g, Fáng Jǐ (Radix Stephaniae Tetrandrae) 30 g, Gān Cǎo (Radix et Rhizoma Glycyrrhizae) 15 g, Xìng Rén (Semen Armeniacae Amarum) 15 g, Bǎi Hé (Bulbus Lilii) 15 g, and Huáng Qí (Radix Astragali) 45 g; grind into coarse powder, decoct 12 g/time with 5 pieces of Shēng Jiāng (Rhizoma Zingiberis Recens) to treat lung abscess, vomiting and coughing of pus and blood, qi stagnation in the chest, thirst, vexation, swollen feet, and deep yellow urine.

[Precautions] Jié Gěng (Radix Platycodonis), up-lifting in nature, is contraindicated in cases of qi counterflow and deficiency-fire flaming upward. It may cause gastric mucosa irritation and therefore should be used cautiously in patients with gastric hemorrhage and stomach ulcer. Taking overdose raw plant will result in poisoning manifested as oral mucosa burning pain and swelling, profuse saliva, vomiting, nausea, abdominal pain, diarrhea, and even convulsion, unconsciousness, and difficulty of breath in serious case.

Daily practices

1. Bái Fù Zǐ (Rhizoma Typhonii), Bái Jiè Zǐ (Semen Sinapis), and Jié Gěng (Radix Platycodonis) are all medicinals that dissolve phlegm, what are the similarities and differences among them in terms of actions and indications?
2. What are the major differences among Bái Fù Zǐ (Rhizoma Typhonii), Bái Jiè Zǐ (Semen Sinapis), Jié Gěng (Radix Platycodonis), Bàn Xià (Rhizoma Pinelliae), and Tiān Nán Xīng (Rhizoma Arisaematis) in terms of actions?

瓜蒌 **Guā Lóu** *fructus trichosanthis snakegourd fruit*

[Addendum] 天花粉 Tiān Huā Fěn Radix Trichosanthis Snakegourd Root

The source is from the ripe fruit of perennial herbaceous liana *Trichosanthes kirilowii* Maxim. or *T. uniflora* Hao, family Cucurbitaceae. Alternate names include 栝楼 Guā Lóu and 地楼 Dì Lóu. Sweet in flavor and cold in nature. The whole fruit is called 全瓜蒌 Quán Guā Lóu, the skin 瓜蒌皮 Guā Lóu Pí, and the semen 瓜蒌子 Guā Lóu Zi or 瓜蒌仁 Guā Lóu Rén.

[Actions] Clear heat and dissolve phlegm, expand the chest and dissipate masses, and moisten the intestine and promote defecation. Its peel is considered more effective in clearing heat, dissolving phlegm, expanding the chest, and regulating qi; and the semen is more potent in moistening dryness, dissolving phlegm, moistening the intestine and promoting defecation. Modern research has indicated that it contains active ingredients that can inhibit bacteria, fight against cancer, and treat coronary heart disease.

[Quality] Good quality is large and orange-yellow with a sugary taste, has bright-colored, aromatic, and pungent skin without carpopodium, thin, and full and oily seeds even in size.

[Indications]

1. Cough due to phlegm heat: Guā Lóu (Fructus Trichosanthis) is suitable for cough induced by heat phlegm and dry phlegm. It is combined with Huáng Qín (Radix Scutellariae), Zhǐ Shí (Fructus Aurantii Immaturus), and Dǎn Nán Xīng (Arisaema cum Bile) for dry phlegm cough manifested as yellow and sticky sputum difficult to expectorate, thirst, yellow tongue coating, and rapid pulse; and with Bèi Mǔ (Bulbus Fritillaria), Tiān Huā Fěn (Radix Trichosanthis), Jié Gěng (Radix Platycodonis), and Shā Shēn (Radix Adenophorae seu Glehniae) for cough marked by nonproductive choking cough without sputum or sticky sputum that is difficult to expectorate, and scanty and dry tongue coating.

   For pulmonary abscess with expectoration of purulent sputum, it is combined with Yú Xīng Cǎo (Herba Houttuyniae), Bài Jiàng Cǎo (Herba Patriniae), Dōng Guā Rén (Semen Benincasae), and Lú Gēn (Rhizoma Phragmitis) to clear the lung and expel pus.

2. Chest *bì* and thoracic accumulation: chest *bì* is a disorder that qi movement stagnates in the chest manifested as chest *pǐ* and oppression or chest pain radiating to the back. It commonly occurs in coronary heart disease and gastric disorders. Thoracic accumulation is defined as a disease that phlegm and qi binding in the chest cause pain. It is commonly sees in gastritis and liver and gallbladder diseases. If that is the case, Guā Lóu (Fructus Trichosanthis) is suitable because of its properties of benefiting qi, dissipating masses, and directing phlegm and turbidity downward. It is usually combined with Guì Zhī (Ramulus Cinnamomi), Xiè Bái (Bulbus Allii Macrostemi), and Bàn Xià (Rhizoma Pinelliae for chest *bì*; and with Bàn Xià (Rhizoma Pinelliae) and Huáng Lián (Rhizoma Coptidis) for thoracic accumulation.
3. Constipation: oily Guā Lóu Zǐ (Semen Trichosanthis) can moisten the intestines to promote defecation and is therefore effective for constipation caused by intestinal fluid insufficiency. It is usually combined with Má Rén (Fructus Cannabis), Yù Lǐ Rén (Semen Pruni), Xuán Shēn (Radix Scrophulariae), and Bǎi Zǐ Rén (Semen Platycladi).

This substance can also be applied externally. For instance, it can be ground into powder and mixed with vinegar for external application to relieve erysipelas and red swellings.

[Usage and Dosage] Use raw in general, 10–15 g in decoction.

[Mnemonics] Guā Lóu (Fructus Trichosanthis, Snakegourd Fruit): sweet and cold; moisten and dissolve hot phlegm and effective for chest *bì* and heat-cough.

[Simple and Effective Formulas]

1. 瓜蒌薤白白酒汤 Guā Lóu Xiè Bái Bái Jiǔ Tāng — Trichosanthes, Chinese Chive and White Wine Decoction from *Treatise on Cold Damage* (伤寒论, Shāng Hán Lùn): one Guā Lóu (Fructus Trichosanthis) (pounded), Xiè Bái (Bulbus Allii Macrostemi) 10 g, and white wine 20 ml; decoct in water for oral administration to treat chest *bì*, pain in the chest and back, wheezing, and shortness of breath. Also

used for coronary heart disease and pain of gastric disease with manifestations above.

2. 栝楼散 Guā Dì Sǎn — Melon Stalk Powder from *Formulas for Universal Relief* (普济方, Pǔ Jì Fāng): two Guā Lóu (Fructus Trichosanthis) and jujube-sized Míng Fán (Alumen); put Míng Fán (Alumen) into Guā Lóu (Fructus Trichosanthis), burn but preserve their medical nature, grind into powder, cook radish until soft, and take the radish with radish soup after dipping into the powder to treat wheezing.

[Precautions] Guā Lóu (Fructus Trichosanthis), cold and slippery in nature, is contraindicated in cases of diarrhea due to deficiency-cold of the spleen and stomach, cold-phlegm, and damp-phlegm.

[Addendum] 天花粉 Tiān Huā Fěn Radix Trichosanthis Snakegourd Root.

The source is from the root of *Trichosanthes kirilowii* Maxim, sweet and slightly bitter in flavor and cold in nature. It can clear heat, engender fluids, moisten the lung, transform phlegm, relieve swelling, and expel pus. It is applicable for thirst due to fluid consumption in febrile disease, wasting-thirst, dry cough with scanty sputum, and sores. Use 10–15 g for oral administration.

贝母 Bèi Mǔ *bulbus fritillaria fritillary bulb*

It has two types, namely Chuān Bèi Mǔ (Bulbus Fritillariae Cirrhosae) and Zhè Bèi Mǔ (Bulbus Fritillariae Thunbergii). The former comes from the bulb of the herbaceous perennial *Fritillaria cirrhosa* D. Don, *F. unibracteata* Hsiao et K. C. Hsia, and *F. delavayi* Franch., family Liliaceae. Bitter and sweat in flavor and cold in nature. Whereas the latter is the bulb of herbaceous perennial *Frillaria thunbergii* Miq., family Liliaceae. Alternate names include 浙贝 Zhè Bèi and 象贝母 Xiàng Bèi Mǔ. Bitter in flavor and cold in nature.

[Actions] Chuān Bèi Mǔ (Bulbus Fritillariae Cirrhosae) and Zhè Bèi Mǔ (Bulbus Fritillariae Thunbergii) both can arrest cough, dissolve phlegm, clear heat and dissipate masses, and are applicable for cough and wheezing caused by phlegm obstruction in the lungs. The former, however, is believed more potent in moistening the lung and is more appropriate for chronic cough with scanty sputum and dry throat due to lung deficiency, and the latter is more effective in clearing heat and dissipating masses and more suitable for lung-heat cough and phlegm accumulation. Modern research has demonstrated that it contains a variety of alkaloids and saponins.

[Quality] Chuān Bèi Mǔ (Bulbus Fritillariae Cirrhosae) is divided by production area and spieces into 白炉贝 Bái Lú Bèi, 黄炉贝 Huáng Lú Bèi, 松贝 Sōng Bèi, and 青贝 Qīng Bèi, good quality is firm, powdery, and white. When, Zhè Bèi Mǔ (Bulbus Fritillariae Thunbergii) is big in size, it is called 大贝 Dà Bèi or 元宝贝 Yuán Bǎo Bèi, while the small-sized bulb is known as 珠贝 Zhū Bèi. Good quality is fleshy, thick, white, and powdery with a white cross-section, and 元宝贝 Yuán Bǎo Bèi is superior to 珠贝 Zhū Bèi.

[Indications]

1. Cough due to phlegm heat: Bèi Mǔ (Bulbus Fritillaria) is mainly used for cough caused by phlegm heat or dryness heat in the lung. It is combined with Guā Lóu (Fructus Trichosanthis), Zhī Mǔ (Rhizoma Anemarrhenae), and Sāng Bái Pí (Cortex Mori) for lung heat cough with yellow and thick sputum; with Shā Shēn (Radix Adenophorae seu Glehniae), Mài Dōng (Radix Ophiopogonis), and Bǎi Hé (Bulbus Lilii) for chronic cough with dry throat due to lung yin deficiency; with Yú Xīng Cǎo (Herba Houttuyniae), Jīn Qiáo Mài (Rhizoma Fagopyri Dibotryis), and Jié Gěng (Radix Platycodonis) for phlegm heat accumulation; and with Lú Gēn (Rhizoma Phragmitis), Yì Yǐ Rén (Semen Coicis), Bài Jiàng Cǎo (Herba Patriniae), Yú Xīng Cǎo (Herba Houttuyniae), and Táo Rén (Semen Persicae) for pulmonary abscess with expectoration containing pus and blood.

2. Carbuncles, furuncles, and scrofula: Bèi Mǔ (Bulbus Fritillaria), especially Zhè Bèi Mǔ (Bulbus Fritillariae Thunbergii), is regarded fairly effective in dissipating masses. It is combined with Xuán Shēn (Radix Scrophulariae) and Mǔ Lì (Concha Ostreae) for scrofula (tuberculosis of lymph nodes); and with Tiān Huā Fěn (Radix Trichosanthis), Jīn Yín Huā (Flos Lonicerae Japonicae), Lián Qiào (Fructus Forsythiae), and Zǐ Huā Dì Dīng (Herba Violae) for carbuncles and swellings in the early stage.

[Usage and Dosage] Used raw in general, 3–10 g in decoction. Chuān Bèi Mǔ (Bulbus Fritillariae Cirrhosae) is expensive and therefore most commonly used as powder, 1–1.5 g when taken as a powder.

[Mnemonics] Bèi Mǔ (Bulbus Fritillaria, Fritillary Bulb): cold; relieve phlegm and dissipate masse; Chuān Bèi Mǔ (Bulbus Fritillariae Cirrhosae) is sweet and moistening, while Zhè Bèi Mǔ (Bulbus Fritillariae Thunbergii) is bitter and draining.

[Simple and Effective Formulas]

1. 贝母丸 Bèi Mǔ Wán — Fritillary Bulb Pill from *Comprehensive Recording of Divine Assistance* (圣济总录, Shèng Jì Zǒng Lù): Bèi Mǔ (Bulbus Fritillaria) (plumule removed) 45 g, Gān Cǎo (Radix et Rhizoma Glycyrrhizae) (roasted) 0.9 g, and Xìng Rén (Semen Armeniacae Amarum) (peel and kernel removed, stir-fried) 45 g; grind into powder, make into hoodle-sized pill with honey, and dissolve one pill/time in the mouth and swallow it with saliva for lung-heat cough with profuse sputum and dry throat.

2. 贝母化痰丸 Bèi Mǔ Huà Tán Wán — Fritillary Bulb Phlegm-Transforming Pill from *Advancement of Medicine* (医级, Yī Jí): Chuān Bèi Mǔ (Bulbus Fritillariae Cirrhosae) 30 g, Tiān Zhú Huáng (Concretio Silicea Bambusae) 3 g, Péng Shā (Borax) 3 g, and Wén Gé (Clam) (stir-fried with vinegar) 1.5 g; grind into powder, clean and honey-fry Pí Pá Yè (Folium Eriobotryae), make into Qiàn Shí (Semen Euryales)-sized pill, and dissolve in the mouth for pulmonary abscess, and lung *wěi* (痿, atrophy).

[Precautions] Bèi Mǔ (Bulbus Fritillaria) is contraindicated in cases of cold-phlegm and damp-phlegm. According to "eighteen antagonisms", this herb is incompatible with Wū Tóu (Aconite Main Tuber), but still needs experimental proof.

竹沥 Zhú Lì *succus bambusae bamboo sap*

The source is from the dried sap of the stem of *Bambusa breviflora* Munro or other congeneric plants, family Gramineae. Alternate names include 竹油 Zhú Yóu. Sweet in flavor and cold in nature.

[Actions] Clear heat and eliminate phlegm, and clear the heart and relieve spasm. It is applicable for unconsciousness in febrile disease, wind-stroke with phlegm confounding the orifices, and childhood fright epilepsy and convulsion due to phlegm heat. Animal experiments reveal it has significant antibechic and expectorant effects.

[Quality] Good quality is yellowish white, clear, and without sediment and impurities.

[Indications]

1. Phlegm heat blocking the orifices: Zhú Lì (Succus Bambusae), capable of clearing and dissolving phlegm heat, is applicable for loss of consciousness with delirious speech, phlegm rale in the throat caused by phlegm clouding the heart orifice. It is often used together with Peaceful Palace Bovine Bezoar Pill (安宫牛黄丸, Ān Gōng Niú Huáng Wán) that clear the heart and open the orifices.
2. Phlegm obstruction on the channels and collaterals: Zhú Lì (Succus Bambusae) is taken with small amount of Shēng Jiāng (Rhizoma Zingiberis Recens) juice for numbness and muscle contracture of the limbs or hemiplegia due to phlegm obstruction In the channels and collaterals.
3. Phlegm heat accumulating the lung: Zhú Lì (Succus Bambusae) is combined with Huáng Qín (Radix Scutellariae), Bèi Mǔ (Bulbus Fritillaria), and Bàn Xià (Rhizoma Pinelliae) for cough and wheezing with sticky thick and yellow sputum, chest oppression, and thirst caused by phlegm heat accumulating in the lung.

It can also be applied externally for eye droppings to treat pediatric pinkeye.

[Usage and Dosage] Use raw, alone or mixed with the decoction of other herbs, 30–60 g/ time.

[Mnemonics] Zhú Lì (Succus Bambusae, Bamboo Sap): sweet and cold; clear heat, eliminate phlegm, unblock the collaterals, open the orifices, and relieve cough and wheezing.

[Simple and Effective Formulas]

竹沥汤 Zhú Lì Tāng — Bamboo Sap Decoction from *Important Formulas Worth a Thousand Gold Pieces* (千金要方, Qiān Jīn Yào Fāng): Zhú Lì (Succus Bambusae) 60 g, raw Gé Gēn (Radix Puerariae Lobatae) juice 30 g, and Shēng Jiāng (Rhizoma Zingiberis Recens) juice

10 g; mix up, stew with warm water, and take warm for hemiplegia, lack of consciousness, inability to recognize people, and inability to speak. Also applicable for the sequelae of stroke and other diseases, like unconsciousness and paralysis of limbs with profuse phlegm in the throat.

[Precautions] Zhú Lì (Succus Bambusae), cold in nature, is contraindicated in cases of deficiency-cold of the spleen and stomach and when cough is caused by cold phlegm and wind-cold.

Besides the above-mentioned medicinals, others that commonly used for dissolving phlegm include Xuán Fù Huā (Flos Inulae), Kūn Bù (Thallus Laminariae), Hǎi Zǎo (Sargassum), Zào Jiá (Fructus Gleditsiae), Zhú Rú (Caulis Bambusae in Taenia), Tiān Zhú Huáng (Concretio Silicea Bambusae), Bí Qi (Rhizoma Eleocharitis), Pàng Dà Hǎi (Semen Sterculiae Lychnophorae), Mù Hú Dié (Semen Oroxyli), Méng Shí (Chlorite-schist), Hǎi Fú Shí (Pumex), Hǎi Gé Qiào (Concha Meretricis seu Cyclinae), and Huáng Yào Zǐ (Rhizoma Dioscoreae Bulbiferae).

Daily practices

1. What are the major actions and indications of Guā Lóu (Fructus Trichosanthis), what are the difference between its peel and semen in terms of actions?
2. How many types of Bèi Mǔ (Bulbus Fritillaria) and what are they? What are the similarities and differences between them in terms of actions and indications?
3. What are the similarities and differences between Bèi Mǔ (Bulbus Fritillaria) and Zhú Lì (Succus Bambusae) in terms of actions and indications?

MEDICINALS THAT ARREST COUGH AND WHEEZING

Those herbs are primarily used to stop coughing and wheezing.

The lung is referred to as the major source of cough and panting. These disorders is caused by either lung qi failing to descend and disperse and phlegm qi obstructing the lung caused by externally-contracted six pathogenic factors invading the lungs; or lung qi failing to disperse and descend with obstruction of phlegm-damp in the lung due to internal spleen deficiency and food accumulation. These cough-arresting and wheezing-calming herbs work through a variety of pathways, namely diffusing, draining, clearing, descending, moistening, astringing of the lung, and dissolving phlegm.

The selection of herbs for cough and wheezing is based on the etiology and nature of the disease. Also they should be combined with other herbs that treat the root cause of the problem and improve their abilities of arresting cough and wheezing. For this reason, for the externally-contracted wind-cold cough and wheezing, they are combined with herbs that scatter and dissipate wind-cold; for exterior wind-heat cough, they are used in conjunction with herbs that scatter and dissipate wind-heat; for spleen deficiency producing phlegm-dampness that disturbs the lung, medicinals that tonify the spleen and relieve dampness are added; for pathogenic heat boiling body fluid into phlegm that obstructs the lung, heat-clearing medicinals are included in the prescription; for lung dryness and lack of moisture, substances that moisten the lung are also used; for coldness in the lung, medicinals that warm the lung are combined; and for enduring cough and panting with accompanying lung qi deficiency in most cases, herbs that boost the lung and astringe the lung must be added. Descending and dispersing lung qi and dissolving phlegm are two major approaches for the treatment of cough and panting, however, medicinals that move qi should also be used as smooth qi flow is helpful for phlegm dispersion and cough and panting relief.

Indeed, herbs that arrest cough and wheezing are also among many other categorizes, such as Má Huáng (Herba Ephedrae) in chapter exterior-releasing herbs, Shè Gān (Rhizoma Belamcandae) in heat-clearing herbs, and Lái Fú Zǐ (Semen Raphani) in food stagnation-relieving herbs. Especially most of herbs that dissolve phlegm have an effect of arrest cough and calm wheezing.

杏仁 Xìng Rén *semen armeniacae amarum apricot kernel*

The source is from the ripe semen of deciduous arbor *Prunus armeniaca* L., or *P. armeniaca* L. var. ansu Maxim, family Rosaceae. Alternate names include 杏核仁 Xìng Hé Rén, 苦杏仁 Kǔ Xìng Rén, and 杏梅仁 Xìng Méi Rén. Bitter in flavor and warm in nature with mild toxicity.

[Actions] Arrest cough and relieve wheezing, and moisten the intestine and promote defecation. It is applicable for cough in common cold, asthma, pharyngitis, and constipation due to intestinal dryness. Experiments show that its ingredient almond glycosides are decomposed into virulent hydrocyanic acid, and that ingesting a tiny amount of which has antibechic and antiasthmatic effects. Its amygdalin can fight against cancer and promote hemotopoietic function.

[Quality] Good quality is even-sized, full, fleshy, bitter, and non-oily. Tián Xìng Rén (Semen Armeniacae Dulce), relatively big in size containing less almond glycosides, is generally taken as food.

[Indications]

1. Cough and wheezing: Xìng Rén (Semen Armeniacae Amarum), as a principal medicinal for arresting cough and relieving wheezing, is applicable for different types of cough and wheezing. It is combined with Má Huáng (Herba Ephedrae), Jié Gěng (Radix Platycodonis), and Gān Cǎo (Radix et Rhizoma Glycyrrhizae) for cough and wheezing due to externally-contracted wind-cold; with Sāng Yè (Folium Mori), Jú Huā (Flos Chrysanthemi), and Niú Bàng Zǐ (Fructus Arctii) for the symptoms caused by wind-heat; and with Shí Gāo (Gypsum Fibrosum), Má Huáng (Herba Ephedrae), and Gān Cǎo (Radix et Rhizoma Glycyrrhizae) for cough and wheezing due to lung heat.
2. Constipation due to intestinal dryness: Xìng Rén (Semen Armeniacae Amarum), moistening and oily in nature, is combined with other medicinals that moistening 下 and promoting defecation such as Táo Rén (Semen Persicae), Bǎi Zǐ Rén (Semen Platycladi), and Má Rén (Fructus Cannabis) for constipation due to intestinal fluid insufficiency.

[Usage and Dosage] Traditional sources indicate that it is better to remove the skin and tip before using. However, some resources indicate peel is a rich source of active ingredients and should be included. Use raw in general, stir-fried for constipation. Use 5–10 g in decoction, pounded into pieces prior to decocting, and often added near the end. Reduce the dosage as in pill and powder. Modern research suggest decocting or stir-frying over a long period of time is not recommended as high temperature can easily destroy its active ingredients.

[Mnemonics] Xìng Rén (Semen Armeniacae Amarum, Apricot Kernel): bitter and warm; diffuse the lung to relieve cough, direct qi downward to relieve wheezing, and relieve constipation.

[Simple and Effective Formulas]
杏仁煎 Xìng Rén Jiān — Apricot Kernel Decoction from *Secret Formulas of the Yang Family* (杨氏家藏方, Yáng Shì Jiā Cáng Fāng): Xìng Rén (Semen Armeniacae Amarum) (peel and tip removed, slightly stir-fried) 15 g and Hú Táo Ròu (Semen Juglandis) (peel removed) 15 g; add small amount of raw honey, grind into very fine powder, make 30 g into ten pills, and chew and take one pill/time with Shēng Jiāng (Rhizoma Zingiberis Recens) decoction after meal and at bedtime for persistent cough and wheezing that affect sleep at night.

[Precautions] Xìng Rén (Semen Armeniacae Amarum), oily and slippery, is contraindicated in cases of loose stool and diarrhea. Over-dose use is not recommended as it has certain toxicity.

白前 Bái Qián *rhizoma et radix cynanchi stauntonii cynanchum root and rhizome*

The source is the root and rhizome of *Cynanchum stauntonii* (Decne.) Schltr. ex levl. or *C. glaucescens* (Decne.) Hand.-Mazz., family Asclepiadaceae. Pungent and sweet in flavor and neutral in nature.

[Actions] Dispel phlegm, redirect the qi downward, and arrest cough. It is applicable for lung qi stagnation, cough with profuse sputum, and wheezing due to qi counterflow. It contains saponin that can dispel phlegm.

[Quality] Good quality is thick with long rootlets and without soils and impurities.

[Indications] Bái Qián (Rhizoma et Radix Cynanchi Stauntonii) is mainly used for cough and wheezing with sputum and usually combined with other medicinals in accordance with the state of illness. It is combined with Má Huáng (Herba Ephedrae), Bàn Xià (Rhizoma Pinelliae), and Xìng Rén (Semen Armeniacae Amarum) for the cold-natured symptoms;

with Sāng Bái Pí (Cortex Mori), Dì Gǔ Pí (Cortex Lycii), Huáng Qín (Radix Scutellariae) for the heat-natured symptoms; and with Jīng Jiè (Herba Schizonepetae), Fáng Fēng (Radix Saposhnikoviae), Zǐ Wǎn (Radix et Rhizoma Asteris), Jié Gěng (Radix Platycodonis) for externally-contracted wind-cold. This substance is considered more effective in descending qi and dissolving phlegm, and is particularly suitable for cases of cough and wheezing with phlegm rale in the throat. It is combined with Zǐ Wǎn (Radix et Rhizoma Asteris), Bàn Xià (Rhizoma Pinelliae), and Jīng Dà Jǐ (Radix Euphorbiae Pekinensis) when accompanied with edema.

[Usage and Dosage] Use raw in general, processing with honey to improve its effect of dissolving phlegm and arresting cough. Use 5–10 g in decoction.

[Mnemonics] *Bái Qián* (Rhizoma et Radix Cynanchi Stauntonii, Cynanchum Root and Rhizome): pungent and sweet; specialized in dispelling phlegm, and capable of directing qi downward to relieve coughing, phlegm, and wheezing.

[Simple and Effective Formulas]
久嗽方 Jiǔ Sòu Fāng — Chronic Cough-arresting Formula from *Effective Formulas* (近效方, Jìn Xiào Fāng): Bái Qián (Rhizoma et Radix Cynanchi Stauntonii) 90 g, Sāng Bái Pí (Cortex Mori) 60 g, Jié Gěng (Radix Platycodonis) 60 g, and Gān Cǎo (Radix et Rhizoma Glycyrrhizae) 30 g; chop up and decoct in water until only a third remains, and take on an empty stomach for chronic cough or with hemoptysis.

[Precautions] Bái Qián (Rhizoma et Radix Cynanchi Stauntonii), capable of dispelling pathogen, is contraindicated when cough and wheezing is caused by deficiency.

前胡 **Qián Hú** *radix peucedani hogfennel root*

The source is from the root of *Peucedanum praeruptorum* Dunn and *P. decurisivum* Maxim., family Umbelliferae. Bitter and pungent in flavor and slightly cold in nature.

[Actions] Redirect the qi downward, expel phlegm, and release wind-heat. It is applicable for cough and wheezing caused by externally-contracted wind-heat and lung qi failing to descend.

[Quality] Good quality is dry, full, tender, thick, firm, and strongly aromatic with a yellowish white cross section.

[Indications]

1. Cough with profuse sputum: Qián Hú (Radix Peucedani), capable of descending qi and dissolving phlegm, is applicable for cough and wheezing, thick sputum, and chest oppression due to lung qi failing to descend and commonly combined with Bèi Mǔ (Bulbus Fritillaria), Sāng Bái Pí (Cortex Mori), and Xìng Rén (Semen Armeniacae Amarum). Qián Hú (Radix Peucedani) is similar to Jié Gěng (Radix Platycodonis) in terms of dissolving phlegm, but the former is descending in nature while the latter is ascending. Qián Hú (Radix Peucedani) and Bái Qián (Rhizoma et Radix Cynanchi Stauntonii) both can dissolve phlegm and arrest cough, the former is cold in nature while the latter is warm, in the clinic, however, these two herbs are usually prescribed together to arrest different types of cough.
2. Externally-contracted wind-heat: Qián Hú (Radix Peucedani) is combined with Bò He (Herba Menthae), Jú Huā (Flos Chrysanthemi), Jié Gěng (Radix Platycodonis), and Niú Bàng Zǐ (Fructus Arctii) for cough with scanty sputum and thirst caused by externally-contracted wind-heat with lung failing to diffuse and govern descent.

Its fresh root can be pounded and applied externally to relieve innominate swellings and toxins.

[Usage and Dosage] Use raw in general, honey-fry to reinforce its ability of dissolving phlegm and arresting cough. Use 5–10 g in decoction, decrease the amount in pill and powder.

[Mnemonics] Qián Hú (Radix Peucedani, Hogfennel Root): cold, bitter, pungent, and dispersing; clear wind-heat and relieve cough, and dissolve phlegm.

[Simple and Effective Formulas]

前胡饮 Qián Hú Yǐn — Hogfennel Root Beverage from *Formulas from Benevolent Sages* (圣惠方, Shèng Huì Fāng): Qián Hú (Radix Peucedani) 30 g, Mài Mén Dōng (Radix Ophiopogonis) (plumule removed) 45 g, Bèi Mǔ (Bulbus Fritillaria) (roasted until light yellow) 30 g, Sāng Gēn Bái Pí (Cortex Mori) (filed) 30 g, Xìng Rén (Semen Armeniacae Amarum) (soaked in water, tip and peel removed, stir-fried with bran until light yellow) 15 g, and Gān Cǎo (Radix et Rhizoma Glycyrrhizae) (roasted until reddish, filed) 3 g; grind into fine powder, decoct 12 g/time with Shēng Jiāng (Rhizoma Zingiberis Recens) in water for oral administration to treat cough with sticky sputum, discomfort in the chest, and paroxysmal vexing heat. Also applicable for cough with thirst and sticky sputum difficult to expectorate attributed to lung heat.

[Precautions] Qián Hú (Radix Peucedani), pungent and dispersing in nature, is contraindicated in cases of non-externally-contracted cough and lung yin deficiency induced cough.

Daily practices

1. What precautions should be taken when using medicinals that arrest cough and wheezing?
2. What are the similarities and differences among Xìng Rén (Semen Armeniacae Amarum), Bái Qián (Rhizoma et Radix Cynanchi Stauntonii), and Qián Hú (Radix Peucedani) in terms of actions and indications?

紫菀 Zǐ Wǎn *radix et rhizoma asteris tatarian aster root*

The source is from the root and rhizome of herbaceous perennial *Aster talaricus* L., family Compositae. It is so called as its root is purple, soft, and pliable and alternate names include 青菀 Qīng Wǎn, 返魂草根 Fǎn Hún Cǎo Gēn, and 紫菀茸 Zǐ W ǎn Rōng. Bitter and sweet in flavor and slightly warm in nature.

[Actions] Moisten the lungs and redirect the qi downward, and dispel phlegm and arrest cough. It is applicable for cough and wheezing with inhibited expectoration of sputum or chronic cough with blood in sputum caused by lung deficiency. Experiment shows its decoction and extractives have expectorant, antibechic, and certain antibacterial effect on animals.

[Quality] Good quality is long, purplish red, and flexible; difficult to break off.

[Indications]

1. Externally-contracted and internally-induced cough: Zǐ Wǎn (Radix et Rhizoma Asteris), warm and moistening in nature, can diffuse but not dissipate lung qi and therefore is applicable for different types of cough. It is combined with Jīng Jiè (Herba Schizonepetae), Jié Gěng (Radix Platycodonis), and Bǎi Bù (Radix Stemonae) for externally-contracted wind-cold cough; with Xìng Rén (Semen Armeniacae Amarum) in a pill form for chronic and intractable cough in children; and with Ē Jiāo (Colla Corii Asini), Zhī Mǔ (Rhizoma Anemarrhenae), and Bèi Mǔ (Bulbus Fritillaria) for hectic fever and chronic cough with blood in sputum.
2. Urinary obstruction: Zǐ Wǎn (Radix et Rhizoma Asteris) can diffuse and unblock lung qi to free and regulate the waterways and is therefore applicable for urinary obstruction, either alone or together with medicinals that promote urination.

[Usage and Dosage] Use raw in general. Honey-fry to strengthen its action of supplementing and moistening the lung. Use 5–10 g in decoction.

[Mnemonics] Zǐ Wǎn (Radix et Rhizoma Asteris, Tatarian Aster Root): moisten the lungs, redirect the qi downward, dispel phlegm, and arrest coughing.

[Simple and Effective Formulas]

1. 紫菀散 Zǐ Wǎn Sǎn — Tatarian Aster Root Powder from *Comprehensive Recording of Divine Assistance* (圣济总录, Shèng Jì Zǒng Lù): Zǐ Wǎn (Radix et Rhizoma Asteris) 30 g, Xìng Rén (Semen Armeniacae Amarum) (peel and tip removed) 3 g, Xì Xīn (Radix et Rhizoma Asari) 3 g, and Kuǎn Dōng Huā (Flos Farfarae) 3 g; grind into fine powder and take 2 g/time for

two or three-year-old children with rice soup, three times a day for child-hood cough and wheezing with phlegm rale in the throat.

2. 紫菀丸 Zǐ Wǎn Wán — Tatarian Aster Root Pill from *Ji Feng Formulas for Universal Relief* (鸡峰普济方, Jī fēng Pǔ Jì Fāng): Zǐ Wǎn (Radix et Rhizoma Asteris) and Qiàn Cǎo (Radix et Rhizoma Rubiae) in equal dosage; grind into powder, make into cherry-sized pill with honey, and dissolve one pill/time in the mouth for hematemesis and hemoptysis.

[Precautions] Zǐ Wǎn (Radix et Rhizoma Asteris), relatively warm in nature, is contraindicated in cases of cough due to excess heat.

款冬花 Kuǎn Dōng Huā *flos farfarae common coltsfoot flower*

The source is from the flower bud of herbaceous perennial *Tussilago farfara* L., family Compositae. It literally means welcome winter flower as it grows and blooms in winter. Alternate names include 冬花 Dōng Huā, 款冬 Kuǎn Dōng, 九九花 Jiǔ Jiǔ Huā, and 看灯花 Kàn Dēng Huā. Pungent in flavor and warm in nature.

[Actions] Moisten the lungs and arrest cough, and eliminate phlegm and redirect the qi downward. It is applicable for cough and wheezing with profuse sputum and taxation cough with hemoptysis. Experiments reveal that its decoction has antibechic, expectorant, and antiasthmatic effect.

[Quality] Good quality is dry, large, firm, and fresh purplish red with short pedicle and without soils and sands.

[Indications]
Different types of cough: Kuǎn Dōng Huā (Flos Farfarae) is a commonly-used herb that relieve cough and applicable for different types of cough when prescribed together with other herbs. It is combined with Má Huáng (Herba Ephedrae) and Shēng Jiāng (Rhizoma Zingiberis Recens) for cough due to lung cold; with Shā Shēn (Radix Adenophorae seu Glehniae) and Mài Dōng (Radix Ophiopogonis) for cough caused by lung dryness and heat; with Bǎi Hé (Bulbus Lilii), Bèi Mǔ (Bulbus Fritillaria), and Qīng Dài (Indigo Naturalis) for cough and wheezing with blood-streaked sputum; and with Jié Gěng (Radix Platycodonis),

Dōng Guā Rén (Semen Benincasae), Yì Yǐ Rén (Semen Coicis), and Bài Jiàng Cǎo (Herba Patriniae) for pulmonary abscess with pus-streaked sputum.

Kuǎn Dōng Huā (Flos Farfarae) and Zǐ Wǎn (Radix et Rhizoma Asteris) have similar actions, but the former is considered more effective in arresting cough, and the latter is potent in dissolving phlegm. These two herbs are very commonly used together in the clinic.

Research in recent years indicates its preparation of ethonal extract can relieve asthma; its decoction and injection can increase blood pressure and are therefore applicable for shock.

[Usage and Dosage] Use raw in general; honey-frying is to enhance its ability to moisten the lungs. Use 2–9 g in decoction.

[Mnemonics] Kuǎn Dōng Huā (Flos Farfarae, Common Coltsfoot Flower): pungent and warm; arrest coughing, moisten the lungs, redirect the qi downward, supplementary with Zǐ Wǎn (Radix et Rhizoma Asteris).

[Simple and Effective Formulas]

1. 款冬花汤 Kuǎn Dōng Huā Tāng — Common Coltsfoot Flower Decoction from *Comprehensive Recording of Divine Assistance* (圣济总录, Shèng Jì Zǒng Lù): Kuǎn Dōng Huā (Flos Farfarae) 60 g, Sāng Bái Pí (Cortex Mori) (filed) 15 g, Bèi Mǔ (Bulbus Fritillaria) (plumule removed) 15 g, Wǔ Wèi Zǐ (Fructus Schisandrae Chinensis) 15 g, Gān Cǎo (Radix et Rhizoma Glycyrrhizae) (roasted, filed) 15 g, Zhī Mǔ (Rhizoma Anemarrhenae) 10 g, and Xìng Rén (Semen Armeniacae Amarum) (peel and tip removed, stir-fried) 30 g; grind into powder and decoct 6 g/time in water, and remove dregs for oral administration to treat sudden onset of cough.

2. 百花膏 Bǎi Huā Gāo — Common Coltsfoot Flower Decocted Extract from *Formulas to Aid the Living* (济生方, Jì Shēng Fāng): Kuǎn Dōng Huā (Flos Farfarae) and Bǎi Hé (Bulbus Lilii) (steamed, baked) in equal dosage; grind into powder, make into longan-sized pill with honey, and take one pill/time after meal and at bedtime with Shēng Jiāng (Rhizoma Zingiberis Recens) soup for enduring cough and wheezing or with sputum containing blood.

[Precautions] Kuǎn Dōng Huā (Flos Farfarae), pungent and warm, is contraindicated in cases of excess heat in the lungs.

葶苈子 Tíng Lì Zǐ *semen lepidii pepperweed seed*

The source is from the semen of herbaceous annual or biennial *Descurainia Sophia* (L.) Webb ex Prantl (Beitinglizi) or *Lepidum apetalum* Willd. (Nantinglizi), family Cruciferae. The former is called 北葶苈 Běi Tíng Lì (also known as 苦葶苈 Kǔ Tíng Lì), and the latter is 南葶苈 Nán Tíng Lì (also known as 甜葶苈 Tián Tíng Lì). Bitter and pungent in flavor and cold in nature.

[Actions] Drain the lungs and alleviate asthma, and promote urination, and relieve swelling. It is applicable for phlegm-drool exuberance, cough and wheezing with profuse sputum, edema, and inhibited urination. Experiments display that it has a cardiotonic effect.

[Quality] Good quality is dry body, full seeds, reddish brown, and without soils, sands, and impurities.

[Indications]

1 Cough and wheezing due to phlegm rheum: for cough and wheezing unable to lie flat and facial and eye edema, Tíng Lì Zǐ (Semen Lepidii) can drain phlegm rheum in the lung to relieve cough and wheezing. It is very often prescribed together with Dà Zǎo (Fructus Jujubae) to protect stomach qi.

2 Chest and abdominal water retention: Tíng Lì Zǐ (Semen Lepidii), effective in freeing and regulating the waterways, promoting urination, and reducing swelling, is combined with Xìng Rén (Semen Armeniacae Amarum), Dà Huáng (Radix et Rhizoma Rhei), Fáng Jǐ (Radix Stephaniae Tetrandrae), and Jiāo Mù (Semen Zanthoxyli) for chest and abdominal water retention and inhibited urination.

[Usage and Dosage] The raw herb is strong in action, while stir-fried is moderate. 苦葶苈 Kǔ Tíng Lì is regarded as a potent purgative, whereas 甜葶苈 Tián Tíng Lì is a mild purgative without tendency to injure stomach qi. Use 3–10 g in decoction.

[Mnemonics] Tíng Lì Zǐ (Semen Lepidii, Pepperweed Seed): bitter and pungent; drain the lungs, resolve fluid retention, promote urination, alleviate wheezing, and eliminate hydrothorax and ascites.

[Simple and Effective Formulas]
葶苈散 Tíng Lì Sǎn — Pepperweed Seed Powder from *Effective Formulas from Generations of Physicians* (世医得效方, Shì Yī Dé Xiào Fāng): Tián Tíng Lì (Semen Lepidii) 75 g (stir-fried on paper until purple); grind into powder, decoct 6 g/time in water for oral administration to treat lung qi stagnation, cough and wheezing with inability to lie flat or vomiting blood and pus.

[Precautions] Tíng Lì Zǐ (Semen Lepidii), capable of attacking the pathogen, is contraindicated in cases of cough and wheezing due to lung and kidney qi deficiency and edema caused by spleen and kidney qi deficiency.

Daily practices

1. What are the similarities and differences between Zǐ Wǎn (Radix et Rhizoma Asteris) and Kuǎn Dōng Huā (Flos Farfarae) in terms of nature, flavor, actions and indications? what are the difference among Zǐ Wǎn (Radix et Rhizoma Asteris), Kuǎn Dōng Huā (Flos Farfarae), Xìng Rén (Semen Armeniacae Amarum), Bái Qián (Rhizoma et Radix Cynanchi Stauntonii), and Qián Hú (Radix Peucedani) in terms of indications?
2. What are the similarities and differences between Tián Tíng Lì (Semen Lepidii) and other medicinal that arrest cough and wheezing in terms of actions and indications?

百部 Bǎi Bù *radix stemonae stemona root*

The source is from the tuber of herbaceous perennial *Stemona sessilifolia* (Miq.) Miq., *S. japonica* (Bl.) Miq., and *S. tubeosa* Lour., family Stemonaleae. It is so called its roots are numerous, and hundreds (*Bǎi*) of roots are arranged in typical battle formation (*Bù*). Sweet and bitter in flavor and slightly warm in nature.

[Actions] Moisten the lungs and arrest cough, and kill lice and parasites. It is applicable for different types of acute and chronic cough, whooping cough, pulmonary tuberculosis, pinworm, head louse, and body louse. Experiments has shown that its alkaloid has antiasthmatic, antibechic, antalgic, and antibacterial effects and can kill certain parasites.

[Quality] Good quality is full, yellowish white, fleshy, moist, strong, and solid.

[Indications]

1. Different types of cough: Bǎi Bù (Radix Stemonae) is applicable for different types of cough when appropriate compatibility is implemented. It is combined with Jīng Jiè (Herba Schizonepetae), Jié Gěng (Radix Platycodonis), Zǐ Wǎn (Radix et Rhizoma Asteris), Chén Pí (Pericarpium Citri Reticulatae), Bái Qián (Rhizoma et Radix Cynanchi Stauntonii) for cough caused by wind-cold invading the lung; with Shā Shēn (Radix Adenophorae seu Glehniae), Mài Dōng (Radix Ophiopogonis), Bèi Mǔ (Bulbus Fritillaria), Bǎi Hé (Bulbus Lilii) for hectic cough due to yin deficiency; with Huáng Qí (Radix Astragali), Shā Shēn (Radix Adenophorae seu Glehniae), and Mài Dōng (Radix Ophiopogonis) for chronic cough with fluid and qi consumption. It can be used alone or together with Bèi Mǔ (Bulbus Fritillaria), Guā Lóu Pí (Pericarpium Trichosanthis), Bái Qián (Rhizoma et Radix Cynanchi Stauntonii), and Dì Lóng (Pheretima) for whooping cough. In recent years, it has been used successfully in the treatment of chronic bronchitis and pulmonary tuberculosis.
2. Different types of parasite: Bǎi Bù (Radix Stemonae) can kill intestinal parasites, especially pinworm. Its decoction retention enema is used in the evening before going to bed. External application of its decoction or ethanol extraction is used in the treatment of head louse, body louse, and crab louse.

External application of this herb has been widely used. For instance, it has been prepared into tincture for external wash to treat tinea.

[Usage and Dosage] This medicinal can kill worms, raw substance tastes bitter with mild toxicity and can easily injure stomach qi, therefore honey-fired is more commonly used. It is more effective in moistening the lungs and arresting cough and particularly suitable for chronic cough due to yin deficiency. Use 5–10 g in decoction, up to 10–15 g when use honey-fried, and decrease the amount as in pill and powder.

[Mnemonics] Băi Bù (Radix Stemonae, Stemona Root): bitter and sweet; arrest coughing and kill lice, especially pinworm.

[Simple and Effective Formulas]
止嗽散 Zhǐ Sòu Săn-Cough Stopping Powder from *Medical Revelations* (医学心悟, Yī Xué Xīn Wù): Zhì Gān Căo (Radix et Rhizoma Glycyrrhizae Praeparata cum Melle) 1.5 g, Bái Qián (Rhizoma et Radix Cynanchi Stauntonii) 4.5 g, Băi Bù (Radix Stemonae) 4.5 g, Zǐ Wăn (Radix et Rhizoma Asteris) 4.5 g, Jié Gěng (Radix Platycodonis) 4.5 g, and Jú Hóng (Exocarpium Citri Rubrum) 3 g; decoct in water for oral administration to treat cough caused by lung failing to diffuse and descent when cold pathogens invade the lung.

[Precautions] Băi Bù (Radix Stemonae) should not be used long-term or over-dosage.

枇杷叶 **Pí Pá Yè** *folium eriobotryae loquat leaf*

The source is from the leaf of evergreen subarbor *Eriobotrya japonica* (Thunb.) Lindl., family Rosaceae. Bitter in flavor and slightly cold in nature.

[Actions] Dissolve phlegm and arrest wheezing, and harmonize the stomach and redirect rebelling stomach qi downward. It is applicable for cough and wheezing with thick sputum, thirst due to stomach heat, and vomiting. Experiments indicate hydrocyanic acid decomposed by its amygdalin has cough-arresting effect, its oily substance has expectorant effect, and its ursolic acid has anti-inflammatory effect.

[Quality] Good quality is dry with large and intact leaves.

[Indications]

1. Lung heat cough: Pí Pá Yè (Folium Eriobotryae), cold in nature, is combined with Sāng Bái Pí (Cortex Mori), Mă Dōu Líng (Fructus Aristolochiae), and Huáng Qín (Radix Scutellariae) for lung heat

cough; and with Sāng Yè (Folium Mori), Mài Dōng (Radix Ophiopogonis), Shí Gāo (Gypsum Fibrosum), and Ē Jiāo (Colla Corii Asini) for dry-heat cough. It has recently been prepared into syrup or decocted extract to treat different types of cough.

2. Qi counterflow due to stomach heat: Pí Pá Yè (Folium Eriobotryae), bitter in flavor and descending in nature, is applicable for vomiting and hiccup due to ascending counterflow of stomach qi. It is combined with Zhú Rú (Caulis Bambusae in Taenia), Huáng Lián (Rhizoma Coptidis), and Chén Pí (Pericarpium Citri Reticulatae) for vomiting due to stomach heat.

[Usage and Dosage] Use raw in general, process with honey to strengthen its cough-arresting quality, or in ginger juice to increase its ability to stop vomiting and hiccup. Use 5–9 g in decoction.

[Mnemonics] Pí Pá Yè (Folium Eriobotryae, Loquat Leaf): bitter; redirect rebelling stomach qi downward to arrest vomiting, specialized in relieving coughing, but more attention should be paid to combination.

[Simple and Effective Formulas]
枇杷叶汤 Pí Pá Yè Tāng — Loquat Leaf Decoction from *Comprehensive Recording of Divine Assistance* (圣济总录, Shèng Jì Zŏng Lù): Pí Pá Yè (Folium Eriobotryae) (roasted, hair removed) 120 g, Chén Pí (Pericarpium Citri Reticulatae) (soaked in water, white inner surface of exocarp removed, baked) 150 g, and Gān Cǎo (Radix et Rhizoma Glycyrrhizae) (roasted, filed) 90 g; grind into crude powder, decoct 6 g/time with Shēng Jiāng (Rhizoma Zingiberis Recens) in water, and take warm after removing dregs when necessary for unremitting hiccup with inability to eat and drink.

[Precautions] Pí Pá Yè (Folium Eriobotryae), cold in nature, is contraindicated in cases of vomiting due to stomach cold and wind-cold.

紫苏子 Zǐ Sū Zǐ *fructus perillae perilla fruit*

The source is from the ripe fruit of herbaceous *Perilla frutescens* (L.) Britt., family Labiatae. Alternate names include *Sū Zǐ*. Pungent in flavor and warm in nature.

[Actions] Redirect the qi downward and dissolve phlegm, arrest coughing and wheezing, and moisten the intestines and promote the bowel movement. It is applicable for cough and wheezing with profuse phlegm, and constipation due to intestinal dryness.

[Quality] Good quality is full, round, in even size, grayish brown, fragrant, and without impurities.

[Indications]

1. Cough and wheezing with profuse sputum: Sū Zǐ (Fructus Perillae) is combined with Bàn Xià (Rhizoma Pinelliae), Chén Pí (Pericarpium Citri Reticulatae), and Hòu Pò (Cortex Magnoliae Officinalis) for cough and wheezing with profuse sputum, phlegm accumulation in the throat, and chest and diaphragm fullness and oppression; and with Bái Jiè Zǐ (Semen Sinapis) and Lái Fú Zǐ (Semen Raphani), for spleen deficiency failing to transport in the elderly, food accumulation with phlegm, and cough and wheezing with profuse sputum.
2. Constipation due to intestinal dryness: Sū Zǐ (Fructus Perillae), oily and effective in descending qi, is suitable for intestinal dryness and qi of *fu* organ failing to descend and combined with Má Rén (Fructus Cannabis), Bǎi Zǐ Rén (Semen Platycladi), and Táo Rén (Semen Persicae).

[Usage and Dosage] Use raw in general; stir-frying to moderate its effect. Use 5–10 g in decoction.

[Mnemonics] Zǐ Sū Zǐ (Fructus Perillae, Perilla Fruit): pungent and warm; moisten the intestines, arrest cough and wheezing, and relieve phlegm.

[Simple and Effective Formulas]

1. 苏子散 Sū Zǐ Sǎn — Perilla Fruit Powder from *Materia Medica of South Yunnan* (滇南本草, Diān Nán Běn Cǎo): Sū Zǐ (Fructus Perillae) 3 g, Bā Dá Xìng Rén (Semen Armeniacae Amarum) (peel and tip removed) 30 g, and add Bái Mì (Mel) 6 g for the elderly; grind into powder and take 9 g/time for adult or 3 g/time for child with boiled water to treat chronic and persistent cough in children or the elderly with wheezing and throat phlegm that sounds like a drag saw.
2. 紫苏麻仁粥 Zǐ Sū Má Rén Zhōu — Perilla Fruit and Hemp Seed Congee from *Formulas to Aid the Living* (济生方, Jì Shēng Fāng): Zǐ Sū Zǐ (Fructus Perillae) and Má Rén (Fructus Cannabis); cook until

soft, remove dregs, use the medicated liquid to prepare congee for oral administration to treat difficult defecation.

[Precautions] Sū Zǐ (Fructus Perillae), descending and slippery in nature, is contraindicated in cases of cough and wheezing due to deficiency pattern and loose stool caused by spleen deficiency.

Besides the above-mentioned medicinals, others that also used for arresting cough and relieving wheezing include Mǎ Dōu Líng (Fructus Aristolochiae), Sāng Bái Pí (Cortex Mori), Bái Guǒ (Semen Ginkgo), Yáng Jīn Huā (Flos Daturae), and Nán Tiān Zhú Zǐ (南天竹子). Some medicinals in previous chapters can also arrest cough and asthma, it is important for the learners to review those substances. In addition, Mǎ Dōu Líng (Fructus Aristolochiae) should be used with cautions as its ingredient aristolochic acid has renal toxicity.

Daily practices

1. Summarize the actions and indications of cough and wheezing-arresting medicinals that we learn before?
2. What are the similarities and differences among Bǎi Bù (Radix Stemonae), Pí Pá Yè (Folium Eriobotryae), and Sū Zǐ (Fructus Perillae) in terms of arresting cough and wheezing? what are their other actions and indications?

CHAPTER 11

Eleventh Week

1

MEDICINALS THAT CALM THE SPIRIT

These substances are used primarily to calm the mind.

The heart governs the mind and disturbances of the sprit may lead to such problems as palpitations, insomnia, depressive psychosis, and even some forms of insanity. Causes for restlessness of heart spirit are heart blood deficiency failing to nourish the heart, heart qi deficiency failing to astringe, dysfunction of heart due to blood stasis or phlegm obstruction, and pathogenic heat harassing the interior. Therefore, mind-calming herbs work through a variety of pathways. There are three major categories of substances that calm the spirit:

(1) Those that anchor, settle, and calm the spirit are either minerals or shells. Traditionally their function has been related to their heavy-weight, descending, and subduing properties. They are used to weigh upon the heart so as to calm the spirit.

(2) Those that nourish the heart to calm the spirit are primarily used for nourish and enrich heart blood or boost heart qi.

(3) Those that clear and drain heart heat to protect heart spirit from disturbance and calm the spirit.

While all of the herbs in this section are useful in treating restless heart spirit, each of them is especially suited for a particular aspect of the problem. However, its etiology is very often a complex of heart deficiency and pathogenic excess, the combination of herbs is based on the differentiation of pathogenesis (primary and secondary). For instance, medicinals that nourish the heart and calm the spirit should be prescribed together with those that suppress and calm the spirit in the cases of heart qi deficiency and heart spirit failing to restrain; substances that clear the heart or clear phlegm heat are used together with those that suppress and calm the spirit in cases of restlessness of heart spirit due to pathogenic heat or phlegm heat accumulating in the heart.

Hence, a comprehensive treatment should not only include medicinals of calming the mind but also those that relieve the underlying conditions. If restless heart spirit is due to heart blood deficiency, herbs that supplement blood should also be used; if the problem is caused by heart qi deficiency, herbs that supplement and boost heart qi should be added; if restless heart spirit is resulting from fulminant desertion of heart yang, herbs that supplement the heart and rescue yang should also be prescribed; if the problem is attributable to intense heart fire, herbs that clear the heart and drain fire should be added; if the problem is associated with internal obstruction of blood stasis, herbs invigorate blood and dissolve stasis should be included; if the restless heart spirit is due to phlegm and water retention, herbs that dissolve phlegm and dispel water retention should also be used; and if the trouble is caused by kidney yin (water) deficiency failing to nourish heart (fire), herbs that tonify and nourish kidney yin should be included in the treatment plan.

Minerals should be crushed and cooked before adding other ingredients. They really injure stomach qi, for this reason, they should not be taken long-term as pill and powder. A few of these substances contain toxicity, such as Zhū Shā (Cinnabaris); caution should be used in their processing method and dosage. To minimize toxicity they should also not be taken long-term.

酸枣仁 Suān Zǎo Rén *Semen ziziphi spinosae Spiny date seed*

The source is from the ripe semen of deciduous shrub or arbor *Ziziphus Spinosa* Hu, family Rhamnaceae. It is so called because it looks like Jujube (枣, Zǎo) and sour (酸, Suān) and alternate names include 枣仁 Zǎo Rén and 酸枣核 Suān Zǎo Hé. Sweet in flavor and neutral in nature.

[Actions] Tranquilize the heart and quiet the mind, and restrain abnormal sweating and generate fluid. It is applicable for insomnia with deficiency-vexation, palpitations due to fright, dreaminess, profuse sweating due to general debility, and thirst caused by fluid consumption. Experiments has shown that it has sedative and hypnotic effects on animal and that its active ingredient is jujuboside.

[Quality] Good quality is large, intact, full, lustrous, reddish brown, and without kernel and shell.

[Indications]

1. Insomnia and palpitations: Suān Zǎo Rén (Semen Ziziphi Spinosae), effective in nourishing and enriching yin and blood, is capable of nourishing blood to tranquilize the mind and therefore suitable for disorders caused by heart blood insufficiency. It is combined with Zhī Mǔ (Rhizoma Anemarrhenae), Fú Líng (Poria), and Chuān Xiōng (Rhizoma Chuanxiong) for deficiency-vexation insomnia caused by heart and liver blood deficiency resulting in yin deficiency with yang hyperactivity; and with Rén Shēn (Radix et Rhizoma Ginseng), Bái Zhú (Rhizoma Atractylodis Macrocephalae), and Lóng Yǎn Ròu (Arillus Longan) for palpitations due to fright, restlessness, and insomnia due to overstrain injuring the heart and spleen.
2. Sweating due to weak constitution: Suān Zǎo Rén (Semen Ziziphi Spinosae) is combined with Rén Shēn (Radix et Rhizoma Ginseng), Nuò Dào Gēn Xū (Radix Oryzae Glutinosae), and Wǔ Wèi Zǐ (Fructus Schisandrae Chinensis) for spontaneous sweating and night sweating due to weak constitution.

[Usage and Dosage] Traditionally use raw for somnolence and cooked for insomnia. However, modern research has shown that the raw and cooked both have sedative effects, and that the raw is more significant and over stir-frying will consume its oily substances and result in invalidity. Experiment demonstrates that over-dose can affect sleep or cause lethargy. Use 6–15 g in decoction, crush before decocting, or as a powder with a dosage of 2 g/time.

[Mnemonics] Suān Zǎo Rén (Semen Ziziphi Spinosae, Spiny Date Seed): sweet; nourish the blood, tranquilize the mind, specialized in cure insomnia, and arrest sweating.

[Simple and Effective Formulas]

1. 酸枣仁汤 Suān Zǎo Rén Tāng — Sour Jujube Decoction from *Essentials from the Golden Cabinet* (金匮要略, Jīn Guì Yào Lüè): Suān Zǎo Rén (Semen Ziziphi Spinosae) 10 g, Gān Cǎo (Radix et Rhizoma Glycyrrhizae) 5 g, Zhī Mǔ (Rhizoma Anemarrhenae) 10 g, Fú Líng (Poria) 10 g, and Chuān Xiōng (Rhizoma Chuanxiong) 10 g; decoct in water for oral administration to treat deficiency-consumption, deficiency-vexation, and inability to fall into sleep. Also applicable for different types of insomnia.

2. 盗汗方 Dào Hàn Fāng — Night Sweating-reducing Formula for *Formulas for Universal Relief* (普济方, Pǔ Jì Fāng): Suān Zǎo Rén (Semen Ziziphi Spinosae), Rén Shēn (Radix et Rhizoma Ginseng), and Fú Líng (Poria) in equal dosage; grind into fine powder and take 6 g/time with rice soup for night sweating.

[Precautions] Suān Zǎo Rén (Semen Ziziphi Spinosae), slippery in nature, is contraindicated in cases of diarrhea, spontaneous seminal emission, and insomnia and palpitations due to heat exuberance in the liver and gallbladder.

柏子仁 **Bǎi Zǐ Rén** *Semen platycladi Oriental arborvitael*

The source is from the ripe semen of evergreen arbor *Biota orientalis* (L.) Endl., family Cupressaceae. Alternate names include 柏仁 Bǎi Rén, 柏子 Bǎi Zǐ, 柏实 Bǎi Shí, and 侧柏子 Cè Bǎi Zǐ. In the opinion of the ancients, different from other trees, the branches of cypress grow towards west direction, which corresponds to white (Bǎi) in five element theory; and its flat leaves grow laterally (Cè Bǎi). Sweet in flavor and neutral in nature.

[Actions] Nourish the heart and tranquilize the mind, and moisten the intestine and unblock the bowels. It is applicable for insomnia with deficiency-vexation, palpitations, severe palpitations, night sweating due to yin deficiency, and constipation due to intestinal dryness.

[Quality] Good quality is large, full, yellowish white, oily, and without skin, shell and impurities.

[Indications]

1. Insomnia and palpitations: Bǎi Zǐ Rén (Semen Platycladi), capable of nourishing the heart and tranquilizing the spirit, is prescribed together with Dāng Guī (Radix Angelicae Sinensis), Shú Dì Huáng (Radix Rehmanniae Praeparata), and Shí Chāng Pú (Rhizoma Acori Tatarinowii) for palpitations or severe palpitations, insomnia, and forgetfulness caused by heart blood insufficiency failing to store heart spirit; and with Huáng Qí (Radix Astragali), Dān Shēn (Radix et Rhizoma Salviae Miltiorrhizae), Dāng Guī (Radix Angelicae Sinensis), and Suān Zǎo Rén (Semen Ziziphi Spinosae) for the above-mentioned manifestations due to qi and blood deficiency.
2. Dry and hard stools: Oily Bǎi Zǐ Rén (Semen Platycladi) can nourish blood, moisten dryness, and increase intestinal fluid to promote defecation, and therefore is often combined with Má Zǐ Rén (Fructus Cannabis), Xìng Rén (Semen Armeniacae Amarum), Yù Lǐ Rén (Semen Pruni), and Sōng Zǐ Rén (Semen Pini Koraiens).

It is also applicable for night sweating in a combination with Mǔ Lì (Concha Ostreae), Má Huáng Gēn (Radix et Rhizoma Ephedrae), Bái Zhú (Rhizoma Atractylodis Macrocephalae), Rén Shēn (Radix et Rhizoma Ginseng), and Dà Zǎo (Fructus Jujubae).

[Usage and Dosage] Use raw in general, Bǎi Zǐ Shuāng (Platycladi Praeparatum) is preferred in cases of constitutionally loose stool and diarrhea as it is oily and slippery. Use 6–15 g in decoction.

[Mnemonics] Bǎi Zǐ Rén (Semen Platycladi, Oriental Arborvitael): neutral and sweet; relieve insomnia, unblock the bowels, and tranquilize palpitations due to fright.

[Simple and Effective Formulas]

1. 通便丸 Tōng Biàn Wán — Constipation Removing Pill from *Extension of the Materia Medica* (本草衍义, Běn Cǎo Yǎn Yì): Bǎi Zǐ Rén

(Semen Platycladi), Dà Má Zǐ Rén (Fructus Cannabis), and Sōng Zǐ Rén (Semen Pini Koraiens) in equal dosage; grind into powder, make into phoenix tree seed-sized pill, and take 20 or 30 pills/dose before meal for constipation due to general debility in the elderly.

2. 柏子养心丸 Bǎi Zǐ Yǎng Xīn Wán — Oriental Arborvitael Heart Nourishing Pill from *A Compilation of Benevolent Formulas* (体仁汇编, Tǐ Rén Huì Biān): Bǎi Zǐ Rén (Semen Platycladi) (steamed, dried under sunshine, shell removed) 120 g, Gǒu Qǐ Zǐ (Fructus Lycii) (washed with wine, dried under sunshine) 60 g, Mài Dōng (Radix Ophiopogonis) (plumule removed) 60 g, Dāng Guī (Radix Angelicae Sinensis) (soaked in wine) 60 g, Shí Chāng Pú (Rhizoma Acori Tatarinowii) (unhaired, washed clean) 60 g, Fú Shén (Sclerotium Poriae Pararadicis) (peel and kernel removed) 60 g, Xuán Shēn (Radix Scrophulariae) 60 g, Shú Dì Huáng (Radix Rehmanniae Praeparata) (soaked in wine) 60 g, and Gān Cǎo (Radix et Rhizoma Glycyrrhizae) (coarse layer of bark removed) 15 g; grind into powder, make into phoenix tree seed-sized pill with honey, and take 40–50 pills/time with Dēng Xīn (Medulla Junci) decoction or Guì Yuán (Arillus Longan) decoction for oral administration to treat overstrain, deficiency of heart blood, absent-minded, frequent nightmares, palpitations, forgetfulness, and seminal emission.

[Precautions] Bǎi Zǐ Rén (Semen Platycladi), oily and slippery in nature, should be used with caution in cases of loose stool and phlegm exuberance.

Daily practices

1. What are the actions of medicinals that calm the spirit? What precautions should be taken when using it?
2. What are the similarities and differences between Suān Zǎo Rén (Semen Ziziphi Spinosae) and Bǎi Zǐ Rén (Semen Platycladi) in terms of actions and indications?

龙骨 Lóng Gǔ *Os draconis Dragon bones*

The source is from the fossil skeleton of ancient animals. Sweet and acrid in flavor and neutral in nature.

[Actions] Suppress fright and tranquilize the mind, calm the liver and subdue yang, astringent and retain the essence, and generate flesh and cure the nonhealing sores when used topically. It is applicable for convulsion, epilepsy, and mania, palpitation, forgetfulness, insomnia, dreaminess, spontaneous sweating, night sweating, seminal emission, strangury with turbid discharge, hematemesis, epistaxis, profuse uterine bleeding, prolonged scanty uterine bleeding of variable intervals abnormal vaginal discharge, diarrhea and dysentery with prolapse of anus, and enduring open non-healing ulcer.

[Quality] It is divided into 五花龙骨 Wǔ Huā Lóng Gǔ and 白龙骨 Bái Lóng Gǔ. The former is also known as 花龙骨 Huā Lóng Gǔ, good quality is brittle and laminate with a strong and moisture-absorbing quality; whereas for the latter, good quality is hard and white with a strong, moisture-absorbing quality. The former is superior to the latter.

[Indications]

1. Restlessness of heart spirit: Lóng Gǔ (Os Draconis), heavyweight and suppressing in nature, can subdue and calm heart spirit and is applicable for a variety of disorders caused by restlessness of heart spirit. It is combined with Mǔ Lì (Concha Ostreae) and Guì Zhī (Ramulus Cinnamomi) for paitent with vexation, agitation, and palpitations due to fright; with Dǎn Nán Xīng (Arisaema cum Bile), Tiān Zhú Huáng (Concretio Silicea Bambusae), and Hǔ Pò (Succinum) for freight, depressive psychosis, and mania caused by phlegm-heat; and with Shí Chāng Pú (Rhizoma Acori Tatarinowii), Yuǎn Zhì (Radix Polygalae), and Suān Zǎo Rén (Semen Ziziphi Spinosae) for insomnia, dreaminess, palpitations, and forgetfulness attributed to heart qi insufficiency.
2. Vertigo and dizziness: Lóng Gǔ (Os Draconis) is combined with medicinals that calm the liver and subdue yang such as Mǔ Lì (Concha Ostreae), Bái Sháo (Radix Paeoniae Alba) and Dài Zhě Shí (Haematitum) for vertigo and dizziness caused by ascendant hyperactivity of liver yang through calming and extinguishing liver wind.
3. Efflux desertion patterns: Lóng Gǔ (Os Draconis), astringent in flavor, is capable of consolidating and astringing and therefore suitable for different disorders caused by efflux desertion. It is prescribed

together with Mǔ Lì (Concha Ostreae) and Fú Xiǎo Mài (Fructus Tritici Levis) for spontaneous and night sweating due to body fluid failing to stay in the interiro; with Rén Shēn (Radix et Rhizoma Ginseng) and Fù Zǐ (Radix Aconiti Lateralis Praeparata) for profuse cold sweating caused by original qi collapse and desertion; with Shān Zhū Yú (Fructus Corni), Mǔ Lì (Concha Ostreae), Qiàn Shí (Semen Euryales), and Jīn Yīng Zǐ (Fructus Rosae Laevigatae) for kidney deficiency with seminal emission; with Mǔ Lì (Concha Ostreae) and Hǎi Piāo Xiāo (Endoconcha Sepiae) for abnormal vaginal discharge, profuse uterine bleeding, and prolonged scanty uterine bleeding of variable intervals; and with Chì Shí Zhī (Halloysitum Rubrum), Fú Líng (Poria), and Bì Xiè (Rhizoma Dioscoreae Hypoglaucae) for cloudy urine.

4. Non-healing wound of sores: Lóng Gǔ (Os Draconis), astringent in nature and good at consolidating and astringing, is applicable for different types of sores and ulcers with complete pus discharge and open enduring and non-healing wound and often combined with Chì Shí Zhī (Halloysitum Rubrum), Hǎi Piāo Xiāo (Endoconcha Sepiae), and Wǔ Bèi Zǐ (Galla Chinensis) in a powdered form. It is ground together with Kū Fán (Alumen Dehydratum) into fine powder and applied externally to treat eczema with exudate and itching.

[Usage and Dosage] Use raw to settle and calm the spirit, calcined as an astringent to restrain and consolidate. Topical application to generate the flesh. Use 9–15 g in decoction and reduce the amount in pill and powder.

[Mnemonics] Lóng Gǔ (Os Draconis, Dragon Bones): sweet and pungent; suppress fright and calm the mind, astringent and retain the essence, and relieve vertigo and dizziness.

[Simple and Effective Formulas]

1. 龙骨散 Lóng Gǔ Sǎn — Dragon Bones Powder from *The Complete Works of Jing-yue* (景岳全书, Jǐng Yuè Quán Shū) :calcined Lóng Gǔ (Os Draconis) 30 g, Dāng Guī (Radix Angelicae Sinensis) 30 g, Xiāng Fù (Rhizoma Cyperi) (stir-fried) 30 g, and Zōng Lǚ Tàn (Petiolus Trachycarpi Carbonisatus) 15 g; grind into fine powder and

take 12 g/time with rice soup on an empty stomach rice soup for persistent profuse uterine bleeding.

2. 产后虚汗方 Chǎn Hòu Xū Hàn Fāng — Postpartum Deficiency Sweating Relieving Formula from *Formulas from Benevolent Sages* (圣惠方, Shèng Huì Fāng): Lóng Gǔ (Os Draconis) 30 g and Má Huáng Gēn (Radix et Rhizoma Ephedrae) 30 g; grind into fine powder and take 6 g/time with rice soup when necessary for postpartum persistent sweating due to deficiency.

[Precautions] Lóng Gǔ (Os Draconis), astringent in nature, is contraindicated in cases of unresolved excess pathogens such as fire-heat, damp-turbidity, and phlegm-rheum.

磁石 Cí Shí *Magnetitum magnetite*

It is the natural magnetic iron ore magnetite. It is so called because it attracts iron just like an attractive mother and alternate names include 吸铁石 Xī Tiě Shí. Pungent in flavor and cold in nature.

[Actions] Subdue yang and grasp qi, and suppress fright and calm the mind. It is applicable for vertigo, dizziness, blurred vision, tinnitus, deafness, palpitations due to fright, insomnia, and wheezing due to kidney deficiency. Modern researches reveal that magnetized water can improve blood viscosity and change certain properties of water, which is conducive to human health.

[Quality] Good quality is black, shiny, and strongly attracts iron.

[Indications]

1. Restlessness of heart spirit: Cí Shí (Magnetitum), heavyweight and suppressing in nature to calm the spirit, is applicable for palpitations, fright, insomnia, vexation and agitation, depressive psychosis, and mania caused by heart spirit restlessness and often prescribed together with medicinals that calm the spirit and dissolve phlegm such as Shè Xiāng (Moschus), Lóng Gǔ (Os Draconis), Mǔ Lì (Concha Ostreae), and Qīng Méng Shí (Lapis Chloriti).

2. Yang qi hyperactivity: yang qi exuberance or yin fluid insufficiency failing to control yang qi may cause hyperactivity of yang qi. Cí Shí (Magnetitum), heavyweight and capable of suppressing yang, is combined with other medicinals to relieve this problem. It is combined with medicinals that calm the liver and subdue yang such as Bái Sháo (Radix Paeoniae Alba), Shí Jué Míng (Concha Haliotidis), and Jú Huā (Flos Chrysanthemi) for vertigo, headache, and tinnitus due to ascendant hyperactivity of liver yang; with Dì Huáng (Radix Rehmanniae), Jú Huā (Flos Chrysanthemi), and Gŏu Qǐ Zǐ (Fructus Lycii) for blurred vision and vertigo due to liver and kidney yin deficiency with hyperactivity of deficient yang; and with Shú Dì Huáng (Radix Rehmanniae Praeparata), Shān Zhū Yú (Fructus Corni), Fú Líng (Poria), and Wǔ Wèi Zǐ (Fructus Schisandrae Chinensis) for tinnitus and deafness attributed to kidney yin deficiency.
3. Wheezing due to kidney deficiency: the kidney governs qi reception and kidney qi insufficiency may cause shortness of breath and wheezing, especially upon exertion. Cí Shí (Magnetitum) can assist the kidney and receive qi, and is therefore used together with Rén Shēn (Radix et Rhizoma Ginseng), Shú Dì Huáng (Radix Rehmanniae Praeparata), and Wǔ Wèi Zǐ (Fructus Schisandrae Chinensis).

Its application in the treatment of impotence and senile cataract has been reported in recent years.

[Usage and Dosage] Use raw, or calcine prior to decocting to facilitate active ingredient extraction. Use 10–30 g in decoction, crush before using in decocting; or use as a powder with a dosage of 1–3 g/time.

[Mnemonics] Cí Shí (Magnetitum, Magnetite): pungent and cold; subdue the yang, relieve wheezing, and suppressing palpitations due to fright with heavy sedatives.

[Simple and Effective Formulas]

1. 神曲丸 Shén Qū Wán — Medicated Leaven Pill from *Important Formulas Worth a Thousand Gold Pieces* (千金要方 Qiān Jīn Yào Fāng,): Cí Shí (Magnetitum) 60 g, Yè Míng Shā (Faeces Vespertilionis)

30 g, and Shén Qū (Massa Medicata Fermentata) 120 g; grind into powder, make into phoenix tree seed-sized pill with honey, and take 30
pills/time with rice soup, three times a day for kidney deficiency, mus-
cae volitantes, and hypopsia.

2. 磁石酒 Cí Shí Jiǔ — Magnetite Wine from *Comprehensive Recording
   of Divine Assistance* (圣济总录 Shèng Jì Zǒng Lù,): Cí Shí (Magnetitum)
   (pounded into pieces) 15 g, Mù Tōng (Caulis Akebiae) 250 g, and Shí
   Chāng Pú (Rhizoma Acori Tatarinowii) (soaked in rice-washed water
   for one or two days, cut, baked) 250 g; pack in bag, soak in 1000 ml
   wine for seven days in winter or three days in summer, and drink the
   medicated wine for deafness and tinnitus.

[Precautions] Cí Shí (Magnetitum), heavyweight and suppressing in nature,
is difficult to digest and should therefore be used with caution in cases of
weak spleen and stomach. Long-term use of pill and powder is discouraged.

远志 **Yuǎn Zhì** *Radix polygalae Thin-Leaf milkwort root*

The source is from the root of herbaceous perennial *Polygala tenuifolia*
Wild. and *P. sibirica* L., family Polygalaceae. It is so called as it is capable
of improving wisdom (志 Zhì). Bitter and pungent in flavor and warm in
nature.

[Actions] Calm the mind and benefit the brain, and dispel phlegm and reduce
swelling. It is applicable for patterns of restless heart spirit, such as insomnia, dreaminess, forgetfulness, palpitations due to fright, absent-minded,
cough, profuse sputum, sores, ulcers, swelling, and toxins. Experiments have
demonstrated that it can improve the effect of hypnotic medicine on animal,
and has anticonvulsant and significant expectorant effects.

[Quality] Good quality is thick and has a thick cortex.

[Indications]

1. Restlessness of heart spirit: Yuǎn Zhì (Radix Polygalae) is applicable for
   a variety of disorders due to heart spirit restlessness through combining
   with other medicinals. It is combined with Rén Shēn (Radix et Rhizoma

Ginseng), Dāng Guī (Radix Angelicae Sinensis), Huáng Qí (Radix Astragali), Fú Shén (Sclerotium Poriae Pararadicis), and Lóng Yǎn Ròu (Arillus Longan) for palpitations and insomnia caused by heart and spleen qi and blood insufficiency; with Shè Xiāng (Moschus), Qīng Lóng Chǐ (Dens Draconis), and Fú Shén (Sclerotium Poriae Pararadicis) for palpitations and insomnia due to fright; and with Rén Shēn (Radix et Rhizoma Ginseng), Fú Líng (Poria), and Shí Chāng Pú (Rhizoma Acori Tatarinowii) for forgetfulness attributed to heart qi insufficiency.

2. Cough with profuse sputum: owing to its property of dissolving phlegm, Yuǎn Zhì (Radix Polygalae) is often combined with medicinals that diffuse the lung and dissolve phlegm such as Jié Gěng (Radix Platycodonis), Bàn Xià (Rhizoma Pinelliae), Chén Pí (Pericarpium Citri Reticulatae), and Xìng Rén (Semen Armeniacae Amarum) for externally or internally-contracted cough with profuse sputum.

   It is also used in the treatment of disturbance of consciousness due to phlegm confounding the heart orifice as it can dissolve phlegm.

3. Carbuncles and swellings with pain: Yuǎn Zhì (Radix Polygalae), capable of dispersing and relieving carbuncles and swellings, can be used for oral administration or/and external application. It can be decocted with wine, drinking the wine and using the dreg for external application to treat breast swelling and pain.

It can be ground into fine powder to treat headache as a snuff.

[Usage and Dosage] Use raw. Process with Gān Cǎo (Radix et Rhizoma Glycyrrhizae) to reduce its dry nature and moderate its medicinal property; honey-fry to improve its phlegm-dissolving and cough-arresting ability, and reduce its stimulation to the stomach. Use 3–9 g in decoction, decrease the amount in pill and powder.

[Mnemonics] Yuǎn Zhì (Radix Polygalae, Thin-leaf Milkwort Root): bitter and pungent; benefit the brain, clam the heart, expel phlegm, arrest cough, and dissipate sore and swelling.

[Simple and Effective Formulas]

1. 定志小丸 Dìng Zhì Xiǎo Wán — Mind-tranquilizing Small Pill from *Ancient and Modern Records of Proven Formulas* (古今录验方, Gǔ Jīn Lù Yàn Fāng): Shí Chāng Pú (Rhizoma Acori Tatarinowii) 6 g, Yuǎn

Zhì (Radix Polygalae) (plumule removed) 6 g, Fú Líng (Poria) 6 g, and Rén Shēn (Radix et Rhizoma Ginseng) 90 g; grind into pill, make into phoenix tree seed-sized pill with honey, and take six or seven pills/time, five times a day for heart qi deficiency, paroxysmal sadness and depression, and forgetfulness.

2. 远志汤 Yuǎn Zhì Tāng — Thin leaf Milkwort Root Decoction from *Comprehensive Recording of Divine Assistance* (圣济总录 Shèng Jì Zǒng Lù,): Yuǎn Zhì (Radix Polygalae) (plumule removed) 30 g and Shí Chāng Pú (Rhizoma Acori Tatarinowii) (cut into thin pieces) 30 g; grind into powder, decoct 6 g/time in water, and take the liquid after removing dregs for oral administration to treat persistent stomachache.

[Precautions] Yuǎn Zhì (Radix Polygalae) may cause gastric mucosal irritation. Overdose (for example taken 6 g of powder) will lead to vomiting. It should not be used alone in cases of restlessness of heart spirit due to deficiency.

Besides the above-mentioned medicinals, others that also used for tranquilizing the mind such as Hǔ Pò (Succinum), Hé Huān Pí (Cortex Albiziae), Shè Xiāng (Moschus), Qīng Lóng Chǐ (Dens Draconis), Mǔ Lì (Concha Ostreae), and Yè Jiāo Téng (Caulis Polygoni Multiflori). Some medicinals in other chapters can also calm the spirit, learners are supposed to sum them up to facilitate the study.

Daily practices

1. What are the similarities and differences among Lóng Gǔ (Os Draconis), Cí Shí (Magnetitum), and Yuǎn Zhì (Radix Polygalae) in terms of tranquilizing the spirit?
2. Lóng Gǔ (Os Draconis), Cí Shí (Magnetitum), and Yuǎn Zhì (Radix Polygalae) all can tranquilize the spirit, what are their other actions?

MEDICINALS THAT CALM THE LIVER AND EXTINGUISH WIND

The liver governs the free flow of qi, stores blood, and commands the sinew-membranes of the body. Yin and yang of the liver must maintain relative balance. Liver qi hyperactivity and ascendant hyperactivity of liver yang are usually caused by over ascending and dispersing of liver qi, or heat exuberance of liver yang, or liver yin blood failing to nourish and contain liver yang. Manifestations include headache, vertigo, and vomiting and usually occur in patients with internal miscellaneous diseases. While, interior movement of liver wind can arise from exuberant heat stirring wind or yin deficiency generating wind (water failing to nourish wood), the former is due to hyperactivity of intense yang heat in the liver channel or even burning the sinews in some cases, and the latter is caused by liver yin and blood deficiency failing to nourish and restraining yang qi and liver yang and nourishing the sinews with a subsequent hyperactivity of deficiency-yang or malnourish of the sinews with muscle contracture. Manifestations include spasms, contracture, and convulsion of the sinews and tremor of the limbs and often occur not only in internal *miscellaneous* diseases, but also in febrile diseases when there is heat exuberance or yin consumption.

Herbs that calm the liver and extinguish wind are primarily used to calm liver qi, subdue ascendant hyperactivity of liver yang, and extinguish interior movement of liver wind.

These substances, capable of subduing the adverse or over-flow, calming the liver, anchoring yang, extinguishing wind, arresting spasms, and clearing the liver, are further divided by function character into four classes, namely

(1) heavyweight shell and mineral substances that have pronounced effect in anchoring and suppressing yang and are used for ascendant hyperactivity of liver yang;
(2) worms that are potent in extinguishing wind and are applicable for internal movement of liver wind;
(3) herbs that cool the liver and extinguish wind are often used in cases of ascendant hyperactivity of liver yang and intense liver heat stirring wind. The medicinals that clear liver heat that discussed in chapter three and four (medicinals that clear heat) are commonly used in these cases; and
(4) herbs that nourish yin to extinguish wind are mainly applied to treat liver yin deficiency generating wind.

There are many reasons behind hyperactive liver qi, ascendant hyperactivity of liver yang, and internal stirring of liver wind. The herbs that calm the liver and extinguish wind should be combined with other herbs that treat the root cause of the problem. For hyperactive liver qi, they are combined with herbs that sooth liver qi; for ascendant hyperactivity of liver yang; herbs that clear and drain liver heat are added; for liver and kidney yin deficiency with hyperactivity of yang, herbs that supplement the liver and kidney are included in the treatment plan; for intense liver heat stirring wind, herbs that clear heat and drain fire are added; for yin deficiency stirring wind, herbs that nourish yin are also used. Additional herbs for concurrent symptoms and signs should also be included in the prescription. For ascendant hyperactivity of liver yang with accompanying palpitations and insomnia, herbs that calm the mind are added; for internal movement of liver wind with accompanying pathogen blocking the pericardium and loss of consciousness, herbs that open the orifices are also used.

Some of the substances in this chapter are shell and stone minerals and should be crushed and cooked first. Some of them are animal products with certain toxicity, overdose is discouraged. Some of these substances are warm and drying and patients with yin or blood deficiency should not be given hot substances.

羚羊角 Líng Yáng Jiǎo *Cornu saigae tataricae Antelope horn*

The source is from the horn of adult male *Saiga tatarica* L., family Bovidae. Salty in flavor and cold in nature.

[Actions] Calm and extinguish the liver wind, clear the liver and improve vision, and clear heat and relieve toxin. It is applicable for convulsion caused by exuberant heat stirring wind in febrile diseases, headache and vertigo due to ascendant hyperactivity of liver yang, red, swollen, and painful eyes with blurred eyesight resulting form the liver fire flaming upward, as well as macules, papules, carbuncles, swellings, sores, and toxins in febrile diseases.

[Quality] Good quality is tender, white, shiny, lustrous and smooth like jade, and translucent with visible small capillaries and without cracks.

A variety of counterfeit goods are found in the market such as Cornu Procaprae Gutturosae, long-tail Cornu Procaprae Gutturosae, and Tibetan antelope horn, and more attentions should be paid to identification.

[Indications]

1. Internal stirring of liver wind: pathogenic heat exuberance and intense liver heat in febrile diseases may cause liver wind that manifested as high fever, spasm of the extremities, lock-jaw; or liver heat exuberance in internal miscellaneous diseases may lead to liver wind that manifested as headache, vomiting, and spasm or numbness of the limbs. Owning to its property of clearing liver heat and extinguishing liver wind, Líng Yáng Jiǎo (Cornu Saigae Tataricae) is often prescribed together with medicinals that clear heat and calm liver wind such as Shēng Dì (Radix Rehmanniae), Gōu Téng (Ramulus Uncariae Cum Uncis), Bái Sháo (Radix Paeoniae Alba), Dì Lóng (Pheretima), and Shí Jué Míng (Concha Haliotidis).

2. Ascendant hyperactivity of liver yang: manifestations include headache, vertigo, dizziness, and tinnitus. Líng Yáng Jiǎo (Cornu Saigae Tataricae), cold in nature and capable of calming liver yang, is often combined with Gōu Téng (Ramulus Uncariae Cum Uncis), Tiān Má (Rhizoma Gastrodiae), Dài Zhě Shí (Haematitum), and Bái Sháo (Radix Paeoniae Alba).

3. Liver fire flaming upward: manifestations include red, swollen, and painful eyes, or with nebula. Líng Yáng Jiǎo (Cornu Saigae Tataricae) can drain liver fire to bright the vision and is therefore commonly combined with Lóng Dǎn Cǎo (Radix et Rhizoma Gentianae), Xià Kū Cǎo (Spica Prunellae), Huáng Qín (Radix Scutellariae), and Shí Jué Míng (Concha Haliotidis). It is used together with medicinals that nourish and enrich liver and kidney yin fluid such as Gǒu Qǐ Zǐ (Fructus Lycii), Shēng Dì (Radix Rehmanniae), and Shí Hú (Caulis Dendrobii) for deficiency-heat flaming upward resulting from liver and kidney yin deficiency.

4. Blood heat exuberance: Líng Yáng Jiǎo (Cornu Saigae Tataricae) is good at clearing heat in blood level and often prescribed together other medicinals that clear blood heat for disorders caused by blood heat. It

is combined with medicinals that clear heat and cool blood such as Xī Jiǎo (Cornu Rhinocerotis), Shēng Dì (Radix Rehmanniae), Mǔ Dān Pí (Cortex Moutan), Chì Sháo (Radix Paeoniae Rubra), and Shí Gāo (Gypsum Fibrosum) for pathogen invading blood level in febrile diseases, intense heat, purplish dark macules and papules, unconsciousness, and delirious speech; with medicinals that clear heat and resolve toxins such as Pú Gōng Yīng (Herba Taraxaci), Jīn Yín Huā (Flos Lonicerae Japonicae), Lián Qiào (Fructus Forsythiae), and Mǔ Dān Pí (Cortex Moutan) for sores and carbuncles with intensive heat-toxin.

[Usage and Dosage] Use raw in general, 2–3 g in powders or pills taken directly. When used in decoction, cut 2–3 g into slices, cook for one hour and take the strained decoction with that of the other ingredients. Due to the high cost of this substance, it is usually prescribed in powder or juice form to be taken after mixing with water, 0.3–0.5 g/time. Or use as pill or powder.

[Mnemonics] Líng Yáng Jiǎo (Cornu Saigae Tataricae, Antelope Horn): cold; calm and extinguish the liver wind, cool the blood, subdue fire, and relieve vertigo, pain, and spasm.

[Simple and Effective Formulas]

1. 羚羊角丸 Líng Yang Jiǎ Wán — Antelope Horn Pill from *Comprehensive Recording of Divine Assistance* (圣济总录, Shèng Jì Zǒng Lù): Líng Yáng Jiǎo (Cornu Saigae Tataricae) (cut into a very thin slices with a special knife called Bàng Dāo) 30 g, Xī Jiǎo (Cornu Rhinocerotis) (cut into a very thin slices with a Bàng Dāo) 0.9 g, Qiāng Huó (Rhizoma et Radix Notopterygii) 45 g, Fáng Fēng (Radix Saposhnikoviae) 45 g, stir-fried Yì Yǐ Rén (Semen Coicis) 60 g, Qín Jiāo (Radix Gentianae Macrophyllae) 60 g; grind into fine powder, make into phoenix tree seed-sized pill with the paste of honey, and take 20 pills or gradually up to 30 pills with Zhú Yè (Folium Phyllostachydis Henonis) decoction for post-stroke tremor of hands and feet and sluggish speech. Now, Xī Jiǎo (Cornu Rhinocerotis) is replaced with 10 times of Shuǐ Niú Jiǎo (Cornu Bubali).

2. 羚羊角散 Líng Yang Jiǎ Sǎn — Antelope Horn Powder from *Formulas from Benevolent Sages* (圣惠方 Shèng Huì Fāng,): Líng Yáng Jiǎo (Cornu Saigae Tataricae) scrapes 30 g, Zé Xiè (Rhizoma Alismatis) 15 g, Gān Jú Huā (Flos Chrysanthemi) 30 g, Yù Zhú (Rhizoma Polygonati Odorati) 15 g, and Tù Sī Zǐ (Semen Cuscutae) (soaked in wine for 3 days, dried under sunshine, pounded into powder) 15 g; grind into fine powder, decoct 9 g/time in water, remove dregs, and take liquid for sudden onset of nebula in the eyes.

[Precautions] Líng Yáng Jiǎo (Cornu Saigae Tataricae), cold in nature, is contraindicated in cases of cold congestion and qi stagnation in the liver channel.

石决明 Shí Jué Míng *Concha haliotidis Sea-ear shell*

The source is from the shell of *Haliotis diversicolor* Reeve (光底石决明, Guāng Dǐ Shí Jué Míng) and *H. gigantean* discus Reeve (毛底石决明, Máo Dǐ Shí Jué Míng), family Haliotidae. It is so called because of its ability of relieving eye problems and alternate names include 千里光 Qiān Lǐ Guāng (but not Qiān Lǐ Guāng-Herba Senecionis Scandentis). Salty in flavor and slightly cold in nature.

[Actions] Calm the liver and subdue yang, and clear the liver and improve vision. It is applicable for vertigo, red, swollen and painful eyes, nebula with vision obstruction, and blurred vision.

[Quality] Good quality is thick and have a shiny, multicolored inner surface and clean outer surface without moss, soils, sands, and impurities.

[Indications]

1. Ascendant hyperactivity of liver yang: Shí Jué Míng (Concha Haliotidis), a shell medicinal that calm the liver, is applicable for headache, vertigo, and dizziness caused by ascendant hyperactivity of liver yang and therefore often combined with medicinals that nourish yin and calm the liver such as Shēng Dì (Radix Rehmanniae), Bái Sháo (Radix Paeoniae

Alba), Mǔ Lì (Concha Ostreae), and Dài Zhě Shí (Haematitum); and with Xià Kū Cǎo (Spica Prunellae), Jú Huā (Flos Chrysanthemi), Gōu Téng (Ramulus Uncariae Cum Uncis), and Lóng Dǎn Cǎo (Radix et Rhizoma Gentianae) for intense liver heat.

2. Eye problems due to liver fire: for red, swollen and painful eyes with nebula, cateract, gloucoma, and night blindness caused by liver fire flaming upward, Shí Jué Míng (Concha Haliotidis) can clear the liver and improve vision. It is combined with medicinals that clear and drain liver heat such as Huáng Lián (Rhizoma Coptidis), Jú Huā (Flos Chrysanthemi), and Jué Míng Zǐ (Semen Cassiae) for excess fire of the liver; with medicinals that nourish and enrich liver blood and yin such as Shú Dì Huáng (Radix Rehmanniae Praeparata), Shān Zhū Yú (Fructus Corni), Tù Sī Zǐ (Semen Cuscutae), and Bái Sháo (Radix Paeoniae Alba) for deficiency fire flaming upward resulting from liver blood deficiency; and with Bò He (Herba Menthae), Bái Jí Lí (Fructus Tribuli), Jīng Jiè (Herba Schizonepetae), and Xià Kū Cǎo (Spica Prunellae) for external visual obstruction due to liver heat.

[Usage and Dosage] Use raw in general, calcined one is crisp that can facilitate crushing and active ingredient extraction. Use 15–30 g in decoction, crush before using in decoction and cook before adding other ingredients. Decrease the amount as in pill and powder.

[Mnemonics] Shí Jué Míng (Concha Haliotidis, Sea-ear Shell): salty; calm the liver primarily, clear fire to improve vision, and subdue the liver yang.

[Simple and Effective Formulas]
千里光汤 Qiān Lǐ Guāng Tāng — Sea Ear Shell Decoction from *Longmu's Ophthalmology* (眼科龙木论, Yǎn Kē Lóng Mù Lùn): Qiān Lǐ Guāng (Concha Haliotidis) (Shí Jué Míng), Hǎi Jīn Shā (Spora Lygodii), Gān Cǎo (Radix et Rhizoma Glycyrrhizae), and Jú Huā (Flos Chrysanthemi) in equal dosage; grind into fine powder, decoct 24 g/time into water, remove dregs, and take after meal for oral administration to treat photophobia.

[Precautions] Shí Jué Míng (Concha Haliotidis), cold in nature, is contraindicated in cases of cold congestion and qi stagnation in the liver. It is said to be incompatible with Xuán Fù Huā (Flos Inulae), just for the reference.

Daily practices

1. What are the causes of disorders cured by medicinals that calm the liver and extinguish wind? What are the actions of these medicinals?
2. What are the similarities and differences between Líng Yáng Jiǎo (Cornu Saigae Tataricae) and Shí Jué Míng (Concha Haliotidis) in terms of actions and indications?

珍珠 Zhēn Zhū *Margarita pearl*

[Addendum]: 珍珠母 Zhēn Zhū Mǔ Concha Margaritiferae Usta Mother-of-pearl

The source is from granular secretion of *Pteria margaritifera* (L.), *P. martensii* (Dunker), *Hydiopsis* cumingii (Lea), *Cristaria plicala* (Leach), family Pteriidae and Unionidae. Alternate names include真珠 Zhēn Zhū. Sweet and salty in flavor and cold in nature.

[Actions] Sedate the heart and calm the mind, extinguish wind and fright, clear the liver and remove nebula, and astringent and generate flesh. It is applicable for palpitations due to fright, depressive psychosis, infantile convulsions, red, swollen and painful eyes due to liver heat, nebula and pterygium, and chronic open non-healing sore when applied externally.

[Quality] Good quality is large, round, smooth, coloured light, and lustrous with distinct striations on cross-section.

[Indications]

1. Restlessness of heart spirit: Zhēn Zhū (Margarita) can subdue the heart and tranquilize the spirit and is applicable for different types of disorder caused by restlessness of heart spirit restlessness. It can be used alone or together with other medicinals that nourish the heart and calm the mind such as Shè Xiāng (Moschus), Fú Shén (Sclerotium Poriae

Pararadicis), and Suān Zǎo Rén (Semen Ziziphi Spinosae) for palpitations, or severe palpitations, and insomnia.

2. Wind-stirring and convulsive syncope: Zhēn Zhū (Margarita), capable of relieving convulsion and extinguishing wind, is combined with medicinals that clear and dissolve phlegm heat and relieve convulsion such as Niú Huáng (Calculus Bovis), Bīng Piàn (Borneolum Syntheticum), Dǎn Nán Xīng (Arisaema cum Bile), and Shè Xiāng (Moschus) for infantile convulsions, depressive psychosis, or exuberant heat stirring wind in febrile diseases.

3. Eye problems due to liver heat: Zhēn Zhū (Margarita), effective in clearing the liver to improve vision and relieve nubela and cataract, is combined with Bīng Piàn (Borneolum Syntheticum), Péng Shā (Borax), and Zhū Shā (Cinnabaris) for external application on the eyes to relieve red, swollen and painful eyes with nebula and cataract caused by liver heat harassing the eyes.

4. Erosive sores: Zhēn Zhū (Margarita), capable of astringing and generating flesh and resolving toxins, is suitable for different types of chronic open non-healing sores and ulcers or swollen, painful and erosive throat, and ulcer in the mouth and tongue in a combination with Niú Huáng (Calculus Bovis), Lóng Gǔ (Os Draconis), and Bīng Piàn (Borneolum Syntheticum).

It is also used as an important cosmetic either for oral administration or external application because of its tonic effect on the skin.

[Usage and Dosage] Use raw in general, but often grind with water before being ground into very fine powder. Nowadays its hydrolysate is most commonly used for a better absorption. Generally used as is or in pill and powder form for oral administration, 0.3–1.5 g/time.

[Mnemonics] Zhēn Zhū (Margarita, Pearl): sweet and cold; cure sore, clear the liver, sedate the heart, calm the mind, and extinguish palpitations due to fright.

[Simple and Effective Formulas]

1. 真珠丸 Zhēn Zhū Wán — Pearl Pill from *Comprehensive Recording of Divine Assistance* (圣济总录 Shèng Jì Zǒng Lù,): Zhēn Zhū (Margarita) powder 0.1 g, Fú Lóng Gān (Terra Flava Usta) (Zào Xīn Tǔ) 0.1 g, Dān

Shā (Cinnabaris) 0.1 g, and Shè Xiāng (Moschus) 3 g; grind into powder, make into green-bean sized pill with honey, and take one pill/time with warm water for oral administration to treat childhood fright cry and persistent night cry.

2. 珍宝散 Zhēn Bǎo Sǎn — Treasure Powder from *Famous Doctors' Life-saving Medical Recordings in Ming Dynasty* (丹台玉案, Dān Tái Yù àn): Zhēn Zhū (Margarita) 9 g, Péng Shā (Borax) 3 g, Qīng Dài (Indigo Naturalis) 3 g, Bīng Piàn (Borneolum Syntheticum) 1.5 g, Huáng Lián (Rhizoma Coptidis) 6 g, and Rén Zhōng Bái (Human Urinary Sediment) (calcined) 6 g; grind into fine powder and apply externally to the affected areas for ulcers in the mouth.

[Precautions] Zhēn Zhū (Margarita), cold, heavyweight and suppressing in properties, is not recommended to be taken over a long period of time.

[Addendum] 珍珠母 Zhēn Zhū Mǔ Concha Margaritiferae Usta Mother-of-pearl
The source is from the nacre of mussel, salty in flavor and cold in nature. Owning to its effect of calming the liver, subduing yang, clearing the liver, and improving vision, it is applicable to headache, vertigo, dizziness, tinnitus, vexation, insomnia due to liver-yin deficiency and ascendant hyperactivity of liver yang, as well as red, swollen, and painful eyes caused by liver heat. It can also relieve acidity and astringe and therefore its calcined preparation has recently been ground into powder for oral administration to relieve hyperchlorhydria and ulcer or external application to cure eczema and itching.

牡蛎 **Mǔ Lì** *Concha ostreae* *Oyster shell*

The source is from the shell of *Ostrea gigas* Thunberg, *O. talienwhanensis* Crosse, or *O. rivularis* Gould, family Ostreidae. Salty in flavor and slightly cold in nature.

[Actions] Calm the liver and subdue yang, soften hardness and dissipate nodule, and restrain and consolidate. It is applicable for headache, vertigo, tinnitus, palpitations, insomnia, vexation, and agitation caused by either ascendant hyperactivity of liver yang or yin deficiency with yang hyperactivity, scrofula and phlegm node due to binding constraint of phlegm fire, sweating resulting from deficiency, seminal emission, abnormal vaginal discharge, profuse uterine bleeding, and prolonged scanty uterine bleeding of variable intervals.

[Quality] Good quality is large and well-shaped with a clean and shiny inner side and without soils, sands, and impurities.

[Indications]

1. Ascendant hyperactivity of liver yang: Mǔ Lì (Concha Ostreae) can suppress and subdue yang and is therefore applicable for headache, head distention, vertigo, dizziness, and hot flashes in the face caused by ascendant hyperactivity of liver yang. It is combined with Jú Huā (Flos Chrysanthemi), Xià Kū Cǎo (Spica Prunellae), and Gōu Téng (Ramulus Uncariae Cum Uncis) for liver heat exuberance; with Bái Sháo (Radix Paeoniae Alba), Guī Bǎn (Plastrum Testudinis), and Shēng Dì (Radix Rehmanniae) for yin deficiency with yang hyperactivity; and with Biē Jiǎ (Carapax Trionycis), Guī Bǎn (Plastrum Testudinis), and Ē Jiāo (Colla Corii Asini) for wriggling and tremor of fingers due to yin deficiency generating wind in the late stage of febrile diseases.
2. Restlessness of heart spirit: Mǔ Lì (Concha Ostreae), heavyweight and suppressing to calm the spirit, is applicable for palpitations, insomnia, and freight caused by heart spirit restlessness and often prescribed together with Lóng Gǔ (Os Draconis), Dài Zhě Shí (Haematitum), Zhēn Zhū Mǔ (Concha Margaritiferae Usta), and Suān Zǎo Rén (Semen Ziziphi Spinosae).
3. Efflux desertion patterns: Mǔ Lì (Concha Ostreae), astringent in nature especially after charcination, is appropriate for a variety of efflux desertion. It can be ground into powder for external application or together with Huáng Qí (Radix Astragali), Má Huáng Gēn (Radix et Rhizoma Ephedrae), Fú Xiǎo Mài (Fructus Tritici Levis), and Nuò Dào Gēn Xū (Radix Oryzae Glutinosae) for oral administration to treat spontaneous and night sweating; with Shā Yuàn Jí Lí (Semen Astragali Complanati), Qiàn Shí (Semen Euryales), Lián Xū (Stamen Nelumbinis), and Jīn Yīng Zǐ (Fructus Rosae Laevigatae)

for seminal emission; and with consolidating and astringing medicinals such as calcined Lóng Gǔ (Os Draconis) and calcined Hǎi Piāo Xiāo (Endoconcha Sepiae) for frequent and profuse abnormal vaginal discharge, profuse uterine bleeding, and prolonged scanty uterine bleeding of variable intervals.

4. Phlegm and blood stagnation masses: Mǔ Lì (Concha Ostreae) can soften hardness and dissipate masses and therefore is applicable for accumulations, gatherings, and masses such as scrofula and phlegm node. It is combined with Xuán Shēn (Radix Scrophulariae) and Bèi Mǔ (Bulbus Fritillaria) for scrofula; with Dāng Guī (Radix Angelicae Sinensis), Chái Hú (Radix Bupleuri), and Tǔ Biē Chóng (Eupolyphaga seu Steleophaga) for hepatosplenomegaly; and with Bái Jiè Zǐ (Semen Sinapis), Bàn Xià (Rhizoma Pinelliae), and Zhì Tiān Nán Xīng (Rhizoma Arisaematis praeparatum) for phlegm node.

It has been recently used to relieve acidity for hyperchlorhydria and ulcers.

Mǔ Lì (Concha Ostreae) and Lóng Gǔ (Os Draconis) have similar actions and are commonly used together in the treatment of ascendant hyperactivity of liver yang, heart spirit restlessness, profuse sweating, healthy qi external desertions, frequent and profuse white leukorrhea, profuse uterine bleeding, prolonged scanty uterine bleeding of variable intervals, hyperchlorhydria, and infantile calcium deficiency.

[Usage and Dosage] Use raw to calm the liver, subdue yang, tranquilize the spirit, and dissipate masses; and calcined to restrain and astringe discharge. Use 15–30 g in decoction, up to above 90 g when used for scrofula, 3–6 g/time when taken as powder or used in pill and powder.

[Mnemonics] Mǔ Lì (Concha Ostreae, Oyster Shell): salty and cold; subdue the yang, calm the liver, restrain and consolidate incontinence and prolapse, soften hardness, and dissipate nodule.

[Simple and Effective Formulas]

1. 牡蛎散 Mǔ Lì Sǎn — Oyster Shell Powder from *Important Formulas Worth a Thousand Gold Pieces* (千金要方 Qiān Jīn Yào Fāng,): Mǔ Lì

(Concha Ostreae) 90 g, Bái Zhú (Rhizoma Atractylodis Macrocephalae) 90 g, and Fáng Fēng (Radix Saposhnikoviae) 90 g; grind into fine powder and take 4 g/time with wine for oral administration to treat night sweating and headache upon wind.

2. 止晕汤 Zhǐ Yūn Tāng — Dizziness Relieving Decoction from *Shandong Province Chinese Herbal Medicine Handbook* (山东省中草药手册 Shān Dōng Shěng Zhōng Cǎo Yào Shǒu Cè,): Mǔ Lì (Concha Ostreae) 18 g, Lóng Gǔ (Os Draconis) 18 g, Jú Huā (Flos Chrysanthemi) 9 g, Gǒu Qǐ Zǐ (Fructus Lycii) 12 g, and Hé Shǒu Wū (Radix Polygoni Multiflori) 12 g; decoct in water for oral administration to treat vertigo and dizziness.

[Precautions] Mǔ Lì (Concha Ostreae), cold in nature, should be used with caution in cases of coldness or together with other medicinals when necessary.

代赭石 **Dài Zhě shí** *Haematitum hematite*

The source is from the hematite. It is so called because back to ancient times the best quality was found in Daijun area. Bitter in flavor and cold in nature.

[Actions] Calm the liver and strongly redirect rebellious qi downward, and tranquilize the mind and stanch bleeding. It is applicable for headache and vertigo due to ascendant hyperactivity of liver yang, vomiting and hiccup caused by ascending counterflow of stomach qi, cough and wheezing resulting from ascending counterflow of lung qi, palpitations and insomnia attributed to restlessness of heart spirit, and hemorrhagic disorders.

[Quality] Good quality is brownish red, has a distinct striated section and nail-heads.

[Indications]

1. Ascendant hyperactivity of liver yang: Dài Zhě Shí (Haematitum), heavyweight, suppressing, and cold in nature, can clear liver heat and is used together with medicinals that calm the liver and subdue yang such as Cí Shí (Magnetitum), Shí Jué Míng (Concha Haliotidis), Gōu

Téng (Ramulus Uncariae Cum Uncis), and Niú Xī (Radix Achyranthis Bidentatae) for headache and vertigo caused by ascendant hyperactivity of liver yang; with medicinals that clear liver fire such as Zhī Zǐ (Fructus Gardeniae), Jú Huā (Flos Chrysanthemi), and Xià Kū Cǎo (Spica Prunellae) for intense liver fire; and with medicinals that supplement the liver and kidney such as Shēng Dì (Radix Rehmanniae), Guī Bǎn (Plastrum Testudinis), and Bái Sháo (Radix Paeoniae Alba) when accompanied with liver and kidney insufficiency.

2. Counterflow of qi: Dài Zhě Shí (Haematitum) can direct counterflow downward and applicable for a variety of disorders caused by qi counterflow. It is prescribed together with Bàn Xià (Rhizoma Pinelliae) and Xuán Fù Huā (Flos Inulae) for vomiting and hiccup due to ascending counterflow of stomach qi; with Sāng Bái Pí (Cortex Mori), Guā Lóu (Fructus Trichosanthis), and Huáng Qín (Radix Scutellariae) for cough and wheezing due to lung heat with ascending counterflow of lung qi; with Bàn Xià (Rhizoma Pinelliae), Chén Pí (Pericarpium Citri Reticulatae), and Xuán Fù Huā (Flos Inulae) for qi counterflow attributed to phlegm-damp; and with Rén Shēn (Radix et Rhizoma Ginseng), Shān Yào (Rhizoma Dioscoreae), Shān Zhū Yú (Fructus Corni), and Bǔ Gǔ Zhī (Fructus Psoraleae) for the problem associated with kidney failing to receive qi. It is also applicable for hyperactivity of liver yang due to its effect of directing counterflow downward.

3. Restlessness of heart spirit: Dài Zhě Shí (Haematitum) is capable of suppressing the heart and calming the spirit and used together with medicinals that calm the spirit such as Cí Shí (Magnetitum), Shè Xiāng (Moschus), and Lóng Gǔ (Os Draconis) for palpitations and insomnia.

4. Owing to its cold nature and capacity of clearing blood heat to stanch bleeding and directing counterflow downward, Dài Zhě Shí (Haematitum) is considered more suitable for bleeding caused by counterflow of qi and fire. It is combined with Shēng Dì (Radix Rehmanniae), Mǔ Dān Pí (Cortex Moutan), Huáng Qín (Radix Scutellariae), Dà Jì (Herba Cirsii Japonici), and Xiǎo Jì (Herba Cirsii) for bleeding due to blood heat; with Huái Huā (Flos Sophorae) and Dì Yú (Radix Sanguisorbae) for stool containing blood; with ài Yè Tàn (Folium Artemisiae Argyi Carbonisatum), Pú Huáng (Pollen Typhae), and aged Zōng Lǚ Tàn (Petiolus Trachycarpi Carbonisatus) for profuse uterine

bleeding and prolonged scanty uterine bleeding of variable intervals; and with consolidating and astringing medicinals that supplement the liver and kidney such as Chì Shí Zhī (Halloysitum Rubrum), Wǔ Líng Zhī (Faeces Trogopterori), Shān Zhū Yú (Fructus Corni), calcined Lóng Gǔ (Os Draconis), and calcined Mǔ Lì (Concha Ostreae) for insecurity of the *chong* and *ren mai* with profuse uterine bleeding and prolonged scanty uterine bleeding of variable intervals.

[Usage and Dosage] Use raw in general, calcined to stanch bleeding. Use 15–30 g in decoction, cook first before adding other ingredients. Use 3 g/ time when ground into powder for oral administration.

[Mnemonics] Dài Zhě Shí (Haematitum, Hematite): bitter and cold; redirect rebellious qi downward, calm the liver, arrest bleeding, and tranquilize the heart spirit.

[Simple and Effective Formulas]

1. 代赭石汤 Dài Zhě Shí Tāng — Hematite Decoction from *Formulas from Royal Institute of Medicine* (御药院方, Yù Yào Yuàn Fāng): Dài Zhě Shí (Haematitum) (broken in pieces) 90 g, Chén Pí (Pericarpium Citri Reticulatae) 60 g, Táo Rén (Semen Persicae) 15 g, and Guì Wú Zhū Yú (Fructus Evodiae) 15 g; add ginger and decoct in water for oral administration to treat counterflow qi rushing up to the chest and blocked air passage.
2. 旋覆代赭汤 Xuán Fù Dài Zhě Tāng — Inula and Hematite Decoction from *Treatise on Cold Damage* (伤寒论, Shāng Hán Lùn): Xuán Fù Huā (Flos Inulae) 10 g, Rén Shēn (Radix et Rhizoma Ginseng) 6 g, Shēng Jiāng (Rhizoma Zingiberis Recens) 10 g, Dài Zhě Shí (Haematitum) 15 g, Gān Cǎo (Radix et Rhizoma Glycyrrhizae) 6 g, Bàn Xià (Rhizoma Pinelliae) 9 g, and Dà Zǎo (Fructus Jujubae) six pieces; decoct in water for oral administration to treat stomach qi deficiency, and belching, vomiting, and hiccup due to ascending counterflow of stomach qi.

[Precautions] Dài Zhě Shí (Haematitum), cold in nature, is contraindicated in cases of deficiency-cold. Use with caution during pregnancy as it is heavyweight, suppressing, and dropping in nature.

Daily practices

1. What are the similarities and differences among Zhēn Zhū (Margarita), Mǔ Lì (Concha Ostreae), and Dài Zhě Shí (Haematitum) in terms of actions and indications?
2. What are the actions of Zhēn Zhū (Margarita), Mǔ Lì (Concha Ostreae), and Dài Zhě Shí (Haematitum) beside calming the liver? What are their indications?

天麻 Tiān Má *Rhizoma gastrodiae Tall gastrodis tuber*

The source is from the tuber of parasitic herbaceous perennial *Gastrodia elata* Bl., family Orchidaceae. Alternate names include 赤箭 Chì Jiàn and 明天麻 Míng Tiān Má. Sweet in flavor and neutral in nature.

[Actions] Extinguish wind and arrest spasm, calm the liver and subdue yang, and smooth the channels and collaterals. Modern research has shown that it has sedative and anti-convulsive syncope effects and can increase cerebral blood flow, improve immunity, and induce interferon.

[Quality] Good quality is hard, solid, and heavy with parrot-hook like reddish-brown withered bud and a bright cross-section and without hole in the middle; poor quality is lightweight and spongy with residue caudex and a gloomy cross section.

[Indications]

1. Vertigo and headache: combination of herbs is based on the root cause for vertigo and headache. Tiān Má (Rhizoma Gastrodiae) can calm the liver and subdue yang and is combined with Niú Xī (Radix Achyranthis Bidentatae), Shí Jué Míng (Concha Haliotidis), and Gōu Téng (Ramulus Uncariae Cum Uncis) for ascendant hyperactivity of liver yang; and with Dāng Guī (Radix Angelicae Sinensis) and Bái Sháo (Radix Paeoniae Alba) for blood deficiency with hyperactivity of deficiency yang. This substance is also effective in dispelling wind and dissolving phlegm and can be used together with Bái Zhú (Rhizoma Atractylodis Macrocephalae), Bàn Xià (Rhizoma Pinelliae), and Chén Pí (Pericarpium

Citri Reticulatae) for headache caused by wind-phlegm. It can also be prescribed together with Chuān Xiōng (Rhizoma Chuanxiong), Bàn Xià (Rhizoma Pinelliae), and Fù Zǐ (Radix Aconiti Lateralis Praeparata) for migraine and headache.

2. Internal stirring of liver wind: major manifestations include spasm of the extremities, Tiān Má (Rhizoma Gastrodiae) can enter the liver to dispel wind and arrest spasm. It is prescribed together with medicinals that cool the liver and extinguish wind such as Líng Yáng Jiǎo (Cornu Saigae Tataricae), Gōu Téng (Ramulus Uncariae Cum Uncis), and Lóng Dǎn Cǎo (Radix et Rhizoma Gentianae) for extremely heat generating wind; with Rén Shēn (Radix et Rhizoma Ginseng), Bái Zhú (Rhizoma Atractylodis Macrocephalae), and Bái Jiāng Cán (Bombyx Batryticatus) for spasms and convulsions of the extremities in chronic infantile convulsions; and with Tiān Nán Xīng (Rhizoma Arisaematis), Bái Fù Zǐ (Rhizoma Typhonii), and Fáng Fēng (Radix Saposhnikoviae) for tetanus with locked jaw and opisthotonos.

3. *Bì* pain of the extremities: owning to its properties of soothing and unblocking the channels and collaterals, Tiān Má (Rhizoma Gastrodiae) is effective in the treatment of numbness and pain of the extremities with limited range of mobility. It is combined with medicinals that dispel wind-damp such as Qín Jiāo (Radix Gentianae Macrophyllae), Yì Yǐ Rén (Semen Coicis), Qiāng Huó (Rhizoma et Radix Notopterygii), and Dú Huó (Radix Angelicae Pubescentis) for pain caused by wind-damp; and with medicinals that supplement blood and nourish the liver such as Dāng Guī (Radix Angelicae Sinensis), Chuān Xiōng (Rhizoma Chuanxiong), Niú Xī (Radix Achyranthis Bidentatae), and Dù Zhòng (Cortex Eucommiae) for pain due to blood deficiency.

[Usage and Dosage] Use raw in general, stir-fry or roast to moderate its nature. Use 3–9 g in decoction, 1–1.5 g/time when taken as pill and powder.

[Mnemonics] Tiān Má (Rhizoma Gastrodiae, Tall Gastrodis Tuber): sweet and neutral; extinguish wind, arrest spasm, relieve vertigo and pain, and soothe the channels and collaterals.

[Simple and Effective Formulas]

1. 天麻丸 Tiān Má Wán — Tall Gastrodis Tuber Pill from *Secret Formulas of the Wei Family* (魏氏家藏方, Wèi Shì Jiā Cáng Fāng): Tiān Má (Rhizoma Gastrodiae) 15 g, Quán Xiē (Scorpio) (toxicity removed, stir-fried) 30 g, Tiān Nán Xīng (Rhizoma Arisaematis) (blast-fried, peel removed) 15 g, and Bái Jiāng Cán (Bombyx Batryticatus) (stir-fried to remove silk-thread) 6 g; grind into fine powder, make into tall gastrodia fruit-sized pill with wine-treated pastry, and take 10–15 pills/time/year of age with Jīng Jiè (Herba Schizonepetae) decoction for oral administration to treat convulsions and spasms, especially infantile convulsions.

2. 天麻酒 Tiān Má Jiǔ — Tall Gastrodis Tuber Wine from *Complete Fine and Convenient Formulas* (十便良方, Shí Biàn Liáng Fāng): Tiān Má (Rhizoma Gastrodiae) (cut) 60 g, Niú Xī (Radix Achyranthis Bidentatae) 60 g, Dù Zhòng (Cortex Eucommiae) 60 g, and Fù Zǐ (Radix Aconiti Lateralis Praeparata) 60 g; grind into fine powder, pack in kiginu bag, soak in wine 3 kg for seven days, and take small cup of warm wine/time for oral administration to treat wind *bì* in women and limited range of motion of hands and feet.

[Precautions] Tiān Má (Rhizoma Gastrodiae), effective in dispelling wind, neutral but relatively warm and dry in nature, should not use alone in cases of stirring of wind due to yin and blood deficiency and should combined with medicinals that nourish the blood.

钩藤 Gōu Téng *Ramulus uncariae cum uncis Gambir plant*

The source is from the hooked woody liana of *Uncaria rhynchophylla* (Miq.) Jacks. and other congeneric plants, family Rubiaceae. Alternate names include 钓藤 Diào Téng, 双钩藤 Shuāng Gōu Téng, and 钩钩 Gōu Gōu. Sweet in flavor and slightly cold in nature.

[Actions] Clear heat and calm the liver, extinguish wind and arrest spasm, and decrease blood pressure. It is applicable for headache, vertigo, common cold with convulsion and fright, eclampsia during pregnancy, and hypertension. Animal experiment demonstrates that it has a moderate and prolonged antihypertensive and certain sedative effect, and can reduce heart rate and dilate blood vessels.

[Quality] Good quality is lightweight, tough and firm, glossy, and purplish red with double thorns like anchors, thin stems and without dessicated stems.

[Indications]

1. Ascendant hyperactivity of liver yang: Gōu Téng (Ramulus Uncariae Cum Uncis) is applicable for vertigo and dizziness caused by ascendant hyperactivity of liver yang in a combination with Tiān Má (Rhizoma Gastrodiae), Jú Huā (Flos Chrysanthemi), Shí Jué Míng (Concha Haliotidis), Cí Shí (Magnetitum), and Dài Zhě Shí (Haematitum). It is combined with Xià Kū Cǎo (Spica Prunellae), Huáng Qín (Radix Scutellariae), Zhī Zǐ (Fructus Gardeniae), and broadleaf holly leaf for exuberant liver fire.

2. Internal stirring of liver wind: Gōu Téng (Ramulus Uncariae Cum Uncis) is applicable for different disorders caused by internal stirring of liver wind. It is often combined with medicinals that clear heat, cool the liver, and extinguish wind such as Líng Yáng Jiǎo (Cornu Saigae Tataricae), Shí Jué Míng (Concha Haliotidis), and Tiān Má (Rhizoma Gastrodiae) for high fever with convulsive syncope; and with Bái Jiāng Cán (Bombyx Batryticatus), Dì Lóng (Pheretima), Sāng Yè (Folium Mori), and Chán Tuì (Periostracum Cicadae) for infantile convulsions. However, this substance is moderate in clearing heat and should be prescribed together with medicinals that clear heat, drain fire, and cool the liver for exuberant liver heat.

[Usage and Dosage] Use raw in general, 5–9 g in decoction, up to 30 g. If used in decoctions, it should be added near the end of decocting as experiments display boiling 20 minutes would significantly reduce the active ingredients of lowering blood pressure.

[Mnemonics] Gōu Téng (Ramulus Uncariae Cum Uncis, Gambir Plant): sweet and cold; clear heat, calm the liver, extinguish vertigo and spasm, and decrease blood pressure.

[Simple and Effective Formulas]

1. 钩藤饮子 Gōu Téng Yǐn Zǐ — Uncaria Drink from *Formulas for Universal Relief* (普济方, Pǔ Jì Fāng): Gōu Téng (Ramulus Uncariae Cum Uncis) 15 g, Chán Tuì (Periostracum Cicadae) 15 g, Huáng Lián (Rhizoma Coptidis) 30 g, Gān Cǎo (Radix et Rhizoma Glycyrrhizae) 30 g, Dà Huáng (Radix et Rhizoma Rhei) (slightly blast-fried) 30 g, and Tiān Zhú Huáng (Concretio Silicea Bambusae) 30 g; grind into fine powder, mix 1.5–3 g/time with small amount of Shēng Jiāng (Rhizoma Zingiberis Recens) and Bò He (Herba Menthae), and decoct in water for oral administration to treat convulsion in children.

2. 天麻钩藤饮 Tiān Má Gōu Téng Yǐn — Gastrodia and Uncaria Decoction from *Revision on Diagnosis, Treatment, and Categorized Formulas of Miscellaneous Diseases* (杂病证治新义, Zá Bìng Zhèng Zhì Xīn Yì): Tiān Má (Rhizoma Gastrodiae), Gōu Téng (Ramulus Uncariae Cum Uncis), raw Shí Jué Míng (Concha Haliotidis), Zhī Zǐ (Fructus Gardeniae), Huáng Qín (Radix Scutellariae), Chuān Niú Xī (Radix Cyathulae), Dù Zhòng (Cortex Eucommiae), Yì Mǔ Cǎo (Herba Leonuri), Sāng Jì Shēng (Herba Taxilli), Yè Jiāo Téng (Caulis Polygoni Multiflori), and Zhū Fú Shén (Sclerotium Poriae Pararadicis); decoct in water for oral administration to treat headache, vertigo, tinnitus, blurred vision, tremor, insomnia, and hypertension associated with ascendant hyperactivity of liver yang.

[Precautions] Gōu Téng (Ramulus Uncariae Cum Uncis), relatively cool in nature, should be used use with caution in cases of the absence of fire-heat. Overdose and long-term use is discouraged as it contains toxic rhynchophylline.

决明子 Jué Míng Zǐ *Semen cassiae Cassia seed*

The source is from the ripe semen of herbaceous annual *Cassia obtusifolia* L. or *C. tora* L., family Leguminosae. Alternate names include 草决明 Cǎo Jué Míng and 马蹄决明 Mǎ Tí Jué Míng. Bitter and sweet in flavor and slightly cold in nature.

[Actions] Clear the liver and improve vision, and moisten the intestine and promote the bowel movement. It is applicable for red, swollen, and painful eyes and photophobia with profuse tears due to liver heat and constipation caused by intestinal dryness. Modern research has shown that it has a relatively good hypolipidemic effect.

[Quality] Good quality is dry, full, yellowish brown, and without impurities.

[Indications]

1. Liver heat exuberance: Jué Míng Zǐ (Semen Cassiae), capable of clearing liver heat, is combined with Gōu Téng (Ramulus Uncariae Cum Uncis), Tiān Má (Rhizoma Gastrodiae), and Shí Jué Míng (Concha Haliotidis) for headache and dizziness due to ascendant hyperactivity of liver yang; with liver-clearing medicinals such as Jú Huā (Flos Chrysanthemi), Xià Kū Cǎo (Spica Prunellae), Zhī Zǐ (Fructus Gardeniae), and Huáng Qín (Radix Scutellariae) for liver fire exuberance; and with Jú Huā (Flos Chrysanthemi), Gǔ Jīng Cǎo (Flos Eriocauli), and Mǔ Dān Pí (Cortex Moutan) for red, swollen, and painful eyes, tearing and photophobia due to liver fire flaming upward to the eyes.

   This substance can improve vision and is applicable for blurred vision due to liver yin insufficiency in a combination with other medicinals that supplement the liver and kidney.

2. Constipation due to intestinal dryness: Jué Míng Zǐ (Semen Cassiae), moisturizing in nature, can be decocted alone for oral administration, taken as a tea, or used in the formula to moisten the intestines to promote defecation.

It can also be combined with Shān Zhā (Fructus Crataegi) and Zé Xiè (Rhizoma Alismatis) for hyperlipdemia.

[Usage and Dosage] Use raw. Stir-fry until yellow when used alone as tea. Use 10–15 g in decoction, up to 30 g/day if used alone.

[Mnemonics] Jué Míng Zǐ (Semen Cassiae, Cassia Seed): bitter; clear liver fire, cure eye problems, and promote bowel movements.

[Simple and Effective Formulas]

1. 决明子散 Jué Míng Zǐ Sǎn — Cassia Seed Powder from *Formulas from Benevolent Sages* (圣惠方, Shèng Huì Fāng): Jué Míng Zǐ (Semen Cassiae) and Màn Jīng Zǐ (Fructus Viticis) (cooked with good wine, dried under sunshine) in equal dosage; grind into fine powder and take 6 g/time with warm water after meal and at bedtime for oral administration to treat blurred vision.

2. 治眼煎 Zhì Yǎn Jiān — Eyes Curing Decoction from *Hebei Handbook of Chinese Medicinal Medica* (湖北中医药手册, Hú Běi Zhōng Yī Yào Shǒu Cè,): Jué Míng Zǐ (Semen Cassiae) 9 g, Jú Huā (Flos Chrysanthemi) 9 g, Màn Jīng Zǐ (Fructus Viticis) 6 g, and Mù Zéi (Herba Equiseti Hiemalis) 6 g; decoct in water for oral administration to treat acute conjunctivitis.

[Precautions] Jué Míng Zǐ (Semen Cassiae) is effective in promoting defecation and therefore contraindicated in cases of loose stool.

Daily practices

1. What are the similarities and differences among Tiān Má (Rhizoma Gastrodiae), Gōu Téng (Ramulus Uncariae Cum Uncis), and Jué Míng Zǐ (Semen Cassiae) in terms of actions and indications?
2. What are the similarities and differences between shell and mineral medicinals that calm the liver and extinguish wind and those plant medicinals that calm the liver and extinguish wind in terms of actions?

全蝎 Quán Xiē *Scorpio Scorpion*

The source is from the whole dried body of *Buthus martensi* Karsch, family Buthidae. Alternate names include 全虫 Quán Chóng and 虿 Chài. Its tail is called *Xiē Wěi* (Cauda Scorpionis) when used as a medicinal. Pungent in flavor and neutral in nature.

[Actions] Extinguish wind and stop spasms, attack toxins and dissipate nodules, and unblock the collaterals and arrest pain. It is applicable for infantile convulsions, depressive psychosis, wind-stroke, hemiplegia, deviated eyes and mouth, migraine, wind-damp *bì* pain, tetanus, tuberculosis of lymph nodes, rubella, sores, and swellings. Modern researches indicate it has anticonvulsant, vasodilator, antihypertensive, and sedative effects.

[Quality] Good quality is whole, intact, yellowish brown, and little salt efflorescence.

[Indications]

1. Stirring wind with convulsive syncope: Wú Gōng (Scolopendra), a commonly-used medicinal for extinguishing wind and arresting convulsion, is applicable for exuberant heat stirring wind in febrile diseases, acute and chronic infantile convulsions, post-stroke, depressive psychosis, and tetanus. It is combined with medicinals that cool the liver and extinguish wind such as Líng Yáng Jiǎo (Cornu Saigae Tataricae), Lóng Dǎn Cǎo (Radix et Rhizoma Gentianae), Shí Gāo (Gypsum Fibrosum), and Shuǐ Niú Jiǎo (Cornu Bubali) for high fever stirring wind; with spleen-supplementing medicinals that Rén Shēn (Radix et Rhizoma Ginseng) and Bái Zhú (Rhizoma Atractylodis Macrocephalae) for chronic infantile convulsions caused by spleen deficiency; with Bái Fù Zǐ (Rhizoma Typhonii), Dì Lóng (Pheretima), Chuān Xiōng (Rhizoma Chuanxiong), and Chì Sháo (Radix Paeoniae Rubra) for post-stroke hemiplegia; and with Tiān Nán Xīng (Rhizoma Arisaematis), Fáng Fēng (Radix Saposhnikoviae), and Chán Tuì (Periostracum Cicadae) for tetanus.

2. Pain due to channels and collaterals obstruction: Wú Gōng (Scolopendra), capable of searching and scraping pathogens in the channels and collaterals, is effective in relieving pain or numbness in the extremities caused by obstruction in the channels and collaterals. It is combined with Chuān Xiōng (Rhizoma Chuanxiong), Bái Zhǐ (Radix Angelicae Dahuricae), and Xì Xīn (Radix et Rhizoma Asari) for migraine and headache due to wind-phlegm obstruction in the upper part of body; and with Dì Lóng (Pheretima), Bái Jiè Zǐ (Semen Sinapis), Táo Rén (Semen Persicae), and Bái Huā Shé (Agkistrodon) for pain *bì* pattern caused by wind-damp-phlegm-blood stagnation in the channels, collaterals, and joints.

3. Sores, ulcers, swellings, and masses: Wú Gōng (Scolopendra), effective in resolving toxins, dissipating masses, unblocking the collaterals, and relieving pain, is commonly used for sores, ulcers, swellings, toxins, scrofula, and phlegm node. It also has been used as an important medicinal in the treatment of tuberculosis of lymph nodes and cancer.

[Usage and Dosage] Use the whole body in general, the tail is preferred in a powder form for critical and severe cases due to violent medical property, the whole body should be used when the condition of patient is improved. Use 2–6 g in decoction, decrease the amount when just the tail is used. It should not be decocted for a long time to avoid the evaporation of active ingredients. Use 1.5–2 g when given in pill or powder form.

[Mnemonics] Quán Xiē (Scorpio, Scorpion): extinguish wind, stop spasms, relieve toxins, dissipate nodules, and arrest *bì* pain.

[Simple and Effective Formulas]

1. 止痉散 Zhǐ Jìng Sǎn — Spasm-Relieving Powder from *Hu Bei Chinese Traditional Herbal Medicine Experience Exchange* (湖北中草医药经验交流, Hú Běi Zhōng Cǎo Yī Yào Jīng Yàn Jiāo Liú): Quán Xiē (Scorpio) 30 g, Wú Gōng (Scolopendra) 30 g, Tiān Má (Rhizoma Gastrodiae) 30 g, and Bái Jiāng Cán (Bombyx Batryticatus) 60 g; grind into fine powder and take 1–1.5 g/time for oral administration to treat convulsion in Japanese encephalitis and other febrile diseases.

2. 麝香散 Shè Xiāng Sǎn — Musk Powder from *Formulas for Universal Relief* (普济方, Pǔ Jì Fāng): Shè Xiāng (Moschus) (ground) 0.1 g and dried Quán Xiē (Scorpio) 0.1 g; grind into powder and apply externally to the wound for tetanus.

[Precautions] Quán Xiē (Scorpio), relatively dry in nature, cannot be used long-term in cases of blood deficiency and yin consumption, is contraindicated to cases of deficiency stirring wind, and should be used with caution during pregnancy.

蜈蚣 Wú Gōng *Scolopendra Centipede*

The source is from the dried whole body of *Scolopendra subspinipes mutilans* L., Koch., family Scolopendrae. Alternate names include 百脚 Bǎi Jiǎo and 天龙 Tiān Lóng. Pungent in flavor and warm in nature with toxicity.

[Actions] Extinguish wind and stop spasms, relieve toxins and dissipate masses, and unblock the collaterals and arrest pain. It is applicable for acute and chronic infantile convulsions, tetanus induced convulsion, sores, ulcers, swellings, toxins, and erosive scrofula. Modern researches indicate it has certain anticonvulsant and antitumor effects.

[Quality] Good quality is dry, long, intact, and clean with a red head and blackish green body.

[Indications]

1. Stirring wind with convulsive syncope: Wú Gōng (Scolopendra), similar to Quán Xiē (Scorpio) in terms of extinguishing wind and arresting spasms, is applicable for exuberant heat stirring wind in febrile diseases, acute and chronic infantile convulsions, post-stroke, depressive psychosis, and tetanus. These two herbs are often used together and combined with other herbs in accordance with the state of illness. They are prescribed together with Líng Yáng Jiǎo (Cornu Saigae Tataricae), Gōu Téng (Ramulus Uncariae Cum Uncis), Bái Jiāng Cán (Bombyx Batryticatus), Huáng Lián (Rhizoma Coptidis), and Lóng Dǎn Cǎo (Radix et Rhizoma Gentianae) for infantile high fever with convulsions; with Tiān Zhú Huáng (Concretio Silicea Bambusae) and Bèi Mǔ (Bulbus Fritillaria) for depressive psychosis with intense fire; with Tiān Nán Xīng (Rhizoma Arisaematis), Fáng Fēng (Radix Saposhnikoviae), and Chán Tuì (Periostracum Cicadae) for tetanus; and with Bái Fù Zǐ (Rhizoma Typhonii), Tiān Nán Xīng (Rhizoma Arisaematis), Dì Lóng (Pheretima), and Chì Sháo (Radix Paeoniae Rubra) for post-stroke hemiplegia.
2. Pain due to channels and collaterals obstruction: Wú Gōng (Scolopendra), similar to Quán Xiē (Scorpio) in terms of searching and scraping

pathogens in the channels and collaterals, is effective in relieving pain or numbness in the extremities caused by obstruction in the channels and collaterals. It is combined with Chuān Xiōng (Rhizoma Chuanxiong), Bái Zhǐ (Radix Angelicae Dahuricae), and Xì Xīn (Radix et Rhizoma Asari) for migraine and headache due to wind-phlegm obstruction in the upper part of body; and with Dì Lóng (Pheretima), Bái Jiè Zǐ (Semen Sinapis), Táo Rén (Semen Persicae), and Bái Huā Shé (Agkistrodon) for painful *bì* pattern caused by wind-damp-phlegm-blood stagnation in the channels, collaterals, and joints.

3. Sores, ulcers, swellings, and masses: Wú Gōng (Scolopendra), effective in resolving toxins, dissipating masses, unblocking the collaterals, and relieving pain, is commonly used for sores, ulcers, swellings, toxins, scrofula, and phlegm node. It can be used alone for oral administration and ground into powder for external application to treat scrofula and poisonous snake bites. This medicinal can be ground with Xióng Huáng (Realgar) into powder and mixed with pig bile for external application to treat sores, carbuncles, swellings, and toxins.

Recently, it has been prepared into injection to treat infectious hepatitis with good therapeutic effects.

[Usage and Dosage] The raw substance is strong in action, while toasted one is moderate. Tradition requires removing the head, feet, and tail, modern research however indicates these parts are rich with active ingredients and should not be removed. Use 1–5 g or 1–3 pieces in decoction, decrease the amount as in pill and powder.

[Mnemonics] Wú Gōng (Scolopendra, Centipede): warm and pungent; extinguish wind to arrest spasms, relieve toxins, dissipate nodules, and eliminate *bì* pain.

[Simple and Effective Formulas]

1. 万金散 Wàn Jīn Sǎn — Gold Powder from *Formulas from Benevolent Sages* (圣惠方, Shèng Huì Fāng): one Wú Gōng (Scolopendra) (feet removed, roasted, ground into powder), and equal dosage of Zhū Shā (Cinnabaris) and Qīng Fěn (Calomelas); grind into powder, mix evenly,

prepare into green-bean sized pill with breast milk, and take one pill/ year of age with breast milk for acute convulsions in children.

2. 蜈蚣星风散 Wú Gōng Xīng Fēng Sǎn — Centipede, Jackinthepulpit Tuber, and Siler Powder from *Golden Mirror of the Medical Tradition* (医宗金鉴, Yī Zōng Jīn Jiàn): two Wú Gōng (Scolopendra), Jiāng Biào (Swim Bladder) 9 g, Nán Xīng (Rhizoma Arisaematis) 7.5 g, and Fáng Fēng (Radix Saposhnikoviae) 7.5 g; grind into fine powder and take 6 g/ time with yellow wine, twice a day for tetanus in early stage, exterior pattern with alternating chills and fever, muscle contracture, and locked jaw.

[Precautions] Wú Gōng (Scolopendra), warm and dry in nature, is contraindicated in cases of blood deficiency and yin consumption. It should not be used during pregnancy, overdose and over a long period of time because of its violent property.

地龙 Dì Long *pheretima earth worm*

The source is from the dried body of *Pheretima aspergillum* (Perrier) and *Allolobophora caliginosa* (Savigny) trapezoids (Ant. Duges), family Megascolecidae. The former is called 广地龙 Guǎng De Lóng and the latter 土地龙 Tǔ Dì Lóng, and alternate names include 蚯蚓 Qiū Yǐn and 曲蟮 Qū Shàn. Salty in flavor and cold in nature.

[Actions] Clear heat and stop convulsions, and relieve wheezing and unblock the collaterals. It is applicable for convulsive syncope with high fever, fright, epilepsy, numbness of the limbs, hemiplegia, joint *bì* pain, wheezing and cough due to lung heat, edema with scanty urine, and hypertension. Experiments show that it has antihypertensive, antiasthmatic, antipyretic, sedative, and anticonvulsant effects. An anticoagulant compound obtained from this herb has been recently used for treating cardiovascular diseases.

[Quality] Good quality is large, long, thick, and clean.

[Indications]

1. Internal stirring of liver wind: Dì Lóng (Pheretima), cold in nature, can clear liver heat, is combined with medicinals that clear heat and cool

the liver such as Gōu Téng (Ramulus Uncariae Cum Uncis), Dà Qīng Yè (Folium Isatidis), Shēng Dì (Radix Rehmanniae), and Shí Gāo (Gypsum Fibrosum) for exuberant heat stirring wind in febrile diseases; with medicinals that clear and drain liver fire such as Lóng Dǎn Cǎo (Radix et Rhizoma Gentianae), Dài Zhě Shí (Haematitum), Dǎn Nán Xīng (Arisaema cum Bile), and Zhī Zǐ (Fructus Gardeniae) for depressive psychosis, mania, and epilepsy due to exuberance of liver fire; and with Shí Jué Míng (Concha Haliotidis), Jú Huā (Flos Chrysanthemi), and Mǔ Lì (Concha Ostreae) for headache and vertigo attributed to ascendant hyperactivity of liver yang.

2. Channels and collaterals *bì* obstruction: Dì Lóng (Pheretima) is good at scattering and unblocking the channels and collaterals. It is prescribed together with Rěn Dōng Téng (Caulis Lonicerae Japonicae), Chì Sháo (Radix Paeoniae Rubra), Luò Shí Téng (Caulis Trachelospermi), and Zhī Mǔ (Rhizoma Anemarrhenae) hot-natured pain in the sinews, bones, and joints caused by wind-damp-phlegm-blood stagnation obstruction in the channels and collaterals; with Chuān Wū (Radix Aconiti), Guì Zhī (Ramulus Cinnamomi), and Rǔ Xiāng (Olibanum) for the cold-natured; and with Huáng Qí (Radix Astragali), Dāng Guī (Radix Angelicae Sinensis), and Táo Rén (Semen Persicae) for hemiplegia due to post-stroke qi deficiency and blood stagnation.

3. Cough and wheezing: Dì Lóng (Pheretima) is capable of arresting wheezing and especially suitable for cough and wheezing caused by lung heat. It can be ground into powder or used together with Má Huáng (Herba Ephedrae), Xìng Rén (Semen Armeniacae Amarum), and Shí Gāo (Gypsum Fibrosum) in the formula of arresting cough and wheezing.

4. Inhibited urination: Dì Lóng (Pheretima), effective in clearing heat and promoting urination, is applicable for inhibited urination and anuresis caused by heat accumulation in the bladder and is combined with medicinals that clear heat and promote urination.

5. Hypertension: Dì Lóng (Pheretima), potent in lowering blood pressure, can be used in the formula of controlling blood pressure and is significantly effective in treating hypertension type I and II.

It is also effective in clearing heat and resolving toxins and applicable for a variety of disorders caused by heat-toxin. Putting live Dì Lóng (Pheretima) into white sugar, obtaining its secretion, and applying externally can treat epidemic parotitis, scalding, ulcer in the lower extremities, and herpes zoster.

[Usage and Dosage] Use raw in general or fresh for external pattern. Use 6–12 g in decoction, 1–2 g when taken as powder.

[Mnemonics] Dì Long (Pheretima, Earth Worm): salty and cold; extinguish wind, clear the liver, unblock the collaterals, stop spasms and convulsions, promote urination, and relieve wheezing.

[Simple and Effective Formulas]

1. 地龙散 Dì Long Săn — Earth Worm Powder from *Comprehensive Recording of Divine Assistance* (圣济总录, Shèng Jì Zŏng Lù): Dì Lóng (Pheretima) (soil removed, stir-fried) 15 g, Bàn Xià (Rhizoma Pinelliae) (processed with ginger juice) 15 g, and Chì Fú Ling (Poria Rubra) (black skin removed) 15 g; grind into powder and take 3 g/ time with Shēng Jiāng (Rhizoma Zingiberis Recens) and Jīng Jiè (Herba Schizonepetae) decoction for oral administration to treat wind headache, postpartum headache, and angioneurotic headache.
2. 治赤眼方 Zhì Chì Yăn Fāng — Red Eyes Curing Formula from *Formulas from Benevolent Sages* (Shèng Huì Fāng, 圣惠方): Dì Lóng (Pheretima) (roasted); grind into fine powder and take 6 g/day with tea at bedtime for oral administration to treat prolonged red, swollen, and painful eyes.

[Precautions] Dì Lóng (Pheretima), relatively cold in nature, is contraindicated in cases of loose stool due to constitutionally deficiency-cold of the spleen and stomach.

白僵蚕 Bái Jiāng Cán *Bombyx batryticatus Silkworm*

The source is from the larva of *Bombyx mori* L. (family Bombycidae) before its spinning of silk infected by *Beauveria* (Bals.) Vuill. Alternate names include 僵蚕 Jiāng Cán and 天虫 Tiān Chóng. Salty and pungent in flavor and neutral in nature.

[Actions] Extinguish wind and arrest spasms, dissolve phlegm, disperse wind-heat, and relieve toxin and dissipate accumulation. It is applicable for convulsions due to exuberant heat stirring wind, headache and vertigo caused by wind-heat or liver heat, swollen and painful throat, scrofula, phlegm node, boils, sores, and erysipelas. Experiment results has shown that it has hypnotic and anticonvulsant effects.

[Quality] Good quality is solid and white with a lustrous brownish black cross-section.

[Indications]

1. Convulsion, freight, and epilepsy: Bái Jiāng Cán (Bombyx Batryticatus), capable of extinguishing wind and dissolving phlegm, is applicable for convulsions and freight caused by internal stirring of liver wind or phlegm heat exuberance. It is combined with Sāng Yè (Folium Mori), Jú Huā (Flos Chrysanthemi), and Gōu Téng (Ramulus Uncariae Cum Uncis) for infantile convulsions caused by externally-contracted high fever; and with Rén Shēn (Radix et Rhizoma Ginseng), Bái Zhú (Rhizoma Atractylodis Macrocephalae), Fú Líng (Poria), and Tiān Má (Rhizoma Gastrodiae) for chronic infantile convulsions due to spleen deficiency. It can be used alone or prepared into Defatted Bombyx Batryticatus Tablet for epilepsy.
2. Wind-heat: externally-contracted wind-heat may cause headache, swollen and painful throat, red eyes, rubella, and itching, if that is the case, Bái Jiāng Cán (Bombyx Batryticatus) is commonly used as it is capable of scattering and dissipating wind-heat. It is combined with Jú Huā (Flos Chrysanthemi), Shí Gāo (Gypsum Fibrosum), and Bái Jí Lí (Fructus Tribuli) for wind-heat or liver-heat induced headache; with Sāng Yè (Folium Mori), Mù Zéi (Herba Equiseti Hiemalis), and Chán Tuì (Periostracum Cicadae) for red eyes and tearing on exposure to wind caused by wind-heat; and with Bò He (Herba Menthae), Chán Tuì (Periostracum Cicadae), and Bái Xiān Pí (Cortex Dictamni) for skin itching due to wind-heat.

3. Phlegm congestion into masses: Bái Jiāng Cán (Bombyx Batryticatus), good at dissipating masses, is applicable for scrofula and phlegm node, and often used together with Xuán Shēn (Radix Scrophulariae), Xià Kū Cǎo (Spica Prunellae), Bèi Mǔ (Bulbus Fritillaria), and Mǔ Lì (Concha Ostreae).

It can be prepared into pill for oral administration to treat diabetes or prepared with Wū Méi (Fructus Mume) into pill to relieve stools containing blood.

This substance can be ground into powder and mixed with mature vinegar for external application to treat acute mastitis.

[Usage and Dosage] Use raw for dispersing wind-heat, fry with wheat bran to reduce its gamey smell and improve its effectiveness in other cases. Use 3–10 g in decoction, 1–2 g/dose as in powder.

[Mnemonics] Bái Jiāng Cán (Bombyx Batryticatus, Silkworm): pungent and salty; resolve toxins, dissipate masses, extinguish wind, relieve pain, and arrest spasms and convulsions.

[Simple and Effective Formulas]

1. 白僵蚕散 Bái Jiāng Cán Sǎn — Silkworm Powder from *Secret Formulas of the Wei Family* (魏氏家藏方 Wèi Shì Jiā Cáng Fāng,): Bái Jiāng Cán (Bombyx Batryticatus) (baked until light yellow) 30 g and Tiān Nán Xīng (Rhizoma Arisaematis) (coarse layer of bark removed, filed) 30 g; grind into fine powder, mix 2 g/time with small amount of Shēng Jiāng (Rhizoma Zingiberis Recens) juice, and take with warm water for oral administration to treat entwining throat wind and swollen and painful throat.
2. 治惊风散 Zhì Jīng Fēng Sǎn — Infantile Convulsion Relieving Powder from *Extension of the Materia Medica* (本草衍义 Běn Cǎo Yǎn Yì,): Bái Jiāng Cán (Bombyx Batryticatus), Xiē Wěi (Cauda Scorpionis), tip of Tiān Xióng (Aconiti Tuber Laterale Tianxiong), and tip of Fù Zǐ (Radix Aconiti Lateralis Praeparata) (slightly blast-fried) in equal dosage; grind into fine powder, mix 2–3 g/time with Shēng Jiāng (Rhizoma Zingiberis Recens) juice, and take with warm water for oral administration to treat convulsions in children.

[Precautions] Bái Jiāng Cán (Bombyx Batryticatus) is contraindicated in cases of stirring wind due to deficiency.

Besides the above-mentioned medicinals, others that also used for calming the liver and extinguishing wind are included in the previous chapters, such as exterior-releasing medicinal Chán Tuì (Periostracum Cicadae), mind-calming medicinal Cí Shí (Magnetitum), Bái Jí Lí (Fructus Tribuli), Luó Bù Má Yè (Folium Apocyni Veneti), Guī Bǎn (Plastrum Testudinis), and Biē Jiǎ (Carapax Trionycis).

Daily practices

1. Quán Xiē (Scorpio), Wú Gōng (Scolopendra), Dì Lóng (Pheretima), and Bái Jiāng Cán (Bombyx Batryticatus) are all animal medicinals that calm the liver and extinguish wind; what are the similarities and differences among them in terms of actions and indications?
2. Among the medicinals that calm the liver and extinguish wind, what are these herbs that can both calm liver yang and subdue liver wind?
3. Summarize actions and indications of these medicinals that calm the liver and extinguish wind?

CHAPTER 12

Twelfth Week

1

MEDICINALS THAT OPEN ORIFICES

The heart stores the spirit, which is said to reside in the heart orifices. When pathogenic influences envelop and veil the clear sensory orifices, the spirit is locked up and the patient becomes comatose with delirious speech. This usually occurs in patients with intense pathogenic heat obstructing the pericardium in febrile disease, or phlegm-damp confounding the pericardium in damp-heat disorders; or phlegm-heat, phlegm-turbidity, and phlegm-blood stasis clouding the pericardium in such internal miscellaneous diseases as stroke, infantile convulsions, and depressive psychosis. The orifices-opening substances are used to open up the heart orifices and awaken the spirit.

Most of these substances are aromatic and scattering by nature, also known as aromatic herbs that open the orifices. They are used for opening the orifices to remove pathogenic heat, phlegm turbidity, and blood stasis blocked in the heart orifices so as to revive the heart spirit to open the orifices and restore the consciousness. Blockage of heart orifice is caused by many reasons and can be differentiated into different patterns, and medicinals that open the orifices act in different ways. For instance, closed disorders may be further subdivided into hot closed and cold closed disorders; for the former, orifice-opening herbs that clear the heart are used for the former type, and herbs that warm and open the orifices are applied for the latter. Clinically, orifice-opening substances are always combined with other herbs to treat the root cause of disorder and achieve the optimal effect: for exuberant heat, substances that clear and drain pathogenic heat are also used; for phlegm-damp internal obstruction, herbs that dissolve phlegm and dispel dampness are added; for phlegm heat exuberance, substances that clear and dissolve phlegm heat are included in the prescription; for binding of phlegm and blood stasis with pathogenic heat, substances that clear and dissolve phlegm heat and invigorate blood and dissolve stasis are also applied; and for cases with accompanying stirring wind and convulsions, treatment should include wind-extinguishing medicinals.

The substances that open the orifices should not be used for treating desertion disorders, which has a similar presentation of delirium and coma. However, it is deficient in nature and orifice blockage is excess; their treatment principles are completely different. In such cases, substances that supplement deficiency (see chapters 12 and 13) and rescue from desertion with astringency (see chapter 14) would be appropriate. However for patients with both internal block and external desertions, the orifice-opening and desertion-rescuing substances are used together.

These substances, scattering in nature, are used for relieving symptoms during first-aid, not the root of the disorder. They should only be used for short periods of time. Long-term use can drain the original qi. Most of these substances are aromatic, when ingested they are almost always taken in pill or powder form to prevent evaporation of the active ingredients, make them portable, and for the convenience of first-aid.

麝香 Shè Xiāng *moschus musk*

[Addendum:] 牛黃 Niú Huáng Calculus Bovis Cow Bezoar

The source is from the dried secretion obtained from the fragrant sac of the male *Moschus moschiferus* L., *Moschus sifanicus* Przewalski or *Moschus berezovskii* Flerov, family Cervidae. Alternate names include 当门子 Dāng Mén Zi and 元寸香 Yuán Cùn Xiāng. Pungent in flavor and warm in nature.

[Actions] Open the orifices and revive the spirit, invigorate blood and dissipate masses, arrest pain, and hasten delivery of stillborns or the placenta. It is applicable for unconsciousness, stroke, phlegm syncope, and convulsion caused by heat entering the pericardium in warm febrile disease, severe pain in the chest and abdomen, injuries from falls, fractures, contusions and strains, *bì* pain, sores, ulcers, swellings, and toxins. Modern researches indicate it has an anti-inflammatory effect and can improve beta-adrenergic, rise blood pressure, excite respiration, and contract the uterine.

[Quality] 毛壳麝香 Máo Ké Shè Xiāng refers to the whole sachet and good quality is full, thin-skinned, elastical, and intensely aromatic; 麝香仁 Shè Xiāng Rén refers to the dried secretion from the sachet, also known as 当门子 Dāng Mén Zi, good quality is soft and moist with many granules and strong aroma. A variety of counterfeit goods are found in the market and attentions should be paid to identification.

[Indications]

1. Orifice blockage with unconsciousness: Shè Xiāng (Moschus), intensely pungent, warm and penetrating in nature, can unblock the collaterals and is therefore widely used for different types of orifice blockage with unconsciousness. It is combined with Xī Jiǎo (Cornu Rhinocerotis), Niú Huáng (Calculus Bovis), and Bīng Piàn (Borneolum Syntheticum) for heat block pattern caused by heat blocking the pericardium in febrile diseases; and with Sū Hé Xiāng (Styrax), Dīng Xiāng (Flos Caryophylli), and Chén Xiāng (Lignum Aquilariae Resinatum) for phlegm-damp or cold pathogen blocking the pericardium.

2. Pain due to blood stasis: Shè Xiāng (Moschus), good at scattering and unblocking the channels, has a good pain-relieving effective in the treatment of a variety of pain caused by blood stagnation. It is combined with medicinals that disperse blood stasis, move qi, and relieve pain such as Táo Rén (Semen Persicae), Mù Xiāng (Radix Aucklandiae), Rǔ Xiāng (Olibanum), and Sū Hé Xiāng (Styrax) for chest *bì* with heart pain. It has been recently used in treating coronary heart disease and is included in many Chinese patent medicines for curing coronary heart disease. This substance is combined with medicinals that nourish blood and dissolve blood stasis such as Dāng Guī (Radix Angelicae Sinensis), Chuān Xiōng (Rhizoma Chuanxiong), Xiāng Fù (Rhizoma Cyperi), and Yì Mǔ Cǎo (Herba Leonuri) for dysmenorrheal and abdominal pain caused by postpartum blood stasis; with medicinals that dispel wind,

dissolve dampness, and unblock the collaterals for pain of wind-damp *bì*; and with Rǔ Xiāng (Olibanum), Mò Yào (Myrrha), and Sū Mù (Lignum Sappan) for pain attributed to injuries from falls, fractures, contusions and strains.

3. Sores, ulcers, swellings, and toxins: Shè Xiāng (Moschus), pungent and dispersing to invigorate blood, is combined with Xióng Huáng (Realgar), Niú Huáng (Calculus Bovis), Rǔ Xiāng (Olibanum), and Rěn Dōng Téng (Caulis Lonicerae Japonicae) for the early stage of carbuncles, furuncles, sores, and swellings either through oral administration or external application.

Owning to its effect of scattering and unblocking the collaterals, it is also applicable for asthma, chest oppression, and gastric and abdominal either through oral administration or topical application of plaster on acupuncture point.

[Usage and Dosage] Should not be decocted or processed, use 0.03–0.1 g/time in pill and powder when taken directly. Due to the endangered status of this animal and its great expense, almost all of the commercially available products are synthesized muscone with similar actions.

[Mnemonics] Shè Xiāng (Moschus, Cow Bezoar): pungent and warm; best for opening the orifices, reviving the spirit, invigorating the blood, and arresting pain.

[Simple and Effective Formulas]

1. 麝香汤 Shè Xiāng Tāng — Musk Decoction from *Comprehensive Recording of Divine Assistance* (圣济总录, Shèng Jì Zǒng Lù): Shè Xiāng (Moschus) (ground, used in decoction), Mù Xiāng (Radix Aucklandiae) 30 g, Táo Rén (Semen Persicae) 35 pieces (stir-fried with bran), and Wú Zhū Yú (Fructus Evodiae) (soaked in water for one night, dried by stir-frying) 30 g; pound the latter 3 herbs with a pestle into fine powder, decoct 6 g/time in water and small cup of urine of boy under 12, remove dregs, and mix the liquid with Shè Xiāng (Moschus) 1 g for oral administration to treat sudden onset of heart pain.

2. 麝香散 Shè Xiāng Sǎn — Musk Powder from *Compilation in Treating External Sores* (疡科遗编, Yáng Kē Yí Biān): Shè Xiāng (Moschus)

0.3 g, Yuè Shí (Borax) and Yá Zào (Fructus Gleditsiae Abnormalis) 3 g, Míng Fán (Alumen) 3 g, and Xióng Jīng (Realgar) 3 g; grind into fine powder and take 1.5 g/time for oral administration to treat phlegm confounding the heart orifices and lack of consciousness.

[Precautions] Shè Xiāng (Moschus), pungent, fragrant, and volatile, is strong in scattering and may consume healthy qi when applied inappropriately. It is contraindicated during pregnancy, and in patterns of original qi deficiency and debilitation and qi and blood depletion. This substance is for first-aid and is not allowed for use when when the patient is revived. Use with caution in cases of hypertension as it can raise blood pressure according to modern report.

[Addendum]: 牛黄 Niú Huáng Calculus Bovis Cow Bezoar

The source is from the gallbladder stone of *Bos Taurus domesticus* Gmelin., family Bovidae. Alternate names include 犀黄 Xī Huáng. It, sweet and bitter in flavor and cool in nature, can clear the heart, open the orifices, stop tremors, and relieve toxins. This medicinal is applicable for febrile diseases, loss of consciousness, phlegm confounding in windstoke, fright, spasm, epilepsy, maniac, swollen and painful throat, ulcers in the mouth and tongue, sores, swelling, and carbuncles. Use 0.15–0.3 g, only in pills or powders.

Niú Huáng (Calculus Bovis) and Shè Xiāng (Moschus) both are principal medicinals that open the orifices and similar in terms of indications and administration. They are commonly prescribed together for orifice blockage with unconsciousness, sores, ulcers, swellings, and toxins. However, the former, cool in nature, is considered more effective in clearing heat and resolving toxins, capable of relieving spasm, and most commonly used for sores, ulcers, swellings, and erosions; the latter, warm in nature, is more potent in opening blockage, capable of invigorating blood, and effective in dispersing the sores and ulcers in the early stage.

冰片 Bīng Piàn *borneolum syntheticum borneol*

The source is from the evergreen arbor *Dryobalanops aromatic* Gaertn. f., family Dyptercarpaceae. Alternate names include 龙脑冰片 Lóng Nǎo

Bīng Piàn, 梅花脑 Méi Huā Nǎo, 梅片 Méi Piàn, and 片脑 Piàn Nǎo. Pungent and bitter in flavor and slightly cold in nature.

[Actions] Open the orifices and revive the spirit, clear heat and arrest pain, and improve vision and dissipate nebula. It is applicable for unconsciousness, convulsive syncope, sores, ulcers, swollen and painful throat, aphtha, and red eyes with nebula.

[Quality] Good quality is large, thin, pure white, brittle, and intensely aromatic. Its substitutes are commonly-used, such as 艾片 Ài Piàn, extracted from herbaceous *Blumea virens* DC., family Compositae; and 机制冰片 Jī Zhì Bīng Piàn prepared by taking turpentine and camphor as raw materials. The latter is most commonly found at the market.

[Indications]

1. Orifice blockage with unconsciousness: owning to its pungent and scattering nature, Bīng Piàn (Borneolum Syntheticum) is combined with other medicinals that open the orifices such as Shè Xiāng (Moschus) and Niú Huáng (Calculus Bovis) for a variety of orifice blockage with unconsciousness.
2. Heat-toxin swelling and pain: Bīng Piàn (Borneolum Syntheticum) can clear heat and resolve toxins due to its cold nature and its dispersing property of dissipating swellings and toxins. It is commonly used in the treatment of various types of carbuncles, swellings, boils, toxins, and throat swelling and pain. This substance is combined with Shè Xiāng (Moschus), Niú Huáng (Calculus Bovis), and Zhēn Zhū (Margarita) for different types of heat-toxin swelling and pain; with Péng Shā (Borax), Xuán Míng Fěn (Natrii Sulfas Exsiccatus), and Shè Xiāng (Moschus) for swollen and painful throat when blowed externally; and with Huáng Lián (Rhizoma Coptidis), Kū Fán (Alumen Dehydratum), and Lóng Gǔ (Os Draconis) in a powdered form for purulent discharge in ear when blowed externally.
3. Red eyes with nebula: Bīng Piàn (Borneolum Syntheticum) is combined with Zhēn Zhū (Margarita), Shè Xiāng (Moschus), and Lú Gān Shí (Calamina) and ground into fine powder for red, swollen and painful eyes or with nebula caused by heat-toxin attacking the eyes when applied externally.

Applying tincture of 6% Bīng Piàn (Borneolum Syntheticum) externally to the area of pain for relieving cancer swelling and pain has been reported recently.

[Usage and Dosage] Use raw only, should not be used in decoction. Use 0.03–0.1 g/time as in pill and powder.

[Mnemonics] Bīng Piàn (Borneolum Syntheticum, Borneol): pungent and cold; revive the spirit, open the orifices, clear heat, toxins, and swelling, arrest pain, and cure eye problems.

[Simple and Effective Formulas]
冰硼散 Bīng Péng Săn — Borneol and Borax Powder from *Orthodox Lineage of External Medicine* (外科正宗, Wài Kē Zhèng Zōng): Bīng Piàn (Borneolum Syntheticum) 1.5 g, Shè Xiāng (Moschus) 1.6 g, Xuán Míng Fĕn (Natrii Sulfas Exsiccatus) 15 g, and Péng Shā (Borax) 15 g; grind into very fine powder; blow powder to affected area, and 3 or 5 times/day for acute and chronic throat, mouth, and gum swelling and pain, prolonged cough, hoarseness, painful throat, acute and chronic inflammation of the throat, and fungus infection of the mouth and vagina.

[Precautions] Bīng Piàn (Borneolum Syntheticum), pungent, dispersing and scattering in property, should be used with caution in cases of qi and blood insufficiency and during pregnancy. Long-term use is not recommended as it may consume healthy qi or affect the fetus.

石菖蒲 Shí Chāng Pú *rhizoma acori tatarinowii* *grassleaf sweetflag rhizome*

The source is from the rhizome of the perennial Herbage *Acorus tatarinowii* Schott., family Araceae. Alternate names include 菖蒲 Chāng Pú. Pungent in flavor and warm in nature.

[Actions] Open the orifices and quiet the spirit, vaporize dampness and dispel phlegm, and move qi and harmonize the stomach. It is applicable for loss of consciousness, forgetfulness, and tinnitus caused by damp-turbidity clouding the clear orifices, chest and abdominal distention, oppression, and pain due to dampness obstruction and qi stagnation, and wind-cold-damp *bì*, injuries from falls, fractures, contusions and strains, carbuncles, boils, and scabies. Modern researches show it has certain sedative, antibechic, expectorant, choleretic, and anticonvulsant effects and can promote gastric juice secretion and alleviate smooth muscle spasm.

[Quality] Good quality is thick and aromatic with a reddish brown outer surface and white cross section. It is also named 九节菖蒲 Jiǔ Jié Chāng Pú as originally good quality refers to one cun of this medicinal (1/3 decimeter) consisting of nice segments (九节, Jiǔ Jié), however the Jiǔ Jié Chāng Pú available nowadays is the rhizome of herbaceous *Anemone altaica* Fisch., family Ranunculaceae, and misuse should be avoided.

[Indications]

1. Phlegm-damp clouding the clear orifices: generally, the clear orifices refers to the heart orifice, damp-phlegm or turbidity confounding the clear orifices may cause disturbance of consciousness, manifested as delirium speech and disturbance of consciousness that can fluctuate over the course of a disease. The clear orifices additionally means the orifices in the head and face, phlegm-damp can obstruct the ascending of clear yang qi and lead to problem in the head and face, such as heaviness of the head, tinnitus, and deafness. If that is the case, fragrant Shí Chāng Pú (Rhizoma Acori Tatarinowii) is capable of dissolving dampness and dispelling phlegm and therefore applicable. It is combined with Yù Jīn (Radix Curcumae), Zhī Zǐ (Fructus Gardeniae), and Lián Qiào (Fructus Forsythiae) for damp-heat phlegm clouding the pericardium in damp-warm disease; with Yù Jīn (Radix Curcumae) and Míng Fán (Alumen) for depressive psychosis and mania due to binding of phlegm and qi; with Yuǎn Zhì (Radix Polygalae) and Fú Líng (Poria) for forgetfulness; and with pig kidney and Cōng Bái (Bulbus Allii Fistulosi) for tinnitus and deafness.
2. Dampness obstruction in the spleen and stomach: Shí Chāng Pú (Rhizoma Acori Tatarinowii) is applicable for various disorders caused by dampness obstruction in the spleen and stomach. It is combined with Cāng Zhú (Rhizoma Atractylodis), Hòu Pò (Cortex Magnoliae Officinalis), and Chén Pí (Pericarpium Citri Reticulatae) for cheat and gastric *pǐ*, oppression, and distention, and reduced appetite caused by

dampness obstruction in the middle *jiao*; with Bái Zhú (Rhizoma Atractylodis Macrocephalae), Chén Pí (Pericarpium Citri Reticulatae), and Bàn Xià (Rhizoma Pinelliae) for vomiting and diarrhea due to dampness encumbering in the middle *jiao*; and with Huáng Lián (Rhizoma Coptidis), Shí Lián Zǐ (Caesalpinia), and Chén Pí (Pericarpium Citri Reticulatae) for dysentery without desire for food attributed to gastrointestinal damp-heat exuberance and depleted stomach qi.

It also can be pounded and applied externally to relieve carbuncles, swellings, phlegmon, and injuries from falls, fractures, contusions and strains. It can be combined with Kǔ Shēn (Radix Sophorae Flavescentis) for external wash to treat eczema.

[Usage and Dosage] Use raw in general, do not overcook when used in decoction to protect its aromatic ingredients. Use 5–10 g, up to 10–25 g when used fresh or large-dose. However, some people think the recommended dosage should not exceed 7.5 g, and up to 10 g when used for unblock urination and defecation.

[Mnemonics] Shí Chāng Pú (Rhizoma Acori Tatarinowii, Grassleaf Sweetflag Rhizome): pungent and warm; relieve dampness, open the orifices, improve hearing and vision, and harmonize the heart spirit.

[Simple and Effective Formulas]

1. 菖蒲饮 Chāng Pú Yǐn — Grassleaf Sweetflag Rhizome Beverage from *Comprehensive Recording of Divine Assistance* (圣济总录, Shèng Jì Zǒng Lù): Shí Chāng Pú (Rhizoma Acori Tatarinowii) (cut, baked) 30 g, Gāo Liáng Jiāng (Rhizoma Alpiniae Officinarum) 30 g, Qīng Jú Pí (Pericarpium Citri Reticulatae Viride) (white inner surface of exocarp removed, baked) 30 g, Bái Zhú (Rhizoma Atractylodis Macrocephalae) 15 g, and Gān Cǎo (Radix et Rhizoma Glycyrrhizae) (roasted) 15 g; grind into crude powder and decoct 6 g/time in water for oral administration to treat cholera with persistent vomiting and diarrhea.

2. 菖蒲郁金汤 Chāng Pú Yù Jīn Tāng — Grassleaf Sweetflag Rhizome and Turmeric Root Tuber Decoction from *Complete Treatise on Warm Diseases* (温病全书, Wēn Bìng Quán Shū): fresh Shí Chāng Pú (Rhizoma Acori Tatarinowii) 9 g, stir-fried Shān Zhī (Fructus Gardeniae)

9 g, fresh Zhú Yè (Folium Phyllostachydis Henonis) 9 g, Mǔ Dān Pí (Cortex Moutan) 9 g, Yù Jīn (Radix Curcumae), Lián Qiào (Fructus Forsythiae) 6 g, Mù Tōng (Caulis Akebiae) 5 g, Zhú Lì (Succus Bambusae) 15 g, and Jade Pivot Powder (玉枢丹, Yù Shū Dān) 1.5 g (infused); decoct in water for oral administration for damp-heat phlegm clouding pericardium in damp-warm disease with consciousness disturbance having a fluctuating course.

[Precautions] Shí Chāng Pú (Rhizoma Acori Tatarinowii), fragrant and dry in nature, is contraindicated in cases of yin and blood deficiency and should be used with caution for hematemesis and spontaneous seminal emission.

Daily practices

1. What are the major indication of medicinals that open orifices? What precautions should be taken when using it?
2. What are the similarities and differences between Shè Xiāng (Moschus) and Bīng Piàn (Borneolum Syntheticum) in terms of actions and indications?
3. What are the actions of Shí Chāng Pú (Rhizoma Acori Tatarinowii) beside opening the orifices? What are the differences among Shí Chāng Pú (Rhizoma Acori Tatarinowii), Shè Xiāng (Moschus), and Bīng Piàn (Borneolum Syntheticum) in treating unconsciousness?

MEDICINALS THAT SUPPLEMENT QI

Tonifying herbs are used in treating patterns of deficiency of the qi, blood, yin, and yang. Also known as tonics (补养药, Bǔ Yǎng Yào) and medicinals that supplement deficiency (补虚药, Bǔ Xū Yào). They supplement and boost to treat deficiency and also reinforce strengthen the body's healthy qi against pathogenic factors. These substances are generally subdivided by function into qi-supplementing, blood-nourishing, yin-enriching, and yang-strengthening categories.

Qi-supplementing herbs are used to tonify and boost original qi and qi of different *zang-fu* organs and increase the functional aspects of the body. Original qi is known as the root of life and is of great importance for the maintaining of vitality and health. The spleen is the foundation of acquired (postnatal) constitution, and the lung is the governor of qi throughout the body. For this reason, the key of tonifying qi is to strengthen spleen and lung qi. These herbs, generally sweet warm or sweet neutral in nature, can reinforce qi of various *zang-fu* organs and improve vitality.

The major symptoms of spleen qi deficiency are fatigue, lack of strength, decreased appetite, loose stool, even dropsy of the extremities. If allowed to progress to the stage of sinking of center qi, patients may present with chronic diarrhea with prolapse of anus, gastroptosis, hepatoptosis, and hysteroptosis. The major symptoms of lung qi deficiency are shortness of breath, no desire to speak, shallow breathing, weak voice, and spontaneous sweating. Moreover, because spleen and lung deficiency often occur at the same time, these symptoms are often combined with others.

Qi deficiency exerts great influence on different organs and tissues of the body. It may cause failure to generate blood, sluggish blood flow, water-damp retention generating phlegm and turbidity, and enduring bleeding due to qi deficiency failing to control blood. The patterns of blood deficiency, yang deficiency, phlegm-damp accumulation, and blood stasis obstruction may also involve or aggravate qi deficiency. Therefore, these herbs are used not only in the treatment of spleen and lung qi deficiency, but also often other patterns of deficiency.

These herbs are generally neutral in nature, but if applied in cases of the absence of qi deficiency, the qi movement would be obstructed. For this reason, the practitioner must be cautious with the indications when using these herbs. These substances should be combined with herbs that regulate qi to prevent congestion of qi movement, and also potentiate their absorption and digestion to achieve the optimal effect.

人参 Rén Shēn *radix et rhizoma ginseng ginseng*

The source is from the root of herbaceous perennial *Panax ginseng* C.A. Mey., family Araliaceae. It is so called because this medicinal looks very much like human body. There are many varieties of Rén Shēn (Radix et Rhizoma Ginseng), which are differentiated according to where and how it is grown and prepared. That grown in the wild is called 野山参 Yě Shān Shēn, the wild one that cultivated artificially is called 移山参 Yí Shān

Shēn, the cultivated one is called 园参 Yuán Shēn. Sweet and slightly bitter in flavor and warm in nature.

[Actions] Strongly tonify the original qi, strengthen the heart and prevent the prolapse, and calm the spirit and generate fluids. It is applicable to treat deficiency, overstrain, poor appetite, lassitude, vomiting, loose stool, cough and wheezing due to deficiency, spontaneous sweating, collapse, palpitations due to fright, forgetfulness, vertigo, headache, impotence, frequent urination, wasting-thirst, profuse uterine bleeding, prolonged scanty uterine bleeding of variable intervals, chronic convulsion in children. It is also applicable for poor recovery of different types of chronic deficiency, and qi, blood and body fluid insufficiency. Nowadays there is a great deal of ongoing research. This substance has been found to contain multiple active ingredients such as ginsenoside, indicating it has "adaptogen" effect and can increase body's defense against harmful stimulations, relieve strain and fatigue, excite the central nervous system, promote sexual gland and adrenal function, stimulate hemopoietic organ, lower blood sugar, reinforce cardio function, and regulate cholesterol metabolism. It also has shown antiallergic and antidiuretic effects.

[Quality] Wild 野山参 Yě Shān Shēn is of the best quality and most expensive; good quality is large, thick, firm, intact, juicy, thin striation, long and round residue of rhizome with dense bowl-shaped stem marks, fibrous root containing profuse pearl-like spots. For the cultivated ginseng, 园参 Yuán Shēn, good quality is long, thick, hard, and with long residue of rhizome, cultivated ginseng that is cured by steaming turns red in color is called 红参 Hóng Shēn, (Radix et Rhizoma Ginseng Rubra; the one that fumed by Liú Huáng (Sulphur) and dried under sunshine is called 生晒参 Shēng Shài Shēn, 白干参 Bái Gān Shēn, and 皮尾参 Pí Wěi Shēn; and the one that cured in rock candy and dried under sunshine is called 白参 Bái Shēn, 白抄参 Bái Chāo Shēn, and 糖参 Táng Shēn. Modern research has found that its fibrous lateral roots contain abundant active ingredients and its medical values should never be underestimated.

[Indications]

1. Original qi deficiency and debilitation: Rén Shēn (Radix et Rhizoma Ginseng) can be used alone or together with other medicinals that

rescue from desertion when sudden external desertion of debilitated original qi occur with symptoms and signs of pallid complexion, feeble minute or no pulse, and decreased blood pressure. It is combined with Mài Dōng (Radix Ophiopogonis) and Wǔ Wèi Zǐ (Fructus Schisandrae Chinensis) to boost qi and restrain yin for profuse sweating, thirst, and scattered big pulse resulting form external desertion of qi and yin; with Fù Zǐ (Radix Aconiti Lateralis Praeparata), calcined Lóng Gǔ (Os Draconis), and calcined Mǔ Lì (Concha Ostreae) for cold limbs, profuse cold sweating, and feeble pulse caused by external desertion of yang qi; and with medicinals that supplement qi such as Huáng Qí (Radix Astragali) and Bái Zhú (Rhizoma Atractylodis Macrocephalae) for lassitude, lack of strength, dispirited, and deficient powerless pulse due to long duration of illness with weak constitution or original qi debilitation.

2. Spleen and stomach qi deficiency: Rén Shēn (Radix et Rhizoma Ginseng) is combined with Bái Zhú (Rhizoma Atractylodis Macrocephalae), Fú Líng (Poria), and Shān Yào (Rhizoma Dioscoreae) for lassitude, lack of strength, loose stool, and reduced appetite due to spleen and stomach qi deficiency.

3. Lung qi deficiency and debilitation: to tonify the lungs and restrain qi, Rén Shēn (Radix et Rhizoma Ginseng) is combined with Huáng Qí (Radix Astragali) and Wǔ Wèi Zǐ (Fructus Schisandrae Chinensis) for wheezing, shortness of breath, and faint low voice caused by lung qi insufficiency.

4. Fluid and qi consumption: Rén Shēn (Radix et Rhizoma Ginseng) is combined with Zhī Mǔ (Rhizoma Anemarrhenae) and Shí Gāo (Gypsum Fibrosum) to clear heat pathogen and nourish fluid and qi for thirst, profuse sweating, and lassitude caused by pathogenic heat consuming fluid and qi in febrile diseases; with Tiān Huā Fěn (Radix Trichosanthis), Shí Hú (Caulis Dendrobii), and Shēng Dì (Radix Rehmanniae) to clear the stomach and nourish fluid and qi for thirst and polydipsia due to fluid and qi insufficiency in wasting-thirst disease.

5. Qi failing to contain blood: Use large doses of Rén Shēn (Radix et Rhizoma Ginseng) to boost qi to contain blood for hemorrhagic disorders caused by qi deficiency failing to contain blood. Clinically, it is commonly combined with Huáng Qí (Radix Astragali), Bái Zhú

(Rhizoma Atractylodis Macrocephalae), and Dāng Guī (Radix Angelicae Sinensis). Also applicable for palpitations, forgetfulness, and insomnia associated with qi and blood insufficiency; impotence, seminal emission, profuse uterine bleeding, prolonged scanty uterine bleeding of variable intervals, abnormal vaginal discharge resulting from kidney qi insufficiency; and blood deficiency due to qi deficiency failing to generate blood. Nowadays, it has been prepared into oral solution and capsule as a major health-preservation product and often combined with royal jelly. This substance is also used as raw material for cosmetics.

[Usage and Dosage] Use 1.5–9 g in decoction, up to 15–20 g in cases of supplementing and boosting original qi to rescue from desertion, 1–3 g/time as in pill and powder; and cut 1–3 g/day into slices and melt in the mouth when necessary for regulating and supplementing chronic and debilitated patient.野山参 Yě Shān Shēn (Radix et Rhizoma Ginseng Indici) and 移山参 Yí Shān Shēn are expensive and therefore is usually decocted separately in small amounts of water and then mix with decoction of other herbs.

[Mnemonics] Rén Shēn (Radix et Rhizoma Ginseng, Ginseng): sweet and bitter; strongly tonify the original qi, promote fluid production, supplement qi, and restrain prolapse and collapse.

[Simple and Effective Formulas]

1. 四君子汤 Sì Jūn Zǐ Tāng — Four Gentlemen Decoction from *Formulas from the Imperial Pharmacy* (局方, Jú Fāng): Rén Shēn (Radix et Rhizoma Ginseng) (the residue of rhizome removed), Fú Líng (Poria) (peel removed), Bái Zhú (Rhizoma Atractylodis Macrocephalae), and Zhì Gān Cǎo (Radix et Rhizoma Glycyrrhizae Praeparata cum Melle) in equal dosage; grind into fine powder, decoct 6 g/time in water for oral administration for deficiency of *zang-fu* organs, chest and abdominal distention and fullness, poor appetite, borborygmus, diarrhea, vomiting, and wheezing.
2. 参附汤 Shēn Fù Tāng — Ginseng and Aconite Decoction from *Formulas to Aid the Living* (济生方, Jì Shēng Fāng): Rén Shēn (Radix et Rhizoma Ginseng) 15 g and Shú Fù Zǐ (Radix Aconiti Lateralis Praeparata) 30 g; divide into four equal doses, and decoct each dose

with Shēng Jiāng (Rhizoma Zingiberis Recens) ten pieces in water for oral administration for wheezing due to yang deficiency, spontaneous sweating, night sweating, shortness of breath, and vertigo. Also applicable to collapse of yang qi with manifestations of pale complexion, cold limbs, feeble pulse, and decreased blood pressure.

3. 玉壶丸 Yù Hú Wán — Jade Pot Pill from *Ren-zhai's Direct Guidance on Formulas* (仁斋直指方, Rén Zhāi Zhí Zhǐ Fāng): Rén Shēn (Radix et Rhizoma Ginseng) and Tiān Huā Fěn (Radix Trichosanthis) in equal dosage; use raw, grind into powder, make into phoenix tree seed-sized pill with honey, and take 30 pills/time with Mài Dōng (Radix Ophiopogonis) decoction for diabetes with thirst and polydipsia.

[Precautions] Rén Shēn (Radix et Rhizoma Ginseng), as one of the most commonly used tonics, is effective for various types of deficiency, but should not be abused. It, warm in nature, may assist fire and generate heat when misused for the cases of yin deficiency resulting in vigorous fire and fluid consumption resulting in internal dryness. In a bid to reduce its adverse reactions, more attention should be paid to choose appropriate type of Rén Shēn (Radix et Rhizoma Ginseng) in line with different conditions: Hóng Shēn (Radix et Rhizoma Ginseng Rubra) and Gāo Lì Shēn (Radix et Rhizoma Ginseng) (Bié Zhí Shēn), relatively warm in nature, are suitable for cases of yang qi insufficiency or with deficiency-cold but contraindicated in cases of yin deficiency resulting in vigorous fire; and Shēng Shài Shēn (Radix et Rhizoma Ginseng Cruda) and 皮尾参 Pí Wěi Shēn, relatively neutral and moderate in nature, are appropriate for thirst due to qi deficiency but inappropriate for cases of edema and difficult and painful urination due to damp-heat internal exuberance. Overdose or long-term use is discouraged as it may unnecessary waste this precious medicinal resource and most importantly induce some side effects, such as "Ginseng abuse syndrome" occurred in recent years. This syndrome is defined by insomnia, irritability, higher blood pressure, or depressed emotion, reduced appetite, decreased blood pressure, and allergic reactions. It has been reported that ingesting 0.3 g/day Rén Shēn (Radix et Rhizoma Ginseng) powder over a long period of time may cause the syndrome mentioned above. For chronic disease, it is better to use in winter instead of summer as it may fuel heat and generate fire. This substance is often used together with medicinals that regulate qi such as Chén Pí (Pericarpium Citri Reticulatae) and Mù Xiāng (Radix Aucklandiae) to reduce its negative tendency of stagnating and blocking qi movement. It cannot be used alone in cases of dampness internal exuberance patterns and should be combined with medicinals that relieve dampness for dampness exuberance resulting from qi deficiency.

According traditional literature, this herb antagonizes Wǔ Líng Zhī (Faeces Trogopterori) and is incompatible with Lí Lú (Radix et Rhizoma Veratri Nigri). However, there has no report of adverse effect when Rén Shēn (Radix et Rhizoma Ginseng) and Wǔ Líng Zhī (Faeces Trogopterori) are used together in the treatment of qi deficiency with blood stasis.

Daily practices

1. What are the actions of medicinals that supplement qi? what precautions should be taken when using it?
2. What are the major actions and indications of Rén Shēn (Radix et Rhizoma Ginseng)?
3. What precautions should be taken when using Rén Shēn (Radix et Rhizoma Ginseng)?

西洋参 **Xī Yáng Shēn** *radix panacis quinquefolii* *american ginseng*

the source is from the root of *Panax Quinquefolium*, L., family Araliaceae. Alternate names include 洋参 Yáng Shēn and 花旗参 Huā Qí Shēn. Sweet and slightly bitter in flavor and cold in nature.

[Actions] Tonify qi and nourish yin, and clear heat and generate fluid. It is applicable for thirst and vexing heat in the chest, palms and soles caused by qi and yin deficiency, hemoptysis, and listlessness. Its major active ingredients are ginsenoside and its pharmacologic action is similar to that of Rén Shēn (Radix et Rhizoma Ginseng).

[Quality] Wild Xī Yáng Shēn (Radix Panacis Quinquefolii) is more expensive, good quality is even in size, hard, lightweight, and aromatic with a strong taste and dense striations on the surface.

[Indications] Xī Yáng Shēn (Radix Panacis Quinquefolii) and Rén Shēn (Radix et Rhizoma Ginseng) have similar actions, but the former is relatively cold in nature and most effective in engendering fluid production. Therefore it is most appropriate for cases of qi and yin consumption but contraindicated to warm medicinals.

1. Yin deficiency with vigorous fire: Xī Yáng Shēn (Radix Panacis Quinquefolii), cold in nature and effective in promoting fluid production, is combined with Mài Dōng (Radix Ophiopogonis), Bèi Mǔ (Bulbus Fritillaria), Dì Gǔ Pí (Cortex Lycii), Zhī Mǔ (Rhizoma Anemarrhenae), and Shēng Dì (Radix Rehmanniae) for hemoptysis, vexing heat in the five centers (chest, palms and soles), thirst, and vexation caused by yin deficiency resulting in vigorous fire.
2. Qi and yin consumption in febrile diseases: heat pathogen can easily consume qi and yin during the process of febrile diseases with the manifestations of fever, thirst, red tongue, and thin fast pulse, especially in the summer when summerheat pathogen invades that body and cause heat exuberance and yin consumption. Xī Yáng Shēn (Radix Panacis Quinquefolii), capable of supplementing qi and promoting fluid production, is suitable for qi and yin consumption in febrile diseases and is usually combined with Shēng Dì (Radix Rehmanniae), Shí Hú (Caulis Dendrobii), Tiān Huā Fěn (Radix Trichosanthis), and Mài Dōng (Radix Ophiopogonis).
3. Lung and stomach yin deficiency: to enrich and nourish lung and stomach yin, Xī Yáng Shēn (Radix Panacis Quinquefolii) is prescribed together with Mài Dōng (Radix Ophiopogonis), Shí Hú (Caulis Dendrobii), Shān Yào (Rhizoma Dioscoreae), and Shā Shēn (Radix Adenophorae seu Glehniae) for dry mouth, nonproductive cough, dry tongue, epigastric upset, or belching caused by yin fluid deficiency of the lungs and stomach in the later stage of febrile diseases and miscellaneous diseases of internal medicine.

[Usage and Dosage] Use in decoction, but often decoct separately from other herbs, dissolve into decoction of other herbs for oral administration, 3–6 g/time. Also applicable in pill and powder, 1–2 g/time; cut into slices and melt in the mouth when necessary, 1–2 g/day for debilitated patients with chronic disease who need to take over a long period of time.

[Mnemonics] Xī Yáng Shēn (Radix Panacis Quinquefolii, American Ginseng): cold; promote fluid production, moisten dryness, and cure exhausted qi and yin.

[Simple and Effective Formulas]
治肠红方 Zhì Cháng Hóng Fāng — Stool Containing Blood Resolving Formula from *Categorized Collection of Important Formulas* (类聚要方, Lèi Jù Yào Fāng): Xī Yáng Shēn (Radix Panacis Quinquefolii) 5 g and Guì Yuán Ròu (Arillus Longan) 20 g; steam together and take the decoction for oral administration to treat frequent stool containing blood, fatigue, and yellow complexion.

[Precautions] Xī Yáng Shēn (Radix Panacis Quinquefolii), cold in nature, is contraindicated in cases of loose stool and decreased appetite due to deficiency-cold of the spleen and stomach.

党参 Dǎng Shēn *radix codonopsis codonopsis root*

The source is from the root of herbaceous perennial *Codonopsis pilosula* (Franch.) Nannf. and various congeneric plants, family Campanulaceae. Alternate names include 上党人参 Shàng Dǎng Rén Shēn and 黄参 Huáng Shēn. Sweet in flavor and slightly warm in nature.

[Actions] Tonify the middle *jiao* and augment qi, and generate fluid and nourish blood. It is applicable for poor appetite, loose stool and lassitude of limbs due to center qi deficiency, shortness of breath, cough, wheezing, and faint low voice caused by lung qi deficiency, and sallow complexion, vertigo, and palpitations resulting from qi deficiency failing to generate blood. Modern research has shown that it contains such major active ingredients as saponin and polysaccharide, and can excite the nervous system, improve body's resistance against disease, reinforce hematopoietic function, lower blood pressure, and raise low white blood cell counts caused by chemotherapy and radiotherapy.

[Quality] The best quality is found in Luzhou, Shanxi and known as 潞党参 Lù Dǎng Shēn, good quality is thick, firm, soft, moist, strong-smelling, slightly sweet, and tight-skinned with many striations and without residue left upon chewing, and has lion head-shaped residue of rhizome. 明党参 Míng Dǎng Shēn, the root of herbaceous perennial 明党参, family

Umbelliferae, is effective in moistening the lung, dissolving phlegm, tonifying the stomach, and harmonizing the middle *jiao*. It is different from Dăng Shēn (Radix Codonopsis) and cannot be used as a substitute.

[Indications] The indication of Dăng Shēn (Radix Codonopsis) is similar to but not as strong as that of Rén Shēn (Radix et Rhizoma Ginseng). Clinically, it is often used in place of Rén Shēn (Radix et Rhizoma Ginseng) in ancient formulas. It, mild in nature and moderate in strength, is more effective in supplementing qi and generating blood and therefore is commonly used in relieving general spleen and lung qi deficiency and qi and blood insufficiency. It is combined with medicinals that enrich blood such as Dāng Guī (Radix Angelicae Sinensis), Shú Dì Huáng (Radix Rehmanniae Praeparata), and Bái Sháo (Radix Paeoniae Alba) for qi and blood insufficiency. Rén Shēn (Radix et Rhizoma Ginseng) is preferred for the more serious disorder of collapsed qi with devastated yang.

It can also be applied externally, for instance combining with Huáng Băi (Cortex Phellodendri Chinensis) and ground into powder for childhood aphtha.

[Usage and Dosage] Use raw in most cases, stir-fry or liquid-fry to improve its ability of supplement the middle *jiao* and boost qi. Use 9–15 g in decoction, up to 30–90 g for severe and emergency cases, and decrease the amount as in pill and powder.

[Mnemonics] Dăng Shēn (Radix Codonopsis, Codonopsis Root): sweet and warm; supplementary to Rén Shēn (Radix et Rhizoma Ginseng), tonify the middle *jiao*, augment qi, and assist blood production.

[Simple and Effective Formulas]

1. 上党参膏 Shàng Dăng Shēn Gāo — Codonopsis Root Decocted Extract from *Materia Medica of Combinations* (得配本草, Dé Pèi Běn Căo): Dăng Shēn (Radix Codonopsis) 500 g (cut into slices), Shā Shēn (Radix Adenophorae seu Glehniae) 250 g (cut into slices), and Guì Yuán Ròu (Arillus Longan) 120 g; prepare into decocted extract, infuse one small cup of extract/time into boiling water or other medical liquid for oral administration to treat qi deficiency of the spleen and lungs with faint voice and lassitude.

2. 参芪安胃散 Shēn Qí Ān Wèi Sǎn — Codonopsis Root and Astragalus Stomach Regulating Powder from Zǐ Jīn Collection for Laryngology (喉科紫金集, Hóu kē Zǐ Jīn Jí): Dǎng Shēn (Radix Codonopsis) (baked) 6 g, Huáng Qí (Radix Astragali) (roasted) 6 g, Fú Líng (Poria) 3 g, Gān Cǎo (Radix et Rhizoma Glycyrrhizae) 1.5 g, and Bái Sháo (Radix Paeoniae Alba) 2.1 g; decoct in water for oral administration to treat ulcers in the mouth and tongue occurred when the spleen and stomach are damaged by taking cold and violent medicinals. It is suitable for recurrent aphtha without fire-heat manifestations, and contraindicated for that with fire-heat signs.

[Precautions] Similar to Rén Shēn (Radix et Rhizoma Ginseng), Dǎng Shēn (Radix Codonopsis) is contraindicated in cases of damp-turbidity exburance and stagnation of qi movement to prevent assisting dampness and obstructing qi movement. According to some resources, it should not be used for hypotension and collapse due to its effect of lowering blood pressure, instead Rén Shēn (Radix et Rhizoma Ginseng) is preferred.

太子参 **Tài Zǐ Shēn** *radix Pseudostellariae heterophylly false satarwort root*

The source is form the tuberous root of herbaceous perennial *Pseudostellaria heterophylla* (Miq.) Pax ex Pax et Hoffm., family Caryophyllaceae. Alternate names include 孩儿参 Hái Ér Shēn and 童参 Tóng Cān. Sweet and slightly bitter in flavor and neutral in nature.

[Actions] Nourish the lungs and strengthen the spleen, and augment qi and generate fluid. It is applicable for spleen deficiency with poor appetite, thirst, and shortness of breath.

[Quality] Good quality is dry, full, yellowish white, and without small rootlets.

[Indications]

1. Spleen and lung qi deficiency: Tài Zǐ Shēn (Radix Pseudostellariae), Rén Shēn (Radix et Rhizoma Ginseng), and Dǎng Shēn (Radix Codonopsis) all supplement and boost the spleen and lung, but the first

one is less significant. It is combined with Bái Zhú (Rhizoma Atractylodis Macrocephalae), Shān Yào (Rhizoma Dioscoreae), and Fú Líng (Poria) for decreased appetite, lassitude, and lack of strength caused by spleen deficiency; and with Bǎi Hé (Bulbus Lilii), Shān Yào (Rhizoma Dioscoreae), and Huáng Qí (Radix Astragali) for shortness of breath and faint low voice due to lung deficiency. This substance can strengthen the spleen and lungs and therefore arrest sweating, dissolve phlegm, and reduce swelling.

2. Qi deficiency and fluid consumption: Tài Zǐ Shēn (Radix Pseudostellariae), moistening in nature and sweet in flavor, can not only supplement qi but also promote fluid production. It is combined with Shā Shēn (Radix Adenophorae seu Glehniae) and Mài Dōng (Radix Ophiopogonis) for cough with scanty sputum due to lung dryness with fluid consumption; with Shí Hú (Caulis Dendrobii), Tiān Huā Fěn (Radix Trichosanthis), and Mài Dōng (Radix Ophiopogonis) for thirst and red tongue without coating caused by stomach yin consumption; and with Wǔ Wèi Zǐ (Fructus Schisandrae Chinensis), Suān Zǎo Rén (Semen Ziziphi Spinosae), and Dān Shēn (Radix et Rhizoma Salviae Miltiorrhizae) for palpitations and insomnia associated with heart qi and yin insufficiency.

[Usage and Dosage] Use raw in general, large dose is preferred due to its moderate property, 15–30 g in decoction, up to 60 g when necessary.

[Mnemonics] Tài Zǐ Shēn (Radix Pseudostellariae, Heterophylly False Satarwort Root): sweet; strengthen the spleen and lungs, promote fluid production, and moisten dryness to arrest thirsty.

[Simple and Effective Formulas]
治自汗方 Zhì Zì Hàn Fāng — Spontaneous Sweating Relieving Formula from Shaanxi Journal of Traditional Chinese Medicine (陕西中草药, Shǎnnxī Zhōng Cǎo Yào): Tài Zǐ Shēn (Radix Pseudostellariae) 9 g and Fú Xiǎo Mài (Fructus Tritici Levis) 15 g; decoct in water for oral administration to treat spontaneous sweating.

[Precautions] According to "eighteen antagonisms", Tài Zǐ Shēn (Radix Pseudostellariae) is incompatible with Lí Lú (Radix et Rhizoma Veratri Nigri).

Daily practices

1. What are the similarities and differences among Xī Yáng Shēn (Radix Panacis Quinquefolii), Dǎng Shēn (Radix Codonopsis), and Rén Shēn (Radix et Rhizoma Ginseng) in terms of actions?
2. Why Tài Zǐ Shēn (Radix Pseudostellariae) is considered a substitute of Rén Shēn (Radix et Rhizoma Ginseng) or Dǎng Shēn (Radix Codonopsis)?

黄芪 Huáng Qí *radix astragali astragalus root*

The source is from the root of herbaceous perennial *Astragalus membranaceus* (Fisch.) Bunge var. *mongholicus* (Bunge) Hsiao or *Astragalus membranaceus* (Fisch.) Bunge, family Leguminosae. It is so called as 耆 Qí refers to the senior and this yellow-colored medicinal is among the top tonics. Alternate names include 黄耆 Huáng Qí and 绵黄耆等 Mián Huáng Qí. Sweet in flavor and slightly warm in nature.

[Actions] Boost qi to consolidate the exterior, promote urination to reduce edema, expel toxin and promote discharge of pus, and generate flesh. It is applicable for shortness of breath, lack of strength, poor appetite, loose stool, chronic diarrhea with prolapse of anus due to sinking of center qi, sallow complexion, dry mouth with thirst, profuse uterine bleeding, prolonged scanty uterine bleeding of variable intervals abnormal vaginal discharge, spontaneous sweating due to exterior deficiency, edema caused by qi deficiency, carbuncle and boils difficult to rupture or non-healing enduring erosive sore. Nowadays, this substance is widely used in the treatment of diabetes and chronic nephritis with proteinuria. Modern researches display it contains a variety of active ingredients such as polysaccharide and has immunological function-improving, body-strengthening, cardiotonic, diuretic, antihypertensive, hypoglycemic, and white blood cell counts-rising effects.

[Quality] Good quality is long, thick, sweet, and powdery with a yellowish white cross-section.

[Indications]

1. Spleen and stomach qi deficiency: Huáng Qí (Radix Astragali) is combined with Rén Shēn (Radix et Rhizoma Ginseng) or Dǎng Shēn

(Radix Codonopsis) instead, Bái Zhú (Rhizoma Atractylodis Macrocephalae), and Fú Líng (Poria) for lassitude, lack of strength, decreased appetite, and loose stool due to spleen and stomach deficiency; with Fù Zǐ (Radix Aconiti Lateralis Praeparata) and Ròu Guì (Cortex Cinnamomi) for chilly limbs, bland taste in the mouth, and undigested food in the stool due to spleen and stomach yang qi debilitation; and with medicinals that supplement qi and raise up such as Shēng Má (Rhizoma Cimicifugae), Chái Hú (Radix Bupleuri), Dǎng Shēn (Radix Codonopsis), and Bái Zhú (Rhizoma Atractylodis Macrocephalae) for chronic diarrhea and dysentery with prolapse of anus and other organs attributed to middle *jiao* qi deficiency and sinking.

2. Lung deficiency and weak exterior: the lung governs the *wei* qi and exterior, lung qi deficiency may cause cough, wheezing, shortness of breath, and *wei* qi failing to consolidate the exterior with frequent common cold or spontaneous sweating. Huáng Qí (Radix Astragali) is combined with Rén Shēn (Radix et Rhizoma Ginseng), Gé Jiè (Gecko), and Wǔ Wèi Zǐ (Fructus Schisandrae Chinensis) for cough and wheezing due to lung deficiency through consolidating and astringing lung qi; with calcined Mǔ Lì (Concha Ostreae), Má Huáng Gēn (Radix et Rhizoma Ephedrae), Fú Xiǎo Mài (Fructus Tritici Levis), and Nuò Dào Gēn Xū (Radix Oryzae Glutinosae) for exterior-deficiency with spontaneous sweating by consolidating the exterior and arresting sweating; and with Fáng Fēng (Radix Saposhnikoviae) and Bái Zhú (Rhizoma Atractylodis Macrocephalae) for exterior-deficiency with higher susceptibility to common cold via boosting qi to consolidate the exterior.

   Its action in stabilizing the exterior may be used to produce a therapeutic sweat when diaphoretics doe not work.

3. Edema due to spleen deficiency: Huáng Qí (Radix Astragali) can supplement the spleen and drain water and is applicable for water-dampness retention due to spleen deficiency. It is combined with Bái Zhú (Rhizoma Atractylodis Macrocephalae) and Fáng Jǐ (Radix Stephaniae Tetrandrae) for edema of the limbs and inhibited urination through fortifying the spleen and promoting urination.

4. Hemorrage due to qi deficiency: to enrich the qi to control blood and stanch bleeding, Huáng Qí (Radix Astragali) is combined with

medicinals that supplement qi such as Rén Shēn (Radix et Rhizoma Ginseng), Dāng Guī (Radix Angelicae Sinensis), and Bái Zhú (Rhizoma Atractylodis Macrocephalae) for intractable bleeding due to qi deficiency failing to control blood.

5. Channels and collaterals *bì* obstruction: owning to supplementing qi to promoting qi and blood circulation, Huáng Qí (Radix Astragali) is combined with Táo Rén (Semen Persicae), Hóng Huā (Flos Carthami), and Dì Lóng (Pheretima) for numbness of the limbs and hemiplegia for qi deficiency and blood stagnation.

6. Carbuncles and deep-rooted ulcers difficult to ulcerate: Huáng Qí (Radix Astragali), capable of promoting toxin expression through supplementing qi, is applicable for un-ruptured carbuncles due to qi deficiency failing to expressing toxin, and combined with medicinals invigorate blood and dissipate masses that Dāng Guī (Radix Angelicae Sinensis) and Zào Jiǎo Cì (Spina Gleditsiae) to facilitate toxin expression to early rupture of carbuncles.

[Usage and Dosage] The raw medicinal is considered more effective in benefiting *wei* qi, consolidating the exterior, promoting urination, reducing swelling, expelling pus, and expressing toxins. It is commonly used in exterior-deficiency pattern, edema, sores, and ulcers; liquid-fried Medicinal is more potent in supplementing qi and is applicable for different types of deficiency patterns; and using Huáng Qí Pí (Cortex Astragali) alone is to consolidate the exterior and boost *wei* qi. Use 10–15 g in decoction; increase the amount when used alone or for certain diseases, up to 30–60 g for chronic nephritis with proteinuria, and up to 120 g (five times of the total amount of other herbs) in Yang-Supplementing and Five-Returning Decoction (补阳还五汤, Bǔ Yáng Huán Wǔ Tāng) from *Correction of Errors in Medical Works* (医林改错, Yī Lín Gǎi Cuò).

[Mnemonics] Huáng Qí (Radix Astragali, Astragalus Root): sweet and warm; augment qi to consolidate wei qi, contain blood in the vessel, promote urination, and relieve abscesses and carbuncle.

[Simple and Effective Formulas]

1. 玉屏风散 Yù Píng Fēng Sǎn — Jade Wind-Barrier Powder from *Formulas from the Imperial Pharmacy* (局方, Jú Fāng): Fáng Fēng

(Radix Saposhnikoviae) 30 g, Huáng Qí (Radix Astragali) 30 g, and Bái Zhú (Rhizoma Atractylodis Macrocephalae) 60 g; grind into powder and decoct 9 g/time with Shēng Jiāng (Rhizoma Zingiberis Recens) 3 pieces in water for oral administration for spontaneous sweating.

2. 透脓散 Tòu Nóng Săn-Pus-Expelling Powder from *Orthodox Lineage of External Medicine* (外科正宗, Wài Kē Zhèng Zōng): Huáng Qí (Radix Astragali) 120 g, Chuān Shān Jiǎ (Squama Manitis) (stir-fried, ground into powder) 3 g, Zào Jiǎo Cì (Spina Gleditsiae) 4.5 g, Dāng Guī (Radix Angelicae Sinensis) 6 g, and Chuān Xiōng (Rhizoma Chuanxiong) 9 g; decoct in water for oral administration for carbuncles, sores, and ulcers in which pus is formed but not erupted yet.

3. 黄芪汤 Huáng Qí Tāng — Astragalus Decoction from *Important Formulas Worth a Thousand Gold Pieces* (千金要方, Qiān Jīn Yào Fāng): Huáng Qí (Radix Astragali) 120 g, Guā Lóu (Fructus Trichosanthis) 90 g, Zhì Gān Cǎo (Radix et Rhizoma Glycyrrhizae Praeparata cum Melle) 90 g, Fú Shén (Sclerotium Poriae Pararadicis) 90 g, and Gān Dì Huáng (Radix Rehmanniae Recens) 150 g; put into slices, decoct in water, divide decoction into three doses, and take one dose every day for ten days for oral administration to treat wasting-thirst or diabetes.

[Precautions] Huáng Qí (Radix Astragali), capable of supplementing qi, is contraindicated in cases of pathogen excess and qi congestion. It should not be used by patients with ascendant hyperactivity of liver yang, yin deficiency with internal heat, or chest and abdominal discomfort, *pǐ* and distention as it may fuel pathogen excess and worsen qi congestion. This substance cannot be overdosed since it is warm in nature and may turn into fire to injure yin if applied inappropriately as "superabundance of qi gives rise to fire".

白术 Bái Zhú *rhizoma Atractylodis macrocephalae* *white Atractylodes rhizome*

The source is from the rhizome of herbaceous perennial *Atractylodes macrocephala* Koida, family Compositae. Alternate names include 冬白术 Dōng Bái Zhú. Sweet and bitter in flavor and warm in nature.

[Actions] Tonify the spleen and augment qi, dry dampness and promote urination, and arrest sweating and calm the fetus. It is applicable for spleen deficiency with poor appetite, abdominal distention and diarrhea, vertigo or palpitations due to phlegm rheum, edema, spontaneous sweating, and restless fetus. Modern research has shown that it contains multiple active ingredients such as atractylon and has diuretic, hypoglycemic, liver-protecting, and immunity-regulating effects. This substance has recently been shown to be an inhibitor of mutation.

[Quality] Good quality is large, firm, solid, aromatic, and has a yellowish white cross-section. The one produced in Yuqian of Zhejiang is called 于术 Zhú, becomes less dry in nature, is more effective in supplementing spleen qi with a good quality.

[Indications]

1. Spleen and stomach qi deficiency: Bái Zhú (Rhizoma Atractylodis Macrocephalae) is combined with Rén Shēn (Radix et Rhizoma Ginseng), Fú Líng (Poria), and Gān Cǎo (Radix et Rhizoma Glycyrrhizae) for decreased appetite with loose stool, gastric and abdominal distention and fullness, lassitude, and lack of strength due to spleen and stomach qi deficiency; with Gān Jiāng (Rhizoma Zingiberis) and Rén Shēn (Radix et Rhizoma Ginseng) when accompanied with deficiency-cold pattern manifested as cold extremities and gastric and abdominal cold pain; with Zhǐ Shí (Fructus Aurantii Immaturus) for spleen deficiency with accompanying food accumulation through both attacking and supplementing; for constipation due to qi deficiency, it can be used alone, or in the formulas that moisten the intestines and promote defecation, a large dose is preferred.

2. Edema due to spleen deficiency: Bái Zhú (Rhizoma Atractylodis Macrocephalae), capable of supplementing qi, fortifying the spleen, drying dampness, and draining water retention, is often combined with Fú Líng (Poria), Zhū Líng (Polyporus), and Zé Xiè (Rhizoma Alismatis).

3. Wind-damp *bì* pain: Bái Zhú (Rhizoma Atractylodis Macrocephalae), dry in nature, can remove dampness and dispel wind-damp pathogen in the joint and muscle and is therefore applicable for different types of *bì* pattern. It is combined with Fù Zǐ (Radix Aconiti Lateralis Praeparata)

and Guì Zhī (Ramulus Cinnamomi) for cold-damp *bì* pain; and with Zhī Mǔ (Rhizoma Anemarrhenae) and Fáng Jǐ (Radix Stephaniae Tetrandrae) for damp-heat *bì* pain.

4. Spontaneous sweating due to qi deficiency: owing to its effect of supplementing qi and consolidating the exterior, Bái Zhú (Rhizoma Atractylodis Macrocephalae) can be used alone or together with Huáng Qí (Radix Astragali) and Fú Xiǎo Mài (Fructus Tritici Levis) for unremitting spontaneous sweating.

5. Restless fetus due to qi deficiency: Bái Zhú (Rhizoma Atractylodis Macrocephalae), as a principal medicinal that calm the fetus, is mainly used for restless fetus due to qi deficiency. It is combined with Huáng Qín (Radix Scutellariae) for fetal heat caused by spleen deficiency; and with Ē Jiāo (Colla Corii Asini) and Shēng Dì (Radix Rehmanniae) for vaginal bleeding during pregnancy attributed to blood heat.

It is also applicable for dizziness due to phlegm rheum in a combination with Fú Líng (Poria), Guì Zhī (Ramulus Cinnamomi), and Gān Cǎo (Radix et Rhizoma Glycyrrhizae). Ingesting large dose of this substance to promote defecation and treat constipation has been reported.

[Usage and Dosage] Use raw to dry dampness and promote urination, stir-fried to moderate its property with a better effect on strengthening the spleen and stomach; stir-fry with soil to supplement and boost the spleen and stomach; and scorch to stop diarrhea. Use 5–10 g in decoction, up to 60–90 g when necessary.

[Mnemonics] Bái Zhú (Rhizoma Atractylodis Macrocephalae, White Atractylodes Rhizome): bitter and sweet; tonify the spleen, calm the fetus, and promote urination to arrest spontaneous sweating, vertigo, and palpitation.

[Simple and Effective Formulas]

1. 白术丸 Bái Zhú Wán — Atractylodes Macrocephalae Pill from *Teachings of [Zhu] Dan-xi* (丹溪心法, Dān Xī Xīn Fǎ): Bái Zhú (Rhizoma Atractylodis Macrocephalae) 30 g and Sháo Yào (Radix Paeoniae) 30 g (in winter replace Sháo Yào (Radix Paeoniae) with Ròu

Dòu Kòu (Semen Myristicae), stir-fry for patient with diarrhea); grind into powder and make into pill with the paste of congee for oral administration to treat diarrhea due to spleen deficiency.

2. 术附汤 Zhú Fù Tāng — Atractylodes Macrocephalae and Aconite Decoction from *Effective Formulas* (近效方, Jìn Xiào Fāng): Bái Zhú (Rhizoma Atractylodis Macrocephalae) 60 g, Fù Zǐ (Radix Aconiti Lateralis Praeparata) 1 and 1/2 pieces (blast-fried, peel removed), and Zhì Gān Cǎo (Radix et Rhizoma Glycyrrhizae Praeparata cum Melle) 30 g; grind into fine powder, decoct 9 g/dose with Shēng Jiāng (Rhizoma Zingiberis Recens) five pieces and Dà Zǎo (Fructus Jujubae) one piece in water for oral administration to treat heaviness of the head, vertigo, poor appetite, qi deficiency, and weakness.

[Precautions] Bái Zhú (Rhizoma Atractylodis Macrocephalae), relatively dry in nature, is contraindicated in cases of yin deficiency with internal heat and fire-heat internal exuberance. It cannot be used alone for patients with chest and gastric distention and fullness caused by stagnation of qi movement, and should be combined with qi-regulating medicinals.

山药 Shān Yào *rhizoma Dioscoreae common yam Rhizome*

The source is from the tuberous root of sprawling herbaceous perennial Dioscorea Opposite Thunb., family Dioscoreaceae. Alternate names include 薯蓣 Shǔ Yù and 山芋 Shān Yù. Sweet in flavor and neutral in nature.

[Actions] Tonify and nourish the spleen and stomach, generate fluid and nourish the lungs, strengthen the kidneys and stabilize the essence. It is applicable for poor appetite and persistent chronic diarrhea due to spleen deficiency, cough and wheezing caused by lung deficiency, seminal emission, abnormal vaginal discharge, and frequent urination attributed to kidney deficiency, and wasting-thirst with deficiency heat.

[Quality] Good quality is thick, firm, powdery, and pure white. The best quality is found in Xinxiang, Henan (known as Huanqin in ancient China) and called 怀山药 Huái Shān Yào.

[Indications]

1. Spleen and stomach deficiency: Shān Yào (Rhizoma Dioscoreae), sweet in flavor and moistening in nature, is effective in supplementing spleen qi and enriching spleen yin, and therefore is widely used in a variety of disorders caused by spleen and stomach deficiency. It is combined with Rén Shēn (Radix et Rhizoma Ginseng), Bái Zhú (Rhizoma Atractylodis Macrocephalae), and Fú Líng (Poria) for loose stool, chronic diarrhea, edema, poor appetite, lassitude, malnutrition in children, abnormal vaginal discharge attributed to spleen deficiency and wasting-thirst due to spleen qi and yin deficiency.

2. Lung and kidney yin deficiency: Shān Yào (Rhizoma Dioscoreae), moistening in nature and capable of nourishing yin fluid, is combined with Mài Dōng (Radix Ophiopogonis) and Wǔ Wèi Zǐ (Fructus Schisandrae Chinensis) for chronic cough and wheezing caused by lung yin deficiency or lung and kidney deficiency; and with Shú Dì Huáng (Radix Rehmanniae Praeparata), Shān Zhū Yú (Fructus Corni), and Tù Sī Zǐ (Semen Cuscutae) for seminal emission and frequent urination due to kidney yin insufficiency.

[Usage and Dosage] Use raw, or stir-fry to improve its ability of fortifying the spleen (on the contrary, some physicians believe the raw one is better in fortifying the spleen). Use 9–15 g in decoction, up to above 60 g when used alone or as a principal herb. As a commonly-used herb and food, it is often used in a variety of health-care food.

[Mnemonics] *Shān Yào* (Rhizoma Dioscoreae, Common Yam Rhizome): sweet and neutral; tonify the spleen, moisten the lungs and kidneys, and relieve thirsty and frequent urination.

[Simple and Effective Formulas]

1. 山芋丸 Shān Yù Wán — Common Yam Rhizome Pill from *Comprehensive Recording of Divine Assistance* (圣济总录, Shèng Jì Zǒng Lù): Shān Yào (Rhizoma Dioscoreae) 30 g, Bái Zhú (Rhizoma Atractylodis Macrocephalae) 30 g, and Rén Shēn (Radix et Rhizoma Ginseng) 0.9 g; grind into fine powder, make into small-bean sized pill with the paste

of flour, and take 30 pills/time with rice soup before meal on an empty stomach for spleen and stomach deficiency with poor appetite.

2. 山药酒 Shān Yào Jiǔ — Common Yam Rhizome Wine from *The Grand Compendium of Materia Medica* (本草纲目, Běn Cǎo Gāng Mù): Shān Yào (Rhizoma Dioscoreae), Shān Zhū Yú (Fructus Corni), Wǔ Wèi Zǐ (Fructus Schisandrae Chinensis), and Rén Shēn (Radix et Rhizoma Ginseng); soak in wine and decoct for oral administration for vertigo caused by deficiency of the spleen, stomach, liver and kidneys.

[Precautions] Shān Yào (Rhizoma Dioscoreae), although neutral in nature, is contraindicated in cases of unresolved excess pathogens, indigested food accumulation, and damp-turbidity exuberance.

Daily practices

1. What are the major actions and indications of Huáng Qí (Radix Astragali)? what are the similarities and differences between Huáng Qí (Radix Astragali) and Rén Shēn (Radix et Rhizoma Ginseng) in terms of actions and indications?
2. Bái Zhú (Rhizoma Atractylodis Macrocephalae), Rén Shēn (Radix et Rhizoma Ginseng), and Huáng Qí (Radix Astragali) all are medicinals that supplement qi, what are the differences among them in terms of actions?
3. What are the similarities and differences among Huáng Qí (Radix Astragali), Bái Zhú (Rhizoma Atractylodis Macrocephalae), and Shān Yào (Rhizoma Dioscoreae) in terms of actions and indications?

粉甘草 Gān Cǎo *radix et rhizoma glycyrrhizae licorice root*

The source is from the root and rhizome of herbaceous perennial *Glycyrrhiza uraleusis* Fisch., *G. inflata* Batal. or *G. grabra* L., family Leguminosae. It is so called as it is sweet in flavor and neutral in nature, and capable of moderating the characteristics and relieving toxin of other herbs. Alternate names include Guó Lǎo 国老, Fěn Gān Cǎo 粉甘草, and Fěn Cǎo 粉草. Sweet in flavor and neutral in nature.

[Actions] Harmonize the middle *jiao* and alleviate the spasm, moisten the lungs, tonify the spleen, nourish the heart, relieve the toxin, and moderate and harmonize the characteristics of other herbs. It is applicable for spleen and stomach deficiency, lassitude, lack of strength, palpitations, shortness of breath, cough with profuse sputum, spasms and pain in the stomach cavity, abdomen, and limbs, carbuncles, swellings, sores, and toxins. Modern researches show its active ingredients include glycyrrhizin and glycyrrhizic acid, it has an effect similar to adrenocortical hormone and can inhibit gastric acid secretion and relieve smooth muscle spasms. This substance also has anti-inflammatory, antiallergic, antibechic, antasmatic, antalgic effects. Recent research reveals it has shown anti-tumor, anti-HIV, anti-liver fibrosis, and liver-protecting effects.

[Quality] Good quality is reddish brown, solid, powdery, and sweet with tight thin outer skin and a yellowish white cross section.

[Indications]

1. Heart and spleen deficiency: Gān Cǎo (Radix et Rhizoma Glycyrrhizae) is used together with Guì Zhī (Ramulus Cinnamomi), Mài Dōng (Radix Ophiopogonis), Wǔ Wèi Zǐ (Fructus Schisandrae Chinensis), and Bái Sháo (Radix Paeoniae Alba) for palpitations with knotted or intermittent pulse due to heart qi insufficiency; and with Dǎng Shēn (Radix Codonopsis) and Bái Zhú (Rhizoma Atractylodis Macrocephalae) for tirdness, lack of strength, and faint low voice caused by spleen and stomach deficiency.

2. Cough with sputum: Gān Cǎo (Radix et Rhizoma Glycyrrhizae), effective in moistening the lung, arresting cough, and dissolving phlegm, is applicable for different types of cough when prescribed together with other herbs. For instance, it is combined with Má Huáng (Herba Ephedrae) and Xìng Rén (Semen Armeniacae Amarum) for cough caused by wind-cold invading the lung through scattering and dissipating wind-cold and diffusing and unblocking lung qi; with Má Huáng (Herba Ephedrae), Shí Gāo (Gypsum Fibrosum), and Xìng Rén (Semen Armeniacae Amarum) for cough and wheezing due to lung heat via diffusing the lung and clearing heat; with Bèi Mǔ (Bulbus Fritillaria), Shā Shēn (Radix Adenophorae seu Glehniae), and Xìng Rén (Semen

Armeniacae Amarum) for cough resulting from lung dryness by moistening the lung to arrest cough; and with Gān Jiāng (Rhizoma
Zingiberis) for lung *wěi* (痿, atrophy) with expectoration of drool-
spittle attributed to deficiency cold in the lung through warming the
lung to arrest cough.

3. Spasms and pain: Gān Cǎo (Radix et Rhizoma Glycyrrhizae) is applicable for pain resulting from muscle spasm in the gastrium, abdomen,
and extremities, such as stomachache, abdominal pain, and musculus
gastrocnemius spasm and pain, and often combined with Bái Sháo
(Radix Paeoniae Alba).

4. Heat-toxin patterns: Gān Cǎo (Radix et Rhizoma Glycyrrhizae), capable of clearing heat and resolving toxins, is combined with medicinals
that clear heat and resolve toxins such as Jīn Yín Huā (Flos Lonicerae
Japonicae) and Lián Qiào (Fructus Forsythiae) for sores, ulcers, carbuncles, swellings, and swollen and painful throat caused by heat-
toxin. This substance can also relieve toxins and moderate the
characteristics of other herbs, therefore it is often used as an antidote
and included in a formula to mitigate the violent properties of or harmonize other herbs.

[Usage and Dosage] The raw substance is considered more effective in
clearing heat, relieving toxicity, moistening the lungs, and arresting cough,
while honey-fired one is used to warm the stomach, supplement the middle *jiao* and boost qi. The thick and big one is known as 粉甘草 Fěn Gān
Cǎo and more potent in tonifying; the thin without red skin is more effective in clearing heat and draining fire and therefore is more suitable for
heat-toxin pattern; and the tip, known as 甘草梢 Gān Cǎo Shāo, good
at draining fire in the bladder and is therefore most commonly used in
the treatment of difficult, painful, and frequent urination. Use 2–6g in
decoction, up to 30–60g when used as principal herb or in first-aid for
poisoning.

[Mnemonics] Gān Cǎo (Radix et Rhizoma Glycyrrhizae, Licorice Root):
alleviate spasms, supplement the spleen, lungs, and heart, moderate and
harmonize the characteristics of other herbs, and relieve heat toxins.

[Simple and Effective Formulas]

1. 甘草干姜汤 Gān Cǎo Gān Jiāng Tāng — Licorice and Dried Ginger Decoction from *Essentials from the Golden Cabinet* (金匮要略, Jīn Guì Yào Lüè): Zhì Gān Cǎo (Radix et Rhizoma Glycyrrhizae Praeparata cum Melle) 12 g and Gān Jiāng (Rhizoma Zingiberis) 6 g (blast-fried); chop and decoct in water for oral administration for lung atrophy marked by vomiting drool but without cough.

2. 甘麦大枣汤 Gān Mài Dà Zǎo Tāng — Licorice, Wheat and Jujube Decoction from *Essentials from the Golden Cabinet* (金匮要略, Jīn Guì Yào Lüè): Gān Cǎo (Radix et Rhizoma Glycyrrhizae) 9 g, Xiǎo Mài (Fructus Tritici Levis) 20 g, and Dà Zǎo (Fructus Jujubae) ten pieces; decoct in water for oral administration for visceral agitation in woman featured by loss of self-control over emotion, crying for no apparent reason, and frequent yawning.

[Precautions] Gān Cǎo (Radix et Rhizoma Glycyrrhizae), although neutral in nature, cannot be used overdose or long-term to prevent water-sodium retention and edema. It is contraindicated in cases of damp-turbidity exuberance and stagnation of qi movement due to its sweet flavor and tendency of assisting dampness and obstructing qi movement. According to "eighteen antagonisms", this herb is incompatible with Dà Jǐ (Radix Euphorbiae Pekinensis), Yuán Huā (Flos Genkwa), and Gān Suì (Radix Kansui).

大枣 **Dà Zǎo** *fructus jujubae chinese date*

The source is from ripe fruit of deciduous shrub or subarbor *Ziziphus jujuba* Mill. Var. *inermis* (Bge.) Rehd., family Rhamnaceae. Alternate names include 红枣 Hóng Zǎo. Sweet in flavor and warm in nature.

[Actions] Tonify and nourish the qi and blood of the spleen and stomach, and moderate and harmonize the harsh properties of other herbs. It is applicable for different diseases caused by deficiency of the spleen and stomach and insufficiency of qi and blood. Modern research has indicated that this nutritious herb can protect the liver, increase muscle strength, and regulate immunologic function.

[Quality] Good quality is red, thick, and sweet and has a small seed.

[Indications]

1. Spleen and stomach and qi and blood deficiency: owning to its property
   of supplementing the spleen and stomach and boosting qi and blood, Dà
   Zăo (Fructus Jujubae) is often combined with Rén Shēn (Radix et
   Rhizoma Ginseng) or Dăng Shēn (Radix Codonopsis), Bái Zhú (Rhizoma
   Atractylodis Macrocephalae), Dāng Guī (Radix Angelicae Sinensis),
   Huáng Qí (Radix Astragali), and Bái Sháo (Radix Paeoniae Alba) to cure
   a viarity of disorders caused by spleen and stomach insufficiency and qi
   and blood deficiency. It is also commonly used in tonic dietary therapy.
2. Disharmony between *ying* and *wei* qi: Dà Zăo (Fructus Jujubae) is prescribed together with Shēng Jiāng (Rhizoma Zingiberis Recens) and
   other medicinals that release the exterior to regulate and harmonize
   ying and *wei* qi to relieve aversion to wind-cold and spontaneous sweating caused by externally-contracted pathogen invasion with disharmony between *ying* and *wei* qi.

This herb, effective in moderating the characteristics of other herbs,
reduces side effects of formula with violent properties and protects spleen
and stomach qi. Its application in the treatment of allergic purpura and
hepatitis has been reported recently.

Can also be crushed and decocted for external wash to relieve non-
healing chronic sores.

[Usage and Dosage] Use 10–15 g or 3–5 pieces/dose in decoction, also
applicable in pill–form.

[Mnemonics] Dà Zăo (Fructus Jujubae, Chinese Date): sweet and warm;
tonify the spleen and stomach, nourish the qi and blood, and harmonize
ying and *wei* levels.

[Simple and Effective Formulas]

1. 枣参丸 Zăo Shēn Wán — Jujube and Ginseng Pill from *Food and
   Drink Records* (醒园录, Xǐng Yuán Lù): Dà Zăo (Fructus Jujubae) ten
   pieces (steamed until soft, kernel removed) and Rén Shēn (Radix et

Rhizoma Ginseng) 3 g; steam until soft and pound into hoodle-sized pill for oral administration to treat various patterns of qi deficiency and weakness.

2. 二灰散 Èr Huī Sǎn — Two Charred Substances Powder from *Treatise on Diseases, Patterns, and Formulas Related to the Unification of the Three Etiologies* (三因方, Sān Yīn Fāng): Dà Zǎo (Fructus Jujubae) (burned but medical nature preserved) and Bǎi Yào Jiān (Chinese Gall Leaven) in equal dosage; grind into fine powder and take 6 g/time with rice soup for oral administration to treat hematemesis and hemoptysis.

[Precautions] Dà Zǎo (Fructus Jujubae), although neutral in nature, is contraindicated in cases of abdominal distention caused by stagnated qi movement.

蜂蜜 Fēng Mì *mel honey*

The source is the saccharides engendered by Apis cerana or Apis mellifera, family Apidae. Alternate names include 白蜜 Bái Mì and 蜜糖 Mì Táng. Sweet in flavor and neutral in nature.

[Actions] Tonify the middle *jiao* to alleviate spasms, moisten the lungs to relieve cough, and moisten the intestines to promote the bowel movement. It is applicable for lassitude, shortness of breath, poor appetite, loose stool, and gastric and abdominal pain due to spleen and stomach deficiency, chronic cough caused by lung deficiency, nonproductive cough and dry throat resulting from lung dryness, constipation attributed to intestinal dryness, toxins, as well as sores, ulcers, and scalding when applied externally.

[Quality] Production areas, climate, and sources of plant can influence the quality. For summer honey such as pagoda tree flower honey, clover flower honey, jujube flower honey, and cole flower honey, good quality is light-colored, sticky, and sweet with intense fragrances; for autumn honey, good quality is waterless, oily, grease-like, and pure sweet without stinking smell and impurities, the honey flows down continuously to fold up while stirred up with a stick; poor quality is deep-colored and sour in taste with mild fragrance or bad odors.

[Indications]

1. Deficiency in the middle *jiao* with spasm and tension: Fēng Mì (Mel),
   sweet and moistening, is capable of not only nourishing and tonifying
   but also relieving tension and pain, and therefore often prescribed
   together with other medicinals that supplement the spleen and stomach
   and relieve tension for gastric and abdominal pain caused by deficiency
   in the middle *jiao* and spleen and stomach deficiency. It is used together
   with Guì Zhī (Ramulus Cinnamomi), Bái Sháo (Radix Paeoniae Alba),
   and Gān Cǎo (Radix et Rhizoma Glycyrrhizae) for stomachache due to
   deficiency-cold in the middle *jiao*.
2. Lung fluid dryness: Fēng Mì (Mel) is combined with medicinals that
   moisten the lung such as Shēng Dì (Radix Rehmanniae), Bǎi Hé
   (Bulbus Lilii), and Rén Shēn (Radix et Rhizoma Ginseng) and medicinals that arrest cough such as Kuǎn Dōng Huā (Flos Farfarae), Zǐ Wǎn
   (Radix et Rhizoma Asteris), Bǎi Bù (Radix Stemonae), and Pí Pá Yè
   (Folium Eriobotryae) to relieve cough and dry throat attributed to lung
   dryness.
3. Constipation due to intestinal dryness: Fēng Mì (Mel), nourishing and
   moistening in nature to promote defecation, can be infused alone for
   oral administration, or prepared into turunda for external application, or
   prescribed together with other medicinals that moisten the intestines to
   remove constipation associated with intestinal fluid dryness and center
   qi insufficiency.

This substance can resolve toxins and promote wound healing to cure
sores, ulcers, and scalding when applied externally.

Fēng Mì (Mel) is capable of moderating the characteristics of other
herbs and reducing side effects of a variety of toxic substances. It is also
used as an excipient for different types of tonic pill, not only to modify the
taste and help prepare the pill into a desired shape, but also to increase its
ability of tonifying. During the preparation process, adding this herb can
reinforce tonic effect or mitigate the violent properties of other herbs.

[Usage and Dosage] Use raw in general, or cook on slow fire for a long
period of time. If used in decoction, infuse or dissolve in the decoction of
other herbs, use 15–30 g/time.

[Mnemonics] Fēng Mì (Mel, Honey): sweet; moisten the intestines to promote bowel movements, relieve spasm to arrest pain, and decocted with Gān Cǎo (Radix et Rhizoma Glycyrrhizae).

[Simple and Effective Formulas]

1. 治咳嗽方 Zhì Ké Sòu Fāng — Cough Arresting Formula from *Important Formulas Worth a Thousand Gold Pieces* (千金要方, Qiān Jīn Yào Fāng): Bái Mì (Mel) 500 g and Shēng Jiāng (Rhizoma Zingiberis Recens) 1000 g (juice); decoct on slow fire until 500 g left and take jujube-sized medicinal/dose for oral administration, three times a day to treat chronic cough.
2. 蜜麻散 Mì Má Sǎn — Honey and Black Sesame Powder from *Modern Practical Chinese Materia Medica* (现代实用中药, Xiàn Dài Shí Yòng Zhōng Yào): Fēng Mì (Mel) 54 g and Hēi Zhī Ma (Semen Sesami Nigrum) 45 g; first steam Zhī Ma (Semen Sesami) until cooked, pound and mix with Fēng Mì (Mel), take after dissolve into hot water for oral administration, twice a day to treat hypertension and chronic constipation.

[Precautions] Fēng Mì (Mel), sweet in flavor, can assist dampness to readily induce fullness in the middle *jiao* when applied inappropriately and is therefore contraindicated in cases of phlegm-damp internal exuberance, damp-heat internal accumulation, and intestinal efflux with loose stool.

Daily practices

1. What are the similarities and differences among Gān Cǎo (Radix et Rhizoma Glycyrrhizae), Dà Zǎo (Fructus Jujubae), and Fēng Mì (Mel) in terms of actions and indications? What precautions should be taken when using them?
2. What are the indications of "sweet and moderate" Gān Cǎo (Radix et Rhizoma Glycyrrhizae), Dà Zǎo (Fructus Jujubae), and Fēng Mì (Mel)?

MEDICINALS THAT NOURISH BLOOD

Blood is an important substance that nourishes the body and moistens the *zang-fu* organs. From the perspective of traditional Chinese medicine, blood disorders include blood deficiency, bleeding, and blood stasis. Among them, blood deficiency refers to a lack of blood and may cause dysfunction of *zang-fu* organs in mild cases or death in severe cases.

Blood deficiency may arise from a variety of problems including insufficient resources of generation and transformation due to decreased food intake or failure to transport and transform, blood loss over much caused by hemorrhagic disorders, and excessive consumption of qi and blood in patients who have been ill with serious or chronic disorders.

Blood deficiency affects the whole body, the common and primary symptoms are sallow complexion, pale tongue, and lusterless nails. It may involve different *zang-fu* organs and tissues with diversified clinical manifestations; the organs most affected by this disorder are the heart and liver. The major manifestations of heart blood deficiency include palpitations, insomnia, and dreaminess; the major symptoms of liver blood deficiency are vertigo and dizzy vision. Blood deficiency in women is identified by scanty menstruation, amenorrhea, infertility, or lack of breast milk.

Blood-nourishing herbs are used in treating blood deficiency patterns. They are generally sweet warm or sweet neutral in nature with cloying texture. Blood deficiency may result from a variety of causes, therefore the selection and combination of herbs for blood deficiency are based on the root reason. For instance, for blood deficiency caused by qi deficiency, herbs that supplement qi are also used; for blood deficiency due to bleeding, herbs that stanch bleeding are added; and for case with accompanying yin deficiency, herbs that enrich yin are included in the prescription.

Most of the blood-nourishing herbs are cloying in nature and therefore should not be abused when excess pathogens such as fire heat and damp turbidity are still in exuberance to prevent the occurrence of lingering and difficult-to-resolve pathogens. The cloying substances may readily inure stomach and lead to congestion of qi movement. To counteract this effect, herbs that move qi and strengthen the spleen are often added to prescriptions of tonifying blood.

熟地黄 Shú Dì Huáng *radix rehmanniae Praeparata* *prepared rehmannia root*

The source is from the root of herbaceous perennial *Rehmannia glutinosa* Libosch., family Scrophulariaceae. Alternate names include 熟地黄 Shú Dì Huáng. Sweet in flavor and slightly warm in nature.

[Actions] Nourish blood and enrich yin fluid of the liver and kidneys. It is applicable for a variety of disorders caused by blood deficiency and liver-kidney insufficiency.

[Quality] Good quality is soft, sweet, pitch-black inside and outside, and glutinous with a moist cross-section.

[Indications]

1. Blood deficiency: Shú Dì Huáng (Radix Rehmanniae Praeparata) is a principal herb of enriching blood and usually combined with Dāng Guī (Radix Angelicae Sinensis) and Bái Sháo (Radix Paeoniae Alba) for sallow complexion, vertigo, dizziness, palpitations, insomnia, scanty menstruation, amenorrhea, profuse uterine bleeding, and prolonged scanty uterine bleeding of variable intervals due to blood deficiency.
2. Liver and kidney yin deficiency: Shú Dì Huáng (Radix Rehmanniae Praeparata), also known as an important herb to supplement the kidney and generate essence, is often used in the formula of enriching and nourishing the liver and kidney and frequently prescribed together with Shān Zhū Yú (Fructus Corni) and Shān Yào (Rhizoma Dioscoreae) for soreness and weakness of the waist and knee, vertigo, dizziness, seminal emission, and wasting-thirst due to kidney deficiency.

[Usage and Dosage] Use 10–30 g in decoction; also applicable in pill and powder.

[Mnemonics] Shú Dì Huáng (Radix Rehmanniae Praeparata, Prepared Rehmannia Root): sweet and warm; specialized in strengthening the kidneys, primary herb for gynecological problems, and good at nourishing blood.

[Simple and Effective Formulas]

1. 四物汤 Sì Wù Tāng — Four Substances Decoction from *Formulas from the Imperial Pharmacy* (局方, Jú Fāng): Shú Dì Huáng (Radix Rehmanniae Praeparata), Dāng Guī (Radix Angelicae Sinensis), Chuān Xiōng (Rhizoma Chuanxiong), and Bái Sháo (Radix Paeoniae Alba) in equal dosage; grind into crude powder and decoct 9 g/dose in water for oral administration to treat blood deficiency and stagnation with

menstrual irregularities, abdominal umbilical pain, profuse uterine bleeding, prolonged scanty uterine bleeding of variable intervals, dizziness, and palpitations.

2. 地黄饮子 Dì Huáng Yǐn Zǐ — Rehmannia Drink from *An Elucidation of Formulas* (宣明论方, Xuān Míng Lùn Fāng): Shú Dì Huáng (Radix Rehmanniae Praeparata), Bā Jǐ Tiān (Radix Morindae Officinalis) (plumule removed), Shān Zhū Yú (Fructus Corni), Shí Hú (Caulis Dendrobii), Ròu Cōng Róng (Herba Cistanches) (soaked in wine, baked), Fù Zǐ (Radix Aconiti Lateralis Praeparata) (blast-fried), Wǔ Wèi Zǐ (Fructus Schisandrae Chinensis), Guān Guì Bái (Cortex Cinnamomi), Fú Líng (Poria), Mài Mén Dōng (Radix Ophiopogonis) (plumule removed), Shí Chāng Pú (Rhizoma Acori Tatarinowii), and Yuǎn Zhì (Radix Polygalae) in equal dosage; grind into powder, decoct 9 g/time with Shēng Jiāng (Rhizoma Zingiberis Recens) five pieces, Dà Zǎo (Fructus Jujubae) one piece and Bò He (Herba Menthae) for oral administration to treat post-stroke hemiplegia and sluggish speech.

3. 六味地黄丸 Liù Wèi Dì Huáng Wán — Six-Ingredient Rehmannia Pill from *Key to Diagnosis and Treatment of Children's Diseases* (小儿药证直诀, Xiǎo Ér Yào Zhèng Zhí Jué): Shú Dì Huáng (Radix Rehmanniae Praeparata) 24 g, Shān Yú Ròu (Fructus Corni) 12 g, Shān Yào (Rhizoma Dioscoreae) 12 g, Zé Xiè (Rhizoma Alismatis) 9 g, Fú Líng (Poria) 9 g, and Mǔ Dān Pí (Cortex Moutan) 9 g; grind into powder, make into pill with honey, and take 6–9 g/time with warm water for oral administration to treat kidney yin deficiency with soreness and weakness of the waist and knee, vertigo, dizziness, tinnitus, deafness, night sweating, seminal emission, wasting and thirst, steaming bone fever, consumptive fever, dry tongue and throat, pain in the heel, continuous dribbling urination, and red tongue with scanty coating.

[Precautions] Shú Dì Huáng (Radix Rehmanniae Praeparata), greasy and cloying in nature, is contraindicated in cases of damp exuberance. Combining with Shā Rén (Fructus Amomi) and Chén Pí (Pericarpium Citri Reticulatae) helps to counteract regulate qi and fortify the stomach and is applicable for patients with spleen and stomach deficiency.

当归 Dāng Guī *Radix Angelicae Sinensis Chinese angelica*

The source is from the root of herbaceous perennial *Angelica sinensis* (Oliv.) Diels, family Umbelliferae. It is so called because it is a principal medicinal for various gynecological problems just like a woman who yearns for a reunion with her husband; or it can redirect qi and blood flow. Sweet and pungent in flavor and warm in nature.

[Actions] Nourish and regulate blood, harmonize menses to arrest pain, relieve cough and wheezing, and moisten the intestines to promote the bowel movement. It is applicable for blood deficiency, sallow complexion, vertigo, palpitations, menstrual irregularities, amenorrhea, dysmenorrhea, deficiency-cold abdominal pain, constipation due to intestinal dryness, wind-damp bì pain, injuries from falls, fractures, contusions and strains, carbuncles, sores, ulcers, cough, and wheezing. Modern research has shown that it can repel malignant anemia, increase coronary artery blood flow volume, reduce myocardial oxygen consumption, improve immunologic function, protect liver cell, inhibit bacteria, and arrest asthma.

[Quality] Good quality is fragrant and has large axial root, long body, few branches, and a yellowish white cross section. Herbs that produced in Gansu province is of high quality, whereas 东当归 Dōng Dāng Guī, 粉绿当归 Fěn Lǜ Dāng Guī, and 欧当归 Ōu Dāng Guī are of poor quality and should not be used.

[Indications]

1. Blood deficiency and blood stasis: Dāng Guī (Radix Angelicae Sinensis), capable of supplementing and invigorating blood, is well-known as "sagacious medicinal curing blood problems" as it can realize movement within tonification and tonification within movement and has been widely used in the patterns of blood deficiency and blood stasis. It is combined with Shú Dì Huáng (Radix Rehmanniae Praeparata), Chuān Xiōng (Rhizoma Chuanxiong), and Bái Sháo (Radix Paeoniae Alba) for vertigo, dizzy vision, palpitations, forgetfulness, and insomnia caused by blood deficiency; and with Rén Shēn (Radix et Rhizoma Ginseng) or Dǎng Shēn (Radix Codonopsis), Huáng

Qí (Radix Astragali), and Bái Zhú (Rhizoma Atractylodis Macrocephalae) when accompanied with qi deficiency.

This herb is used as a principal herb for menstrual irregularities, dysmenorrhea, amenorrhea, and postpartum abdominal pain caused by blood deficiency or with accompanying blood stasis. It is combined with Xiāng Fù (Rhizoma Cyperi), Táo Rén (Semen Persicae), and Hóng Huā (Flos Carthami) for qi stagnation and blood stasis; with Ròu Guì (Cortex Cinnamomi), and ài Yè (Folium Artemisiae Argyi) for cold congestion and blood stasis; and with Mǔ Dān Pí (Cortex Moutan), Shēng Dì (Radix Rehmanniae), and Chì Sháo (Radix Paeoniae Rubra) for blood heat and blood stagnation.

Dāng Guī (Radix Angelicae Sinensis), capable of dissipating cold with acrid-warm property, is combined with other medicinals that warm and unblock for pain caused by cold congealing and blood stagnation. For instance, it is often used together with Chuān Xiōng (Rhizoma Chuanxiong), Xì Xīn (Radix et Rhizoma Asari), and Bái Zhǐ (Radix Angelicae Dahuricae) for headache; with Chái Hú (Radix Bupleuri), Yù Jīn (Radix Curcumae), Zhǐ Qiào (Fructus Aurantii), and Yán Hú Suǒ (Rhizoma Corydalis) for pain in the chest and rib-side; with Guì Zhī (Ramulus Cinnamomi), Bái Sháo (Radix Paeoniae Alba), and Mù Xiāng (Radix Aucklandiae) for deficiency-cold abdominal pain; and with Qiāng Huó (Rhizoma et Radix Notopterygii), Guì Zhī (Ramulus Cinnamomi), Hǎi Fēng Téng (Caulis Piperis Kadsurae), and Jī Xuè Téng (Caulis Spatholobi) for joint and muscle pain due to wind-cold-damp obstruction in the channels and collaterals. This substance is often prescribed with other herbs to treat pain resulting from a variety of causes. For instance, it is combined with medicinals that clear and drain damp-heat such as Bái Sháo (Radix Paeoniae Alba), Huáng Lián (Rhizoma Coptidis), Huáng Qín (Radix Scutellariae), and Mù Xiāng (Radix Aucklandiae) for damp-heat dysentery with abdominal pain; and with Rǔ Xiāng (Olibanum), Mò Yào (Myrrha), and Sū Mù (Lignum Sappan) for pain resulting from injuries from falls, fractures, contusions and strains.

It is also applicable for carbuncles, sores, ulcers, and a variety of tumor caused by blood stasis. It is combined with Jīn Yín Huā (Flos Lonicerae Japonicae), Lián Qiào (Fructus Forsythiae), and Chuān Shān Jiǎ

(Squama Manitis) pieces for sores and ulcers in the early stage; with Huáng Qí (Radix Astragali) and Ròu Guì (Cortex Cinnamomi) for difficult-to-heal carbuncles in the late stage due to qi and blood deficiency; and with Sān Léng (Rhizoma Sparganii) and É Zhú (Rhizoma Curcumae) for different types of tumor.

2. Constipation due to intestinal dryness: Dāng Guī (Radix Angelicae Sinensis), moistening in nature, can promote defecation, especially for the elderly and people with weak constitution after long-duration of illness, and is often prescribed together with Ròu Cōng Róng (Herba Cistanches), Má Rén (Fructus Cannabis), and Bǎi Zǐ Rén (Semen Platycladi).

3. Chronic cough and wheezing: Dāng Guī (Radix Angelicae Sinensis) is combined with Sū Zǐ (Fructus Perillae), Bàn Xià (Rhizoma Pinelliae), and Fú Líng (Poria) for persistent and chronic cough and wheezing. Nowadays, injecting its preparation into acupuncture point for chronic bronchitis has been reported.

This substance can be prepared into injection for arrhythmia, ischemic stroke, joint and muscle pain, neuralgia, and thromboangiitis obliteran, or prepared with Bái Jiāng Cán (Bombyx Batryticatus) into anti-rejection drug with a good therapeutic effect.

[Usage and Dosage] Different functions are ascribed to the head (the uppermost part), the tail (the part deepest in the soil), and the body (the part in-between) of Dāng Guī (Radix Angelicae Sinensis). The head is most commonly used for hemorrhagic disorders of the lower part of the body, such as stool containing blood, hematuria, profuse uterine bleeding, and prolonged scanty uterine bleeding of variable intervals; the body is for enrich and nourish yin blood; the tail is regarded more most effective in invigorating blood and dissolving stasis; and the entire root is usually prescribed for nourishing and invigorating blood. Use raw to enrich blood, regulate menstruation, moisten the intestines, and promote defecation; fry the herb in wine to strengthen its blood-invigorating properties; process with wine to treat facial disorders; carbonize it if used for hemorrhagic disorders; and process it with ginger juice for the treatment of phlegm disorders.

Use 5–10 g in decoction, increase the amount when used to enrich blood, invigorate blood, regulate menstruation, moisten the intestines, and promote defecation. Also used in pill and powder.

[Mnemonics] Dāng Guī (Radix Angelicae Sinensis, Chinese angelica): pungent and warm; nourish and invigorate blood and moisten the intestines to promote defecation.

[Simple and Effective Formulas]

1. 当归丸 Dāng Guī Wán — Chinese Angelica Pill from *Comprehensive Recording of Divine Assistance* (圣济总录, Shèng Jì Zŏng Lù): Dāng Guī (Radix Angelicae Sinensis) (cut, baked) 30 g, Gān Qī (Resina Toxicodendri) (stir-fried until smoking) 15 g, and Chuān Xiōng (Rhizoma Chuanxiong) 15 g; grind into very fine powder, make into phoenix tree seed-sized pill with honey, and take 20 pills with warm wine for oral administration to treat amenorrhea in virgins.

2. 当归散 Dāng Guī Sǎn — Chinese Angelica Powder from *Confucians' Duties to Their Parents* (儒门事亲, Rú Mén Shì Qīn): Dāng Guī (Radix Angelicae Sinensis) 30 g, Lóng Gǔ (Os Draconis) (stir-fried until red-colored) 60 g, Xiāng Fù (Rhizoma Cyperi) (stir-fried) 9 g, and hair ashes of Zōng Lǔ (Petiolus Trachycarpi) 15 g; grind into powder and take 9–12 g/time with rice soup on an empty stomach for profuse uterine bleeding.

3. 当归散 Dāng Guī Sǎn — Chinese Angelica Powder from *Formulas from Benevolent Sages* (Shèng Huì Fāng, 圣惠方): Dāng Guī (Radix Angelicae Sinensis) 30 g, Guì Xīn (Cortex Cinnamomi) 30 g, Dì Lóng (Pheretima) (slightly stir-fried) 30 g, Bái Jiāng Cán (Bombyx Batryticatus) (slightly stir-fried) 30 g, Wēi Líng Xiān (Radix et Rhizoma Clematidis) 30 g, Lòu Lú (Radix Rhapontici) 30 g, Chuān Xiōng (Rhizoma Chuanxiong) 30 g, and Bái Zhǐ (Radix Angelicae Dahuricae) 30 g; grind into fine powder and take 6 g/time with warm wine for oral administration to treat unremitting pain in the joint and muscle all over the body.

[Precautions] Dāng Guī (Radix Angelicae Sinensis), warm in nature, should not be overdosed or used long-term and should be used with caution in cases of excessive internal heat or pathogenic heat exuberance. Owning to its moistening nature, it is contraindicated for loose stools resulting from deficiency-cold of the spleen and stomach. It should be stir-fried with earth or in a combination with medicinals that fortify the spleen when necessary.

Daily practices

1. What are the caused and manifestations of blood deficiency? what precautions should be taken when using medicinals that nourish blood?
2. What are the similarities and differences between Shú Dì Huáng (Radix Rehmanniae Praeparata) and Dāng Guī (Radix Angelicae Sinensis) in terms of actions and indications?

Thirteenth Week

白芍 **Bái Sháo** *radix paeoniae alba white peony root*

The source is from the root of herbaceous perennial *Paeonia Lactiflora* Pall. family Ranunculaceae. It is so called because of its beautiful flowers like charming ladies. Alternate names include 白芍药 Bái Sháo Yào and 金芍药 Jīn Sháo Yào. Bitter and sour in flavor and slightly cold in nature.

[Actions] Nourish blood and soften the liver, and stops spasms and arrest pain. It is applicable for headache, vertigo, chest and rib-side pain, abdominal pain, spasms and pain of the limbs, sallow complexion with blood deficiency, menstrual irregularities, spontaneous sweating, and night sweating. Modern researches display it can inhibit gastrointestinal motility and has sedative, spasmolytic, antibacterial, and immunity-regulatory effects. It also has certain anti-cancer and anti-liver fibrosis effects.

[Quality] Good quality is thick, long, straight, firm, powdery, and with a clean surface.

[Indications]

1. *Ying*-blood insufficiency: Bái Sháo Yào (Radix Paeoniae Alba) has the effect of enriching blood and is therefore combined with other medicinals that enrich blood such as Dāng Guī (Radix Angelicae Sinensis) and Shú Dì Huáng (Radix Rehmanniae Praeparata) for various patterns of blood deficiency. From the perspective of traditional Chinese medicine, *ying* is a major component of blood, *ying* and *wei* must be harmonized to consolidate and astringe the exterior. The disharmony between

ying and *wei* qi may cause sweating with aversion to wind. This herb can also astringe *ying* and harmonize yin and is often combined with Guì Zhī (Ramulus Cinnamomi) to harmonize *ying* and *wei* qi; and with calcined Lóng Gǔ (Os Draconis) and calcined Mǔ Lì (Concha Ostreae) for profuse sweating.

2. Liver yin deficiency with contraction of the sinews: the liver is the unyielding viscus that needs to be softened and nourished by liver yin, and the liver governs the sinew-membranes that also needs to be nourished by liver yin. Pathologically, liver yin insufficiency may cause liver qi stagnation and sinew-membranes contracture and pain. Bái Sháo Yào (Radix Paeoniae Alba) is often prescribed together with Chuān Liàn Zǐ (Fructus Toosendan) and Yán Hú Suǒ (Rhizoma Corydalis) for chest and rib-side pain due to liver yin deficiency; with Gān Cǎo (Radix et Rhizoma Glycyrrhizae) for gastric and abdominal pain and hand and foot contracture and pain; and with Fáng Fēng (Radix Saposhnikoviae) and Bái Zhú (Rhizoma Atractylodis Macrocephalae) for abdominal pain and loose stool resulting from liver qi invading the spleen through strengthening the spleen and softening the liver.

3. Liver yin deficiency with ascendant hyperactivity of liver yang: liver yin failing to nourish may cause hyperactivity of liver yang. Bái Sháo Yào (Radix Paeoniae Alba) is capable of nourishing liver yin to calm the liver and combined with Shēng Dì (Radix Rehmanniae), Chuān Niú Xī (Radix Cyathulae), and Mǔ Dān Pí (Cortex Moutan) for headache, vertigo, tinnitus, and eye distention caused by liver yin deficiency with ascendant hyperactivity of liver yang.

In recent years, it has been combined with Hǎi Piāo Xiāo (Endoconcha Sepiae) and ground into powder for oral administration to treat stomach and duodenum ulcer; and combined with Gān Jiāng (Rhizoma Zingiberis) and ground into powder for oral administration to relieve chronic and unremitting white leucorrhea.

[Usage and Dosage] Use raw in most cases, may stir-fry with wine to pacify its sour and cold nature and reinforce its effect on harmonizing the middle *jiao* and alleviating tension. Use 5–12 g in decoction, increase the amount when used for relaxing tension and arresting pain, and 1–5 g/time in pill and powder.

[Mnemonics] Bái Sháo (Radix Paeoniae Alba, White Peony Root): sour and cold; nourish blood, soften the liver, stop spasms to arrest pain, restrain yin, and arrest sweating.

[Simple and Effective Formulas]

1. 芍药汤 Sháo Yào Tāng — Peony Decoction from *Doctor Zhu's Effective Medical Formulas* (朱氏集验医方 Zhū Shì Jí Yàn Yī Fāng): Zhì Xiāng Fù (Rhizoma Cyperi Praeparata) 120 g, Ròu Guì (Cortex Cinnamomi) 90 g, Yán Hú Suǒ (Rhizoma Corydalis) (stir-fried) 90 g, and Bái Sháo Yào (Radix Paeoniae Alba) 90 g; grind into fine powder and take 6 g with boiled water for oral administration to treat rib-side pain in women.

2. 当归芍药散 Dāng Guī Sháo Yào Sǎn — Chinese Angelica and Peony Powder from *Essentials from the Golden Cabinet* (金匮要略, Jīn Guì Yào Lüè): Dāng Guī (Radix Angelicae Sinensis) 90 g, Sháo Yào (Radix Paeoniae) 500 g, Fú Líng (Poria) 120 g, Zé Xiè (Rhizoma Alismatis) 250 g, and Chuān Xiōng (Rhizoma Chuanxiong) 90 g; grind into powder and take 2 g/time with wine for oral administration to treat abdominal pain during pregnancy and various disorders caused by blood deficiency with static blood.

[Precautions] Bái Sháo (Radix Paeoniae Alba), cold in nature, is contraindicated in cases of pain caused by deficiency-cold. Also should not be used in patients with phlegm-damp internal exuberance to prevent lingering pathogen from assisting dampness. Bái Sháo (Radix Paeoniae Alba) and Chì Sháo (Radix Paeoniae Rubra) are originated from the same plant, however their actions and indications are different. The former is to tonify and astringe, while the latter is to drain and disperse.

何首乌 Hé Shǒu Wū *radix polygoni multiflori fleeceflower root*

The source is from the root of herbaceous perennial *Polygonum multiforum* Thunb., family Polygonaceae. Alternate names include 赤首乌, Chì Shǒu Wū 地精, Dì Jīng and 首乌, Shǒu Wū. It is so called because legends say ingesting this herb can change white hair into black. Bitter, sweet, and astringent in flavor and slightly warm in nature.

[Actions] Tonify the liver and kidney, nourish blood and dispel wind, moisten the intestines to promote bowel movement, prevent attack of malaria and relieve toxins. It is applicable for premature graying of the hair and beard due to liver and kidney yin deficiency, vertigo caused by blood deficiency, soreness and weakness of the waist and knee, soreness and pain in the sinews and bones, seminal emission, profuse uterine bleeding, prolonged scanty uterine bleeding of variable intervals, abnormal vaginal discharge, prolonged dysentery, malaria, carbuncle, swellings, scrofula, and hemorrhoids. Modern researches suggest that it can lower blood lipids, alleviate atherosis, strengthen the nerve system, and promote intestinal mobility.

[Quality] Good quality is heavy, firm, and powdery with reddish brown or purplish brown outer surface. In ancient books, it has been divided into 赤首乌 Chì Shǒu Wū and 白首乌 Bái Shǒu Wū, the former is commonly used, while the latter is from tuberous root of herbaceous *Cynanchum auriculatum* Royle ex Wight or *Cynanchum bungei* Decne., family Asclepiadaceae. These two herbs have similar actions.

[Indications]

1. Blood deficiency and liver-kidney yin deficiency pattern: Hé Shǒu Wū (Radix Polygoni Multiflori) is astringent in flavor and therefore effective not only in tonifying essence and blood but also restraining and consolidating essential qi. It is combined with medicinals that enrich blood such as Dāng Guī (Radix Angelicae Sinensis) and Bái Sháo (Radix Paeoniae Alba) for vertigo, palpitations, and insomnia caused by blood deficiency; and with medicinals that supplement the liver and kidneys such as Dì Huáng (Radix Rehmanniae), Nǚ Zhēn Zǐ (Fructus Ligustri Lucidi), Tù Sī Zǐ (Semen Cuscutae), and Shān Zhū Yú (Fructus Corni) for soreness and weakness of the waist and knee, tinnitus, seminal emission, and premature graying of the hair and beard caused by liver and kidney deficiency.
2. Constipation due to intestinal dryness: Hé Shǒu Wū (Radix Polygoni Multiflori), especially the raw one, is moistening in nature. It can be used alone or combined with other medicinals that moisten the intestines and promote bowel movements such as Dāng Guī (Radix

Angelicae Sinensis), Má Rén (Fructus Cannabis), and Bǎi Zǐ Rén (Semen Platycladi) for constipation caused by blood and intestinal fluid deficiency. Clinically, it can be used to replace raw Dà Huáng (Radix et Rhizoma Rhei) when it is used as a purgative for the elderly or weak suffering from biliary tract infection, gall stones, and jaundice.

3. Persistent and chronic malaria: for chronic and unremitting malaria due to qi and blood deficiency, Hé Shǒu Wū (Radix Polygoni Multiflori) is combined with Rén Shēn (Radix et Rhizoma Ginseng) to boost qi and nourish blood to relieve malaria.

4. Sores and ulcers: Hé Shǒu Wū (Radix Polygoni Multiflori), capable of resolving toxins, is applicable for carbuncles, scrofula, sores, and ulcers by either combining with other herbs for oral administration or decocting the raw for external application. It can also dispel wind through supplementing blood and therefore is combined with Dāng Guī (Radix Angelicae Sinensis), Jīng Jiè (Herba Schizonepetae), Fáng Fēng (Radix Saposhnikoviae), and Chán Tuì (Periostracum Cicadae) for skin itching, sores, and rashes caused by blood dryness stirring wind.

It has recently been reported this substance can be used in the treatment of hyperlipemia and whooping cough.

[Usage and Dosage] Use raw to promote bowel movements, arrest malaria, and relieve sores and ulcers; processed one (known as 熟首乌 Shú Shǒu Wū or 制首乌 Zhì Shǒu Wū) in decoction as a tonic, especially for promoting defecation. Use 10–15 g in general, up to 20–30 g when the raw one is used to promote defecation, and decrease the amount when used in pill and powder for being taken over a long period of time.

[Mnemonics] Hé Shǒu Wū (Radix Polygoni Multiflori, Fleeceflower Root): bitter and sweet; tonify the liver and kidney, nourish blood, dispel wind, moisten the intestines to promote bowel movement, treat malaria, and relieve toxins.

[Simple and Effective Formulas]

1. 乌牛丸 Wū Niú Wán — Fleeceflower Root and Two-toothed Achyranthes Root Pill from *Empirical Formulas* (Jīng Yàn Fāng,

Empirical Formulas (经验方 Jīng Yàn Fāng): Hé Shǒu Wū (Radix Polygoni Multiflori) 500 g and Niú Xī (Radix Achyranthis Bidentatae) (filed) 500 g; soak into 1000 ml good-quality wine for seven days, dry and pound into powder, make into phoenix tree seed-sized pill with honey, and take 30–50 pills/time for oral administration to treat atrophy and weakness of the sinew and bone, soreness and pain in the waist and knee, failure to walk, and itching all over the body.

2. 何首乌散 Hé Shǒu Wū Sǎn — Fleeceflower Root Powder from *Essence of External Medicine* (外科精要, Wài Kē Jīng Yào): Fáng Fēng (Radix Saposhnikoviae), Kǔ Shēn (Radix Sophorae Flavescentis), Hé Shǒu Wū (Radix Polygoni Multiflori), and Bò He (Herba Menthae) in equal dosages; grind into crude powder, boil 15 g/time with wine and water (1:1) for external wash to treat sores, carbuncle, swollen, itching, and pain all over the body.

[Precautions] Raw Hé Shǒu Wū (Radix Polygoni Multiflori), as a mild laxative, should be used with caution in cases of loose stools; while the processed one, as a tonic, is contraindicated in cases of damp-turbidity exuberance. Overdose of raw Hé Shǒu Wū (Radix Polygoni Multiflori) is not recommended to avoid potential poisoning symptoms, even spasms and respiratory paralysis in sever cases.

阿胶 Ē Jiāo *colla corii asini donkey-hide gelatin*

The source is from the donkey hide stewed and concentrated as gelatinous mass of *Equus asinus* L., family Equidae. Alternate names include 驴皮胶 Lǘ Pí Jiāo. Sweet in flavor and neutral in nature.

[Actions] Nourish yin and moisten dryness, and enrich blood and stanch bleeding. It is applicable for blood deficiency with sallow complexion, vertigo, palpitations, vexation insomnia, lung dryness, taxation cough, hemoptysis, hematemesis, epistaxis, ematuria stool with blood, profuse uterine bleeding, prolonged scanty uterine bleeding of variable intervals, and vaginal bleeding during pregnancy. Modern research has shown that it can increase the quantity of red blood cells, white blood cells, and platelets in peripheral blood, improve immunologic function,

facilitate calcareous absorption, and counteract traumatic and hemorrhagic shock.

[Quality] It is so called Ē Jiāo (Colla Corii Asini) as this medicinal mainly
produced in Dong E county of Shandong province is genuine regional
medicinal. Good quality is of uniform color, brittle, and translucent with
a shine cross section and without any foul odor. In recent years, 新阿胶
Xīn Ē Jiāo has been created by preparing pig skin with certain Chinese
medicinals, but its effects still need further researches.

[Indications]

1. Patterns due to blood deficiency: Ē Jiāo (Colla Corii Asini), good at
   enriching blood and nourishing yin, is combined with medicinals that
   supplement qi and blood such as Shú Dì Huáng (Radix Rehmanniae
   Praeparata), Dāng Guī (Radix Angelicae Sinensis), Rén Shēn (Radix et
   Rhizoma Ginseng), and Huáng Qí (Radix Astragali) for sallow complexion, vertigo, palpitations, and insomnia due to blood deficiency; and
   with Chuān Xù Duàn (Radix Dipsaci), Fú Líng (Poria), and Zhù Má
   Gēn (Radix Boehmeriae) for restless fetus caused by blood deficiency.
2. Different types of bleeding: Ē Jiāo (Colla Corii Asini), effective in
   enriching blood and restraining and stanching bleeding, is applicable
   for different types of hemorrhagic disorders. It is stir-fried with Gé Jiè
   powder (Gecko) first and then used together with Bái Jí (Rhizoma
   Bletillae) and Sān Qī (Radix et Rhizoma Notoginseng) for hemoptysis
   and hematemesis; or stir-fired with Pú Huáng (Pollen Typhae) and then
   used together with Shēng Dì (Radix Rehmanniae), Qiàn Cǎo (Radix et
   Rhizoma Rubiae), and Dì Yú (Radix Sanguisorbae) for profuse uterine
   bleeding, prolonged scanty uterine bleeding of variable intervals,
   hematuria, and stools containing blood.
3. Yin deficiency with inner dryness: Ē Jiāo (Colla Corii Asini), capable of
   nourishing yin fluid, is combined with Shā Shēn (Radix Adenophorae
   seu Glehniae), Mài Dōng (Radix Ophiopogonis), Zhī Mǔ (Rhizoma
   Anemarrhenae), and Xìng Rén (Semen Armeniacae Amarum) for dryness cough due to lung yin deficiency; with Huáng Lián (Rhizoma
   Coptidis) and Jī Zi Huáng (Egg Yolk) for deficiency-vexation insomnia
   caused by yin deficiency with vigorous fire; and with Guī Bǎn (Plastrum

Testudinis), Biē Jiǎ (Carapax Trionycis), and Mǔ Lì (Concha Ostreae) for convulsions of the limbs due to yin deficiency stirring wind via nourishing yin to extinguish wind.

It has recently been reported that this substance has been used in the treatment of progressive muscular dystrophy, leukocytopenia, thrombocytopenic purpura, and threatened miscarriage.

[Usage and Dosage] Stir-fry with Pú Huáng (Pollen Typhae) or Gé Lí (Clam) powder (called ē Jiāo Zhū-Colla Corii Asini Pilula) is for different types of hemorrhagic disorders. If used in decoction, it should be melted by steaming in yellow wine or water prior to dissolve into the decoction of other herbs. Use 6–15 g in general.

[Mnemonics] Ē Jiāo (Colla Corii Asini, Donkey-hide Gelatin): sweet and neutral; good at arresting bleeding, and can enrich blood, calm the fetus, moisten dryness, and nourish yin.

[Simple and Effective Formulas]

1. 阿胶饮 Ē Jiāo Yǐn — Donkey-hide Gelatin Beverage from *Comprehensive Recording of Divine Assistance* (圣济总录, Shèng Jì Zǒng Lù): Ē Jiāo (Colla Corii Asini) (roasted) 30 g and Rén Shēn (Radix et Rhizoma Ginseng) 60 g; grind into powder and decoct 8 g/time with Dàn Dòu Chǐ (Semen Sojae Praeparatum) soup and Cōng Bái (Bulbus Allii Fistulosi), and take warm for oral administration upon the onset of cough to treat persistent coughing.
2. 胶艾汤 Jiāo Ài Tāng — Donkey-Hide Gelatin and Mugwort Decoction from *Classical Formulas* (小品方, Xiǎo Pǐn Fāng): Ē Jiāo (Colla Corii Asini) 60 g (roasted) and Ài Yè (Folium Artemisiae Argyi) 60 g; decoct in water for oral administration, divide into three equal doses, one dose one time, to treat restless fetus with vaginal bleeding and abdominal pain during pregnancy.
3. 胶蜜汤 Jiāo Mì Tāng — Donkey-Hide Gelatin and Honey Decoction from *Ren-zhai's Direct Guidance on Formulas* (仁斋直指方, Rén Zhāi Zhí Zhǐ Fāng): Ē Jiāo (Colla Corii Asini) (stir-fried) 6 g, Cōng Bái (Bulbus Allii Fistulosi) with root three pieces, and honey two

spoonfuls; decoct Cōng Bái (Bulbus Allii Fistulosi) first, remove Cōng Bái (Bulbus Allii Fistulosi), add Ē Jiāo (Colla Corii Asini) and honey, and take before meal for oral administration to treat constipation in the weak and elderly.

[Precautions] Ē Jiāo, nourishing and cloying in nature with a side effect of injuring the stomach, should be used with caution in cases of spleen and stomach deficiency, indigestion, *pǐ* (痞) and fullness in the chest and abdomen, and greasy tongue coating.

Daily practices

1. What are the similarities and differences between Bái Sháo (Radix Paeoniae Alba) and Chì Sháo (Radix Paeoniae Rubra) in terms of actions and indications?
2. What are the similarities and differences among Bái Sháo (Radix Paeoniae Alba), Hé Shǒu Wū (Radix Polygoni Multiflori), and Ē Jiāo (Colla Corii Asini) in terms of actions and indications?
3. Among medicinals that nourish blood, which ones can stanch bleeding and which ones can invigorate blood? Among the medicinals that we learn before, which ones can nourish blood and stanch bleeding? Which ones can nourish blood and invigorate blood?

MEDICINALS THAT ENRICH YIN

In traditional Chinese medicine, yin is a general term to describe the various forms of yin fluids in human body, each *zang-fu* organ contains its own yin to coordinate with yang of each. Blood is also considered as part of yin fluid however yin deficiency discussed in this section refers primarily to yin fluid insufficiency of *zang-fu* organs, and correspondingly yin-enriching herbs are used primarily to tonify the yin of each *zang-fu* organs. These herbs are also known as medicinals that nourish yin (养阴药, Yǎng Yīn Yào) and medicinals that nurture or moisten yin (滋阴药, Zī Yīn Yào). These substances generally are sweet cold, salty cold or sour sold in flavor and nature. The organs most affected by this problem are the lungs, stomach, liver, and kidneys. The stomach is considered as the foundation of postnatal constitution, yin fluid in the body primarily relies on its digestion of food and drinks, stomach fluid sufficiency will bring in inexhaustible source of qi and blood production and build up abundant yin fluids all over the body. The stomach and lung are in mutual generation of earth (the stomach) and metal (the lung), stomach yin and lung yin are related to each other, physiologically and pathologically, lung and stomach yin deficiency often occur at the same time, the treatment plan should, therefore, include nourishing both lung yin and stomach yin. The kidney is the foundation of congenital (prenatal) constitution, kidney yin (kidney essence) is essential for the generation of yin fluid. Liver yin comes from kidney yin, yǐ (乙; i.e., liver) and guǐ (癸; i.e., kidney) are from the same source, liver and kidney yin deficiency often occur together, hence the treatment should be based on supplementing yin fluids of both the liver and kidney.

Clinically, lung yin deficiency is manifested as dry cough, hemoptysis, dry throat, and flushed cheeks; stomach yin deficiency is featured by thirst, gastric upset, belching, and smooth bare red tongue; liver yin deficiency has such symptoms and signs as dry eyes, blurred vision, and dizziness; and kidney yin usually presents as vertigo, tinnitus, soreness and weakness of the waist and knee, night sweating, and seminal emission. However, the lung and stomach, and the liver and kidney often suffer from yin deficiency at the same time, these symptoms are often occur together.

Yin deficiency may arise from different causes including constitutionally yin deficiency, poor recovery from a serious disease, enduring blood deficiency, and chronic yang deficiency. The selection and combination of herbs for yin deficiency are based on the *zang-fu* organ, degree, and root reason of yin deficiency. Yin tonics are generally enriching and cloying, inappropriate application may injure the stomach or cause lingering pathogen. For this reason, they should be combined with herbs that supplement the spleen and move qi. These herbs are expected to be used with caution in cases of damp exuberance and unresolved fire-heat.

北沙参 **Běi Shā Shēn** *radix glehniae straight ladybell root*

[Addendum] 南沙参 Nán Shā Shēn Radix Adenophorae Adenophora Root.

The source is from the root of herbaceous perennial *Glehnia littoralis* Fr. Schmidt *ex* Miq., family Umbelliferae. It is so called because it looks like Rén Shēn (Radix et Rhizoma Ginseng) and grows in sandy soil. Alternate names include 银条参 Yín Tiáo Shēn and 北条参 Běi Tiáo Shēn. Sweet and bitter in flavor and slightly cold in nature.

[Actions] Nourish yin and moisten the lung, and tonify the stomach and generate fluids. It is applicable for cough due to lung heat and dryness, taxation cough with bloody sputum, and fluid consumption with thirst in febrile diseases.

[Quality] Good quality is thick, firm, yellowish white, and brittle.

[Indications]

1. Lung yin deficiency: Shā Shēn (Radix Adenophorae seu Glehniae) can be used alone or together with Bèi Mǔ (Bulbus Fritillaria), Mài Dōng (Radix Ophiopogonis), and Bǎi Hé (Bulbus Lilii) for dryness cough and nonproductive cough with scanty sputum due to lung yin deficiency or lung heat, pulmonary tuberculosis with chronic cough, and dry throat and hoarseness caused by lung heat. It is combined with Mǎ Dōu Líng (Fructus Aristolochiae), Jié Gěng (Radix Platycodonis), and Zǐ Wǎn (Radix et Rhizoma Asteris) in cases of severe cough.
2. Stomach yin deficiency: Shā Shēn (Radix Adenophorae seu Glehniae) is prescribed with Mài Dōng (Radix Ophiopogonis), Shí Hú (Caulis Dendrobii), and Yù Zhú (Rhizoma Polygonati Odorati) for stomach yin deficiency manifested as thirst, belching, and red or crimson tongue in febrile diseases and epigastric upset, gastric dull pain, and smooth bare red tongue in internal miscellaneous diseases.

[Usage and Dosage] Use raw and prepare in decoction in most cases. Use 6–15 g in decoction, small amount when used for chronic yin deficiency of the lungs and stomach, and bigger amount in cases of yin consumption with thirst in febrile disease. It should be decocted for a long time to facilitate active ingredient extraction.

[Mnemonics] Shā Shēn (Radix Adenophorae seu Glehniae, Straight Ladybell Root): sweet and bitter; nourish lung yin, supplement stomach yin, and arrest thirsty.

[Simple and Effective Formulas]

1. 沙参麦冬汤 Shā Shēn Mài Dōng Tāng — Straight Ladybell Root and Dwarf Lilyturf Tuber Decoction from *Systematic Differentiation of Warm Diseases* (温病条辨, Wēn Bìng Tiáo Biàn): Shā Shēn (Radix Adenophorae seu Glehniae) 9 g, Mài Dōng (Radix Ophiopogonis) 9 g, Yù Zhú (Rhizoma Polygonati Odorati) 6 g, Gān Cǎo (Radix et Rhizoma Glycyrrhizae) 3 g, Sāng Yè (Folium Mori) 4.5 g, Bái Biǎn Dòu (Semen Lablab Album) 4.5 g, and Tiān Huā Fěn (Radix Trichosanthis) 4.5 g; decoct in water for oral administration to treat dryness damaging the lung and stomach with fluid exhaustion manifested as thirst, dry cough with scanty sputum, and red tongue with scanty coating.

2. 治干咳方 Zhì Gān Ké Tāng — Dry Cough-arresting Decoction from *Simple and Effective Formulas for Health* (卫生易简方, Wēi Shēng Yì Jiǎn Fāng): Běi Shā Shēn (Radix Glehniae) 120 g, Mài Dōng (Radix Ophiopogonis) 120 g, Zhī Mǔ (Rhizoma Anemarrhenae) 120 g, Chuān Bèi Mǔ (Bulbus Fritillariae Cirrhosae) 120 g, Shú Dì Huáng (Radix Rehmanniae Praeparata) 120 g, Biē Jiǎ (Carapax Trionycis) 120 g, and Dì Gǔ Pí (Cortex Lycii) 120 g; make into pill or medicinal paste and take 9 g in the morning with boiled water for oral administration to treat yin deficiency resulting in vigorous fire, cough without sputum, steaming bone fever, dry skin, bitter taste in the mouth, and vexation.

[Precautions] Běi Shā Shēn (Radix Glehniae) is considered more effective in nourishing yin, suitable for cough due to lung dryness, and contraindicated in cases of cough due to exogenous wind-cold invasion. According to "eighteen antagonisms", this herb is incompatible with Lí Lú (Radix et Rhizoma Veratri Nigri).

[Addendum] 南沙参 Nán Shā Shēn Radix Adenophorae Adenophora Root

The source is from the root of herbaceous perennial *Adenophora tetraphylla* (Thunb.) Fisch., *Adenophora stricta* Miq. Shashen, and other congeneric plants, family Campanulaceae. Alternate names include 白沙参 Bái Shā Shēn. It, sweet in flavor and slightly cold in nature, is capable of clearing the lungs, nourishing yin, tonifying the stomach, and generating fluids. It is applicable for dry cough or taxation cough with hemoptysis due to lung-heat and yin deficiency, or febrile diseases with fluid consumption, dry tongue, thirst, and poor appetite. Use 10–15 g in general. Nán Shā Shēn (Radix Adenophorae) and Běi Shā Shēn (Radix Glehniae) are similar in nature and flavor, and both can moisten and nourish the lung and stomach. The former, however, is more potent in dissolving phlegm and arresting cough, and the latter in nourishing yin.

麦冬 Mài Dōng *radix ophiopogonis dwarf lilyturf tuber*

The source is from the tuberous root of herbaceous perennial *Ophiopogon japonicus* (Thunb.) Ker. Gawl., family Liliaceae. It is so called because its leaves are wheat-shaped and non-withering even in winter. Alternate names include 麦门冬 Mài Mén Dōng and 寸冬 Cùn Dōng. Sweet and slightly bitter in flavor and cold in nature.

[Actions] Nourish yin and generate fluids, moisten the lungs and arrest cough, and clear the heart and relieve restlessness. It is applicable for lung dryness with nonproductive cough, deficiency-consumption cough, thirst resulting from fluid consumption, vexation insomnia, wasting-thirst caused by internal heat, and constipation due to intestinal dryness. Modern research has shown that it can improve cardiac contractility and anti-hypoxia ability and regulate immunologic function.

[Quality] Good quality is thick, large, soft, aromatic, chewy, and sweet, and has a light yellowish white outer surface.

[Indications]

1. Lung yin deficiency: Mài Dōng (Radix Ophiopogonis) is frequently combined with Sāng Yè (Folium Mori), Xìng Rén (Semen Armeniacae Amarum), and Ē Jiāo (Colla Corii Asini) for nonproductive cough and wheezing, dry throat, and nose dryness attributed to lung yin deficiency and dryness-heat in the lung; and with Bǎi Hé (Bulbus Lilii), Shā Shēn (Radix Adenophorae seu Glehniae), and Shēng Dì (Radix Rehmanniae) for chronic taxation cough with blood-streaked sputum.

2. Stomach yin deficiency: Mài Dōng (Radix Ophiopogonis) is often combined with Yù Zhú (Rhizoma Polygonati Odorati) and Shā Shēn (Radix Adenophorae seu Glehniae) for thirst, dry tongue and mouth, and red tongue with scanty coating due to stomach yin deficiency; and with medicinals that moisten the intestines and promote bowel movements for constipation caused by yin fluid insufficiency of the intestines and stomach as it is moistening in nature.

3. Heart yin deficiency with hyperactivity of heart fire: Mài Dōng (Radix Ophiopogonis), effective in nourishing heart yin to clear heart fire, is usually combined with Shēng Dì (Radix Rehmanniae), Suān Zǎo Rén (Semen Ziziphi Spinosae), and Huáng Lián (Rhizoma Coptidis) for vexation, palpitations, and insomnia due to heart yin deficiency with hyperactivity of heart fire in miscellaneous diseases; with Ē Jiāo (Colla Corii Asini) and Huáng Lián (Rhizoma Coptidis) for failure of the heart and kidney to interact caused by kidney yin deficiency and heart fire hyperactivity in febrile diseases; and with Shēng Dì (Radix Rehmanniae), Zhú Yè Xīn (Folium Pleioblasti), and Xī Jiǎo (Cornu Rhinocerotis) for unconsciousness and crimson tongue resulting from pathogen entering into the heart and *ying* level in warm febrile disease; with Rén Shēn (Radix et Rhizoma Ginseng) and Wǔ Wèi Zǐ (Fructus Schisandrae Chinensis) for palpitations and scattered and big pulse due to qi and yin insufficiency of the heart through enriching heart qi and yin. It has recently been prepared into oral solution and injection and widely used in the treatment of different types of cardiovascular diseases.

[Usage and Dosage] Use raw in general, process with wine when the herb is used in tonifying formulas, mix with Shè Xiāng (Moschus) for clearing the heart and calming the mind. Frying in wine reduces its cold properties, which is indicated when the herb is used to tonifying formulas. Materia medica literature holds that its kernel should be removed before use as it can drive people restless, but still needs to be proved by modern pharmacological research. Use 6–12 g.

[Mnemonics] Mài Dōng (Radix Ophiopogonis, Dwarf Lilyturf Tuber): sweet and cold; nourish the lungs, moisten dryness, supplement stomach yin, clear the heart, and relieve restlessness.

[Simple and Effective Formulas]

1. 麦门冬饮子 Mài Mén Dōng Yǐn Zǐ — Ophiopogon Drink from *Formulas from Benevolent Sages* (圣惠方, Shèng Huì Fāng): raw Mài Dōng (Radix Ophiopogonis) juice 40 ml, raw Xiǎo Jì (Herba Cirsii) juice 40 ml, and Shēng Dì (Radix Rehmanniae) juice 40 ml; mix together, keep warm, and add Fú Lóng Gān (Terra Flava Usta, Ignited Yellow Earth) 3 g for oral administration to treat persistent hematemesis and epistaxis.

2. 麦门冬汤 Mài Mén Dōng Tāng — Ophiopogon Decoction from *Essentials from the Golden Cabinet* (金匮要略, Jīn Guì Yào Lüè): Mài Dōng (Radix Ophiopogonis) 10 g, Rén Shēn (Radix et Rhizoma Ginseng) 10 g, Bàn Xià (Rhizoma Pinelliae) 5 g, Gān Cǎo (Radix et Rhizoma Glycyrrhizae) 6 g, Jīng Mǐ (Oryza Sativa L.) 100 g, and Dà Zǎo (Fructus Jujubae) five pieces; decoct in water for oral administration, four times a day to treat ascent counterflow of qi resulting from erroneous use of warming therapy and throat discomfort.

[Precautions] Mài Dōng (Radix Ophiopogonis), cold and relatively cloying in nature, is contraindicated in cases with loose stool and abdominal distention due to spleen and stomach deficiency-cold, phlegm-damp internal exuberance, and unresolved externally-contracted wind-cold.

Daily practices

1. What are the major actions of medicinal that enrich yin? What precautions should be taken when using it?
2. What are the similarities and differences between Běi Shā Shēn (Radix Glehniae) and Mài Dōng (Radix Ophiopogonis) in terms of actions and indications?

天冬 Tiān Dōng *radix asparagi asparagus tuber*

The source is the tuberous root of climber herbaceous *Asparagus cochinchinensis* (Lour.) Merr., family Liliaceae. Alternate names include 天门冬 Tiān Mén Dōng and 明天冬 Míng Tiān Dōng. Sweet and bitter in flavor and cold in nature.

[Actions] Nourish yin and generate fluids, moisten the lungs and clear the heart, and enrich the kidney yin. It is applicable for nonproductive cough due to lung dryness, deficiency-consumption cough, thirst caused by fluid consumption, vexation insomnia, wasting-thirst, and constipation attributed to intestinal dryness. Modern research has shown that it can improve immunity.

[Quality] Good quality is thick, strong, yellowish white, and translucent.

[Indications]

1. Cough due to lung dryness: Tiān Dōng (Radix Asparagi) can nourish lung yin and is often combined with Shā Shēn (Radix Adenophorae seu Glehniae), Mài Dōng (Radix Ophiopogonis), Bèi Mǔ (Bulbus Fritillaria), and Bǎi Hé (Bulbus Lilii) for nonproductive cough with scanty sputum or blood in sputum caused by lung yin deficiency.
2. Kidney yin deficiency: Tiān Dōng (Radix Asparagi), effective in nourishing kidney yin and descending fire with its bitter flavor, is commonly combined with Shēng Dì (Radix Rehmanniae) or Shú Dì Huáng (Radix Rehmanniae Praeparata), Zhī Mǔ (Rhizoma Anemarrhenae), and Huáng Bǎi (Cortex Phellodendri Chinensis) for tidal fever, wasting-thirst, and seminal emission attributed to kidney yin deficiency resulting in vigorous fire.
3. Constipation due to intestinal dryness: Tiān Dōng (Radix Asparagi), moistening in nature, is combined with other medicinals that moisten the intestines such as Xuán Shēn (Radix Scrophulariae), Mài Dōng (Radix Ophiopogonis), and Zhī Mǔ (Rhizoma Anemarrhenae).

In recent year, it has been prepared into tablets and injections, and is effective for malignant lymphoma and different types of breast masses like lobular hyperplasia. This medicinal is combined with Bái Huā Shé Shé Cǎo (Herba Hedyotis Diffusae) to treat breast cancer and has certain therapeutic effect.

[Usage and Dosage] Use raw in general, steam with wine to strengthen its effect of enrich and nourish. Use 6–15 g in decoction, up to 60 g when used alone.

[Mnemonics] Tiān Dōng (Radix Asparagi, Asparagus Tuber): sweet and bitter; supplement the lungs and kidneys, relieve deficiency-fire, and moisten the dryness of intestines.

[Simple and Effective Formulas]

1. 三才丸　Sān Cái Wán — Heaven, Human, and Earth Pill from *Confucians' Duties to Their Parents* (儒门事亲 Rú Mén Shì Qīn): Tiān Dōng (Radix Asparagi) (plumule removed), Rén Shēn (Radix et Rhizoma Ginseng), and Shú Dì Huáng (Radix Rehmanniae Praeparata) in equal dosage; grind into fine powder, make into cherry-sized pill, and dissolve in the mouth for cough.

2. 天门冬丸　Tiān Mén Dōng Wán — Asparagus Tuber Pill from *Experiential Formulas for Universal Relief* (普济本事方 Pǔ Jì Běn Shì Fāng): Tiān Dōng (Radix Asparagi) 30 g (soaked in water, plumule removed), Zhì Gān Cǎo (Radix et Rhizoma Glycyrrhizae Praeparata cum Melle) 15 g, Xìng Rén (Semen Armeniacae Amarum) (peel and tip removed, stir-fried until well-done) 15 g, Bèi Mǔ (Bulbus Fritillaria) (plumule removed, stir-fried) 15 g, Bái Fú Líng (Poria) (peel removed) 15 g, Ē Jiāo (Colla Corii Asini) (stir-fried with clam powder into bead) 15 g; grind into fine powder and make into hoodle-sized pill, and dissolve in the mouth, one pill one time, maximum ten pills/day for hematemesis and hemoptysis.

[Precautions] Tiān Dōng (Radix Asparagi), cold and slippery in nature, is contraindicated in cases with diarrhea and loose stool due to deficiency-cold of the spleen and stomach.

石斛 **Shí Hú** *caulis dendrobii dendrobium*

The source is from the stem of evergreen herbaceous perennial *Dendrobium aduncum* Wall ex Lindl., *D. nobil* Lindll., or D. *officinale* Kimura et Migo, and other congeneric plants, family Orchidaceae. Alternate names include 林兰 Lín Lán. Sweet and bland in flavor and slightly cold in nature.

[Actions] Nourish yin and clear heat, and tonify the stomach and generate fluids. It is applicable for dry mouth, vexation, and thirst due to stomach yin deficiency, deficiency-heat as a consequence of an illness, and blurred vision. Modern researches indicate its dendrobine has certain analgesic and antipyretic effect, oral administration of its decoction can promote gastric juice secretion and help digestion.

[Quality] Good quality is golden, shiny, lightweight, pliable, and collected in the autumn. The best 黄草石斛 Huáng Cǎo Shí Hú is produced in Taiwan and Jiading of Sichuan; the best quality of 铁皮石斛 Tiě Pí Shí Hú is 枫斗 Fēng Dòu, processed in Laokou of Hubei. The one produced in Huoshan area of Anhui is also of good quality and called 霍石斛 Huò Shí Hú; and the best quality 金钗石斛 Jīn Chāi Shí Hú is found in Guangxi and Guangdong.

[Indications]

1. Yin consumption in febrile disease: Shí Hú (Caulis Dendrobii) is combined with Shēng Dì (Radix Rehmanniae), Mài Dōng (Radix Ophiopogonis) for thirst, dry mouth and tongue, red tongue with scanty coating, and thin fast pulse due to yin fluid consumption by pathogenic heat in febrile diseases; and with medicinals that cleat pathogenic heat when pathogenic heat is unresolved.
2. Stomach yin insufficiency in miscellaneous diseases: Shí Hú (Caulis Dendrobii) is combined with Mài Dōng (Radix Ophiopogonis), Bái Sháo (Radix Paeoniae Alba), and Zhú Rú (Caulis Bambusae in Taenia) for reduced appetite, gastric discomfort, gastric dull pain or with burning sensation, belching, hiccup, dry mouth and tongue, and smooth bare red tongue or with scanty coating caused by stomach yin consumption in miscellaneous diseases.
3. Liver-kidney deficiency: Shí Hú (Caulis Dendrobii), capable of supplementing the yin fluif of the liver and kidneys, is combined with Qīng Xiāng Zǐ (Semen Celosiae), Tiān Dōng (Radix Asparagi), Shēng Dì (Radix Rehmanniae), Gǒu Qǐ Zǐ (Fructus Lycii), and Jú Huā (Flos Chrysanthemi) for hypopsia, blurred vision, and cataract caused by liver and kidney yin deficiency; and with other medicinals that supplement the liver and kidney for atrophy and weakness of the limbs due to liver and kidney insufficiency.

[Usage and Dosage] Use raw in general, the fresh is considered more potent in nourishing yin fluid. Use 5–15 g in decoction, increase the amount when used fresh. It should be decocted for a comparatively long time.

[Mnemonics] Shí Hú (Caulis Dendrobii, Dendrobium): sweet and bland; specialized in promoting fluid production, red tongue with scanty coating, and cook longer when use fresh.

[Simple and Effective Formulas]

1. 清热保津法 Qīng Rè Bǎo Jīn Fǎ — Heat-Clearing and Fluid-Preserving Method from *Treatise on Seasonal Diseases* (时病论, Shí Bìng Lùn): fresh Shí Hú (Caulis Dendrobii) 9 g, Lián Qiào (Fructus Forsythiae) (plumule removed) 9 g, Tiān Huā Fěn (Radix Trichosanthis) 6 g, fresh Shēng Dì (Radix Rehmanniae) 12 g, Mài Dōng (Radix Ophiopogonis) (plumule removed) 12 g, and Rén Shēn Yè (Folium Ginseng) 2.4 g; decoct in water for oral administration to treat damage to thin fluid in warm febrile disease with black and dry tongue coating.

2. 石斛散 Shí Hú Sǎn-Dendrobium Powder from *Comprehensive Recording of Divine Assistance* (圣济总录, Shèng Jì Zǒng Lù): Shí Hú (Caulis Dendrobii) 30 g, Xiān Líng Pí (Herba Epimedii) 30 g, and Cāng Zhú (Rhizoma Atractylodis) (rice-washed water soaked in water, cut, baked) 15 g; grind into fine powder and take 6 g/time with rice soup, twice a day for night blindness.

[Precautions] Shí Hú (Caulis Dendrobii), cold and clearing-moistening in nature, should be used with caution in cases of loose stool due to spleen and stomach deficiency, pathogenic heat exuberance, and unresolved damp turbidity.

玉竹 Yù Zhú *rhizoma polygonati odorati fragrant solomonseal rhizome*

The source is from the rhizome of herbaceous perennial *Polygonatum odoratum* (Mill.) Druce, family Liliaceae. Alternate names include 萎蕤 Wēi Ruí and 葳蕤 Wēi Ruí. Sweet in flavor and neutral in nature.

[Actions] Nourish yin-fluid in the lungs, stomach, and heart. It is applicable for yin consumption of the lungs and stomach, cough due to dryness-heat, and thirst with dry tongue. Modern research has shown that it contains cardenolide and has shown hypoglycemic and hypolipidemic effects.

[Quality] Good quality is dry, long, full, yellowish white, soft, moist, and non-oily.

[Indications]

1. Lung yin deficiency: Yù Zhú (Rhizoma Polygonati Odorati) is applicable for both lung yin consumption in febrile disease and nonproductive cough due to lung dryness in miscellaneous diseases. It is combined with Shā Shēn (Radix Adenophorae seu Glehniae), Mài Dōng (Radix Ophiopogonis), Bèi Mǔ (Bulbus Fritillaria), and Guā Lóu Pí (Pericarpium Trichosanthis) for dry mouth, thirst, and cough with scanty sputum due to lung yin deficiency.

2. Stomach yin deficiency: Yù Zhú (Rhizoma Polygonati Odorati) is prescribed together with Shēng Dì (Radix Rehmanniae), Shā Shēn (Radix Adenophorae seu Glehniae), and Mài Dōng (Radix Ophiopogonis) for fluid consumption with thirst in febrile diseases or stomach yin insufficiency in miscellaneous diseases.

It can be combined with medicinals that release the exterior such as Bò He (Herba Menthae) and Dàn Dòu Chǐ (Semen Sojae Praeparatum) for fever, aversion to cold, cough, sore throat, dry mouth, and thirst due to yin fluid insufficiency with invasion of exogenous pathogens.

This substance is also capable of nourishing heart yin and is prepared into liquid extract with Dǎng Shēn (Radix Codonopsis) for angina pectoris due to qi and yin deficiency.

[Usage and Dosage] Use raw in general, the raw is considered more effective in clearing-supplementing effect and the steamed (until it turns black) is better at moistening-supplementing. Use 10–15 g in decoction, up to 30 g when used alone or as a cardiotonic.

[Mnemonics] Yù Zhú (Rhizoma Polygonati Odorati, Fragrant Solomonseal Rhizome): sweet, neutral, and moistening; nourish the lung, stomach, and heart.

[Simple and Effective Formulas]

1. 玉竹麦门冬汤 Yù Zhú Mài Mén Dōng Tāng — Fragrant Solomonseal Rhizome and Dwarf Lilyturf Tuber Decoction from *Systematic Differentiation of Warm Diseases* (温病条辨, Wēn Bìng Tiáo Biàn): Yù Zhú (Rhizoma Polygonati Odorati) 9 g, Mài Dōng (Radix Ophiopogonis) 9 g, Shā Shēn (Radix Adenophorae seu Glehniae) 6 g, and raw Gān Cǎo (Radix et Rhizoma Glycyrrhizae) 3 g; decoct in water for oral administration to treat autumn dryness consuming stomach yin.

2. 加减萎蕤汤 Jiā Jiǎn Wēi Ruí Tāng — Solomon's Seal Variant Decoction from *Popular Guide to the 'Treatise on Cold Damage'* (通俗伤寒论, Tōng Sú Shāng Hán Lùn): Wēi Ruí (Rhizoma Polygonati Odorati) 9 g, raw Cōng Bái (Bulbus Allii Fistulosi) 2–3 pieces, Jié Gěng (Radix Platycodonis) 5 g, Bái Wēi (Radix et Rhizoma Cynanchi Atrati) 3 g, Dàn Dòu Chǐ (Semen Sojae Praeparatum) 10 g, Bò He (Herba Menthae) 4 g, Zhì Gān Cǎo (Radix et Rhizoma Glycyrrhizae Praeparata cum Melle) 1.5 g, and Dà Zǎo (Fructus Jujubae) two pieces; decoct in water for oral administration to treat yin deficiency combined with wind-warmth common cold and winter warmth with cough, dry throat, and phlegm.

[Precautions] Yù Zhú (Rhizoma Polygonati Odorati), moistening in nature, is contraindicated in cases of phlegm-damp internal accumulation, deficiency-cold of the spleen and stomach, and cold coagulation with qi stagnation. It should be used with cautions for patients with tachycardia or hypertension since its adrenocortical hormone effect may speed up the heartbeat and raise blood pressure further.

Daily practices

1. What are the similarities and differences between Mài Dōng (Radix Ophiopogonis) and Tiān Dōng (Radix Asparagi) in terms of actions and indications?
2. What are the similarities and differences among Tiān Dōng (Radix Asparagi), Shí Hú (Caulis Dendrobii), and Yù Zhú (Rhizoma Polygonati Odorati) in terms of actions and indications?

黄精 **Huáng Jīng** *rhizoma polygonati siberian*
solomon's seal rhizome

The source is from the rhizome of herbaceous perennial *Polygonatum sibiricum* Red., *P. kingianum* Coll. et Hemsl., and *P. crytonema* Hua, family Liliaceae. It is so called because in the opinion of the ancients, this medicinal is nurtured by the essence of the earth, which corresponds to yellow according to five element theory. Sweet in flavor and neutral in nature.

[Actions] Moisten the lungs and nourish the kidneys, and tonify the spleens and augment qi. It is applicable for cough due to lung deficiency and dryness, vertigo and soreness and weakness of the waist and knee caused by kidney and essence deficiency, and spleen and stomach asthenia. Modern experiments reveal that it has shown certain inhibitory effect against tubercle bacillus.

[Quality] Good quality is dry, large, moist, and sweet.

[Indications]

1. Dryness-cough due to yin deficiency: Huáng Jīng (Rhizoma Polygonati), potent in nourishing and supplementing lung and kidney yin, is applicable for cough caused by lung dryness and chronic and hectic cough resulting form lung and kidney yin deficiency. It is combined with Shā Shēn (Radix Adenophorae seu Glehniae), Mài Dōng (Radix Ophiopogonis), and Bèi Mǔ (Bulbus Fritillaria) for cough with lung dryness; and with Shēng Dì (Radix Rehmanniae), Tiān Dōng (Radix Asparagi), and Bǎi Bù (Radix Stemonae) for taxation and chronic cough due to lung and kidney yin deficiency.
2. Spleen and stomach deficiency: Huáng Jīng (Rhizoma Polygonati), effective in nourishing spleen and stomach yin and boosting spleen and stomach qi, is combined with Rén Shēn (Radix et Rhizoma Ginseng), Bái Zhú (Rhizoma Atractylodis Macrocephalae), and Fú Líng (Poria) for lassitude, lack of strength, and poor appetite attributed to spleen and stomach deficiency; and with Shí Hú (Caulis Dendrobii), Mài Dōng (Radix Ophiopogonis), and Shān Yào (Rhizoma Dioscoreae) for lassitude, lack of strength, decreased appetite, and red tongue with

scanty coating associated with qi and yin deficiency of the spleen and stomach.

3. Kidney yin deficiency: Huáng Jīng (Rhizoma Polygonati), capable of enriching kidney yin, is combined with Gǒu Qǐ Zǐ (Fructus Lycii), Hé Shǒu Wū (Radix Polygoni Multiflori), and Shú Dì Huáng (Radix Rehmanniae Praeparata) for soreness and weakness of the waist and knee, vertigo, blurred vision, and premature graying of the hair and beard caused by kidney yin insufficiency; and with Tiān Huā Fěn (Radix Trichosanthis) and Mài Dōng (Radix Ophiopogonis) for wasting-thirst due to spleen and kidney deficiency.

Due to its moderate nature and effect of nourishing yin and tonifying the spleen, it is commonly used in dietary therapy and can be stewed with pork, chicken, or duct to treat deficiency-consumption and pulmonary tuberculosis. It has been recently reported that ingesting Huáng Jīng (Rhizoma Polygonati) with crystal sugar is effective for pinworm.

[Usage and Dosage] Use raw in general, process with wine for strengthening the sinews and bones. Use 10–20 g in decoction, up to 30 g when used alone.

[Mnemonics] Huáng Jīng (Rhizoma Polygonati, Siberian Solomon's Seal Rhizome): sweet and neutral; enrich and nourish the lungs and kidneys, supplement the spleen, and best for medicated diet.

[Simple and Effective Formulas]

1. 枸杞丸 Gǒu Qǐ Wán — Wolfberry Fruit Pill from *Fine Formulas of Wonderful Efficacy* (奇效良方, Qí Xiào Liáng Fāng): Gǒu Qǐ Zǐ (Fructus Lycii) and Huáng Jīng (Rhizoma Polygonati) in equal dosage; grind into fine powder and make into phoenix tree seed-sized pill with the paste of honey, and take 50 pills/dose with warm water on an empty stomach to tonify essential qi.

2. 补脾方 Bǔ Pí Fāng — Spleen-tonifying Formula from *Empirical Formulas* (经验方, Jīng Yàn Fāng): Huáng Jīng (Rhizoma Polygonati) 30 g, Dǎng Shēn (Radix Codonopsis) 30 g, and Shān Yào (Rhizoma Dioscoreae) 30 g; steam with pullet for fatigue and weakness due to spleen and stomach deficiency.

[Precautions] Huáng Jīng (Rhizoma Polygonati), not as stomach-injuring as other yin-nourishing medicinals but still tonic, is contraindicated in cases of abdominal distention due to qi movement stagnation.

枸杞子 Gǒu Qǐ Zǐ *fructus lycii chinese wolfberry fruit*

The source is from the ripe fruit of deciduous shrub *Lycium barbarum* L., family Solanaceae. It is so called because it has 枸 Gǒu-shaped thorn in the stems and the length of stem matches 杞 Qǐ. Alternate names include 甘杞子 Gān Qǐ Zǐ, 杞子 Qǐ Zǐ, and 狗奶子 Gǒu Nǎi Zǐ. Sweet in flavor and neutral in nature.

[Actions] Nourish and tonify the liver and kidneys, and enrich blood and boost essence to improve vision. It is applicable for deficiency-consumption with essence deficiency, soreness and weakness of the waist and knee, vertigo, tinnitus, wasting-thirst due to internal heat, shallowness due to blood deficiency, and blurred vision. Modern pharmacological research has shown that it can reduce blood sugar, regulate immunological function, promote hematopoietic function, and protect the liver.

[Quality] Good quality is large, fleshy, sweet, red, and soft, and has a small seed. *Lycium chinense* L., known as 土枸杞子, Tǔ Gǒu Qǐ Zǐ has a smaller, lusterless, and thin fruit with many seeds and is regarded as an inferior herb.

[Indications]

1. Liver and kidney yin deficiency: Gǒu Qǐ Zǐ (Fructus Lycii) is combined with Shú Dì Huáng (Radix Rehmanniae Praeparata), Shā Yuàn Jí Lí (Semen Astragali Complanati), and Shān Zhū Yú (Fructus Corni) for soreness and weakness of the waist and knee, seminal emission, and dizziness due to liver and kidney deficiency.
2. Eye disorders: Gǒu Qǐ Zǐ (Fructus Lycii), a principal herb for eye problems, can treat different types of eye disorder such as dizziness, blurred vision, and cataract caused by liver yin insufficiency and is combined with Jú Huā (Flos Chrysanthemi), Bái Sháo (Radix Paeoniae Alba), Shān Zhū Yú (Fructus Corni), and Shēng Dì (Radix Rehmanniae).

This substance can also moisten and nourish lung yin, and is often combined with medicinals that enrich the lungs and stomach for non-productive cough and thirst due to lung dryness.

It is also effective in supplementing blood and is commonly used in the treatment of blood deficiency pattern.

[Usage and Dosage] Prepare into decocted extract, medical wine, or dietary therapy. Use 5–10 g in decoction.

[Mnemonics] Gǒu Qǐ Zǐ (Fructus Lycii, Chinese Wolfberry Fruit): sweet; nourish the liver and kidneys, and relieve eye problems due to yin deficiency.

[Simple and Effective Formulas]

1. 杞菊地黄丸 Qǐ Jú Dì Huáng Wán — Lycium Berry, Chrysanthemum and Rehmannia Pill from *Advancement of Medicine* (医级, Yī Jí): Shú Dì Huáng (Radix Rehmanniae Praeparata), Shān Zhū Yú (Fructus Corni), Fú Líng (Poria), Shān Yào (Rhizoma Dioscoreae), Mǔ Dān Pí (Cortex Moutan), Zé Xiè (Rhizoma Alismatis), Gǒu Qǐ Zǐ (Fructus Lycii), and Jú Huā (Flos Chrysanthemi); grind into fine powder and make into pill for oral administration to treat blurring vision, strabismus, and dry and painful eyes due to liver and kidney insufficiency.
2. 枸杞子散 Gǒu Qǐ Zǐ Sǎn — Wolfberry Fruit Powder from *Formulas from Benevolent Sages* (圣惠方, Shèng Huì Fāng): Gǒu Qǐ Zǐ (Fructus Lycii) 30 g, Huáng Qí (Radix Astragali) 45 g, Rén Shēn (Radix et Rhizoma Ginseng) (the residue of rhizome removed) 30 g, Guì Xīn (Cortex Cinnamomi) 0.9 g, Dāng Guī (Radix Angelicae Sinensis) 30 g, and Bái Sháo (Radix Paeoniae Alba) 30 g; grind into powder and decoct 9 g/time with Shēng Jiāng (Rhizoma Zingiberis Recens) 0.2 g and two Dà Zǎo (Fructus Jujubae) for oral administration to treat deficiency-consumption, kidney qi deficiency, slightly thirst, and frequent urination.

[Precautions] Gǒu Qǐ Zǐ (Fructus Lycii), moderate in nature, is contraindicated when an exterior condition is not cleared and in cases with excessive damp-turbidity, loose stools, diarrhea, and excess heat exuberance.

百合 **Bǎi Hé** *bulbus lilii lily bulb*

The source is from the bulb of herbaceous perennial *Lilium brownii* F.E. Brown var. *colchesteri* Wils., *L. pumilum* DC., or *L. longiflorum* Thunb., family Liliaceae. The name literally means hundred meetings as the root is a gathering of many scales. It is so called also because of its effectiveness in treating lily disease. Alternate names include 白百合 Bái Bǎi Hé. Sweet and slightly bitter in flavor and slightly cold in nature.

[Actions] Nourish yin and moisten the lungs to arrest cough, and clear the heart to tranquilize the mind. It is applicable for non-productive cough due to lung dryness and restlessness of heart spirit caused by heart fire exuberance.

[Quality] Good quality is thick and yellowish white with uniform scales and relatively few striations. The wild herb has thick and small scales with a bitter taste; whereas the cultivated herb has wide and thin scales with a mild bitter taste and moderate medical effect.

[Indications]

1. Dryness-cough due to lung yin deficiency: Bǎi Hé (Bulbus Lilii), capable of nourishing lung yin and clearing lung fire with its bitterness, is applicable for chronic cough due to lung dryness with heat and often combined with Shēng Dì (Radix Rehmanniae), Bèi Mǔ (Bulbus Fritillaria), and Mài Dōng (Radix Ophiopogonis).
2. Restlessness of heart spirit due to hyperactivity of heart fire: Bǎi Hé (Bulbus Lilii) can clear heart fire and is therefore combined with Shēng Dì (Radix Rehmanniae) and Zhī Mǔ (Rhizoma Anemarrhenae) for ascendant hyperactivity of heart fire with kidney yin consumption and residual heat that has not been cleared in the late stage of febrile diseases; and with medicinals that clear the heart and calm the mind for fidget, palpitations, and insomnia due to restlessness of heart spirit in miscellaneous diseases.

Owning to its moderate nature and clearing-supplementing effect, Bǎi Hé (Bulbus Lilii) is commonly used in dietary therapy. Stewing it, for instance, with Lián Zǐ (Semen Nelumbinis) and Dà Zǎo (Fructus Jujubae) is effective in improving qi and blood insufficiency as well as qi and yin deficiency of the spleen, stomach, and lung.

[Usage and Dosage] Use 10–30 g in decoction, increase the amount properly when used alone or in dietary therapy.

[Mnemonics] Bǎi Hé (Bulbus Lilii, Lily Bulb): clearing-supplementing in nature; sweet and slightly bitter; relieve lung dryness and palpitation when cook with Lián Zǐ (Semen Nelumbinis) and Dà Zǎo (Fructus Jujubae).

[Simple and Effective Formulas]

1. 百合固金汤 Bǎi Hé Gù Jīn Tāng — Lily Bulb Metal-Securing Decoction from *Shen Zhai's Bequeathed Book* (慎斋遗书, Shèn Zhāi Yí Shū): Shú Dì Huáng (Radix Rehmanniae Praeparata) 9 g, Shēng Dì (Radix Rehmanniae) 9 g, body of Dāng Guī (Radix Angelicae Sinensis) 9 g, Bái Sháo (Radix Paeoniae Alba) 3 g, Gān Cǎo (Radix et Rhizoma Glycyrrhizae) 3 g, Jié Gěng (Radix Platycodonis) 2.4 g, Xuán Shēn (Radix Scrophulariae) 2.4 g, Bèi Mǔ (Bulbus Fritillaria) 4.5 g, Mài Dōng (Radix Ophiopogonis) 4.5 g, and Bǎi Hé (Bulbus Lilii) 4.5 g; decoct in water for oral administration to treat lung-heat induced sore throat, cough, and hemoptysis.

2. 百合煎 Bǎi Hé Jiān — Lily Bulb Decoction from *Complete Collection of Experience* (经验广集, Jīng Yàn Guǎng Jí): steam or cook Bǎi Hé (Bulbus Lilii) with honey and take at frequent intervals for oral administration to treat lung abscess.

[Precautions] Bǎi Hé (Bulbus Lilii) can be taken over a long period of time due to its moderate nature, and is contraindicated in cases of excessive damp-turbidity and stagnated qi movement.

Daily practices

1. What are the similarities and differences among Huáng Jīng (Rhizoma Polygonati), Gǒu Qǐ Zǐ (Fructus Lycii), and Bǎi Hé (Bulbus Lilii) in terms of actions and indications?

2. What are the similarities and differences between Gǒu Qǐ Zǐ (Fructus Lycii) and medicinals that nourish blood in terms of actions and indications?

山茱萸 Shān Zhū Yú *fructus corni cornus*

The source is from the ripe fruit of deciduous subarbor *Schisandra chinensis* (Turcz.) Baill, family Magnoliaceae. Alternate names include 山萸肉 *Shān* Yú Ròu, 萸肉 Yú Ròu, 蜀枣 Shǔ Zǎo, and 枣皮 Zǎo Pí. Sour and astringent in flavor and slightly warm in nature.

[Actions] Supplement the liver and kidneys, and restrain essence and arrest prolapse. It is applicable for vertigo, tinnitus, soreness and weakness of the waist and knee, impotence, seminal emission, enuresis, frequent urination, profuse uterine bleeding, prolonged scanty uterine bleeding of variable intervals, abnormal vaginal discharge, profuse sweating, collapse, and wasting-thirst due to internal heat. Modern research has shown that it has a significant anti-shock, certain antibacterial and anti-tumor effect.

[Quality] Good quality is dry, thick, soft, moist, purplish red, seedless, and without impurities.

[Indications]

1. Liver and kidney deficiency: Shān Zhū Yú (Fructus Corni), the principal herb that tonify the liver, kidney, and essential qi, is widely used in cases of liver and yang deficiency because it can tonify liver and kidney yin and meanwhile strengthen essence and yang. It is frequently combined with Shú Dì Huáng (Radix Rehmanniae Praeparata) and Shān Yào (Rhizoma Dioscoreae) for soreness and weakness of the waist and knee, vertigo, tinnitus, bone-steaming fever, and tidal fever caused by liver and kidney insufficiency; and with Bǔ Gǔ Zhī (Fructus Psoraleae) and Dāng Guī (Radix Angelicae Sinensis) for impotence, premature ejaculation, seminal emission, and spontaneous seminal emission due to kidney yang debilitation.

2. Efflux desertion patterns: Shān Zhū Yú (Fructus Corni), sour and astringent, is one of the commonly-used astringent herbs. For diseases like seminal emission, spontaneous seminal emission, and enuresis, this substance can not only cure the root by strengthening the kidneys but also treat the branch via consolidating and astringing, and usually is combined with Jīn Yīng Zǐ (Fructus Rosae Laevigatae), Fù Pén Zǐ

(Fructus Rubi), and Sāng Piāo Xiāo (Oötheca Mantidis). It is combined with Wǔ Wèi Zǐ (Fructus Schisandrae Chinensis), Huáng Qí (Radix Astragali), and Fú Xiǎo Mài (Fructus Tritici Levis) for spontaneous sweating and night sweating due to exterior deficiency failing to insecure; and with Rén Shēn (Radix et Rhizoma Ginseng) and Fù Zǐ (Radix Aconiti Lateralis Praeparata) for persistent deficiency-wheezing with profuse sweating and even collapse.

Shān Zhū Yú (Fructus Corni) and Shú Dì Huáng (Radix Rehmanniae Praeparata) both are principal herbs that tonify the liver and kidneys. The former, however, is regarded more potent in supplementing liver yin and capable of assisting yang to consolidate and astringe, the latter is more effective in enriching kidney yin and capable of supplementing the blood. These two herbs are very commonly used together in treating disorders of liver and kidney deficiency.

[Usage and Dosage] Use raw or steam it to improve its ability of nourishing and supplementing the liver and kidneys. Use 4–10 g in decoction, double the amount when used alone, and up to 30–60 g in cases of shock.

[Mnemonics] Shān Zhū Yú (Fructus Corni, Cornus): sour and warm; tonify the kidneys to rescue from desertion, relieve vertigo and dizziness, stop profuse uterine bleeding, arrest vaginal discharge, and resolve wheezing and profuse sweating.

[Simple and Effective Formulas]

1. 地黄丸 Dì Huáng Wán — Rehmannia Pill from *Key to Diagnosis and Treatment of Children's Diseases* (小儿药证直诀, Qián Shì Xiǎo Ér Yào Zhèng Zhí Jué): Shú Dì Huáng (Radix Rehmanniae Praeparata) 24 g, Shān Zhū Yú (Fructus Corni) 12 g, Shān Yào (Rhizoma Dioscoreae) 12 g, Zé Xiè (Rhizoma Alismatis) 9 g, Mǔ Dān Pí (Cortex Moutan), and Bái Fú Líng (Smilax lanceifolia Roxb.) 9 g; grind into powder and make into phoenix tree seed-sized pill with honey, for children infuse three pills/time into warm water, and take it on an empty stomach for infantile kidney deficiency with delayed closure of fontanel, lack of

spirit, and lusterless complexion. Now, it has been widely used to treat various diseases caused by liver-kidney yin deficiency, such as diabetes, arteriosclerosis, soreness and weakness of the waist and knee, and dizziness. Alternate names include Six-Ingredient Rehmannia Pill (六味地黄丸, Liù Wèi Dì Huáng Wán).

2. 治遗尿方 Zhì Yí Niào Fāng — Enuresis Curing Formula from *Fand Long Tan's Family Secret Book* (方龙潭家秘, Fāng Lóng Tán Jiā Mì): Shān Zhū Yú (Fructus Corni) 60 g, Yì Zhì Rén (Fructus Alpiniae Oxyphyllae) 30 g, Rén Shēn (Radix et Rhizoma Ginseng) 24 g, and Bái Zhú (Rhizoma Atractylodis Macrocephalae) 24 g; divide into ten equal doses and decoct in water for oral administration to treat urinary incontinence of the elderly or enuresis.

[Precautions] Shān Zhū Yú (Fructus Corni), tonic and astringent, is contraindicated when excess pathogens are not cleared such as fire-heat, damp-heat, and phlegm-heat. Also not recommended in cases of hyperactivity of ministerial fire with persistent erection of penis because of its effect of assisting kidney yang or when patients present unresolved exterior condition or strangury and difficult urination due to its astringent nature.

旱莲 Mò Hàn Lián *herba ecliptae yerbadetajo*

[Addendum] 女贞子 Nǚ Zhēn Zǐ Fructus Ligustri Lucidi Privet Fruit

The source is from the whole plant of herbaceous annual *Eclipta prostrate* L., family Compositae. Alternate names include 墨旱莲 Mò Hàn Lián, 旱莲草 Hàn Lián Cǎo, and 鳢肠 Lǐ Cháng. Sweet and sour in flavor and cold in nature.

[Actions] Nourish yin and tonify the kidneys, and cool blood and arrest bleeding. It is applicable for vertigo and premature graying of the hair and beard associated with liver and kidney yin deficiency and hematemesis, epistaxis, hematuria, stool with blood, profuse uterine bleeding, prolonged scanty uterine bleeding of variable intervals due to yin deficiency with blood heat.

[Quality] Good quality is dry and blackish green without impurities.

[Indications]

1. Liver and kidney yin deficiency: Mò Hàn Lián (Herba Ecliptae) is clearing and supplementing or neutrally supplementing the liver and kidney and its nature is not cloying. It is usually combined with Nǚ Zhēn Zǐ (Fructus Ligustri Lucidi) for soreness and weakness of the waist and knee, vertigo, tinnitus, and seminal emission caused by liver and kidney yin deficiency.
2. Bleeding due to yin deficiency with blood heat: Mò Hàn Lián (Herba Ecliptae), cold in nature, can cool the blood to stanch bleeding. It can be used alone or in a combination with medicinals that cool the blood and stanch bleeding such as Shēng Dì (Radix Rehmanniae), Ē Jiāo (Colla Corii Asini), Cè Bǎi Yè (Cacumen Platycladi), and Ǒu Jié (Nodus Nelumbinis Rhizomatis) for hemorrhagic disorders caused by yin deficiency with blood heat.

It can be prepared alone into decoction for heat dysentery. Mixing Bái Fán (Alumen) with its decoction for external wash can treat vaginal itching. Twisting the fresh into juice and applying externally can stanch traumatic bleeding.

[Usage and Dosage] Use raw in general, or twist the fresh into juice. Use 10–15 g in decoction, double the amount when used fresh or alone.

[Mnemonics] Mò Hàn Lián (Herba Ecliptae, Yerbadetajo): sweet and sour; enrich and nourish the liver and kidney, cool blood, and arrest bleeding.

[Simple and Effective Formulas]

1. 二至丸 Èr Zhì Wán — Double Supreme Pill from *Medical Formulas Collected and Analyzed* (医方集解, Yī Fāng Jí Jiě): Mò Hàn Lián (Herba Ecliptae) and Nǚ Zhēn Zǐ (Fructus Ligustri Lucidi) in equal dosage; decoct the former into cream, grind the latter into powder, put them together, make into pill with honey, and take 6–12 g/time for oral administration, twice a day, to treat liver and kidney deficiency with vertigo, blurred vision, soreness and pain in the waist and back, and atrophy and weakness in the lower extremities.

2. 血便方 Biàn Xiě Fāng — Stool with blood Relieving Formula from *Empirical Family Formulas* (家藏经验方, Jiā Cáng Jīng Yàn Fāng): Mò Hàn Lián (Herba Ecliptae); dry by roasting and grind into powder, and take 6 g/time with rice soup for oral administration to treat stool containing blood due to intestinal wind.

[Precautions] Mò Hàn Lián (Herba Ecliptae), cold in nature, should be used with caution in cases of deficiency-cold of the spleen and stomach.

[*Addendum*] 女贞子 **Nǔ Zhēn Zǐ** *fructus ligustri lucidi privet fruit*

The source is from ripe fruit of evergreen shrub or subarbor *Ligustrum lucidum* Ait., family Oleaceae. Nǔ Zhēn Zǐ (Fructus Ligustri Lucidi), sweet and bitter in flavor and cool in nature, can nourish the liver-kidney yin and is applicable to vertigo, soreness and weakness of the waist and knee, tinnitus, seminal emission, premature graying of the hair, hypopsia, and blurred eyesight attributed to liver-kidney yin deficiency. Recent research has shown that its ingredient oleanolic acid exerts a significant effect on protecting the liver and decreasing enzyme, and therefore it has been widely used to treat different types of hepatitis. It is commonly combined with Mò Hàn Lián (Herba Ecliptae), Shēng Dì (Radix Rehmanniae), and Gǒu Qǐ Zǐ (Fructus Lycii). Use 10–15 g each time.

黑芝麻 **Hēi Zhī** *Ma semen sesami nigrum black sesame*

The source is from the ripe semen of herbaceous annual *Sesamum indicum* DC, family Pedaliaceae. Alternate names include 芝麻 Zhī Ma, 黑脂麻 Hēi Zhī Ma, 脂麻 Zhī Ma, 巨胜子 Jù Shèng Zi, and 胡麻 Hú Ma. Sweet in flavor and neutral in nature.

[Actions] Tonify the liver and kidneys, and nourish blood and moisten dryness. It is applicable for vertigo, premature graying of the hair and beard, and skin dryness due to liver and kidney deficiency and essence and blood insufficiency, and constipation due to intestinal dryness.

[Quality] Good quality is large, black, and full without impurities.

[Indications]

1. Liver-kidney deficiency and essence-blood insufficiency: Hēi Zhī Ma (Semen Sesami Nigrum) is capable of strengthening the liver, kidneys, essence and blood, and can be taken over a long period of time due to its moderate nature. It is combined with medicinals that supplement the liver, kidney, essence and blood such as Shú Dì Huáng (Radix Rehmanniae Praeparata), Shān Zhū Yú (Fructus Corni), and Bái Sháo (Radix Paeoniae Alba) for vertigo, soreness and weakness of the waist and knee, seminal emission, frequent urination, and premature graying of the hair and beard caused by deficiency of the liver, kidney, essence and blood.
2. Constipation due to intestinal dryness: Hēi Zhī Ma (Semen Sesami Nigrum), oily and moistening, is applicable for the treatment of constipation of intestinal dryness resulting from fluid and blood deficiency. It can be used alone or together with medicinals that moisten the intestines such as Dāng Guī (Radix Angelicae Sinensis) and Má Rén (Fructus Cannabis).

[Usage and Dosage] Stir-fry until well done and grind into powder, use 10–30 g, also use in pill and powder.

[Mnemonics] Hēi Zhī Ma (Semen Sesami Nigrum, Black Sesame): sweet and moistening; supplement the liver and kidneys, nourish blood, moisten dryness, and applicable for medicated diet.

[Simple and Effective Formulas]

1. 桑麻丸 Sāng Ma Wán — Mulberry Leaf and Black Sesame Pill from *Advancement of Medicine* (医级, Yī Jí): Sāng Yè (Folium Mori) (frosted, peduncle and striations removed, withered under sunshine) and Hēi Zhī Ma (Semen Sesami Nigrum) (stir-fried) in equal dosage; grind into powder, pound into pill with glutinous rice soup, or make into pill with honey, and take 12–15 g/day for oral administration to treat liver and kidney deficiency with eye problems, dry skin, and constipation.
2. 治风湿散 Zhì Fēng Shī Sǎn — Wind-damp Relieving Powder from *Fang's Orthodox Lineage of Pulses* (方脉正宗, Fāng Mài Zhèng

Zōng): Hēi Zhī Ma (Semen Sesami Nigrum) 500 g, Bái Zhú (Rhizoma Atractylodis Macrocephalae) 240 g, and Wēi Líng Xiān (Radix et Rhizoma Clematidis) (stir-fried with wine) 120 g; grind into powder, and take 15 g/time with boiled water for oral administration, twice a day, morning and evening to treat wind-damp *bì* with migrating pain over the body and heavy waist and feet.

[Precautions] Hēi Zhī Ma (Semen Sesami Nigrum), slippery in nature, is contraindicated in cases of diarrhea and loose stools.

Daily practices

1. Shān Zhū Yú (Fructus Corni), Mò Hàn Lián (Herba Ecliptae), and Hēi Zhī Ma (Semen Sesami Nigrum) all are medicinals that enrich yin; what are the similarities and differences among them in terms of actions and indications?
2. Among medicinals that enrich yin, which ones can also nourish blood, supplement the spleen, moisten the intestines, calm the spirit, respectively?
3. Among medicinals that enrich yin, which ones are effective in treating eye problems caused by liver and kidney yin deficiency?

龟板 Guī Bǎn *plastrum testudinis tortoise plastron*

The source is from the plastron or carapace (in a few cases) of *Chinemys reevesii*, family Testudinidae. Alternate names include 龟壳 Guī Ké and 龟版 Guī Bǎn. Sweet and salty in flavor and cold in nature.

[Actions] Nourish yin and subdue yang, boost the kidneys and strengthen bones, enrich blood and tranquilize the mind, and consolidate 经 and arrest bleeding. It is applicable for convulsive syncope, vertigo, restlessness, vexing heat in the chest, palms and soles due to yin deficiency with yang hyperactivity or internal stirring of deficiency wind with serious yin consumption in febrile diseases, soreness and weakness of the waist and knee, weakness of the sinews and bones, and delayed fontanel closure caused by kidney deficiency, and palpitations due to fright, insomnia, and forgetfulness resulting from heart deficiency.

[Quality] Good quality is large and clean with bloodstain and without carrion.

[Indications]

1. Yin deficiency with internal heat or stirring of wind: Guī Bǎn (Plastrum Testudinis), capable of nourishing yin and subduing yang, is combined with medicinals that nourish yin and clear heat such as Zhī Mǔ (Rhizoma Anemarrhenae), Huáng Bǎi (Cortex Phellodendri Chinensis), and Shēng Dì (Radix Rehmanniae) for bone-steaming fever, hectic fever, and vexing heat in the chest, palms and soles caused by liver and kidney yin deficiency; with medicinals that nourish yin and extinguish wind such as Shēng Dì (Radix Rehmanniae), Bái Sháo (Radix Paeoniae Alba), Mǔ Lì (Concha Ostreae), and Biē Jiǎ (Carapax Trionycis) for convulsive syncope and wriggling of the extremities due to yin deficiency with stirring of wind; and with medicinals that nourish yin to anchor yang such as Shí Jué Míng (Concha Haliotidis), Chuān Niú Xī (Radix Cyathulae), Mǔ Lì (Concha Ostreae), Jú Huā (Flos Chrysanthemi), and Shēng Dì (Radix Rehmanniae) for vertigo, dizziness, and flashed cheeks in the afternoon due to yin deficiency with yang hyperactivity.

2. Bone atrophy due to kidney deficiency: Guī Bǎn (Plastrum Testudinis), known as a medicinal with an affinity to flesh and blood that can enrich essence, blood, and kidney yin, is applicable for different types of atrophy caused by kidney deficiency. It is combined with Shú Dì Huáng (Radix Rehmanniae Praeparata), Dāng Guī (Radix Angelicae Sinensis), and Suǒ Yáng (Herba Cynomorii) for soreness and weakness of the waist and knees, weakness of the sinews and bones, delayed fontanel closure, retarded dental development, and retardation of walking.

3. Profuse uterine bleeding and prolonged scanty uterine bleeding of variable intervals due to kidney deficiency: Guī Bǎn (Plastrum Testudinis), effective in tonifying the kidney to insecure the the *chong* and *ren mai*, is combined with Shú Dì Huáng (Radix Rehmanniae Praeparata), Shān Zhū Yú (Fructus Corni), and Shān Yào (Rhizoma Dioscoreae) for profuse uterine bleeding, prolonged scanty uterine bleeding of variable intervals, and profuse menstruation caused by kidney deficiency with insecurity of the *chong* and *ren* mai.

4. Restlessness of heart spirit due to blood deficiency: Guī Bǎn (Plastrum Testudinis), capable of nourishing blood and calming the heart spirit, is combined with Lóng Gǔ (Os Draconis), Yuǎn Zhì (Radix Polygalae), and Fú Shén (Sclerotium Poriae Pararadicis) for palpitations due to fright, insomnia, and forgetfulness caused by deficiency of heart blood.

[Usage and Dosage] The herb can be prepared into decocted extract, or dissolved in other medicinal extract, or used in decoction of the other herbs. Use 10–30 g, crush and cook before adding other ingredients to the decoction. Fry in vinegar until brittle before decocting to make it easier to be crushed and to facilitate active ingredient extraction.

[Mnemonics] Guī Bǎn (Plastrum Testudinis, Tortoise Plastron): sweet and salty; supplement kidney essence, stop profuse uterine bleeding, and subdue deficiency-yang.

[Simple and Effective Formulas]

1. 补肾丸 — Bǔ Shèn Wán — Kinedy Tonifying Pill from *Teachings of Dan-xi* (丹溪心法, Dān Xī Xīn Fǎ): Huáng Bǎi (Cortex Phellodendri Chinensis) (stir-fried) 45 g, Guī Bǎn (Plastrum Testudinis) (wine-fried) 45 g, Gān Jiāng (Rhizoma Zingiberis) 6 g, Niú Xī (Radix Achyranthis Bidentatae) 30 g, and Chén Pí (Pericarpium Citri Reticulatae) 15 g; grind into powder, make into phoenix tree seed-sized pill with ginger juice or wine, and take 70 pills/time for oral administration to treat flaccid sinews and bones and deficient qi and blood.
2. 龟柏姜栀丸 — Guī Bǎi Jiāng Zhī Wán — Tortoise Shell, Phellodendron, Dried Ginger, and Gardenia Pill from *Introduction to Medicine* (医学入门, Yī Xué Rù Mén): Guī Bǎn (Plastrum Testudinis) 90 g, Huáng Bǎi (Cortex Phellodendri Chinensis) 30 g, stir-fried Gān Jiāng (Rhizoma Zingiberis) 3 g, and Zhī Zǐ (Fructus Gardeniae) 7.5 g; grind into fine powder, make into pill with the paste of wine, and take with boiled water for oral administration to treat persistent reddish leucorrhea with abdominal pain.

[Precautions] Guī Bǎn (Plastrum Testudinis), cloying and relatively cold in nature, should be used with caution in cases of spleen and stomach deficiency, reduced appetite with loose stool, and internal accumulation of dampness.

鳖甲 Biē Jiǎ *carapax trionycis turtle carapace*

The source is from the shell of *Trionyx sinensis* Wiegmann, family Trionychidae. Salty in flavor and cold in nature.

[Actions] Nourish yin and anchor yang, and soften hardness and dissipate masses. It is applicable for yin consumption with internal stirring of deficiency wind in febrile diseases manifested as convulsive syncope, yin deficiency with internal heat, chronic malaria, malaria with splenomegaly, amenorrhea, and masses.

[Quality] Good quality is large and intact without carrion.

[Indications]

1. Yin deficiency with internal heat or stirring of wind due to yin deficiency: Biē Jiǎ (Carapax Trionycis), capable of nourishing yin and subduing yang, is combined with medicinals that nourish yin and clear heat such as Qīng Hāo (Herba Artemisiae Annuae), Zhī Mǔ (Rhizoma Anemarrhenae), Huáng Bǎi (Cortex Phellodendri Chinensis), and Shēng Dì (Radix Rehmanniae) for bone-steaming fever, hectic fever, and vexing heat in the chest, palms and soles caused by liver and kidney yin deficiency; with medicinals that nourish yin and extinguish wind such as Shēng Dì (Radix Rehmanniae), Bái Sháo (Radix Paeoniae Alba), Mǔ Lì (Concha Ostreae), and Guī Bǎn (Plastrum Testudinis) for convulsive syncope and wriggling of the extremities due to yin deficiency with stirring of wind; and with medicinals that nourish yin to anchor yang such as Shí Jué Míng (Concha Haliotidis), Chuān Niú Xī (Radix Cyathulae), Mǔ Lì (Concha Ostreae), Jú Huā (Flos Chrysanthemi), and Shēng Dì (Radix Rehmanniae) for vertigo, dizziness, and flashed cheeks in the afternoon due to yin deficiency with yang hyperactivity.

2. Accumulations, gatherings and masses: Biē Jiǎ (Carapax Trionycis), potent in softening hardness and dissipating masses, can relieve various

types of accumulations, gatherings, and masses due to stagnation of qi, blood, phlegm, and damp. It is combined with medicinals that sooth the liver and invigorate blood such as Chái Hú (Radix Bupleuri), Qīng Pí (Pericarpium Citri Reticulatae Viride), and Chì Sháo (Radix Paeoniae Rubra) for splenomegaly and hepatosplenomegaly due to chronic malaria; and with medicinals that dissipate masses such as É Zhú (Rhizoma Curcumae) and Sān Léng (Rhizoma Sparganii) for masses in the abdomen.

Biē Jiǎ (Carapax Trionycis) and Guī Bǎn (Plastrum Testudinis) has similar actions. The former, however, is considered more potent in enriching liver yin and relieving dissipate masses, and the latter is more effective in nourishing kidney yin, strengthening the sinews and bones, and consolidating the channels and stanching bleeding

[Usage and Dosage] Use raw in most cases, vinegar-fried until crisp before decocting to make it easier to be crushed and to facilitate active ingredient extraction. Use 10–30 g in decoction.

[Mnemonics] Biē Jiǎ (Carapax Trionycis, Turtle Carapace): salty and cold; enrich yin, subdue yang, calm liver wind, and dispel masses.

[Simple and Effective Formulas]

1. 消积散 — Xiāo Jī Sǎn — Accumulation Relieving Powder from *Formulas of the Zhen Family* (甄氏家乘方, Zhēn Shì Jiā Chéng Fāng): Biē Jiǎ (Carapax Trionycis) (roasted to crisp, ground into fine powder) 30 g, Hǔ Pò (Succinum) (ground into fine powder) 9 g, and Dà Huáng (Radix et Rhizoma Rhei) (mixed and stir-fried with rice wine); grind into fine powder, take 6 g/time with water for oral administration, twice a day, morning and evening to treat abdominal accumulations and masses.

2. 鳖甲散 — Biē Jiǎ Sǎn — Turtle Carapace Powder from *Comprehensive Recording of Divine Assistance* (圣济总录, Shèng Jì Zǒng Lù): Biē Jiǎ (Carapax Trionycis) (filed into pieces) 30 g, Gé Lí (Clam) powder (stir-fried with Biē Jiǎ (Carapax Trionycis) until it turns aromatic and yellow) 30 g, and Shú Dì Huáng (Radix Rehmanniae Praeparata) 45 g

(dried by solarizing); grind into fine powder, take 5 g/time with tea (water) for oral administration to treat persistent hematemesis.

[Precautions] Biē Jiǎ (Carapax Trionycis), cloying and relatively cold in nature, should be used with caution in cases of spleen and stomach deficiency, reduced appetite with loose stools, and internal accumulation of dampness. It is contraindicated during pregnancy because of its effect of dissipating masses.

Daily practices

1. What are the similarities and differences between Guī Bǎn (Plastrum Testudinis) and Biē Jiǎ (Carapax Trionycis) in terms of actions and indications?
2. What are the differences between shell medicinals that enrich yin and plant medicinals that enrich yin in terms of actions?
3. Give some examples of medicinals that nourish lung yin, stomach yin, liver yin, and kidney yin, respectively?

CHAPTER 14

Fourteenth Week

1

MEDICINALS THAT TONIFY YANG

Yang qi is the main source and manifestation of the human vital force, and yang qi deficiency may lead to a variety of disorders. Yang-tonifying herbs are used for supplementing yang qi and applicable for deficient yang patterns. They are also known as herbs that assist yang. Most of these herbs are sweet, warm or acrid, hot in nature, and therefore they are also considered as part of the herbs that warm the interior. The kidneys are the basis of all the body's yang, the most important use of tonifying yang method is to tonify the kidney yang. The herbs described in this chapter are used for tonifying kidney yang, and for descriptions of herbs used for tonifying the yang qi of other *zang-fu* organs see chapter six "medicinals that warm the interior". As you may be aware, some herbs in chapter six can also tonify kidney yang.

Deficient and debilitated yang qi may arise from a variety of causes such as prenatal insufficiency, weakness due to serious or chronic disorders, long-term qi deficiency, and kidney yin insufficiency. The selection and combination of herbs and treatment method for kidney yang deficiency are based on the root reason and secondary pattern of yang deficiency.

Most of these herbs are warm and drying. Use with caution as they can injure yin fluid and assist fire-heat if applied inappropriately.

鹿茸 Lù Róng *cornu cervi pantotrichum deer velvet*

The source is from the horn (non-ossifying and with fine hairs) of male *Cervus Nippon* Temminck or C. *elaphus* L. family Cervidae. Alternate

516

names include 斑龙珠 Bān Lóng Zhū. Sweet and salty in flavor and warm in nature.

[Actions] Generate essence to tonify marrow, boost kidney and augment yang, and strengthen sinews and bones. It is applicable for deficiency-consumption emaciation, lassitude, vertigo, tinnitus, deafness, blurred vision, soreness and weakness of the waist and knee, impotence, spontaneous seminal emission, deficiency-cold in the uterine, profuse uterine bleeding, and prolonged scanty uterine bleeding of variable intervals. Modern research has shown that pantocrine has shown a hormonal effect that can promote growth and development, increase work capacity, improve sleep quality and appetite, decrease the rate of fatigue, improve energy metabolism, and increase red blood cells.

[Quality] Good quality is thick, firm, lightweight, tender, fine hairs, reddish brown (花鹿茸 Huā Lù Róng) or grayish brown (鹿茸 Mǎ Lù Róng), oily, and shiny with round main branch, plump apiculus, and a fine cross-section without ridges in the lower part.

[Indications]

1. Kidney-yang deficiency: manifestations include cold body and limbs, soreness and weakness of the waist and knee, frequent urination, enuresis, impotence with sterility, infertility due to cold in the uterus, wheezing caused by deficient kidney yang failing to receive/grasp qi sent down from the lung, or diarrhea when spleen yang is affected. Lù Róng (Cornu Cervi Pantotrichum) can be ground into a powder or combined with other medicinals that strengthen the kidney and warm yang such as Rén Shēn (Radix et Rhizoma Ginseng), Ròu Cōng Róng (Herba Cistanches), Shā Yuàn Jí Lí (Semen Astragali Complanati), and Bā Jǐ Tiān (Radix Morindae Officinalis).

2. Kidney deficiency and essence-blood insufficiency: Lù Róng (Cornu Cervi Pantotrichum), known as a medicinal with an affinity to flesh and blood that warms yang, nourishes essence and blood, and fills marrows, is applicable for essence and blood deficiency caused by enduring illness and many other chronic and consumptive diseases. It is combined with Shú Dì Huáng (Radix Rehmanniae Praeparata), Dāng Guī (Radix Angelicae Sinensis), and Shān Zhū Yú (Fructus Corni) for timidity,

fatigue, lusterless or darkish complexion, dizziness, forgetfulness, and palpitation attributed to kidney deficiency with blood and essence insufficiency.

3. Atrophy and weakness due to kidney-deficiency: Lù Róng (Cornu Cervi Pantotrichum) is used together with other medicinals that strengthen the kidneys such as Shú Dì Huáng (Radix Rehmanniae Praeparata), Shān Zhū Yú (Fructus Corni), Fú Líng (Poria), and Guī Bǎn (Plastrum Testudinis) for children with physical and/or mental development disorders, delayed fontanel closure, retarded dental development, and retardation of walking attributed to kidney deficiency.

It is also applicable for profuse uterine bleeding, prolonged scanty uterine bleeding of variable intervals, white and clear abnormal vaginal discharge, chronic, suppurative and non-healing yin-type sores and ulcers caused by insecurity of the *chong* and *ren mai*.

It has been recently used in the treatment of various kinds of anemia and thrombopenia.

[Usage and Dosage] Not used for decoction, but taken as a powder or pill form, 0.6–2 g/time; prepared with 20% proof alcohol, as a medicinal wine, 10 ml/time, three times a day; processed into pantocrine injection for intramuscular injection, 2 ml/time, one time one day or every other day.

[Mnemonics] Lù Róng (Cornu Cervi Pantotrichum, Deer Velvet): salty and sweet; warm the kidney to tonify deficiency, supplement essence and blood, and relieve atrophy and weakness.

[Simple and Effective Formulas]

1. 黑丸 Hēi Wán — Black Pill from *Formulas to Aid the Living* (济生方, Jì Shēng Fāng): Lù Róng (Cornu Cervi Pantotrichum) (soaked in wine) and Dāng Guī (Radix Angelicae Sinensis) (soaked in wine) in equal dosage; grind into fine powder, make into phoenix tree seed-sized pill with the paste of Wū Méi (Fructus Mume) decocted extract, and take 50 pills/time with rice soup for oral administration to treat exhaustion of essence and blood with blackish complexion, deafness, blurred vision, dry mouth even after drinking too much water, lumbago,

weakness in the legs, cloudy urine, and hot sensation in the upper part and cold in the lower part of the body.

2. 鹿茸散 Lù Róng Sǎn — Deer Velvet Powder from *Ancient and Modern Records of Proven Formulas* (古今录验方 Gǔ Jīn Lù Yàn Fāng): Lù Róng (Cornu Cervi Pantotrichum) (roasted) 60 g, Dāng Guī (Radix Angelicae Sinensis) 60 g, Gān Dì Huáng (Radix Rehmanniae Recens) 60 g, Kuí Zǐ (Fructus Malvae) 50 g, and Pú Huáng (Pollen Typhae) 50 g; grind into fine powder, take 2 g/time with wine for oral administration, and 3 times a day to treat hematuria.

[Precautions] Lù Róng (Cornu Cervi Pantotrichum), warm in nature and effective in assisting yang, is contraindicated in cases of yin deficiency with yang hyperactivity and excessive heat exuberance. Single or long-term use of high dose is not recommended, as epistaxis and vertigo from taking 5 or 6 g/day this substance everyday for seven days have been reported.

肉苁蓉 Ròu Cōng Róng *herba cistanches desert cistanche*

The source is from the fleshy stem with ramentum of parasitic herbaceous annual *Cistauche deserticola* Y.C. Ma, family Orobanchaceae. It is so called because of its tonic but mild nature and fleshy root. Alternate names include 大芸 Dà Yún and 淡大芸 Dàn Dà Yún. This herb tonifies the yang yet is not drying, its effects are moderate. Sweet and salty in flavor and warm in nature.

[Actions] Tonify the kidney and strengthen yang, and moisten the intestines to facilitate the bowel movement. It is applicable for impotence, infertility, soreness and weakness of the waist and knee, coldness in the lower limbs, weakness of the sinews and bones, and constipation due to intestinal dryness.

[Quality] Good quality is thick, firm, reddish brown, soft, and moist. The one collected in spring is called 甜苁蓉 Tián Cōng Róng, and the one collected in autumn is called 咸苁蓉 Xián Cōng Róng or 盐苁蓉 Yán Cōng Róng.

[Indications]

1. Kidney-yang deficiency: Ròu Cōng Róng (Herba Cistanches), warm but not dry in nature, tonifying but not cloying, is often used together with other medicinals that strengthen the kidneys such as Shú Dì Huáng (Radix Rehmanniae Praeparata), Dāng Guī (Radix Angelicae Sinensis), Tù Sī Zǐ (Semen Cuscutae), Shé Chuáng Zǐ (Fructus Cnidii), Chuān Xù Duàn (Radix Dipsaci), Bā Jǐ Tiān (Radix Morindae Officinalis), and Dù Zhòng (Cortex Eucommiae) for impotence, cold pain in the lower back and knees, sterility, and infertility due to kidney yang deficiency.
2. Constipation due to intestinal dryness: Ròu Cōng Róng (Herba Cistanches), moistening and juicy with an effect of nourishing the intestines and promoting defecation, can be decocted alone or combined with Dāng Guī (Radix Angelicae Sinensis) and Má Rén (Fructus Cannabis) for constipation caused by kidney yang deficiency and intestinal fluid insufficiency, especially in the elderly and weak.

[Usage and Dosage] Use raw in general, salt-treated for frequent urination and spontaneous seminal emission. Use 10–15 g in decoction.

[Mnemonics] Ròu Cōng Róng (Herba Cistanches, Desert Cistanche): sweet and warm; generate essence and blood, warm kidney yang, and facilitate defecation.

[Simple and Effective Formulas]

1. 肉苁蓉丸 Ròu Cōng Róng Wán — Desert Cistanche Pill from *Formulas from Benevolent Sages* (圣惠方 Shèng Huì Fāng): Ròu Cōng Róng (Herba Cistanches) (soaked in wine for one night, peel removed, roasted) 30 g, Shé Chuáng Zǐ (Fructus Cnidii) 30 g, Yuǎn Zhì (Radix Polygalae) 30 g, Wǔ Wèi Zǐ (Fructus Schisandrae Chinensis) 30 g, Fáng Fēng (Radix Saposhnikoviae) (the residue of rhizome removed) 30 g, Fù Zǐ (Radix Aconiti Lateralis Praeparata) (cracked by blast-frying, peel and navel removed) 30 g, Tù Sī Zǐ (Semen Cuscutae) (soaked in wine for three days, dried by solarizing) 30 g, Bā Jǐ Tiān (Radix

Morindae Officinalis, Morinda Root) 30 g, and Dù Zhòng (Cortex Eucommiae) (coarse layer of bark removed, roasted until light yellow) 30 g; grind into powder and make into phoenix tree seed-sized pill with honey, and take 30 pills/day with warm wine or salt solution on an empty stomach for kidney qi and essence deficiency.

2. 润肠丸 Rùn Cháng Wán — Intestine-Moistening Pill from *Formulas to Aid the Living* (Jì Shēng Fāng, 济生方): Ròu Cōng Róng (Herba Cistanches) (soaked in wine, baked) 60 g and Chén Xiāng (Lignum Aquilariae Resinatum) (ground) 30 g; grind into fine powder and make phoenix tree seed-sized pill with Má Rén (Fructus Cannabis) decoction, and take 70 pills with rice soup on an empty stomach to treat constipation due to intestinal dryness in the weak and elderly.

[Precautions] Ròu Cōng Róng, warm in nature and capable of assisting yang and moisten the intestines, is contraindicated in cases of yin deficiency resulting in vigorous fire, internal excessive heat, loose stools, and diarrhea.

冬虫夏草 Dōng Chóng Xià Cǎo *cordyceps chinese caterpillar fungus*

The source is from the stroma of *Cordyceps sinensis* (Berk.) Sacc. Parasitized on the larva of *Hepialus armoricanus* Oberthru and the larva. Alternate names include 虫草 Chóng Cǎo. Sweet in flavor and warm in nature.

[Actions] Tonify the kidneys and nourish the lungs, strengthen the yang and augment the essence, and relieve cough and wheezing. It is applicable for cough and wheezing due to phlegm rheum, deficiency wheezing, hemoptysis, spontaneous sweating, night sweating, impotence seminal emission, soreness and weakness of the waist and knee, and weakness and poor recovery from disease. Experiments reveal it has certain antiasthmatic, anti-tubercle bacillus, antihypertensive, antitumor, and senescence-delaying effects, and can improve immunologic, cardiovascular, and renal function.

[Quality] Good quality is intact with a short stick-like fungus and a bright yellow, fat, full, and round insect part with a bright yellow outside and white inside.

[Indications]

1. Kidney-yang deficiency: Dōng Chóng Xià Cǎo (Cordyceps), warm but not dry, can supplement kidney yang and enrich essence. It can be either soaked alone in wine or combined with Shú Dì Huáng (Radix Rehmanniae Praeparata), Shān Zhū Yú (Fructus Corni), and Xiān Líng Pí (Herba Epimedii) for kidney-deficiency induced impotence and seminal emission; and with Dù Zhòng (Cortex Eucommiae), Chuān Xù Duàn (Radix Dipsaci), and Gǒu Jǐ (Rhizoma Cibotii) for lumbago caused by kidney deficiency.
2. Cough and asthma due to deficiency: Dōng Chóng Xià Cǎo (Cordyceps), tonifying both yin and yang and arresting cough and wheezing, is commonly used in the treatment of different types of cough and wheezing caused by either lung insufficiency or lung and kidney deficiency. It can be used alone or in combination with medicinals that enrich the lungs, dissolve phlegm, and arrest cough and wheezing, such as Shā Shēn (Radix Adenophorae seu Glehniae), Bèi Mǔ (Bulbus Fritillaria), and Gé Jiè (Gecko) for patient with chronic and enduring diseases.
3. Weak constitution with spontaneous sweating: Dōng Chóng Xià Cǎo (Cordyceps) can be used either in combination with other medicinals that tonify deficiency or stewed together with food such as pork, chicken and duck for patients with deficiency and poor recovery from illness, chills, spontaneous sweating, lassitude, and lack of strength.

Recent studies reveal this substance has preventive and therapeutic effects on liver fibrosis, either used alone or together with Huáng Qí (Radix Astragali) and Táo Rén (Semen Persicae).

[Usage and Dosage] Use for regulating-supplementing in general, apply in dietary therapy in most cases, decoction, or grind into powder and take with other decoction, or in pill and powder. Use 5–10 g for stewing or in decoction, 2–3 g/time in powder. However, it is expensive and therefore often replaced by Paecilomyces hepiali Chen in the preparation of Chinese patent medicine such as granules, oral solution, and capsule.

[Mnemonics] Dōng Chóng Xià Cǎo (Cordyceps, Chinese Caterpillar Fungus): sweet and warm; nourish the lung and kidney, relieve deficiency wheezing and spontaneous sweating, and stewed with meat.

[Simple and Effective Formulas]

虫草鸭 Chóng Cǎo Yā — Cordyceps Duck from *Supplement to 'The Grand Compendium of Materia Medica'* (本草纲目拾遗 Běn Cǎo Gāng Mù Shí Yí): one aged male duck, remove haslet, put Dōng Chóng Xià Cǎo (Cordyceps) 3–5 pieces into the head of duck, then tighten with thread, and steam with wine and soy sauce until soft to treat weakness after disease.

[Precautions] Dōng Chóng Xià Cǎo (Cordyceps), warm in nature, is discouraged to be used alone for patient with internal heat resulting from yin deficiency. Due to its moderate effect, it has to be taken over a long period of time to treat deficiency patterns.

Daily practices

1. What are medicinals that tonify yang? What are the indications?
2. What are the differences and similarities between Lù Róng (Cornu Cervi Pantotrichum), Ròu Cōng Róng (Herba Cistanches), and Dōng Chóng Xià Cǎo (Cordyceps) in terms of actions and indications?

仙茅 **Xiān Máo** *rhizoma curculiginis common curculigo rhizome*

The source is the rhizome of herbaceous perennial *Curculigo orchioides* Gaertn., family Amaryllidaceae. It is so called because its leaves are spear-shaped and in the opinion of ancients, long-term use can make people immortal. Pungent in flavor and hot in nature with mild toxicity.

[Actions] Warm the kidneys and fortify yang, strengthen the sinews and bones, and expel cold and dampness. It is applicable for impotence, seminal cold, urinary incontinence, cold pain in the heart and abdomen, and soreness and weakness of the waist and knee.

[Quality] Good quality is dry, thick, firm, hard, and black.

[Indications]

1. Kidney-yang deficiency: Xiān Máo (Rhizoma Curculiginis), hot in nature and capable of tonifying kidney yang, is often combined with medicinals that tonify kidney such as Shú Dì Huáng (Radix Rehmanniae

Praeparata), Dāng Guī (Radix Angelicae Sinensis), Tù Sī Zǐ (Semen Cuscutae), Shé Chuáng Zǐ (Fructus Cnidii), Chuān Xù Duàn (Radix Dipsaci), Bā Jǐ Tiān (Radix Morindae Officinalis), and Dù Zhòng (Cortex Eucommiae) for impotence, premature ejaculation, cold pain in the waist and knee, sterility, infertility, and frequent urination associated with kidney-yang deficiency.

2. Cold-damp *bì* and pain: Xiān Máo (Rhizoma Curculiginis), effective in warming and tonifying kidney yang, dispersing cold-damp, and strengthening the sinews and bones, is combined with Sāng Jì Shēng (Herba Taxilli), Dù Zhòng (Cortex Eucommiae), and Yín Yáng Huò (Herba Epimedii) for painful *bì* pattern, cold pain in the waist and knee, atrophy and weakness of the sinews and bones, and contractures of the lower limbs caused by kidney yang deficiency and cold-damp invasion.

Nowadays, it has been widely used in the treatment of menopausal syndrome and urogenital system disorders attributed to kidney yang deficiency.

[Usage and Dosage] Use raw in general, often soaked in rice-washed water or processed with wine to reduce its hot nature. Use 3–10 g, reduce the amount as in pill and powder.

[Mnemonics] Xiān Máo (Rhizoma Curculiginis, Common Curculigo Rhizome): pungent and hot; warm and supplement the kidney, strengthen the sinew and bone, and expel cold and dampness.

[Simple and Effective Formulas]

1. 神秘散 Shén Mì Sǎn — Mysterious Powder from *Treatise on Diseases, Patterns, and Formulas Related to the Unification of the Three Etiologies* (三因方 Sān Yīn Fāng): Xiān Máo (Rhizoma Curculiginis) (rice-washed water soaked in water for 3 days, dried under sunshine, stir-fried) 15 g, Tuán Shēn (Radix et Rhizoma Ginseng) 0.3 g, Ē Jiāo (Colla Corii Asini) 30.3 g, and Jī Nèi Jīn (Endothelium Corneum Gigeriae Galli) one piece; grind into powder and take 6 g/time with glutinous rice soup for deficiency-type wheezing due to heart-kidney deficiency with qi counterflow.

2. 二仙汤 Èr Xiān Tāng — Two Immortals Decoction from *Compil*ation of *Research on Chinese Medicine* (中医研究工作资料汇编 Zhōng Yī Yán Jiù Gōng Zuò Zī Liào Huì Biān): Xiān Máo (Rhizoma Curculiginis), Xiān Líng Pí (Herba Epimedii), Bā Jǐ Tiān (Radix Morindae Officinalis), Zhī Mǔ (Rhizoma Anemarrhenae), Huáng Bǎi (Cortex Phellodendri Chinensis), and Dāng Guī (Radix Angelicae Sinensis) in equal dosage, decoct 15–30 g in water for oral administration, and take twice a day to treat hypertension caused by disharmony of the *chong* and *ren* mai and menopause disorders.

[Precautions] Due to its properties, Xiān Máo (Rhizoma Curculiginis), relatively dry in nature, can easily damage yin and stir fire. It is contraindicated in cases of yin deficiency with vigorous fire. It is toxic in large doses and reactions such as swelling of the tongue can occur.

淫羊藿 Yín Yáng Huò *herba epimedii aerial part of epimedium*

The source is from the whole plant of herbaceous perennial *Epimedium brevicornu* Maxim. and *E.sagittatum* (Sieb. et Zucc) Maxim., family Berberidaceae. It is so called because legends say that this substance can trigger estrus in sheep and alternate names include 仙灵脾 Xiān Líng Pí. Pungent and sweet in flavor and warm in nature.

[Actions] Warm and tonify kidney yang, strengthen the sinews and bones, and dispel wind-damp. It is applicable for impotence, seminal emission, and atrophy and weakness of the sinews and bones caused by kidney yang debilitation, wind-damp *bì* pain, and spasm and numbness of the limbs. From the perspective of modern pharmacological research, it can increase sexual activity and sexual desire. Animal experiments suggest it has anti-hypertensive, anti-allergic, anti-inflammatory, immune system-regulatory, anti-aging, and antiviral effects.

[Quality] Good quality is dry and yellowish green with many leaves.

[Indications]

1. Kidney yang deficiency and debilitation: Yín Yáng Huò (Herba Epimedii), warm in nature and effective in tonifying kidney yang, is

applicable for impotence, scanty sperm, cold pain in the waist and knee, sterility and infertility, and frequent urination caused by kidney yang deficiency. It can be used alone as medical wine or decocted along with other kidney-supplementing medicinals such as Shú Dì Huáng (Radix Rehmanniae Praeparata), Dāng Guī (Radix Angelicae Sinensis), Tù Sī Zǐ (Semen Cuscutae), Shé Chuáng Zǐ (Fructus Cnidii), Chuān Xù Duàn (Radix Dipsaci), Bā Jǐ Tiān (Radix Morindae Officinalis), and Dù Zhòng (Cortex Eucommiae).

2. Atrophy and *bì* of the sinews and bones: Yín Yáng Huò (Herba Epimedii) can tonify kidney yang and meanwhile unblock the collaterals and dispel wind-damp with acrid-warm properties. Therefore, it is usually combined with Sāng Jì Shēng (Herba Taxilli), Wēi Líng Xiān (Radix et Rhizoma Clematidis), Luò Shí Téng (Caulis Trachelospermi), and Gǒu Jǐ (Rhizoma Cibotii) for chronic wind-damp *bì* and poststroke hemiplegia.

This herb is also applicable for cough and wheezing due to lung and kidney deficiency and toothache caused by kidney deficiency in the elderly. It has been wildly used in the treatment of menopausal syndrome, urogenital system disorders, hypertension, neurasthenia, hyperlipemia, poststroke paralysis, hypertrophic pelvospondylitis, and cervical osteoarthritis with kidney yang deficiency.

In recent years, this substance has been used for treating coronary heart diseases and shown an effect on angina pectoris.

[Usage and Dosage] Use raw in most cases, roasted to moderate its warm and dryness nature and fortify its tonic function. Use 6–12 g in decoction, higher dosage for a short-term use, or prepared into pill, powder, tincture, extract tablet, and injection.

[Mnemonics] Yín Yáng Huò (Herba Epimedii, Aerial Part of Epimedium): warm; warm and supplement the kidney, strengthen the sinew and bone, and relieve atrophy.

[Simple and Effective Formulas]

1. 仙灵脾散 Xiān Líng Pí Sǎn — Epimedium Powder from *Formulas from Benevolent Sages* (圣惠方 Shèng Huì Fāng): Xiān Líng Pí (Herba

Epimedii) 30 g, Wēi Líng Xiān (Radix et Rhizoma Clematidis) 30 g, Chuān Xiōng (Rhizoma Chuanxiong) 30 g, Guì Xīn (Cortex Cinnamomi) 30 g, and Cāng Ěr Zǐ (Fructus Xanthii) 30 g; grind into fine powder, take 3 g/time with warm wine when necessary for oral administration to treat wind-damp *bì* with migrating pain.

2. 固牙散 Gù Yá Sǎn — Teeth Securing Powder from *Fine Formulas of Wonderful Efficacy* (奇效良方 Qí Xiào Liáng Fāng): grind Xiān Líng Pí (Herba Epimedii) into crude powder and decoct to rinse the mouth for toothache.

[Precautions] Yín Yáng Huò (Herba Epimedii), pungent, warm and drying in nature, is contraindicated in cases yin deficiency with internal fire. Taking the herb in large doses or long-term may cause thirst, nausea, vertigo, epistaxis, and abdominal distention.

杜仲 Dù Zhòng *cortex eucommiae eucommia bark*

The source is from the bark of deciduous arbor *Eucommia ulmoides* Oliv., family Eucommiaceae. It is so called because a man named Dù Zhòng took this herb orally and then became "immortal". Alternate names include 木棉 Mù Mián and 思仙 Sī Xian. Sweet and slight pungent in flavor and warm in nature.

[Actions] Tonify the liver and kidneys, strengthen the sinew and bones, calm the fetus, and lower the blood pressure. It is applicable for lumbago and weakness of the sinews and bones caused by kidney deficiency, uterine bleeding during pregnancy, restless fetus, and hypertension. Modern research has shoun that it can lower blood pressure and improve adrenal cortex and immunologic function. This medicinal has shown diuretic, sedative, antalgic, cardiotonic, and anti-inflammatory effect.

[Quality] Good quality is large and thick with a dark purple inside and without coarse layer of bark. When broken, the bark should produce many thin white threads.

[Indications]

1. Sinews and bones atrophy and weakness due to liver and kidney insufficiency: owning to its effect of supplementing the liver and kidneys and

strengthening the sinews and bones, Dù Zhòng (Cortex Eucommiae) is widely used in the treatment of lumbago, soreness and weakness of the waist and knee, atrophy and weakness of the sinews and bones, and paralysis of the limbs. It is commonly combined with Sāng Jì Shēng (Herba Taxilli), Bǔ Gǔ Zhī (Fructus Psoraleae), and Hé Táo Rén (Semen Juglandis) for lumbago caused by kidney deficiency; with Chuān Xù Duàn (Radix Dipsaci), Shú Dì Huáng (Radix Rehmanniae Praeparata), Shān Zhū Yú (Fructus Corni), and Niú Xī (Radix Achyranthis Bidentatae) for atrophy and weakness of the sinews and bones due to liver and kidney insufficiency; and with Shú Dì Huáng (Radix Rehmanniae Praeparata), Tiān Má (Rhizoma Gastrodiae), and Cí Shí (Magnetitum) for tinnitus and vertigo resulting from kidney deficiency.

2. Restless and agitated fetus due to kidney deficiency: Dù Zhòng (Cortex Eucommiae) is often combined with Bái Zhú (Rhizoma Atractylodis Macrocephalae), Chuān Xù Duàn (Radix Dipsaci), and Zhù Má Gēn (Radix Boehmeriae) for agitated fetus, bleeding during pregnancy, and habitual miscarriage caused by kidney deficiency. It is also applicable for impotence, seminal emission, frequent urination, and hypertention due to kidney deficiency. It should be combined with Xià Kū Cǎo (Spica Prunellae), Jué Míng Zǐ (Semen Cassiae), and Huáng Qín (Radix Scutellariae) for hypertensive patients with accompanying liver fire exuberance signs.

[Usage and Dosage] While the herb is usually used in a raw form, it is most effective in supplementing the liver and kidney when stir-fried. Use 6–12 g in decoction, increase the amount when used alone.

[Mnemonics] Dù Zhòng (Cortex Eucommiae, Eucommia Bark): sweet and warm; tonify the liver and kidney, strengthen the sinew and bones, and calm the fetus.

[Simple and Effective Formulas]

1. 思仙散 Sī Xiān Sǎn — Missing Immortal Powder from *Essential Reflections on Safeguarding Life* (活人心统 Huó Rén Xīn Tǒng): Chuān Mù Xiāng (Radix Vladimiriae) 3 g, Bā Jiǎo Huí Xiāng (Fructus Anisi Stellati) 9 g, and Dù Zhòng (Cortex Eucommiae) (stir-fried,

removal of thin white threads) 9 g; decoct in water for oral administration for lumbago.

2. 杜仲饮 Dù Zhòng Yǐn — Eucommia Bark Drink from *Comprehensive Recording of Divine Assistance* (圣济总录 Shèng Jì Zǒng Lù): Dù Zhòng (Cortex Eucommiae) (removal of coarse layer of bark, roasted) 45 g, Chuān Xiōng (Rhizoma Chuanxiong) 30 g, and Fù Zǐ (Radix Aconiti Lateralis Praeparata) (cracked by blast-frying, removal of peel and navel)15 g; grind into crude powder, decoct 10 g/time with Shēng Jiāng (Rhizoma Zingiberis Recens) for oral administration to treat post-stroke tendon and vessel spasms and tension and weakness in the waist and knee.

[Precautions] Dù Zhòng (Cortex Eucommiae), warm in nature, is contraindicated in cases of yin deficiency resulting in vigorous fire.

Daily practices

1. What are the similarities and differences among Xiān Máo (Rhizoma Curculiginis), Yín Yáng Huò (Herba Epimedii), and Dù Zhòng (Cortex Eucommiae) in terms of actions and indications?
2. Among medicinals that tonify yang, which ones are considered more impotent in strengthening yang? Which are more effective in reinforc-
ing the sinews and bones? Which ones are capable of moistening the intestines to promote defecation? Which ones are capable of receiving qi to arrest wheezing?

ASTRINGENT MEDICINALS

In the process of metabolism, qi, blood, fluid, semen, sweat, urine, and stool are physiologically controlled by relative *zang-fu* organs. Disorders in which these bodily substances are circulated, secreted, and discharged abnormally occur when *zang-fu* organs are in dysfunction. These disorders include external desertions of qi, blood, and fluid, profuse sweating, seminal emission, spontaneous seminal emission, profuse and frequent urination, frequent and profuse vaginal discharge, profuse uterine bleeding, prolonged scanty uterine bleeding of variable intervals, chronic diarrhea, chronic cough and wheezing, and open non-healing

sores. If that is the case, treatment method of consolidating and astringing is adopted. Astringency herbs that consolidate and restrain are used primarily for treating disorders of efflux desertion. Also known as consolidating medicinals (固涩药 Gù Sè Yào) and astringing medicinals (收涩药 Shōu Sè Yào).

Most of these herbs are sour and astringent with the effect of stabilization and binding. They can be subdivided by action into different categories, namely herbs that stop sweating to rescue from desertion, restrain the lung to arrest cough, bind the intestines to stop chronic diarrhea, consolidate essence and reduce urination, restrain and stanch bleeding, and close sores with astringency. However, one herb very often has diverse functions and sores funchions it is hard to be classified into just a single category.

These stabilizing and binding herbs are used primarily for treating the branch manifestation and preventing the further scattering of healthy qi. However, such problems are usually associated with healthy qi debilitation, thus herbs that culture and supplement healthy qi should be added according to the root cause of the problem to treat the root and branch simultaneously and optimize the effect. For instance, for spontaneous sweating due to qi deficiency, herbs that supplement qi are added; for night sweating caused by yin deficiency, herbs that nourish yin are also used; for cough and wheezing attributed to lung and kidney deficiency failing to receive qi, herbs that tonify the lung and kidney are included in the prescription; for seminal emission, spontaneous seminal emission, frequent urination, abnormal vaginal discharge, profuse uterine bleeding, prolonged scanty uterine bleeding of variable intervals resulting from kidney deficiency, herbs that supplement kidney are also prescribed; and for chronic diarrhea and dysentery resulting from spleen and kidney yang deficiency, herbs that tonify the spleen and kidney are added. Some of the herbs that consolidate and bind also have the effect of supplementing and boosting, whereas some herbs that supplement and boost also have the effect of consolidating and binding, like Shān Zhū Yú (Fructus Corni). These herbs are preferred as they can treat the root and branch simultaneously even when used alone.

As these herbs restrain and bind they are not suitable for patients whose excess conditions have not fully resolved, such as residual of exterior pathogens, internal exuberance of heat, and internal stagnation of damp-phlegm. If they are used in these situations, the conditions will be prolonged and possibly exacerbated just like "keeping the invader behind closed doors". In such cases, herbs that consolidate and bind with accompanying effect of dispelling pathogens would be appropriate.

五味子 **Wǔ Wèi Zǐ** *fructus schisandrae Chinensis Chinese magnolivine fruit*

The source is from the ripe fruit of perennial deciduous woody liana *Schisandra chinensis* (Tuecz.) Bail. and S. *Sphenanthera* Rehd. Et Wils., family Magnoliaceae. The former is called 北五味子 Běi Wǔ Wèi Zi and the latter is called 南五味子 Nán Wǔ Wèi Zi. It is so called as its skin and pulp have sweet and sour flavors, and the kernel is acrid, bitter, and salty to taste. Sour in flavor and warm in nature.

[Actions] Consolidate and bind, fortify qi and generate fluids, and tonify the kidneys and calm the heart. It is applicable for chronic cough, deficiency wheezing, nocturnal emission, spontaneous seminal emission, enuresis, frequent urination, chronic diarrhea, spontaneous sweating, night sweating, thirst due to fluid consumption, shortness of breath, deficient pulse, wasting-thirst due to internal heat, palpitations, and insomnia. Modern research has shoun that it can reinforce the excitatory and inhibitory process of central nervous system, improve work efficiency, regulate cardiovascular system and blood pressure, strengthen the heart, increase adrenal cortex performance, reduce glutamic-pyruvic transaminase, and exert an inhibitory effect against bacteria and virus.

[Quality] Good quality is dry, large, thick, fleshy, moist, and purplish red skin and 果皮. Běi Wǔ 北五味子 Wèi Zi is considered with better quality, and more effective for nourishing the lung and kidney, engendering fluids, and astringing yin, stopping coughs, and most likely to be used as a tonic; while 南五味子 Nán Wǔ Wèi Zi is regarded less potent in nourishing and tonifying, and is commonly used for cough and wheezing caused by cold fluid retention in the lung.

[Indications]

1. Efflux desertion patterns: Wǔ Wèi Zǐ (Fructus Schisandrae Chinensis) is effective in the treatment of disorders of efflux desertion such as

spontaneous sweating, night sweating, chronic cough and wheezing, persistent diarrhea, seminal emission, and enuresis. It is often combined with Mǔ Lì (Concha Ostreae), Má Huáng Gēn (Radix et Rhizoma Ephedrae), and Fú Xiǎo Mài (Fructus Tritici Levis) for spontaneous sweating and night sweating; with Rén Shēn (Radix et Rhizoma Ginseng) and Mài Dōng (Radix Ophiopogonis) for collapse with profuse sweating; with Gān Jiāng (Rhizoma Zingiberis), Xì Xīn (Radix et Rhizoma Asari), and Má Huáng (Herba Ephedrae) for cough and wheezing due to cold fluid-retention; with Shú Dì Huáng (Radix Rehmanniae Praeparata) and Shān Zhū Yú (Fructus Corni) for cough and wheezing caused by deficiency; with Bǔ Gǔ Zhī (Fructus Psoraleae) and Ròu Dòu Kòu (Semen Myristicae) for chronic diarrhea resulting form spleen and kidney yang deficiency; and with Sāng Piāo Xiāo (Oötheca Mantidis), Lóng Gǔ (Os Draconis), Jīn Yīng Zǐ (Fructus Rosae Laevigatae), and Fù Pén Zǐ (Fructus Rubi) for seminal emission and enuresis attributed to kidney deficiency.

2. Qi and yin consumption: Wǔ Wèi Zǐ (Fructus Schisandrae Chinensis) can boost qi and promote fluid production, especially when in a combination with sweet medicinals as "the combination of sour and sweet medicinals boosts yin". It is used together with Rén Shēn (Radix et Rhizoma Ginseng), Mài Dōng (Radix Ophiopogonis), Zhī Mǔ (Rhizoma Anemarrhenae), and Tiān Huā Fěn (Radix Trichosanthis) for thirst and profuse sweating due to qi and yin consumption in febrile disease or qi and yin deficiency in miscellaneous diseases.

3. Restlessness of heart spirit: Wǔ Wèi Zǐ (Fructus Schisandrae Chinensis), effective in tonifying the kidney and calming the heart, is often combined with Mài Dōng (Radix Ophiopogonis), Suān Zǎo Rén (Semen Ziziphi Spinosae), Fú Shén (Sclerotium Poriae Pararadicis), and Dì Huáng (Radix Rehmanniae) for restlessness of heart spirit caused by heart and kidney deficiency. In recent years, it has been prepared into a syrup to treat neurasthenic palpitations, insomnia and forgetfulness.

Wǔ Wèi Zǐ (Fructus Schisandrae Chinensis) and its schizandrol have been recently applied for various kinds of liver diseases and have shown a reduced impact on enzyme.

[Usage and Dosage] Use raw in general, its powder, pill or tablet forms instead of decoction are preferred when it is used to decrease enzyme, as its active ingredients that may be destroyed under high temperature. Use 1.5–9 g in decoction, crush prior to decocting to facilitate active ingredient extraction from the semen, 2–3 g/time in pill and powder, use small amount for cough and wheezing caused by lung cold, and bigger amount as a tonic.

[Mnemonics] Wŭ Wèi Zĭ (Fructus Schisandrae Chinensis, Chinese Magnolivine Fruit): sour; rescue from desertion and collapse, fortify qi, promote fluid production, and calm the heart spirit.

[Simple and Effective Formulas]

1. 五味细辛汤 Wŭ Wèi Xì Xīn Tāng — Chinese Magnolivine Fruit and Asarum Decoction from *Ji Feng Formulas for Universal Relief* (鸡峰 普济方 Jī Fēng Pŭ Jì Fāng): Bái Fú Líng (Smilax lanceifolia Roxb.) 120 g, Gān Căo (Radix et Rhizoma Glycyrrhizae) 90 g, Gān Jiāng (Rhizoma Zingiberis) 90 g, Xì Xīn (Radix et Rhizoma Asari) 90 g, and Wŭ Wèi Zĭ (Fructus Schisandrae Chinensis) 75 g; grind into fine powder, and decoct 6 g/time in water for oral administration to treat unremitting cough due to wind-cold invasion.

2. 五味子散 Wŭ Wèi Zĭ Săn — Chinese Magnolivine Fruit Powder from *Experiential Formulas for Universal Relief* (普济本事方 Pŭ Jì Běn Shì Fāng): Wŭ Wèi Zĭ (Fructus Schisandrae Chinensis) 60 g and Wú Zhū Yú (Fructus Evodiae) 15 g; stir-fry until cooked and aromatic, grind into powder, and take 6 g/time with aged rice soup for oral administration to treat kidney diarrhea, remitting early morning diarrhea.

[Precautions] Wŭ Wèi Zĭ (Fructus Schisandrae Chinensis), astringent in nature, retains and preserves pathogenic influences when misused and is therefore contraindicated when an exterior condition is not cleared. It should be combined with acrid medicinals that are capable of opening such as Xì Xīn (Radix et Rhizoma Asari) and Gān Jiāng (Rhizoma Zingiberis) for wind-cold and cold fluid retention in the lung.

乌梅 Wū Méi *fructus mume smoked plum*

The source is from smoked unripe fruit of deciduous arbor *Prunus mume* (*Sieb*) Sieb. Et Zucc., family Rosaceae. It is called 乌梅肉 Wū Méi Ròu when the kernel is removed. Sour and astringent in flavor and neutral in nature.

[Actions] Astringe the lungs and bind up the intestines, and generate fluids and expel roundworms. It is applicable for chronic cough due to lung deficiency, protracted dysentery and diarrhea, wasting-thirst due to deficiency heat, roundworm-induced abdominal pain, and roundworm in the biliary tract. From the perspective of modern research, it has an antibiotic, anti-fungus and anti-allergic effect and can stimulate the contraction of bile duct. Modern research has shoun that it has antibacterial, antifungal, and antiallergic effect and can promote biliary tract contraction.

[Quality] Good quality is dry, large, fleshy, soft, moist, and sour with a small seed.

[Indications]

1. Chronic cough due to lung deficiency: Wū Méi (Fructus Mume) is used together with Xìng Rén (Semen Armeniacae Amarum), Hē Zǐ (Fructus Chebulae), and Yīng Sù Qiào (Pericarpium Papaveris) for chronic cough with scanty sputum due to lung deficiency via inhibiting the leakage of lung qi to arrest cough.
2. Unremitting dysentery and diarrhea: Wū Méi (Fructus Mume) is combined with Ròu Dòu Kòu (Semen Myristicae) and Hē Zǐ (Fructus Chebulae) to treat chronic diarrhea and dysenteric with healthy qi deficiency via binding up the intestine to arrest diarrhea; and with Huáng Lián (Rhizoma Coptidis) and Bīng Láng (Semen Arecae) for unresolved damp-heat pathogen through clearing and removing damp-heat. Clinically, it has been reported that this herb has an effect against intestinal double infection and acute bacillary dysentery caused by long-term use of hormone or broad-spectrum antibiotic.
3. Thirst due to fluid consumption: Wū Méi (Fructus Mume) is sour in flavor and effective in restraining yin and engendering fluid especially when in a combination with sweet medicinals as "the combination of sour and sweet medicinals boost yin". It can be used alone or together with Mài Dōng (Radix Ophiopogonis), Shí Hú (Caulis Dendrobii), and Tiān Huā Fěn (Radix Trichosanthis) for summer-heat induced fluid consumption and wasting-thirst.
4. Roundworm induced abdominal pain and roundworm in biliary tract: Wū Méi (Fructus Mume), capable of tranquilizing the movement of

roundworm, is often combined with Huā Jiāo (Pericarpium Zanthoxyli) and Huáng Lián (Rhizoma Coptidis) for abdominal pain due to round-worm and roundworm in biliary tract.

5. Hemorrhagic disorders: owning to its effect of astringency, Wū Méi (Fructus Mume) can be used in the combination with other medicinals that stanch bleeding for different types of hemorrhagic disorders, such as profuse uterine bleeding, prolonged scanty uterine bleeding of vari-able intervals, stool containing blood, and hematuria.

Owning to its strong sour and astringent nature, it can be used topically to treat pterygium and haemorrhoids. Injecting the medical solution contain-ing 5% Wū Méi (Fructus Mume) into hemorrhoids can successfully necrotize the disorder. Grinding into powder or preparing the charred one into powder and applying externally can treat pterygium and open non-healing sores.

[Usage and Dosage] Use raw in general, partially charred when used for diarrhea, dysentery, and hemorrhagic disorders. Use 3–10 g in decoction, and up to more than 15 g when used to treat abdominal pain due to round-worm or roundworm in the biliary tract.

[Mnemonics] Wū Méi (Fructus Mume, Smoked Plum): sour and acrid; cure chronic dysentery and cough, arrest bleeding, calm roundworms, promote fluid production, and relieve thirst.

[Simple and Effective Formulas]

1. 乌梅丸 Wū Méi Wán — Mume Pill from *Formulas from Benevolent Sages* (圣惠方 Shèng Huì Fāng): Wū Méi (Fructus Mume) 20 pieces (roasted) and Huáng Lián (Rhizoma Coptidis) 30 g; grind into fine powder, make into chesspieces-sized pill with wax, prepare into phoe-nix tree seed-sized pill with the paste of honey, take 10–20 pills/time, three times a day for dysentery with no food intake.

2. 治久咳方 Zhì Jiǔ Ké Fāng — Chronic Cough Formula from *The Grand Compendium of Materia Medica* (本草纲目 Běn Cǎo Gāng Mù): Wū Méi (Fructus Mume) flesh (slightly stir-fried) and Yīng Sù Qiào (Pericarpium Papaveris) (removal of striations and membrane, honey-fried) in equal dosage; grind into powder and take 6 g/time with honey at bedtime for oral administration to treat persistent cough.

[Precautions] Wū Méi (Fructus Mume), astringent in nature, is contraindicated in cases caused by invasion of excess pathogens, except for certain infectious diseases in the intestines.

Daily practices

1. What are the nature, flavor, actions, and indications of medicinals that consolidate and astringe? what precautions should be taken when using them?
2. What are the similarities and differences between Wǔ Wèi Zǐ (Fructus Schisandrae Chinensis) and Wū Méi (Fructus Mume) in terms of actions and indications?

诃子 Hē Zzǐ *fructus chebulae medicine terminalia fruit*

The source is from the ripe fruit of the deciduous arbor *Terminalia chebula* Retz, or *T. chebula* Retz. Var. *gangetica* Roxb., family Combretacae. Alternate names include 诃黎勒 Hē Lí Lēi. Bitter, sour and astringent in flavor and neutral in nature.

[Actions] Bind up the intestines to stop diarrhea, astringe the lung to relieve cough, and clear and drain lung-fire. It is applicable for different types of chronic dysentery, persistent diarrhea, and prolonged cough and wheezing. Modern research suggests that it has a strong inhibitory effect against bacteria and dysentery.

[Quality] Good quality is yellowish brown, shiny, solid, and hard.

[Indications]

1. Chronic diarrhea and dysentery: Hē Zǐ (Fructus Chebulae), with a strong sour and astringent nature, is potent in consolidating and astringing the intestines and therefore frequently combined with Yīng Sù Qiào (Pericarpium Papaveris) and Gān Jiāng (Rhizoma Zingiberis) for chronic diarrhea and dysentery even with prolapse of anus caused by efflux desertion of the large intestine. It is used together with medicinals that clear and eliminate damp-heat such as Mù Xiāng (Radix Aucklandiae), Huáng Lián (Rhizoma Coptidis), and Gān Cǎo (Radix et Rhizoma Glycyrrhizae) for chronic dysentery with unresolved damp-heat in the intestines.

2. Cough and wheezing due to lung deficiency: Hē Zǐ (Fructus Chebulae) (without kernel), capable of restraining lung qi, is combined with Xìng Rén (Semen Armeniacae Amarum), Bèi Mǔ (Bulbus Fritillaria), and Wǔ Wèi Zǐ (Fructus Schisandrae Chinensis) for cough and wheezing due to lung deficiency; with Jié Gěng (Radix Platycodonis) and Gān Cǎo (Radix et Rhizoma Glycyrrhizae) for hoarseness caused by lung deficiency with fire; and with Mù Hú Dié (Semen Oroxyli) and Chán Tuì (Periostracum Cicadae) for hoarseness attributed to yin deficiency, wind-cold invasion, and overstrain.

[Usage and Dosage] Use raw for hoarseness due to deficiency fire in the lungs and roasted for chronic cough and diarrhea. Use 3–10 g in decoction.

[Mnemonics] Hē Zzǐ (Fructus Chebulae, Medicine Terminalia Fruit): bitter and sour; astringe the lung and relieve wheezing, bind up the intestines to stop diarrhea, and cure loss of voice.

[Simple and Effective Formulas]

1. 诃子饮 Hē Zǐ Yǐn — Terminalia Fruit Drink from *Formulas to Aid the Living* (济生方 Jì Shēng Fāng): Hē Zǐ (Fructus Chebulae) (without kernel) 30 g, Xìng Rén (Semen Armeniacae Amarum) (soaked and without peel and tip) 30 g, and Tōng Cǎo (Medulla Tetrapanacis) 7.5 g; grind into crude powder, decoct 12 g/time with roasted Shēng Jiāng (Rhizoma Zingiberis Recens) five pieces in water and take warm for oral administration to treat loss of voice due to chronic cough.
2. 诃黎勒散 Hē Lí Lēi Sǎn — Medicine Terminalia Fruit Powder from *Formulas from Benevolent Sages* (圣惠方 Shèng Huì Fāng): Hē Zǐ (Fructus Chebulae) (with peel and roasted) 9 g and Bái Fán (Alumen) (prepared into ashes) 300 g; grind into powder and take 6 g/time with congee for oral administration to treat chronic diarrhea in the elderly.

[Precautions] Hē Zǐ (Fructus Chebulae), as an astringent medicinal, is contraindicated for exterior patterns when an exterior condition is not cleared or where there is stagnation of damp-turbidity and damp-heat. However, nowadays it has been successfully used for treating acute dysentery and sudden loss of voice.

石榴皮 **Shí Liú Pí** *pericarpium granati pomegranate husk*

The source is from the pericarp of deciduous shrub or subarbor *Punica granatum* L, family Punicaceae. Sour and astringent in flavor and warm in nature.

[Actions] Astringe the intestines and arrest diarrhea, retain the essence and stanch excessive vaginal discharge, and kill parasites. It is applicable for chronic diarrhea and dysentery, prolapse of anus, seminal emission, abnormal vaginal discharge, and abdominal pain due to worm accumulation. Modern research has indicated that it has strong antibacterial and anti-dysentery effects.

[Quality] Good quality is large and clean.

[Indications]

1. Chronic diarrhea and dysentery: owning to its sour and astringent potency, Shí Liú Pí (Pericarpium Granati) is often prescribed together with Yīng Sù Qiào (Pericarpium Papaveris), Hē Zǐ (Fructus Chebulae), Ròu Dòu Kòu (Semen Myristicae), and Gān Jiāng (Rhizoma Zingiberis) for chronic diarrhea and dysentery or even with prolapse of anus caused by efflux desertion of the large intestine through consolidating the intestine and astringing; and with medicinals that clear and remove damp-heat such as Mù Xiāng (Radix Aucklandiae), Huáng Lián (Rhizoma Coptidis), and Gān Cǎo (Radix et Rhizoma Glycyrrhizae) for chronic dysentery with unresolved damp-heat in the intestines. Owning to its antibacterial and anti-dysentery property, it has a significant effect on acute bacillary dysentery and often used in the formula of relieving acute bacillary dysentery and acute enteritis.
2. Parasites in intestines: Shí Liú Pí (Pericarpium Granati) can kill worms and is therefore often combined with Bīng Láng (Semen Arecae) for roundworm, pinworm, and tapeworm.
3. Profuse uterine bleeding and prolonged scanty uterine bleeding of variable intervals abnormal vaginal discharge: Shí Liú Pí (Pericarpium Granati), capable of consolidating and astringing the *chong* and *ren* mai, is applicable for chronic profuse uterine bleeding, prolonged scanty uterine bleeding of variable intervals, and abnormal vaginal discharge.

It is also applicable for seminal emission and stool containing blood. Dry-frying until charred, grinding into powder, mixing with sesame oil, and applying externally can treat such skin problems as psoriasis and scalding.

[Usage and Dosage] Use 3–10 g in decoction, use raw in general, and stir-fried can reduce its stimulation to the stomach.

[Mnemonics] Shí Liú Pí (Pericarpium Granati, Pomegranate Husk): sour; astringe and consolidate incontinence and collapse, kill intestinal parasites, and stop diarrhea and dysentery.

[Simple and Effective Formulas]

1. 神授散 Shén Shòu Sǎn — Immortal's Powder from *Formulas for Universal Relief* (普济方 Pǔ Jì Fāng): grind aged Shí Liú (Punica granatum Linn) (roasted) into fine powder and take 9–12 g/time with rice soup for oral administration to treat persistent dysentery.
2. 治脱肛方 Zhì Tuō Gāng Fāng — Rectal Prolapse Relieving Formula from *Medical Literature Arranged by Category* (医钞类编 Yī Chāo Lèi Biān): Shí Liú Pí (Pericarpium Granati), aged wall soil, and small amount of Bái Fán (Alumen); decoct into thick liquid to fumigate and wash, apply topically with fine powder of Wǔ Bèi Zǐ (Galla Chinensis) for prolapse of anus due to severe diarrhea and dysentery.

[Precautions] According to some traditional resources, Shí Liú Pí (Pericarpium Granati) is contraindicated in acute diarrhea and dysentery. However, nowadays it has been proven effective in the treatment of acute dysentery, especially excessive dysentery or with prolapse of anus.

肉豆蔻 Ròu Dòu Kòu *semen myristicae nutmeg*

The source is from the ripe semen of tall arbor *Myristica fragrans* Houtt., family Myristicacene. Alternate names include 肉蔻 Ròu Kòu, 肉果 Ròu Guǒ, and 玉果 Yù Guǒ. Pungent in flavor and warm in nature.

[Actions] Warm the middle *jiao* and move the qi, and bind up the intestine to stop diarrhea. It is applicable for chronic and unremitting diarrhea, deficiency-cold with qi stagnation, gastric and abdominal distending pain, poor appetite, and vomiting.

[Quality] Good quality is large, heavy, solid, hard, oily, and aromatic when crushed.

[Indications]

1. Chronic diarrhea due to spleen and kidney deficiency-cold: Ròu Dòu Kòu (Semen Myristicae), warm and astringent in property, can warm the spleen and stomach and warm the spleen and kidney. It is often combined with Dǎng Shēn (Radix Codonopsis) and Bái Zhú (Rhizoma Atractylodis Macrocephalae) for diarrhea induced by spleen deficiency; with Fù Zǐ (Radix Aconiti Lateralis Praeparata) and Hē Zǐ (Fructus Chebulae) for chronic and unremitting diarrhea caused by spleen and kidney deficiency-cold; and with Wǔ Wèi Zǐ (Fructus Schisandrae Chinensis), Bǔ Gǔ Zhī (Fructus Psoraleae), and Wú Zhū Yú (Fructus Evodiae) for diarrhea before dawn due to kidney yang insufficiency.
2. Spleen and stomach deficiency-cold and qi stagnation: Ròu Dòu Kòu (Semen Myristicae), acrid and warm, can warm the middle *jiao* and move qi, and is combined with Mù Xiāng (Radix Aucklandiae), Bàn Xià (Rhizoma Pinelliae), and Gān Jiāng (Rhizoma Zingiberis) for gastric and abdominal distending pain caused by middle *jiao* deficiency-cold with stagnated qi movement.

[Usage and Dosage] Use raw in most cases, roast the herb to remove oil, moderate its properties, and minimize potential side effects. Use 3–10 g in decoction, 1.5–3.0 g/time in pill and powder.

[Mnemonics] Ròu Dòu Kòu (Semen Myristicae, Nutmeg): pungent and warm; astringe the spleen and kidney, relieve chronic diarrhea due to deficiency cold, and smooth qi in the middle *jiao*.

[Simple and Effective Formulas]

1. 肉豆蔻丸 Ròu Dòu Kòu Wán — Nutmeg Pill from *An Elucidation of Formulas* (宣明论方 Xuān Míng Lùn Fāng): Ròu Dòu Kòu (Semen

Myristicae) 0.3 g, Bīng Láng (Semen Arecae) 0.3 g, Qīng Fěn (Calomelas) 0.3 g, and Hēi Qiān Niú (Silene adenantha Franch) 45 g (first-ground powder); grind into powder, make into green-bean sized pill with the paste, take 10–20 pills/time with Lián Qiào (Fructus Forsythiae) decoction for oral administration, three times a day, to treat internal retention of water-dampness with drum-like abdominal distention but relatively strong body.

2. 四神丸 Sì Shén Wán — Four Spirits Pill from *Summary of Internal Medicine* (内科摘要 Nèi Kē Zhāi Yào): decoct Shēng Jiāng (Rhizoma Zingiberis Recens) 120 g and Dà Zǎo (Fructus Jujubae) 50 pieces together and remove ginger and liquid; grind Ròu Dòu Kòu (Semen Myristicae) 30 g, Wǔ Wèi Zǐ (Fructus Schisandrae Chinensis) 30 g, Bǔ Gǔ Zhī (Fructus Psoraleae) 60 g, and Wú Zhū Yú (Fructus Evodiae) 15 g into powder, make into phoenix tree seed-sized pill with the paste of the above-mentioned Dà Zǎo (Fructus Jujubae), and take 50–70 pills/time on a empty stomach before dawn for diarrhea and poor appetite due to spleen and kidney deficiency.

[Precautions] Ròu Dòu Kòu (Semen Myristicae), as an astringent medicinal, is contraindicated in cases of unresolved excess pathogens. Overdose is discouraged because of its toxicity. Vertigo and delirium from ingesting 7.5 g/dose of the powdered herb have been reported.

莲子 Lián Zǐ *semen nelumbinis lotus seed*

The source is from the ripe semen of aquatic herbaceous perennial *Nelumbo nucifera* Gaertn, family Nymphaeaceae. Alternate names include 莲蓬子 Lián Peng Zi. Sweet and astringent in flavor and neutral in nature.

[Actions] Tonify the spleen to arrest diarrhea, augment the kidneys to restrain the essence, and nourish the heart to calm the mind. It is applicable for chronic diarrhea and poor appetite due to spleen deficiency, seminal emission and spontaneous seminal emission caused by kidney deficiency, deficiency-vexation, restlessness, palpitations due to fright, insomnia, profuse uterine bleeding, prolonged scanty uterine bleeding of variable intervals, and abnormal vaginal discharge.

[Quality] Good quality is dry, large, full, intact, and without damage caused by worms and mildew. 莲子肉 Lián Zǐ Ròu refers to the fresh one without plumule and is more effective in supplementing the middle *jiao* and nourish the heart; 石莲子 Shí Lián Zǐ refers to frosted, ripe, hard herb with pericarp, is more potent in supplementing the spleen and arresting diarrhea, and has been traditionally used to dysentery with inability to eat.

[Indications]

1. Kidney deficiency failing to consolidate: Lián Zǐ (Semen Nelumbinis), capable of supplementing the kidney and consolidating and astringing, is applicable for seminal emission, spontaneous seminal emission, and white-turbid urine caused by kidney deficiency and often used in a combination with Shā Yuàn Jí Lí (Semen Astragali Complanati), Fú Líng (Poria), Lóng Gǔ (Os Draconis), Jīn Yīng Zǐ (Fructus Rosae Laevigatae), and Fù Pén Zǐ (Fructus Rubi).
2. Chronic diarrhea due to spleen deficiency: Lián Zǐ (Semen Nelumbinis), good at fortifying the spleen and capable of astringing, is combined with Bái Zhú (Rhizoma Atractylodis Macrocephalae), Dǎng Shēn (Radix Codonopsis), Fú Líng (Poria), Shān Yào (Rhizoma Dioscoreae), and Biǎn Dòu (Semen Lablab Album) for chronic diarrhea and reduced appetite due to spleen deficiency.
3. Restlessness of heart spirit: Lián Zǐ (Semen Nelumbinis), capable of nourishing the heart to calm the spirit and restoring interaction between the heart and the kidney, is combined with Mài Dōng (Radix Ophiopogonis), Shēng Dì (Radix Rehmanniae), Fú Shén (Sclerotium Poriae Pararadicis), and Bǎi Zǐ Rén (Semen Platycladi) for palpitations, insomnia, forgetfulness, and deficiency-vexation caused by kidney water failing to interact with heart fire or heart qi insufficiency.

It can also be used to stanch profuse uterine bleeding and prolonged scanty uterine bleeding of variable intervals through supplementing and boosting the spleen and kidney.

This substance, neutral and moderate in nature, is commonly used in dietary therapy.

[Usage and Dosage] Use raw in general, 10–15 g in decoction, remove the plumule before use, and applicable for dietary therapy.

[Mnemonics] Lián Zǐ *(Semen Nelumbinis, Lotus Seed): sweet and neutral; good for medicated diet; supplement the kidney, tonify the spleen, nourish the heart, and calm the spirit.

[Simple and Effective Formulas]

1. 莲子六一汤 Lián Zǐ Liù Yī Tāng — Lotus Seed Six-to-One Decoction from *Ren-zhai's Direct Guidance on Formulas* (仁斋直指方 Rén Zhāi Zhí Zhǐ Fāng): Shí Lián Ròu (Semen Nelumbinis) (with kernel) 180 g and Zhì Gān Cǎo (Radix et Rhizoma Glycyrrhizae Praeparata cum Melle) 30 g; grind into fine powder and take 6 g/time with Dēng Xīn Cǎo (Medulla Junci, Juncus) decoction for oral administration to treat cloudy urine.
2. 莲肉散 Lián Ròu Sǎn — Nelumbinis Seed Powder from *Fine Formulas of Wonderful Efficacy* (奇效良方 Qí Xiào Liáng Fāng): Shí Lián Ròu (Semen Nelumbinis), Yì Zhì Rén (Fructus Alpiniae Oxyphyllae), and Lóng Gǔ (Os Draconis) (with five colors) in equal dosage; grind into fine powder and take with rice soup on an empty stomach for cloudy urine, nocturnal emission, and seminal emission.

[Precautions] Lián Zǐ (Semen Nelumbinis), sweet and tonic, should be used with caution in cases of fullness, *pǐ*, and distention of the middle *jiao* with dry stools. Ingesting raw too much may cause gastric and abdominal distention.

Daily practices

1. What are the similarities and differences among Hē Zǐ (Fructus Chebulae), Shí Liú Pí (Pericarpium Granati), Ròu Dòu Kòu (Semen Myristicae), and Lián Zǐ (Semen Nelumbinis) in terms of actions and indications?
2. What are the similarities and differences between Ròu Dòu Kòu (Semen Myristicae) and Bái Dòu Kòu (Fructus Amomi Kravanh) in terms of actions and indications? What precautions should be taken when using them?

芡实 Qiàn Shí *semen euryales euryale seed*

The source is the ripe semen of aquatic herbaceous annual *Euryale ferox* Salisb., family Nymphaeaceae. Alternate names include 鸡头实 Jī Tóu Shí and 鸡头米 Jī Tóu Mǐ. It is so called as it is a substitute food when there is a shortage of food (Qiàn, 欠). This medicinal is also known as 鸡头 Jī Tóu because its flower looks like a chicken head. Sweet and astringent in flavor and neutral in nature.

[Actions] Stabilize the kidneys to retain the essence, strengthen the spleen to arrest diarrhea, and stop profuse vaginal discharge. It is applicable for seminal emission and white-turbid urine due to kidney deficiency, diarrhea caused by spleen deficiency, and white leucorrhea.

[Quality] Good quality is full, in even size, powdery, and without fragments, 碎末 skin and shell 皮壳.

[Indications]

1. Kidney deficiency patterns: Qiàn Shí (Semen Euryales), capable of tonifying the spleen and kidney and consolidating, is combined with Jīn Yīng Zǐ (Fructus Rosae Laevigatae), Fú Líng (Poria), and Fù Pén Zǐ (Fructus Rubi) for seminal emission, white-turbid urine, and frequent urination due to kidney deficiency.
2. Spleen deficiency patterns: Qiàn Shí (Semen Euryales) is combined with Dǎng Shēn (Radix Codonopsis), Bái Zhú (Rhizoma Atractylodis Macrocephalae), and Shān Yào (Rhizoma Dioscoreae) to relieve diarrhea due to spleen deficiency through fortifying the spleen and arresting diarrhea; with Huáng Bǎi (Cortex Phellodendri Chinensis), and Chūn Bái Pí (Cortex Toonae Sinensis Radicis) for frequent white leucorrhea caused by spleen deficiency.

This substance, neutral in nature, is commonly used in dietary therapy.

[Usage and Dosage] 10–15 g in decoction, also applicable for dietary therapy.

[Mnemonics] Qiàn Shí (Semen Euryales, Euryale Seed): sweet and astringent; supplement the spleen and kidney, and relieve seminal emission, diarrhea, and profuse vaginal discharge.

[Simple and Effective Formulas]

玉锁丹 Yù Suǒ Dān — Jade Lock Elixir from *Secret Formulas of the Yang Family* (杨氏家藏方 Yáng Shì Jiā Cáng Fāng): Qiàn Shí (Semen Euryales) 30 g, Lián Huā Ruǐ (Stamen Nelumbinis) 30 g, Lóng Gǔ (Os Draconis) 30 g and Wū Méi (Fructus Mume) flesh (baked) 30 g; grind into powder and make into Qiàn Shí (Semen Euryales)-sized pill with the paste of decocted Shān Yào (Rhizoma Dioscoreae), take one pill/time with warm wine or salt solution on an empty stomach to treat nocturnal emission and spontaneous seminal emission.

[Precautions] Qiàn Shí (Semen Euryales) and Lián Zǐ (Semen Nelumbinis) have similar actions. Both are mild in nature, overdose or long-term use, however, may cause blockage of qi movement.

金樱子 Jīn Yīng Zǐ *fructus rosae laevigatae cherokee rose fruit*

The source is from the ripe fruit of evergreen climber shrub *Rosa laevigata* Michx, family Rosaceae. It is so called because its shape is similar to a container that is called 罂 Yīng (small-mouthed jar). Sour, sweet, and astringent in flavor and neutral in nature.

[Actions] Consolidate essence and reduce urination, astringe the intestines to arrest diarrhea. It is applicable for seminal emission due to kidney deficiency, enuresis and frequent urination, abnormal vaginal discharge, chronic diarrhea and dysentery, prolapse of anus, uterine prolapse, profuse uterine bleeding, and prolonged scanty uterine bleeding of variable intervals. Modern research reveals that it has antibacterial, antiviral, anti-arteriosclerosis, digestive aid, and intestinal secretion-inhibitor effects.

[Quality] Good quality is dry, large, reddish yellow, and without burrs.

[Indications]

1. Kidney deficiency failing to insecure: Jīn Yīng Zǐ (Fructus Rosae Laevigatae), slight sweet to tonify and sour and acrid to astringe, can be used alone or together with medicinals that supplement the kidney and consolidate essence such as Shú Dì Huáng (Radix Rehmanniae

Praeparata), Qiàn Shí (Semen Euryales), and Fù Pén Zǐ (Fructus Rubi) for seminal emission, enuresis, abnormal vaginal discharge, and white-turbid urine caused by kidney deficiency. It is often combined with Bì Xiè (Rhizoma Dioscoreae Hypoglaucae) and Yì Zhì Rén (Fructus Alpiniae Oxyphyllae) for white-turbid urine.

2. Spleen deficiency diarrhea and dysentery: for chronic diarrhea and dysentery due to spleen deficiency, Jīn Yīng Zǐ (Fructus Rosae Laevigatae) can be used alone or in a combination with Dǎng Shēn (Radix Codonopsis), Bái Zhú (Rhizoma Atractylodis Macrocephalae), and Qiàn Shí (Semen Euryales) to fortify the spleen and astringe the intestines.

This medicinal is also applicable for prolapse of anus, hysteroptosis, profuse uterine bleeding, and prolonged scanty uterine bleeding of variable intervals due to its property of consolidate and astringe.

[Usage and Dosage] Use raw in general, 6–15 g in decoction, and prepare into decocted extract for oral administration.

[Mnemonics] Jīn Yīng Zǐ (Fructus Rosae Laevigatae, Cherokee Rose Fruit): sour and sweet; reduce urination, arrest profuse vaginal discharge, and arrest seminal emission, diarrhea, and dysentery with astringency.

[Simple and Effective Formulas]

1. 金櫻子膏 Jīn Yīng Zǐ Gāo — Cherokee Rose Fruit Decocted Extract from *A Handbook of Famous Physicians of the Ming Dynasty* (明医指掌 Míng Yī Zhǐ Zhǎng): Jīn Yīng Zǐ (Fructus Rosae Laevigatae) (removal of hairs and seeds); pound into pieces and cook with water into decocted extract for oral administration to treat nocturnal emission and spontaneous seminal emission.

2. 金櫻猪小肚方 Jīn Yīng Zhū Xiǎo Dù Fāng — Cherokee Rose Fruit and Pig's Bladder Formula from *Quan Zhou Compilation of Materia Medica* (泉州本草 Quán Zhōu Běn Cǎo): Jīn Yīng Zǐ (Fructus Rosae Laevigatae) (removal of thorn and pulp) 10 g and one Zhū Xiǎo Dù (Pig's Bladder); decoct in water for oral administration to treat frequent urination, profuse urine, and urinary incontinence.

[Precautions] Jīn Yīng Zǐ (Fructus Rosae Laevigatae), sour and astringent, is contraindicated in cases of cold in the middle *jiao* and fire due to excess.

覆盆子 Fù Pén Zǐ *fructus rubi chinese raspberry*

The source is from unripe fruit of deciduous shrub *Rubus chingii* Hu, family Rosaceae. Sweet and sour in flavor and slightly warm in nature.

[Actions] Fortify the kidneys and consolidate the essence, and restrain urine and improve vision. It is applicable for seminal emission, spontaneous seminal emission, enuresis, frequent urination and impotence caused by kidney deficiency and blurred vision.

[Quality] Good quality is large, full, granular, round, firm, grayish green, and without leaves and stems.

[Indications]

1. Kidney deficiency failing to insecure: Fù Pén Zǐ (Fructus Rubi), sweet in flavor to tonify and sour in flavor to consolidate, can be used alone or together with medicinals that supplement the kidney and consolidate essence such as Shú Dì Huáng (Radix Rehmanniae Praeparata), Qiàn Shí (Semen Euryales), and Sāng Piāo Xiāo (Oötheca Mantidis) for seminal emission, enuresis, frequent urination, and abnormal vaginal discharge caused by kidney deficiency. It is combined with Shú Dì Huáng (Radix Rehmanniae Praeparata), Yín Yáng Huò (Herba Epimedii), and Xiān Máo (Rhizoma Curculiginis) for impotence due to kidney deficiency.
2. Liver and kidney deficiency and debilitation: owning to its effect of supplementing the liver and kidney, Fù Pén Zǐ (Fructus Rubi) is prescribed together with Bái Sháo (Radix Paeoniae Alba), Shēng Dì (Radix Rehmanniae), and Gǔ Jīng Cǎo (Flos Eriocauli) for blurred vision due to liver and kidney deficiency and debilitation.

[Usage and Dosage] Use raw in general, and steam with (rice) wine is more effective in supplementing the liver and kidneys. Use 10–15 g in decoction.

[Mnemonics] Fù Pén Zǐ (Fructus Rubi, Chinese Raspberry): sweet and sour; fortify the kidney and liver, consolidate essence, reduce urination, and specialized in curing seminal emission.

[Simple and Effective Formulas]
治阳痿方 Zhì Yáng Wěi Fāng — Impotence-curing Formula from *Binhu's Verse on Simple and Effective Formulas* (濒湖集简方 Bīn Hú Jí Jiǎn Fāng): Fù Pén Zǐ (Fructus Rubi); soak into wine, bake to dry, grind into powder, and take 6 g with wine for oral administration every morning to treat impotence.

[Precautions] Fù Pén Zǐ, sour and astringent, is contraindicated in cases of difficult and painful urination with scanty urine due to kidney deficiency with fire.

Daily practices

1. What are the similarities and differences between Qiàn Shí (Semen Euryales) and Lián Zǐ (Semen Nelumbinis) in terms of actions and indications?
2. What are the similarities and differences among Qiàn Shí (Semen Euryales), Jīn Yīng Zǐ (Fructus Rosae Laevigatae), and Fù Pén Zǐ (Fructus Rubi) in terms of actions and indications?

罂粟壳 Yīng Sù Qiào *pericarpium papaveris poppy husk*

The source is from the husk of herbaceous annual or biennial *Papaver somniferum* L., family Papaveraceae. Alternate names include 御米壳 Yù Mǐ Ké. Sour and astringent in flavor and neutral in nature with toxicity.

[Actions] Astringe the intestines to arrest diarrhea, astringe the lung to relieve cough, and arrest pain. It is applicable for different types of incontinence, such as chronic diarrhea and dysentery, protracted cough, different types of pain, and chronic and incessant cough.

[Quality] Good quality is large, yellowish white, hard, and thick.

[Indications]

1. Chronic diarrhea and dysentery: Yīng Sù Qiào (Pericarpium Papaveris), effective in astringing the intestines, can be prescribed alone or together with Hē Zǐ (Fructus Chebulae) and Wū Méi (Fructus Mume) for chronic diarrhea and dysentery without internal accumulation of excess pathogens.
2. Lung deficiency chronic cough: Yīng Sù Qiào (Pericarpium Papaveris), capable of astringing lung qi and relieving cough, can be used along or in a combination with Wū Méi (Fructus Mume) for chronic cough with scanty or no sputum.
3. Pain: Yīng Sù Qiào (Pericarpium Papaveris) has anaesthetic and analgesic effects and therefore is applicable for pain caused by traumatic injury and in the sinews, bones, chest and abdomen.

[Usage and Dosage] Use honey-fired to arrest cough and vinegar-fried to relieve diarrhea and pain. Use 3–6 g in decoction.

[Mnemonics] Yīng Sù Qiào (Pericarpium Papaveris, Poppy Husk): sour and acrid; use with caution as it is toxic; relieve cough, diarrhea, and pain with a strong astringency.

[Simple and Effective Formulas]

1 治水泄方 Zhì Shuǐ Xiè Fāng — Lienteric Diarrhea Relieving Formula from *Empirical Formulas* (经验方 Jīng Yàn Fāng): one Yīng Sù Qiào (Pericarpium Papaveris) (removal of pedicle and membrane), 10 Wū Méi (Fructus Mume) flesh, and 10 Dà Zǎo (Fructus Jujubae) flesh; decoct in water for oral administration to treat prolonged watery diarrhea.
2. 小百劳散 Xiǎo Láo Bǎi Sǎn — Minor Powder from *An Elucidation of Formulas* (宣明论方 Xuān Míng Lùn Fāng): stir-fry and grind Yīng Sù Qiào (Pericarpium Papaveris) into powder, decoct 6 g/time with Wū Méi (Fructus Mume) and take warm for oral administration to treat chronic consumptive wheezing and cough, and profuse spontaneous sweating.

[Precautions] Yīng Sù Qiào (Pericarpium Papaveris) is toxic and a an illegal drug. With a tendency towards addiction, it must be used just temporarily and not regularly used or used as a seasoning. In cases of chronic diarrhea and dysentery, non-toxic herbs such as Hē Zǐ (Fructus Chebulae) and Shí Liú Pí (Pericarpium Granati) are among the first choices. It is contraindicated in patients with unresolved pathogens, especially acute diarrhea and dysentery, as it works only on consolidating and astringing but not dispelling pathogens. It is just used temporarily

桑螵蛸 Sāng Piāo Xiāo *oötheca mantidis mantis egg-case*

The source is from the egg case of the insect *Tenodera sinensis* Saussure, *Statilia maculate* Thunb., or *Hierodula patellifera* Serville, family Mantis. Sweet and salty in flavor and neutral in nature.

[Actions] Tonify the kidneys and assist yang, and consolidate essence and reduce urination. It is applicable for seminal emission, spontaneous seminal emission, enuresis, frequent urination, abnormal vaginal discharge, and impotence caused by kidney deficiency.

[Quality] Good quality is dry, large, yellow, and unhatching. The hatched one cannot be used as a medicinal.

[Indications]

1. Kidney deficiency failing to insecure: Sāng Piāo Xiāo (Oötheca Mantidis), effective in tonifying and consolidating, can be used alone or together with medicinals that supplement the kidney and consolidate essence such as Shú Dì Huáng (Radix Rehmanniae Praeparata), Qiàn Shí (Semen Euryales), and Sāng Piāo Xiāo (Oötheca Mantidis) for seminal emission, enuresis, frequent urination, cloudy urine, and abnormal vaginal discharge caused by kidney deficiency. It is combined with Shú Dì Huáng (Radix Rehmanniae Praeparata), Yín Yáng Huò (Herba Epimedii), and Xiān Máo (Rhizoma Curculiginis) for impotence due to kidney deficiency impotence; and with Yì Zhì Rén (Fructus Alpiniae Oxyphyllae) and Shān Yào (Rhizoma Dioscoreae) to consolidate and astringe profuse urine.

2. Kidney deficiency impotence: Sāng Piāo Xiāo (Oötheca Mantidis), capable of supplementing kidney and assisting yang, is applicable for impotence and premature ejaculation caused by kidney deficiency and often combined with Tù Sī Zǐ (Semen Cuscutae), Bǔ Gǔ Zhī (Fructus Psoraleae), Ròu Cōng Róng (Herba Cistanches), and Shā Yuàn Jí Lí (Semen Astragali Complanati).

[Usage and Dosage] Usually use in stir-fried form as the raw may cause diarrhea, and stir-fry with salt to improve its ability of tonifying kidney and consolidating essence. Use 3–10 g in decoction.

[Mnemonics] Sāng Piāo Xiāo (Oötheca Mantidis, Mantis Egg-case): sweet; specialized in reducing urination, supplement the kidney, assist yang, and consolidate essence.

[Simple and Effective Formulas]
桑螵蛸散 Sāng Piāo Xiāo Sǎn — Mantis Egg Shell Powder from the *Extension of the Materia Medica* (本草衍义 Běn Cǎo Yǎn Yì): Sāng Piāo Xiāo (Oötheca Mantidis) 30 g, Yuǎn Zhì (Radix Polygalae) 30 g, Shí Chāng Pú (Rhizoma Acori Tatarinowii) 30 g, Lóng Gǔ (Os Draconis) 30 g, Rén Shēn (Radix et Rhizoma Ginseng) 30 g, Fú Shén (Sclerotium Poriae Pararadicis) 30 g, Dāng Guī (Radix Angelicae Sinensis) 30 g, and vinegar-treated Guī Bǎn (Plastrum Testudinis) 30 g; grind into powder and take 6 g/time with Rén Shēn (Radix et Rhizoma Ginseng) decoction for oral administration at bedtime to treat forgetfulness and frequent urination.

[Precautions] Sāng Piāo Xiāo (Oötheca Mantidis), warm and astringent in nature, is contraindicated in cases of frequent urination and difficult and painful urination caused by either yin deficiency with internal heat or damp-heat in the bladder.

海螵蛸 Hǎi Piāo Xiāo *endoconcha sepiae cuttlebone*

The source is from the internal shell of the mollusk *sepiella maindroni* de Rochebrunc. or *Sepia esculenta* Hoyle, family Cuttlefish. Alternate names include 乌贼骨 Wū Zéi Gǔ. Salty and astringent in flavor and slightly warm in nature.

[Actions] Restrain and stanch bleeding, consolidate the essence and arrest profuse vaginal discharge, control acidity to alleviate pain, and resolve dampness to promote healing of sore. It is applicable for profuse uterine bleeding, prolonged scanty uterine bleeding of variable intervals, pneumorrhagia, gastrorrhagia, traumatic bleeding, seminal emission, abnormal vaginal discharge, stomachache, acid regurgitation, eczema, and skin ulcers with pus.

[Quality] Good quality is dry, white, and intact.

[Indications]

1. Bleeding: Hǎi Piāo Xiāo (Endoconcha Sepiae), capable of consolidating and stanching bleeding, is applicable for different types of hemorrhagic disorders. It is combined with Qiàn Cǎo (Radix et Rhizoma Rubiae), Ē Jiāo (Colla Corii Asini), and Pú Huáng (Pollen Typhae) for profuse uterine bleeding and prolonged scanty uterine bleeding of variable intervals; with Bái Jí (Rhizoma Bletillae) and Sān Qī (Radix et Rhizoma Notoginseng) for pulmonary hemorrhage and gastric hemorrhage; with Pú Huáng (Pollen Typhae) and Cè Bǎi Yè (Cacumen Platycladi) for hematuria. It can also be ground into powder and applied externally for traumatic bleeding.
2. Kidney deficiency failing to insecure: Hǎi Piāo Xiāo (Endoconcha Sepiae) is combined with Dǎng Shēn (Radix Codonopsis), Bái Zhú (Rhizoma Atractylodis Macrocephalae), Shān Yào (Rhizoma Dioscoreae), and Qiàn Shí (Semen Euryales) for abnormal vaginal discharge caused by kidney deficiency; and with Shān Zhū Yú (Fructus Corni), Jīn Yīng Zǐ (Fructus Rosae Laevigatae), Shā Yuàn Jí Lí (Semen Astragali Complanati), and Tù Sī Zǐ (Semen Cuscutae) for seminal emission due to kidney deficiency.
3. Stomachache and acid regurgitation: Hǎi Piāo Xiāo (Endoconcha Sepiae) can control acid and therefore is combined with Bèi Mǔ (Bulbus Fritillaria) or Bái Sháo (Radix Paeoniae Alba) for stomachache and hyperchlorhydria.

This substance can also consolidate dampness and close sore when applied externally and therefore is applicable for nonhealing sores of long duration or profuse pus in a combination with Duàn Shí Gāo (Gypsum Fibrosum Praeparatum) and Bīng Piàn (Borneolum Syntheticum). Combining with Huáng Bǎi (Cortex Phellodendri Chinensis) and Qīng Dài (Indigo Naturalis) can treat eczema.

Taking its powder orally can treat asthma.

[Usage and Dosage] Use raw in general, 6–12 g in decoction, and 1.5–3 g/ time in pill and power.

[Mnemonics] Hǎi Piāo Xiāo (Endoconcha Sepiae, Cuttlebone): salty; consolidate essence, arrest profuse vaginal discharge, restrain and arrest bleeding, and alleviate pain.

[Simple and Effective Formulas]

1. 治吐衄方 Zhì Tù Nǜ Fāng — Hematemesis and Epistaxis-Arresting Formula from the *Formulas from Benevolent Sages* (圣惠方 Shèng Huì Fāng): Hǎi Piāo Xiāo (Endoconcha Sepiae); grind into fine powder and take 6 g/time with congee for oral administration to treat hematemesis and epistaxis.
2. 治漏下不止方 Zhì Lòu Xià Bù Zhǐ Fāng — Formula for Persistent and Prolonged Scanty Uterine Bleeding of Variable Intervals from the *Important Formulas Worth a Thousand Gold Pieces* (千金要方 Qiān Jīn Yào Fāng): Hǎi Piāo Xiāo (Endoconcha Sepiae) 60 g, Dāng Guī (Radix Angelicae Sinensis) 60 g, Lù Róng (Cornu Cervi Pantotrichum) 90 g, Ē Jiāo (Colla Corii Asini) 90 g, and Pú Huáng (Pollen Typhae) 30 g; grind into fine powder and take 3 g/time with wine on an empty stomach for prolonged and persistent scanty uterine bleeding of variable intervals.

[Precautions] Hǎi Piāo Xiāo (Endoconcha Sepiae) is capable of restraining and stanching bleeding, however comprehensive treatment plan should be based on the root cause of bleeding.

Daily practices

1. List the medicinals that astringe the intestine to arrest diarrhea and the medicinals that supplement kidney to consolidate essence in terms of the name, actions, and indications.

2. What are the similarities and differences among Yīng Sù Qiào (Pericarpium Papaveris), Hē Zǐ (Fructus Chebulae), and Shí Liú Pí (Pericarpium Granati) in terms of actions and indications?
3. What are the similarities and differences between Sāng Piāo Xiāo (Oötheca Mantidis) and Hǎi Piāo Xiāo (Endoconcha Sepiae) in terms of actions and indications?
4. Among medicinals that astringe and consolidate, which ones have certain toxicity? What precautions should be taken when using them?

Index